DAVIDSON'S
DIABETES
MELLITUS

Diagnosis and
Treatment

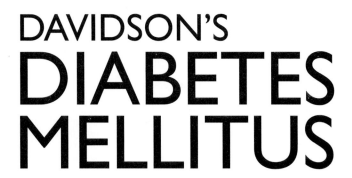

FIFTH EDITION

DAVIDSON'S
DIABETES
MELLITUS

Diagnosis and Treatment

ANNE PETERS HARMEL, M.D.
Division of Endocrinology and Metabolism
Professor of Clinical Medicine
Keck School of Medicine, University of Southern
California
and
Director of USC Clinical Diabetes Programs
USC Westside Center for Diabetes
Los Angles, California

RUCHI MATHUR, M.D.
Division of Endocrinology and Metabolism
Clinical Assistant Professor
Keck School of Medicine, University of Southern
California
Los Angeles, California

SAUNDERS
An Imprint of Elsevier, Inc.

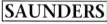

An Imprint of Elsevier, Inc.

The Curtis Center
Independence Square West
Philadelphia, Pennsylvania 19106

NOTICE

Medicine is an ever-changing field. Standard safety precautions must be followed, but as new research and clinical experience broaden our knowledge, changes in treatment and drug therapy may become necessary or appropriate. Readers are advised to check the most current product information provided by the manufacturer of each drug to be administered to verify the recommended dose, the method and duration of administration, and contraindications. It is the responsibility of the licensed prescriber, relying on experience and knowledge of the patient, to determine dosages and the best treatment for each individual patient. Neither the publisher nor the author assumes any liability for any injury and/or damage to persons or property arising from this publication.

Previous editions copyrighted 1998, 1991

Library of Congress Cataloging-in-Publication Data

Davidson's diabetes mellitus : diagnosis and treatment.– 5th ed. / Anne Peters Harmel,
  Ruchi Mathur
     p. ; cm.
   Rev. ed. of: Diabetes mellitus / Mayer B. Davidson. 4th ed. c1998.
   Includes bibliographical references and indexes.
   ISBN 0-7216-9596-5
   1. Diabetes. I. Title: Diabetes mellitus. II. Harmel, Anne Peteres, III. Mathur, Ruchi.
   IV. Davidson, Mayer B. Diabetes mellitus.
   [DNLM: 1. Diabetes Mellitus–diagnosis. 2. Diabetes Mellitus–therapy. WK 810 D2535 2004]
   RC660.D376 2004
   616.4'62–dc22

                                  2003066793

Acquisitions Editor: Todd Hummel
Developmental Editor: Carla L. Holloway
Publishing Services Manager: Joan Sinclair
Project Manager: Mary Stermel

A portion of the proceeds from this book will be donated to the American Diabetes Association Research Foundation to help fund diabetes research

Printed in the United States

Last digit is the print number: 9   8   7   6   5   4   3   2   1

To Max and Mark and the
memory of Alison, with love
A.P.H.

To my parents for their example, to my husband for his support, and to my children for all
their joy
R.M.

CONTRIBUTORS

CHRISTINE A. BEEBE, MS, RD, LD, CDE
Instructor, University of Illinois Chicago
Associate Director, Educational and Scientific Affairs
Takeda Pharmaceuticals North America, Inc.
Lincolnshire, Illinois

EVELYNE FLEURY-MILFORT, MSN, C-RNP, BC-ADM, CDE
Instructor in Clinical Medicine
Division of Diabetes, and Endocrinology
Keck School of Medicine, University of Southern California
Nurse Practitioner
University of Southern California Center for Diabetes
Los Angeles, California

WILLIAM HOWELL
Assistant Clinical Professor of Medicine
Keck School of Medicine, University of Southern California
Los Angeles, California

FRANCINE RATNER KAUFMAN, MD
Professor of Pediatrics
Keck School of Medicine, University of Southern California
Head, The Center for Diabetes, Endocrinology and Metabolism
Childrens Hospital Los Angeles
Los Angeles, California

DAVID M. KENDALL, MD
Associate Professor of Medicine
University of Minnesota
Chief of Clinical Services and Medical Director
International Diabetes Center
Minneapolis, Minnesota

PREFACE

The first edition of this book was published almost 25 years ago, in 1981. As stated then, the book was "intended primarily for physicians and other professionals who provide care for patients with diabetes mellitus" for the purpose of improving the outcomes of these patients. A lot has changed since that time. To mention just a few of the changes: glycated hemoglobin levels are the mainstay of evaluating glycemic control; self-monitoring of blood glucose is widely accepted, especially in those patients requiring insulin; insulin analogues are now available, more closely mimicking beta-cell secretion with another preparation providing a 24-hour basal level; and three new classes of oral drugs—glitazones, alpha glucosidase inhibitors, and meglitinides—have been introduced. Furthermore, the controversy of whether tight control is helpful for the microvascular complications has been laid to rest, with irrefutable intervention trials in both type 1 and type 2 diabetic patients. The increase of macrovascular disease in diabetic patients has been recognized, with impressive intervention trials demonstrating that treatment of the risk factors (lipids, blood pressure) is beneficial for this complication as well. Finally, angiotensin-converting enzyme inhibitors and angiotensin-receptor blockers have been shown to forestall the development of diabetic nephropathy.

In spite of these and other improvements in care, diabetes remains a devastating syndrome. It is still the leading cause of blindness in people between the ages of 20 and 74 years, the most common reason for patients to need dialysis, the cause of over half of all lower-extremity amputations, and the source of three quarters of the deaths in diabetic patients. In the early 1990s, the average glycated hemoglobin was 9.5%, improving to only 8.5% at the end of the decade. In 2002, diabetes cost the United States $132 billion, $98 billion of which was for direct medical care and $34 billion of which was for indirect costs of short- and long-term disability. The American Diabetes Association has promulgated evidence-based standards of care that, if fulfilled, would markedly reduce the morbidity, mortality, and cost of this devastating syndrome. These guidelines are currently met less than half of the time.

In the next 25 years, the problems engendered by diabetes are caloric intakes and sedentary lifestyles of people in industrialized societies. In the minority population with whom I work, type 2 diabetes is commonly seen in people in their 20s and sometimes in their teens. Unless outcomes change, this will mean vision loss, dialysis, amputations, and heart attacks for these people in their 40s, with markedly shortened life expectancies. Hopefully, the principles and techniques enunciated in this 5th edition will help providers caring for diabetic patients improve the outcomes and enhance the lives of those individuals who have entrusted their care to us.

Having issued the challenge, it is time to pass the torch to the next generation. I am fortunate to have Anne Peters Harmel, M.D., and her colleague, Ruchi Mathur, M.D., take over this daunting task. Anne trained with me and has gone on to become an expert in her own right, providing innovative and caring treatment for diabetic patients fortunate enough to be under her care. She and Ruchi have the skills and dedication necessary to improve outcomes in people with diabetes, often not an easy task. They have imparted the knowledge base to accomplish this in this volume. May it prove helpful to readers.

Mayer B. Davidson

ACKNOWLEDGMENTS

We are grateful to Mayer B. Davidson, M.D., for his meticulous review and critique of this edition.

A.P.H., R.M.

I would like to thank Anne Peters Harmel, M.D., for her guidance and mentorship throughout this process.

R.M.

CONTENTS

DIAGNOSIS, CLASSIFICATION, AND EPIDEMIOLOGY OF DIABETES MELLITUS

DEFINITION

Diabetes mellitus is a syndrome consisting of metabolic, vascular, and neuropathic components that are interrelated. It is defined as a group of metabolic diseases that are characterized by hyperglycemia resulting from defects in insulin secretion, insulin action, or both.[1] The lack of effective insulin action leads to alterations in carbohydrate, fat, and protein metabolism. The chronic hyperglycemia of diabetes is associated with long-term dysfunction and damage of organs, including the kidneys, eyes, nerves, heart, and blood vessels.

The majority of cases of diabetes fall into two major categories of pathogenesis. Type 1 diabetes mellitus is caused by an absolute deficiency of insulin secretion. Individuals at risk for developing type 1 diabetes can be identified by serologic markers showing evidence of autoimmune pathologic conditions occurring in the islet cells of the pancreas. In type 2 diabetes, the cause of the disease is a combination of factors including insulin resistance at the level of the muscle and liver, and an inadequate insulin secretory response. The classification of diabetes is described in detail later in this chapter.

Hyperglycemia is the sine qua non of diabetes and is the parameter most closely monitored to make the diagnosis and to judge therapy. Equally important are treatments to lower cardiovascular disease risk. The vascular syndrome that is seen in relation to diabetes consists of abnormalities in both large vessels (macroangiopathy) and small vessels (microangiopathy). The macroangiopathic changes cause cerebrovascular accidents, myocardial infarctions, and peripheral vascular disease. Although these large vessel sequelae may occur in people without diabetes, they appear earlier and are more severe in diabetic patients. The clinical expressions of the microangiopathic changes are diabetic retinopathy and nephropathy. Finally, various abnormalities in the peripheral and autonomic nervous systems are also part of the diabetic syndrome. Most of these neuropathic changes are due to metabolic alterations, although a few of them may be secondary to vascular causes.

DIABETES: A LOCAL AND GLOBAL EPIDEMIC

Each day in the United States, 2200 people are diagnosed with diabetes. Recent data reveal that 6.5% of the U.S. population has diabetes.[2] This amounts to more than 17 million people and reveals an increase in prevalence from 4.9% during the previous 8 years. This increase was observed across all ages, races, educational levels, weights, and geographic distributions throughout the United States.[2] Of these people with diabetes, more than 5 million have the disease and do not know it. The complications resulting from diabetes are significant causes of morbidity and mortality.[3] Diabetes is the leading cause of new cases of blindness in people between the ages of 20 and 74 years, and each year in the United States approximately 20,000 people lose their sight secondary to complications of diabetes. Diabetes is also the leading cause of end-stage renal disease, and accounts for approximately 30,000 patients per year. Diabetes is associated with neuropathy and decreased peripheral blood flow. Both of these factors contribute to diabetes being the most common cause of nontraumatic lower limb amputations. The risk of leg amputation is up to 40 times greater in the diabetic population than others, and more than 56,000 amputations are performed per year in the United States on patients with diabetes. Heart disease and stroke are also more prevalent in people with diabetes. This population is two to four times more likely to suffer heart disease and cerebrovascular accidents than a comparable nondiabetic population.

From an economic perspective, the total annual economic cost of diabetes in 2002 was estimated to be 132 billion dollars in the United States.[4] This includes 91.8 billion dollars in direct treatment costs. The remaining indirect costs were attributed to mortality and disability. In-patient hospital care accounted for 43.9% of the cost, and 15.1% went toward nursing home care. The per capita cost resulting from diabetes in 2002 amounted to $13,243, compared with healthcare costs for people without diabetes, which incurred a per capita cost of $2,560. Overall, almost one out of every five dollars

spent on healthcare in the United States is for a person with diabetes. Remember, these numbers reflect the population in the United States only. Globally, the statistics are staggering.

The prevalence of diabetes in adults worldwide was estimated to be 4.0% in 1995, and is estimated to rise to 5.4% by the year 2025.[5] The absolute numbers translate into 135 million people and 300 million people, respectively. Although diabetes is seen more frequently in developed than in developing countries, the trend is more substantial in the developing world, where the increase in diabetes is projected at 170% by the year 2025. In the near future, the global burden of diabetes will especially affect India, China, and the United States, in part because of their large population base and in part because of the rapidity by which diabetes is increasing in prevalence in these countries. These data, although projected, support earlier predictions of the epidemic nature of diabetes in the world during the first quarter of the 21st century. The repercussions will have a sizable impact both in terms of healthcare resources and utilization and on the quality and quantity of life for afflicted individuals and their families.

INCIDENCE AND PREVALENCE OF DIABETES AMONG SPECIFIC COMMUNITIES

There are a number of factors contributing to the discordant outcomes of diabetes-related morbidity and mortality in different patient populations, including socioeconomic status, genetic predisposition, cultural perceptions of disease, and availability of resources. Although some of these factors are difficult or impossible to change, other factors, such as an increasingly sedentary life style, an increase in obesity, and poor nutritional habits modeled after a Western diet, are modifiable. In the United States, type 2 diabetes is more commonly seen in African American, Latino, and Native American populations. The profile of complications in these subsets of patients are also higher than in their non–Hispanic Caucasian cohorts.[6-13]

African Americans are 1.7 times more likely to have diabetes than non–Hispanic Caucasians. One in four African Americans between the ages of 65 and 74 has diabetes. In addition to these high rates of disease, this population also has higher rates of retinopathy, lower limb amputations, and kidney disease. Hypertension is a common comorbid condition in this population, and further increases the risk of heart disease and renal disease. Of interest is the fact that in African American women, almost 50% of the risk for the development of diabetes is related to modifiable factors such as weight, diet, and activity.[14] In the Latino population of the United States, diabetes is two times higher that in non–Hispanic Caucasians.[15] It is estimated that 10.6% of all Hispanic Americans, or 1.2 million, have type 2 diabetes, and this number increases to 25% between the ages of 45 and 74.[16] The prevalence of retinopathy in the Hispanic American population is 32% to 40%, and up to 21% of this population will develop kidney disease. Among people with diabetes, Hispanic Americans are 4.5 to 6.6 times more likely to suffer from end-stage renal disease. An additional concern in this population is the increase of type 2 diabetes in children and adolescents. In one study, 45% of Hispanic American patients younger than 17 years old who were diagnosed with new-onset diabetes actually had type 2 diabetes.[17] Of note is the fact that the overwhelming majority of these children had a body mass index (BMI) in the obese range, with an average BMI of 32.9 kg/m^2. Type 2 diabetes has reached epidemic proportions in the Native American community. The prevalence of diabetes in this population is 12.2% for those older than 19 years. The complication rates secondary to diabetes are continuing to increase in this population. Retinopathy occurs in 18% to 24% of this population, and kidney disease is occurs in

10% to 21%. Rate of amputations of the lower limb secondary to diabetes is three to four times higher in Native Americans than in the general population.[18]

The resulting discrepancy between populations is remarkable. In general, in the United States there is considerable variation in racial and ethnic healthcare access and utilization for a number of diseases and conditions. For example, African American women and Latino women are less likely to have mammography performed than their age-matched non–Hispanic Caucasian cohorts.[19] For diabetic patients in the United States, variation in healthcare access and outcomes has recently been documented.[20] Based on National Health and Nutrition Examination Survey (NHANES III) data, in which questionnaires and clinical and laboratory data on healthcare access, utilization, and medical outcomes were obtained, there are racial and ethnic differences. Hemoglobin A_{1c} (A1C) levels were statistically lower in non–Hispanic Caucasians than in Hispanic Americans and African Americans, as was clinical proteinuria. Low-density lipoprotein levels and uncontrolled hypertension showed similar trends. The study revealed differences in preferred treatment modalities in these three groups of patients; it also demonstrated that non–Hispanic Caucasians and African Americans had higher rates of health insurance coverage than Hispanic Americans, both younger and older than the age of 65.

Globally, there are more women with diabetes than men. Recent studies put the numbers at 73 million versus 62 million, respectively.[5] This ratio is more pronounced in the developed world. In women, diabetes is the sixth leading cause of death in the United States. In addition to the complications mentioned previously, women with diabetes have an increased risk of vaginal infections and complications during pregnancy. In women who do not have diabetes at the time of conception, gestational diabetes develops in 2% to 5%. Those who do develop gestational diabetes have an increased risk of developing type 2 diabetes within 5 to 10 years, and this risk varies depending on BMI. With confounding obesity, there is a 60% to 70% chance that a woman with a history of gestational diabetes will develop type 2 diabetes.[21] Chapter 11 deals in depth with gestational diabetes.

CURRENT RECOMMENDED CRITERIA FOR THE DIAGNOSIS OF DIABETES MELLITUS

Prior to 1979 there were at least six different sets of criteria used to diagnose diabetes.[22] This meant that a person could have diabetes by one set of criteria, but not by another. As a result, the prevalence of the disease on a population basis varied depending on criteria used. In 1979 the National Diabetes Data Group (NDDG) recommended one set of criteria,[23] which was slightly modified by the World Health Organization (WHO) a year later.[24] These criteria were based on the results of several prospective studies[25-27] using oral glucose tolerance tests (OGTTs) and following the development of retinopathy in these patients for the next 3 to 8 years. The rationale was that the development of this microvascular complication specific for diabetes could serve as the basis for choosing criteria to be used for the diagnosis of diabetes. Based on these studies, a fasting value of greater than 140 mg/dl or a 2-hour value following ingestion of 75 g glucose of 200 mg/dl made the diagnosis. The original and subsequent criteria developed to diagnose "diabetes" were designed to identify individuals who have sufficient hyperglycemia to put them at risk for developing diabetic retinopathy. Lesser degrees of glucose elevation (particularly postglucose challenge glucose elevations) are associated with a high risk for macrovascular disease and are

discussed subsequently in Chapter 8. Regardless of the label used to diagnose the syndrome, elevations in glucose levels, both mild and more severe, are associated with an increased risk of macrovascular and/or microvascular complications.

The criteria for the diagnosis of diabetes have been reevaluated, mainly because the cutoff points of a fasting plasma glucose (FPG) concentration of 140 mg/dl and a 2-hour value in the OGTT of 200 mg/dl are not equivalent.[1] Nearly everyone with an FPG level of 140 mg/dl or higher has a 2-hour OGTT value of 200 mg/dl or higher, whereas fewer than half of those not previously known to have diabetes but with 2-hour OGTT values of 200 mg/dl or higher have FPG concentrations of 140 mg/dl or higher.[28-30] Thus individuals receiving an OGTT are more likely to be diagnosed with diabetes than if only an FPG concentration of 140 mg/dl or higher were used to evaluate glycemic status. Several large studies have determined that the FPG concentration that is equivalent to a 2-hour OGTT value of 200 mg/dl is approximately 7 mmol/L or 126 mg/dl.[1] The new fasting cut-off point of 126 mg/dl was lowered so that the 2-hour value of 200 mg/dl on an OGTT could be retained as a criterion for the diagnosis of diabetes. The lower cut-off point was "in the interest of standardization and also to facilitate field work, particularly where the OGTT may be difficult to perform and where the cost and demands on a participant's time may be excessive."[1] However, OGTTs are inconvenient to administer and unpleasant for patients.[31] The results of the OGTT are also affected by a variety of factors, including the time of day the test is administered, physical activity, preceding carbohydrate intake, and length of time spent fasting prior to the test,[32-34] whereas the FPG concentration has been found to be much more stable. In addition, physicians rarely use OGTTs as a tool for diagnosing diabetes; in actuality, less than 20% of diabetic patients are diagnosed by OGTT.[35] Regardless of the drawbacks, much of the epidemiologic data

TABLE 1-1	OFFICIAL CRITERIA FOR THE DIAGNOSIS OF DIABETES MELLITUS
	1. Symptoms of diabetes plus casual plasma glucose concentration ≥200 mg/dl (11.1 mmol/L). [Casual = any time of day without regard to time since last meal. The classic symptoms of diabetes include polyuria, polydipsia, and unexplained weight loss.] *or* 2. FPG ≥126 mg/dl (7.0 mmol/L). Fasting is defined as no caloric intake for at least 8 hours. *or* 3. 2hPG ≥200 mg/dl during an oral glucose tolerance test (OGTT). The test should be performed as described in reference 3 or 5 using a load of 75 g anhydrous glucose. In the absence of unequivocal hyperglycemia with acute metabolic decompensation, these criteria should be confirmed by repeat testing on a different day. The third measure (OGTT) is not recommended for routine clinical use.

2hPG, 2-hour plasma glucose; FPG, fasting plasma glucose; OGTT, oral glucose tolerance test.

Adapted from Report of the Expert Committee on the Diagnosis and Classification of Diabetes Mellitus. Diabetes Care 20:1183, 1977

on diabetes have been obtained using OGTTs, so it is considered the definitive test for the diagnosis of diabetes. Based on these considerations, new criteria for the diagnosis of diabetes, which rely heavily on FPG concentrations, have been adopted by the American Diabetes Association (ADA) and the WHO (Table 1-1). Note that OGTTs are not recommended for routine clinical use. If one is performed (sampling only before and 2 hours after a 75-g glucose load under conditions described by the NDDG[23] and the WHO,[24] the 2-hour value (Table 1-2) determines the glycemic status.

Given the fact that this new FPG concentration criterion is relatively recent, it remains unclear as to the overall impact of these new guidelines for diagnosis in specific populations. In one study evaluating the impact of the new diagnostic criteria for diabetes, 20,624 subjects were reviewed.[36] These subjects had an OGTT performed per standard methodology. Of these subjects, 31% with a diagnosis of diabetes based on the new FPG criterion did not have diabetes based on their 2-hour OGTT values. In another study of more than 7500 individuals, the baseline FPG concentration was found to be a major predictor of an individual's risk for developing diabetes, and the use of a lower cut of 126 mg/dl led to earlier diagnosis among individuals with risk.[37]

Conversely, a European study (the Diabetes Epidemiology: Collaborative analysis of Diagnostic criteria in Europe [DECODE] study) evaluated data from 29,108 subject and found that 31% of patients would remain undiagnosed if only the new FPG criterion were applied.[38] They also found that the sensitivity and specificity of the FPG concentration in detecting diabetes depended on the individual's BMI. Although the literature remains confusing at this point, it suggests that FPG, 2-hour plasma glucose concentrations, and A1C levels all have a role to play in the diagnosis of diabetes.

The new criteria also identify FPG concentrations that do not meet the criteria for diabetes but are higher than the normal value of less than 110 mg/dl. These individuals are considered to have *impaired fasting glucose* (IFG). IFG is not considered a clinical entity in its own right, but is a risk factor for the future development of diabetes[39] and macrovascular disease.[40] Regarding absolute levels, a cut-off of 104 mg/dl seemed to define a group more similar to the group with impaired glucose tolerance (IGT) with regard to prevalence and the risk of subsequent diabetes.[41] Therefore, if an OGTT is performed and the 2-hour value meets the older criterion for IGT (Table 1-2), this entity is now considered only a risk factor for

TABLE 1-2 PREVIOUS CRITERIA OF THE WORLD HEALTH ORGANIZATION		
	Diabetes Mellitus	**Impaired Glucose Tolerance**
Fasting	≥140 (7.8)*	<140 (7.8)*
	or	*and*
OGTT (2 hour)	≥200 (11.1)	140–199 (7.8-11.1)
	or	
Random	≥200 (11.1)	Not part of criteria

OGTT, oral glucose tolerance test.

*Venous plasma glucose concentrations in mg/dl (mmol/L).

From World Health Organization: Diabetes Mellitus: Report of a WHO Study Group (Tech Rep Series 626). WHO, Geneva, 1980

the development of diabetes and macrovascular disease. The risk for diabetes in individuals who were diagnosed in the past with IGT is approximately 13.8% per year,[41a] although approximately 25% may revert to normal glucose tolerance, and some may remain with IGT. The rate of progression from IGT to diabetes was less than 5% per year in Caucasian populations,[3] but higher in ethnic groups predisposed to type 2 diabetes (discussed later). One would assume that a similar prognosis would hold for IFG, although data to substantiate this statement are not easily available.

ALTERNATIVE APPROACH TO THE DIAGNOSIS OF DIABETES

A1C levels have not yet been included in the diagnostic criteria for diabetes, although it is an invaluable tool for making treatment decisions. Part of the reluctance to use A1C values for screening is based on a lack of standardizations of the assays, although a national standardization process is currently being developed.[42] At this time, the new diagnostic criteria do not reflect treatment goals. For example, 60% of patients diagnosed with an FPG concentration between 126 and 140 mg/dl have an A1C level within the normal range.[43,44] Similarly, two thirds of patients diagnosed with a 2-hour value on an OGTT of 200 to 239 mg/dl have a normal A1C level.[44] Because treatment is based on

A1C goals, how do we treat these patients? Should we treat these patients? What is our goal for follow-up? The following is an approach not sanctioned by the ADA or WHO, but based on a clinical perspective. It uses initial measurements of FPG concentrations and subsequent measurements of A1C levels in selected patients and is based on the following logic.

Except for a very few populations in which the prevalence of diabetes is very high and therefore the distribution of blood glucose concentrations is bimodal,[45,46] a unimodal distribution is the norm.[47,48] Thus there is no clear-cut demarcation between normal and abnormal blood glucose concentrations. In 1979 and 1980 the NDDG and the WHO, respectively, chose a level of glycemia to diagnose diabetes that was associated with the subsequent development of the specific complication of diabetic retinopathy. People who sustain normal A1C levels do not develop this microvascular complication. There have been five studies in several thousand diabetic patients carried out over 6 to 9 years relating the average A1C level to the development and progression of diabetic retinopathy and nephropathy.[49-54] All five demonstrated that if the average A1C level were less than 1% above the upper limit of normal (ULN) for the assay used (e.g., <7% for the assay used in the Diabetes Control and Complications Trial, in which the ULN was 6.0%), there was virtually no development or progression of diabetic retinopathy or nephropathy. Thus individuals with normal A1C levels are not at risk for the microvascular complications of diabetes, even if they are mildly hyperglycemic. Not only are A1C levels tightly linked to diabetic retinopathy, nephropathy, and neuropathy, but recent reports have also demonstrated that blocking the production of advanced glycation end products beyond the formation of A1C (and therefore independent of hyperglycemia) markedly retards the development of these complications.[55-58]

We must balance the advantages of diagnosing diabetes against its potential disadvantages in terms of insurance (both life and medical), employment, and psychosocial implications.[59-61] For instance, people carrying the diagnosis of diabetes are eight times more likely to be unable to obtain medical insurance because of poor health or illness than are those without diabetes.[61]

It is not clear that it would be helpful to label people with FPG concentrations of 126 to 139 mg/dl or 2-h values on an OGTT of 200 to 239 mg/dl, but with normal A1C levels, as having diabetes. Their treatment would be the same nonpharmacologic life style therapies of diet and exercise as would be prescribed for individuals with similar A1C levels and FPG concentrations of 110 to 125 mg/dl, which qualifies them for the diagnosis of IFG.[1] There is little to support the notion that giving individuals with mild degrees of hyperglycemia a diagnosis of diabetes makes them more compliant with the life style changes that are the cornerstone of treatment.

Some argue that the lowered FPG concentrations for the diagnosis of diabetes are justified because there are so many individuals with undiagnosed type 2 diabetes, and at diagnosis approximately 10% of patients already have nephropathy[62] and 20% already have retinopathy.[63] These people remain undiagnosed because they are not evaluated, not because the FPG concentration for the diagnosis remains too high.

Similarly, the ADA committee that decided on the new diagnostic criteria for diabetes included macrovascular disease in its contention that earlier diagnosis and appropriate treatment would decrease the subsequent complications of diabetes.[1] This reasoning may not be valid because the increased risk for coronary artery disease extends all the way down to the highest quartile of normal FPG concentrations[64-66] and even to A1C levels higher than 5.0% compared with lower values.[67] Furthermore, improved glycemic control (unfortunately) has little effect on the morbidity and mortality from cardiovascular disease in people with diabetes.[68] A number of other risk factors for macrovascular disease need to be addressed, but the prevalence of these risk factors are similar in those with IFG (FPG concentrations of 110 to 125 mg/dl) and those in the new cohort of diabetes (FPG concentrations of 126 to 139 mg/dl).[69] Thus, from a macrovascular perspective, there is no advantage in distinguishing between the two groups and labeling people in the latter as having diabetes.

Given the importance of excessive glycation of proteins in the pathogenesis of the diabetic microvascular and neuropathic complications and the principle that the level of glycemia associated with these complications is appropriate for the diagnosis of diabetes, the alternative approach to diagnosis, which takes into account these clinical outcomes, is suggested in Figure 1-1. This diagnostic algorithm uses measurements of FPG concentrations followed by A1C levels in people whose FPG values are neither normal (<110 mg/dl) nor meet the older criterion for the diagnosis of diabetes (≥140 mg/dl). The A1C level determines whether an individual with a FPG concentration of 110 to 139 mg/dl has diabetes or a milder degree of hyperglycemia. An elevated A1C level, if confirmed, makes the diagnosis of diabetes. A normal value makes the diagnosis of IFG, which is a high-risk category for the future development of both diabetes and cardiovascular disease, and warrants

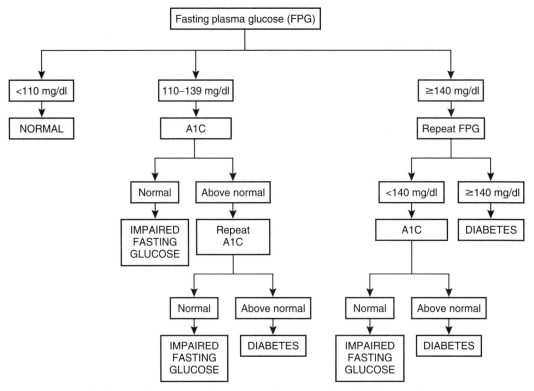

FIGURE 1-1. Algorithm for an alternative, clinically relevant approach to the diagnosis of diabetes mellitus.

close follow-up and aggressive treatment of the risk factors for each.

It has been argued that A1C assays are not yet standardized enough to be used in the diagnosis of diabetes.[6] However, using an assay meeting the recent standards of the National Glycohemoglobin Program to analyze the NHANES III data, Rohlfing and colleagues[70] concluded that A1C levels are both sensitive and specific for detecting diabetes.

If the approach outlined in Figure 1-1 is followed, diabetes will be diagnosed in those at risk for developing the microvascular and neuropathic complications. Individuals with milder degrees of hyperglycemia (who are currently not at risk for these complications) will also be identified so that appropriate measures can be instituted to reduce their chances of developing diabetes or cardiovascular disease. Persons who should be screened for diabetes are listed in Table 1-3.

IMPLICATIONS AND IMPORTANCE OF IMPAIRED GLUCOSE TOLERANCE

IGT has a strong relationship to cardiovascular disease,[71,72] and this is explored in detail in Chapter 8. Because our current diagnostic criteria for diabetes is related to the development of retinopathy (a microvascular complication) and because macrovascular disease (including heart disease and stroke) is the main cause of death in diabetes, there is some controversy over why IGT is not considered a disease entity in its own right. There is a body of literature suggesting that diabetes-associated macrovascular disease develops earlier than microvascular disease when plasma glucose levels are in the "prediabetic" range.[73] With minor controversy,[74] most data on this subject show that IGT is a significant

TABLE 1-3	CRITERIA FOR TESTING FOR DIABETES IN ASYMPTOMATIC, UNDIAGNOSED INDIVIDUALS

1. Testing for diabetes should be considered in all individuals at age 45 years and older. If results are normal, it should be repeated at 3-year intervals.
2. Testing should be considered at a younger age (starting as low as 10 years of age in high-risk individuals) or should be carried out more frequently in individuals who meet one or more of the following criteria:
   - Are obese (≥120% desirable body weight or a body mass index ≥27 kg/m²)
   - Have a first or second-degree relative with diabetes
   - Are members of a high-risk ethnic population (e.g., African American, Hispanic, Native American, Asian American)
   - Delivered a baby weighing >9 pounds or who have been diagnosed with GDM
   - Are hypertensive (≥140/90)
   - Have an HDL-C level ≤35 mg/dl and/or a triglyceride level ≥250 mg/dl
   - Had IFG or IGT on previous testing
   - Have features of insulin resistance such as polycystic ovarian syndrome

The fasting plasma glucose (FPG) test or oral glucose tolerance test (OGTT) may be used to diagnose diabetes; however, the FPG test is greatly preferred because of its ease of administration, convenience, acceptability to patients, and lower cost. The OGTT is not recommended in clinical settings.

GDM, gestational diabetes mellitus; HDL, high-density lipoprotein; IFG, impaired fasting glucose; IGT, impaired glucose testing.

Adapted from Report of the Expert Committee on the Diagnosis and Classification of Diabetes Mellitus. Diabetes Care 20:1183, 1977.

risk factor for the development of cardiovascular disease. In fact, a population-based study using 2583 subjects from the famous Framingham cohort[75] showed that metabolic risk factors for coronary heart disease, including obesity, hypertension, decreased high-density lipoproteins levels, elevated triglyceride levels, and hyperinsulinemia, showed a continuous increase across the spectrum of nondiabetic glucose tolerance. This increase began at the lowest quintiles of normal fasting glucose.[75] A Japanese study looking at 2651 subjects showed a significantly increased risk of death from cardiovascular disease in those with IGT compared with those with normal glucose tolerance.[76] When reanalyzed, these results did not hold true for the IFG group. The authors concluded that postchallenge hyperglycemia is an important predictor for the development of atherosclerosis. These results were echoed in the Chicago Heart study in men[77] and the Rancho Bernardo study in older women.[78] More recently, it has been shown that in the United States there is a gradient of mortality associated with abnormal glucose tolerance

ranging from 40% in those with IGT to 110% in those with overt diabetes.[79] These associations were independent of other established cardiovascular risk factors. The European Investigation into Cancer (EPIC) study showed a 270% increase in cardiovascular events and death in men who were 40 to 74 years of age and whose A1C levels were 5.0% to 5.4%, compared with those less than 5.0% over 4 years.[80] There is no evidence, however, that lowering glycemia improves outcomes of macrovascular disease.

THE ROLE OF SCREENING FOR DIABETES

It is important to realize that methods used for screening and methods used for diagnosis are not necessarily equivalent.[81,82] A screening test is helpful in diseases that are significantly under-diagnosed and when there is a relatively long interval between early warning signs of the disease and more severe disease manifestations. If a disease's outcome of morbidity and mortality can be lessened by early detection, this also makes it appropriate for screening. Type 2 diabetes fits all these criteria and, as such, it makes an ideal candidate for screening, particularly in high-risk populations. Although early detection of type 2 diabetes through screening may be a worthwhile public health strategy, the health benefits of early detection have never been firmly established.[81] In addition, screening itself may lead to misdiagnosis, inappropriate investigation and treatment, and avoidable adverse events and unnecessary costs financially, socially, and emotionally.[82,83] There is also the consideration of the increasing cost of health care and the cost-to-benefit ratio of screening for a particular disease. Although these comments are applicable to any screening process, diabetes itself has particular issues that make it a difficult disease to screen. Variations exist in sensitivity, specificity, and positive predictive value, depending on which test is employed. It is also difficult to physically implement a screening program that necessitates fasting laboratory values on a random population. Fasting and random serum glucose, urine glucose, and A1C levels often lack the sensitivity needed to identify patients early in the course of the disease. Practically, capillary glucose measurements with adjustments for postprandial period and age can be an effective screening strategy.[84] The cost-effectiveness for such screening programs can be improved if limited to high-risk individuals who are younger than 45 years of age.[85] Another important point to make about screening for any disease is that once high-risk subjects are identified, there must be provisions by which to confirm the diagnosis and implement a treatment strategy. These resources must be in place to allow for the ultimate success of any screening endeavor.

CLASSIFICATION OF DIABETES MELLITUS

In 1979 the NDDG, in addition to proposing diagnostic criteria, also classified diabetes and its related disorders.[23] The WHO adopted this classification (with minor modifications) the next year[24] and added malnutrition-related diabetes in 1985.[86] Given the state of knowledge at that time, the classification was based on a combination of clinical manifestations or treatment requirements, for example, insulin-dependent diabetes mellitus (IDDM, type 1), non–insulin-dependent diabetes mellitus (NIDDM, type 2), and pathogenesis (e.g., "other types" [secondary], gestational). When the earlier classification was formulated, a definitive cause of any of the categories of diabetes had not been established except for some of the secondary types (e.g., steroid induced, pancreatitis). Some of the genetic markers for type 1 diabetes had just been discovered, but an in-depth understanding of the immunologic basis for type 1 diabetes was in its infancy.

In the past decade and a half, a much firmer understanding of the pathogenesis and, in some cases, the causes of the various categories of diabetes has been attained. On the basis of these new findings, both the Expert Committee on the Diagnosis and Classification of Diabetes[1] (constituted by the ADA) and the WHO[87] have proposed a new classification of diabetes and its related disorders (Table 1-4). The main features of the changes are as follows:

1. The terms *insulin-dependent diabetes mellitus* and *non–insulin-dependent diabetes mellitus* and their acronyms (IDDM and NIDDM) have been eliminated. Many physicians, allied health professionals, and patients have been confused by this nomenclature and mistakenly classified all individuals receiving insulin as having IDDM. The terms *type 1* and *type 2* diabetes are retained.

2. The category of diabetes named *type 1* includes all forms of diabetes that are either *primarily* caused by autoimmune destruction of the pancreatic β-cells or

TABLE 1-4 ETIOLOGIC CLASSIFICATION OF DIABETES MELLITUS

I. Type 1 diabetes* (β-cell destruction usually leading to absolute insulin deficiency)
  A. Autoimmune
  B. Idiopathic
II. Type 2 diabetes* (insulin resistance with relative insulin deficiency)
III. Other specific types
  A. Genetic defects of β-cell function
    1. Mitochondrial DNA defect
    2. Wolfram's syndrome
    3. Maturity-onset diabetes of the young (MODY)
      a. Chromosome 20q (MODY-1)
      b. Chromosome 7p (MODY-2)
      c. Chromosome 12q (MODY-3)
  B. Genetic defects in insulin action
    1. Type A insulin resistance
    2. Leprechaunism
    3. Rabson-Mendenhall syndrome
    4. Lipodystrophy
  C. Diseases of the exocrine pancreas
    1. Pancreatitis (including fibrocalculous pancreatopathy)
    2. Pancreatectomy
    3. Trauma (severe)
    4. Neoplasia
    5. Cystic fibrosis
    6. Hemochromatosis
  D. Endocrinopathies
    1. Cushing syndrome
    2. Acromegaly
    3. Pheochromocytoma
    4. Glucagonoma
    5. Aldosteronoma
    6. Hyperthyroidism
    7. Somatostatinoma

  E. Drug or chemical induced
    1. Nicotinic acid
    2. Glucocorticoids
    3. Thyroid hormone
    4. β-Adrenergic agonists
    5. Thiazides
    6. Phenytoin (Dilantin)
    7. Pentamidine (intravenous)
    8. Diazoxide
    9. Vacor
    10. Interferon-α
  F. Infections
    1. Congenital rubella
    2. Cytomegalovirus
    3. Coxsackie B
    4. Mumps
    5. Adenovirus
  G. Uncommon forms of immune-mediated diabetes
    1. Anti-insulin receptor antibodies
    2. Stiff-man syndrome
  H. Other genetic syndromes sometimes associated with diabetes
    1. Down syndrome
    2. Klinefelter syndrome
    3. Turner syndrome
    4. Prader-Willi syndrome
    5. Myotonic dystrophy
    6. Laurence-Moon-Biedl syndrome
    7. Friedreich's ataxia
    8. Huntington's chorea
    9. Porphyria
    10. Others
IV. Gestational diabetes mellitus (GDM)

MODY, maturity-onset diabetes of the young.
*Patients with any form of diabetes may require insulin at some stage of their disease. Such use of insulin does not, per se, classify the patient.
Adapted from Report of the Expert Committee on the Diagnosis and Classification of Diabetes Mellitus. Diabetes Care 20:1183, 1997.

caused by a *primary* defect in β-cell function secondary to another (nonautoimmune) cause.

3. The category of diabetes named *type 2* includes the most common form of diabetes, which results from insulin resistance combined with inadequate insulin secretion.

4. IGT is removed as a distinct clinical entity and is considered to be a risk factor only.

5. The category of gestational diabetes is retained but has been defined differently by the Expert Committee on the Classification and Diagnosis of Diabetes[1] (who retained

the criteria of the NDDG[23] and the WHO.[87]

6. Malnutrition-related diabetes has been deleted by the WHO.

It is important to realize that in this new classification, patients with any form of diabetes may require insulin treatment at some stage of their disease. The use of insulin per se does not help to designate which category of diabetes a patient has.

TYPE I DIABETES

The *autoimmune* form of this type of diabetes is by far the most common. It was previously called *type 1 diabetes, IDDM,* or *juvenile-onset diabetes.* It results from a cell-mediated autoimmune destruction of the pancreatic β-cells. The rate of destruction is variable but is generally more rapid in children than in adults. Some patients, particularly children and adolescents, may present with ketoacidosis as the first manifestation of the disease. Others have modest fasting hyperglycemia that can rapidly change to severe hyperglycemia or ketoacidosis in the presence of infection or other stress. Still others, particularly adults, may retain residual β-cell function for many years. When β-cell reserves of insulin are depleted, these patients are ketosis-prone—that is, they develop ketosis and eventually ketoacidosis in the absence of insulin treatment (see Chapter 2) and cannot survive without it. Markers of immune destruction (autoantibodies to islet cells, insulin, glutamic acid decarboxylase [GAD] in the islets, and tyrosine phosphatases in the islets) are present in 85% to 90% of individuals when fasting hyperglycemia is initially detected. The peak incidence of this form of type 1 diabetes occurs in childhood and adolescence. Approximately 75% of individuals who develop type 1 diabetes do so before 30 years of age. The onset in the remaining patients may occur at any age, even in the eighth and ninth decades of life. Autoimmune destruction of β-cells has a genetic predisposition (that can be identified by human leukocyte antigen [HLA] typing) but is also related to environmental factors that are still poorly understood (see Chapter 2). Although these patients are characteristically lean, this form of type 1 diabetes can occasionally occur in obese individuals as well. These patients are also prone to other autoimmune disorders, such as Graves' disease, Hashimoto's thyroiditis, Addison's disease, and vitiligo.

It has been suggested that early childhood immunizations may influence the risk of children developing type 1 diabetes later in life. In particular, diphtheria, tetanus, pertussis vaccinations at 2 months of age were high in suspicion.[88] Data also suggested that administration of the hepatitis B vaccine at birth reduced the incidence of diabetes compared with children given the first dose when older than 6 weeks of age, but more recent studies do not support this finding.[89] A series of *Haemophilus influenzae* B vaccines starting at 3 months was also thought more likely to be a causal factor in the onset of diabetes compared with one shot at 24 months.[90] However, a prospective study of 317 children younger than 12 years old having first-degree relatives with type 1 diabetes showed no difference in the development of diabetes compared with case controls, regardless of actual immunizations received or the dosing regimens used before the age of 9 months.[91] Some forms of type 1 diabetes are *idiopathic.* Only a small minority of patients with type 1 diabetes fall into this category. Of these, not all have permanent insulinopenia and are prone to ketoacidosis. This is a form of type 1 diabetes, most common among African Americans,[92-94] in which patients may present with diabetic ketoacidosis; however, their subsequent requirements for insulin may wax and wane. The lesion seems to be decreased insulin secretion rather than insulin resistance.[95] This form of diabetes is strongly inherited, lacks immunologic evidence for autoimmunity, and is not associated with any particular types of HLA.

Although little is known about this idiopathic form of type 1 diabetes, it is known that the presence of GAD is closely correlated with evidence of insulitis, whereas islet cell antibodies are not (insulitis being a direct result of the autoimmune process). A study looking at 56 Japanese patients with type 1 diabetes identified a subset of patients who did not express GAD, islet cell antibodies, or insulin antibodies.[96] This subset had higher plasma glucose concentration, decreased urinary excretion of C peptide, and a more severe metabolic disorder with ketoacidosis. The authors concluded that some patients with idiopathic type 1 diabetes have a nonautoimmune fulminant disorder with the absence of insulitis and related antibodies. The cause of this disorder is not known, but is hypothesized to be viral because biopsy specimens obtained showed significant lymphocytic infiltration of the involved pancreas.

Approximately 10% of patients diagnosed with type 2 diabetes have circulating autoantibodies to either islet cell cytoplasmic antigens or GAD.[97] This subgroup is referred to as latent autoimmune diabetes in adults (LADA) and has been included in the new WHO classification of diabetes. It is a slow progressive form of type 1 diabetes.[98] There are common features of both type 1 and type 2 diabetes in these patients, and although insulin secretion is present into adulthood, it begins to deteriorate with time. LADA patients do have a component of insulin resistance (discussed in the following section) like their type 2 counterparts. However, they exhibit a more severe defect in maximal stimulated β-cell capacity than patients with type 2 diabetes.[99]

TYPE 2 DIABETES

In type 2 diabetes, (previously called *NIDDM,* or *adult-onset diabetes*), affected individuals have insulin resistance in combination with a relative (rather than an absolute) deficiency of insulin secretion. Initially and sometimes throughout their lifetimes, these patients do not require insulin to achieve satisfactory diabetic control. There are almost certainly many different causes of type 2 diabetes (as defined here), and it is likely that the number of patients in this currently most common form of diabetes will decrease in the future as identification of specific pathogenic processes and genetic defects permits better differentiation and a more definitive classification. Indeed, the major differences between the older classification[100] and this new one (see Table 1-4) reflect just that evolution. Although the specific causes of this form of diabetes are not known, autoimmune destruction of pancreatic β-cells does not occur and patients do not have any other known causes of diabetes or association with other diseases listed in Table 1-4.

Of patients with this form of diabetes, 80% to 90% are obese. Obesity itself adds additional insulin resistance. Even those patients who are not obese by traditional weight criteria—for example, percent of desirable body weight or BMI (kilograms of weight per meters of height^2)—may have an increased percentage of body fat distributed predominantly in the abdominal region (see the discussion of insulin resistance syndrome in Chapter 8). Ketoacidosis can rarely occur in type 2 diabetes, but it is almost always precipitated by the stress of another illness (e.g., infection). Type 2 diabetes is frequently undiagnosed for many years because the elevated glucose concentrations are not high enough to elicit the classic symptoms of uncontrolled diabetes. It has been estimated that the length of time between the onset of hyperglycemia and the diagnosis of type 2 diabetes is 9 to 12 years.[101] Unfortunately, these patients are at increased risk of developing the microvascular, neuropathic, and macrovascular complications of diabetes (see Chapter 8) during this period. This delay in diagnosis explains why approximately 20% of patients have one or more of the microvascular and neuropathic complications when the diagnosis of diabetes is first made.

Although patients with this form of diabetes may have insulin concentrations that appear to be normal or even high, the elevated glucose levels would be expected to result in even higher insulin concentrations if β-cell function were normal. Thus insulin secretion is defective in these patients and is insufficient to compensate for their insulin resistance. Although their insulin resistance diminishes with weight reduction and lowering of glucose concentrations by either non-pharmacologic or pharmacologic means (reversal of glucose toxicity),[102] the genetic component of insulin resistance remains. Because some effective insulin also remains in these patients, they are ketosis resistant; that is, even in the absence of treatment, ketonuria is very unlikely (see Chapter 2 for metabolic explanation).

The risk of developing type 2 diabetes increases with obesity, age, and a sedentary life style. It is estimated that the chances double for every 20% increase over desirable body weight and for each decade after the fourth (the latter regardless of weight). The prevalence of diabetes in persons 65 to 74 years of age is nearly 20% and probably is higher in people in the 9th and 10th decades. Type 2 diabetes is more common in certain ethnic groups. Compared with a 6% prevalence in Caucasians, the prevalence in African Americans and Asians is estimated to be 10%, in Hispanics 15%, and in certain Native American tribes 20% to 50%.[103,104] Finally, it occurs much more frequently in women with prior gestational diabetes mellitus (GDM) (25% to 50%)[105] compared with those going through pregnancy with normal glucose tolerance (see Chapter 10). Type 2 diabetes is often associated with a strong familial, probably genetic predisposition, much more so, in fact, than with the autoimmune form of type 1 diabetes. However, the genetics of type 2 diabetes are complex and are not clearly defined (see Chapter 2). This is at least partly because of the heterogeneity of this form of diabetes, as mentioned earlier.

OTHER SPECIFIC TYPES

Genetic Defects of the β-cell

A point mutation in mitochondrial DNA (deoxyribonucleic acid), which is therefore maternally transmitted, has been found to be associated with diabetes and deafness.[106,107] This occurs at position 3243 in the transfer RNA (ribonucleic acid) of the leucine gene leading to an A-to-G substitution. An identical lesion occurs in the mitochondrial myopathy, encephalopathy, lactic acidosis, and strokelike (MELAS) syndrome; however, diabetes is not part of this syndrome, suggesting different phenotypic expressions of this genetic lesion.

Wolfram's syndrome is an autosomal recessive disorder characterized by insulin-deficient diabetes and the absence of β-cells at autopsy.[108] Other manifestations include diabetes insipidus, hypogonadism, optic atrophy, and neural deafness.

Maturity-onset diabetes of the young (MODY) is characterized by onset of hyperglycemia at an early age (generally before age 25 years).[109] It is inherited in an autosomal dominant pattern. Individuals with MODY have impaired insulin secretion rather than decreased insulin action.[110-112] Abnormalities at five genetic loci in separate families have been identified. The lesion on chromosome 7p (MODY-2) results in a defective glucokinase gene.[113,114] Glucokinase converts glucose to glucose-6-phosphate, the metabolism of which in the β-cell stimulates insulin secretion. Thus glucokinase serves as the glucose sensor for the β-cell. Because of this defect in the glucokinase gene, increased concentrations of glucose are necessary to elicit normal insulin secretion. A second lesion that has been identified is on chromosome 20q (MODY-1) and is tightly linked to the adenosine deaminase locus.[115,116] A third identified lesion is on chromosome 12q (MODY-3) and is linked to microsatellite markers.[117,118] The mechanisms by which the latter two genetic abnormalities cause hyperglycemia are unknown, although both affected genes produce hepatic transcription factors.

Genetic Defects in Insulin Action

Many unusual causes of diabetes result from genetically determined abnormalities of insulin action. The metabolic abnormalities associated with mutations of the insulin receptor[119] may range from hyperinsulinemia and modest hyperglycemia to frank diabetes. Some individuals with these mutations may have acanthosis nigricans. Women may be virilized and have enlarged, cystic ovaries. In the past, this syndrome was termed *type A insulin resistance*.[120] Leprechaunism[121,122] and the Rabson-Mendenhall syndrome[123] are two pediatric syndromes that have mutations in the insulin receptor gene with subsequent alterations in insulin receptor function and extreme insulin resistance. The former is distinguished by characteristic facial features, and the latter is associated with abnormalities of teeth and nails and pineal gland hyperplasia. Patients with these syndromes and other patients with alterations in insulin receptor function may have defects[119] in (1) receptor synthesis, (2) transport of the receptor to the plasma membrane, (3) binding of the receptor to the insulin molecule, (4) transmembrane signaling, or (5) endocytosis-recycling-degradation of the receptor.

Patients with both total[124] and partial[125] congenital lipodystrophy have insulin resistance but normal insulin receptor genes.[126] Therefore it is assumed that the lesions must reside in the postreceptor signal transduction pathways in these conditions.

Diseases of the Exocrine Pancreas

Any process that diffusely injures enough of the pancreas can cause diabetes. Acquired processes include pancreatitis,[127] pancreatec-tomy, and severe trauma. A unique combination of pancreatitis and diabetes, termed *fibrocalculous pancreatic diabetes*[128] or *fibrocalculous pancreatopathy*[129] is a form of diabetes with a high prevalence in tropical and developing countries. It most often affects young and malnourished individuals. It is characterized by abdominal pain radiating to the back, pancreatic calcifications on radiographs, and, frequently, exocrine insufficiency.[130,131] It had been considered part of malnutrition-related diabetes[130] until recently, when that category of diabetes was deleted.[132] Inherited processes include cystic fibrosis[133] and hemochromatosis[134] (bronze diabetes). An exception to the statement that diffuse injury is necessary to cause diabetes is the increased association of diabetes with adenocarcinoma of the pancreas[135,136] (which is usually localized to a small part of the pancreas).

Endocrinopathies[137]

Hormonal secretion by some endocrine tumors can cause diabetes. Excess secretion of glucocorticoids (Cushing's syndrome, in which Cushing's disease is one cause), growth hormone (acromegaly), and catecholamines (pheochromocytoma) impairs insulin action. The main effect of hyperthyroidism is to increase glucose turnover, although insulin action is also mildly impaired.[138] Diabetes does not occur in hyperthyroidism unless β-cell reserve is also decreased. Catecholamines (pheochromocytoma), somatostatinomas,[139] and aldosteronomas (via hypokalemia)[140] impair insulin secretion. Glucagonomas cause mild diabetes by increasing hepatic glucose production. Diabetes generally disappears with successful treatment of the endocrinopathies, although it may persist even after resolution of Cushing's syndrome and acromegaly.

Drug or Chemical Induced[141,142]

Drugs can cause diabetes by either impairing insulin secretion or enhancing insulin resistance. Those that affect insulin secretion are intravenous (not inhaled) pentamidine,[143] Vacor[144] (a rat poison, not a drug), phenytoin (Dilantin), interferon-α[145,146] (probably by an autoimmune mechanism), diazoxide, and thiazides (secondary to potassium deficiency). Those that affect insulin action are nicotinic acid (niacin), glucocorticoids, β-adrenergic agonists, thyroid hormones, and estrogens. Estrogens and thyroid hormones usually precipitate diabetes only in those who have impaired β-cell reserves and who, in the absence of these two drugs, are able to maintain normoglycemia.

Infections

The role of viruses in causing diabetes is controversial.[147] They may be involved in the pathogenesis of diabetes in one of two ways: either by directly infecting and destroying pancreatic β-cells or by precipitating or contributing to the autoimmune process that underlies immune-mediated type 1 diabetes. Although evidence for direct pancreatic involvement has been obtained in several patients[148,149] it has been conspicuously absent in almost all others in which it was sought.[150] Thus the viruses listed in Table 1-4 are most likely to be involved in the pathogenesis of diabetes by participating somehow in the autoimmune process, because circulating autoantibodies are found in the majority of patients whose diabetes has been linked to viruses.

Uncommon Forms of Immune-Mediated Diabetes

Two known conditions are currently categorized as uncommon forms of immune-mediated diabetes. The stiff-man syndrome is an autoimmune disorder involving the central nervous system and is characterized by painful stiffness of the axial muscles and painful spasms.[151] Patients often have high titers of autoantibodies to GAD, and approximately one third develop diabetes.

Autoantibodies to the insulin receptor compete with insulin for binding to the receptor, thereby blocking the action of the hormone and causing diabetes.[152] As in other states of extreme insulin resistance (listed earlier under Genetic Defects of Insulin Action), patients with antibodies to the insulin receptor often have acanthosis nigricans. This syndrome was originally termed *type B insulin resistance*.[153] These antibodies can sometimes activate the insulin receptor, causing hypoglycemia. Antiinsulin receptor antibodies are also occasionally found in other autoimmune states (e.g., systemic lupus erythematosus, Hashimoto's thyroiditis, scleroderma, primary biliary cirrhosis, immune thrombocytopenia purpura) as well as in Hodgkin's lymphoma.[154] In these instances, hypoglycemia is the clinical problem.

Other Genetic Syndromes Sometimes Associated with Diabetes

Many genetic syndromes are accompanied by an increased incidence of diabetes mellitus.[154] The chromosomal abnormalities of only a few have been identified (e.g., Down syndrome, Klinefelter's syndrome, Turner's syndrome). In none of these genetic syndromes, however, has the mechanism of diabetes been elucidated. Other genetic syndromes sometimes associated with diabetes are listed in Table 1-4.

GESTATIONAL DIABETES MELLITUS

Pregnancy presents an exception to the previous discussion about the diagnosis of diabetes. Because even minor abnormalities of glucose tolerance in pregnant women can be associated with increased risk to the fetus at delivery or in the neonatal period, it was previously recommended that screening for GDM be carried out for all pregnant women. This recommendation has been

TABLE 1-5 SCREENING* AND DIAGNOSIS† SCHEME FOR GESTATIONAL DIABETES MELLITUS		
	50-g Screening Test	100-g Diagnostic Test
Fasting	—	105 mg/dl
1 hour	140 mg/dl	190 mg/dl
2 hour	—	165 mg/dl
3 hour	—	145 mg/dl

*Screening for gestational diabetes mellitus (GDM) should *not* be performed in pregnant women who meet *all* of the following criteria: <25 years of age, normal body weight, no first-degree relative with diabetes, *and* not Hispanic, Native American, Asian, or African-American.

†The 100-g diagnostic test is performed on patients who have a positive result of a screening test. The diagnosis of GDM requires any two of the four plasma glucose values obtained during the test to meet or exceed the values shown above.

Adapted from Report of the Expert Committee on the Diagnosis and Classification of Diabetes Mellitus. Diabetes Care 20:1183, 1997.

altered to exclude from screening those women in a low-risk group for GDM because it is unlikely to be very cost-effective.[129] Women in this low-risk group are younger than 25 years, are of normal body weight, have no first-degree relatives with diabetes, and are not members of an ethnic or racial group with a high prevalence of type 2 diabetes (Hispanic, African American, Native American, Asian). Pregnant women who fulfill *all* of these criteria usually do not need to be screened for GDM unless they have other high-risk characteristics for a poor obstetric outcome (see Chapter 11).

Screening is usually carried out between 24 and 28 weeks of gestation (unless other high-risk factors indicate an earlier evaluation). The oral glucose load is 50 g, and the test does not have to be performed in the fasting state. If the glucose concentration measured 1 hour later is 140 mg/dl or higher, a full OGTT should be carried out. This OGTT differs from the OGTT performed in the nonpregnant state in three respects. First, the recommended oral glucose load is 100 g. Second, blood samples are collected before and 1, 2, and 3 hours after the oral challenge. Third—and most importantly—the criteria (Table 1-5) for making the diagnosis of diabetes in pregnancy are much more sensitive than in nongravid women.[100] When screening was carried out in all pregnant women, GDM was found in approximately 2% to 4%.[155] (Diabetes and pregnancy are discussed in Chapter 11.)

REFERENCES

1. Report of the Expert Committee on the Diagnosis and Classification of Diabetes Mellitus. Diabetes Care 20:1183, 1997.
2. Mokdad AH, Ford ES, Bowman BA et al: Diabetes trends in the US 1990-1998. Diabetes Care 23:1278, 2000.
3. Harris MI: Diabetes in America: Epidemiology and scope of the problem. Diabetes Care 21(Suppl 3): C11, 1998.
4. American Diabetes Association. Economic Costs of Diabetes in the U.S. in 2002. Diabetes Care 26:917-932, 2003.
5. King H, Aubert RE, Herman WH: Global burden of diabetes 1995-2025. Prevalence, numerical estimates and projections Diabetes Care 21:1414, 1998.
6. Harris MI, Klein R, Cowie CC et al: Is the risk of diabetes retinopathy greater in non-Hispanic blacks and Mexican Americans than in non-Hispanic whites with type 2 diabetes? Diabetes Care 21:1230, 1998.
7. Haffner SM, Fong D, Stern MP et al: Diabetic retinopathy in Mexican Americans and non-Hispanic whites. Diabetes 37:878, 1988.
8. Franklin GM, Kahn LB, Baxter J et al: Sensory neuropathy in non–insulin-dependent diabetes: The San Luis Valley Diabetes Study. Am J Epidemiol 131:633, 1990.
9. Cowie CC, Port FK, Wolfe RA et al: Disparities in incidence of diabetic end-stage renal disease according to race and type of diabetes. N Engl J Med 321:1074, 1989.
10. Haffner SM, Mitchell BD, Pugh JA et al: Proteinuria in Mexican Americans and non-Hispanic whites with NIDDM. Diabetes Care 12:530, 1989.

11. Nelson RG, Morgenstern H, Bennett PH: An epidemic of proteinuria in Pima Indians with type 2 diabetes mellitus. Kidney Int 54:2081, 1998.

12. Resinick HE, Valsania P, Phillips CL: Diabetes mellitus and nontraumatic lower extremity amputation in black and white Americans: The National Health and Nutrition Examination Survey Epidemiologic Follow-up Study 1971-1992. Arch Intern Med 159:2470, 1999.

13. Lavery LA, van Houtum WH, Ashry HR et al: Diabetes-related lower extremity amputations disproportionately affect blacks and Mexican Americans. South Med J 92:593, 1999.

14. Brancati FL, Keo WH, Folsom AR et al: Incident type 2 diabetes mellitus in African American and white Adults: The Atherosclerosis Risk in Communities Study. JAMA 283:2253, 2000.

15. King H, Rewers M: Global estimates for prevalence of diabetes mellitus and impaired glucose tolerance in adults. WHO Ad Hoc Diabetes Reporting Group. Diabetes Care 16:157, 1993.

16. Diabetes facts and figures among Latinos. www.diabetes.org/main/info/facts/facts_latinos.jsp. Retrieved: 07/06/2003.

17. Neufeld ND, Raffel LJ, Landon C et al: Early presentation of type 2 diabetes in Mexican-American youth. Diabetes Care 21:80, 1998.

18. Nelson RG, Gohdes DM, Everhart JE et al: Lower-extremity amputations in NIDDM. 12-year follow-up study in Pima Indians. Diabetes Care 11:8, 1988.

19. Yood MU, Johnson CC, Blount A et al: Race and differences in breast cancer survival in a managed care population. J Natl Cancer Inst 91:1487, 1999.

20. Harris MI. Racial and ethnic differences in health care access and health outcomes for adults with type 2 diabetes. Diabetes Care 24:454, 2001.

21. Dalfra MD, Lapolla A, Masin M et al: Antepartum and early postpartum predictors of type 2 diabetes development in women with gestational diabetes mellitus. Diabetes Medtab 27:675, 2001.

22. Valleron AJ, Eschwege E, Papoz L et al: Agreement and discrepancy in the evaluation of normal and diabetic oral glucose tolerance test. Diabetes 24(6):585-593, 1975.

23. National Diabetes Data Group: Classification and diagnosis of diabetes mellitus and other categories of glucose intolerance. Diabetes 28:1039, 1979.

24. World Health Organization: WHO expert committee on Diabetes Mellitus: Second report. Geneva, Switzerland: World Health Organization, technical report 646, 1980.

25. Jarrett RJ, Keen H: Hyperglycemia and diabetes mellitus. Lancet 2:1009, 1976.

26. Sayegh HA, Jarrett RJ: Oral glucose tolerance tests and the diagnosis of diabetes mellitus: Results of a prospective study based on the Whitehall survey. Lancet 2:431, 1979.

27. Pettitt DJ, Knowler WC, Lisse JR et al: Development of retinopathy and proteinuria in relation to plasma-glucose concentrations in Pima Indians. Lancet 2:1050, 1980.

28. Harris MI, Hadden WC, Knowler WC et al: Prevalence of diabetes and impaired glucose tolerance and plasma glucose levels in U.S. population aged 20-74 yr. Diabetes 36:523, 1987.

29. Peters AL, Davidson MB, Schriger DL et al: A clinical approach for the diagnosis of diabetes mellitus. JAMA 15:1246, 1996.

30. Modan M, Harris MI: Fasting plasma glucose in screening for NIDDM in the U.S. and Israel. Diabetes Care 17:436, 1994.

31. Stolk RP, Orchard TJ, Grobbee DE: Why use the oral glucose tolerance test? Diabetes Care 18:1045, 1995.

32. Olefsky JM, Reaven GM: Insulin and glucose responses to identical oral glucose tolerance tests performed forty-eight hours apart. Diabetes 23:449, 1974.

33. Kosaka K, Mizuno Y, Kuzuya T: Reproducibility of the oral glucose tolerance test and the rice-meal test in mild diabetes. Diabetes 15:901, 1966.

34. Wang PY, Kaneko T, Wang Y et al: Impairment of glucose tolerance in normal adults following a lowered carbohydrate intake. Tokoku J Exp Med 189(1):59-70, 1999.

35. Melton LJ, Palumbo RJ, Chu CP: Incidence of diabetes mellitus by clinical type. Diabetes Care 6:75, 1983.

36. Shaw JE, de Courten M, Boydo EJ et al: Impact of new diagnostic criteria for diabetes in different populations. Diabetes Care 22:762, 1999.

37. Dinneen SF, Maldonado D, Leibson CL et al: Effects of changing diagnostic criteria on the risk of developing diabetes. Diabetes Care 21:1408, 1998.

38. The DECODE Study group. Is fasting glucose sufficient to define diabetes? Epidemiological data from 20 European studies. Diabetologia 42:647, 1999.

39. Charles MA, Fontbonne A, Thibult N et al: Risk factors for NIDDM in white population. Paris prospective study. Diabetes 40:796, 1991.

40. Charles MA, Balkau B, Vauzelle-Kervroedan F et al: Revision of diagnostic criteria for diabetes (Letter). Lancet 348:1657, 1996.

41. Shaw JE, Zimmet PZ, Hodge AM et al: Impaired fasting glucose: How low should it go? Diabetes Care 23:34, 2000.

41a. Heine RJ, Nijpels G, Mooy JM: New data on the rate of progression of impaired glucose tolerance to NIDDM and predicting factors. Diabet Med 13(3 Suppl 2):S12-S14, 1996.

42. Eckfeldt JH, Burns DE: Another step toward standardization of methods for measuring hemoglobin A1c. Clin Chem 43:1811, 1997.

43. Peters AL: Diagnosing diabetes in 2000. Curr Opin Endocrinol Diabetes 2000 7:31, 2000.

44. Davidson MB, Schriger DL, Peters AL et al: Revisiting the oral glucose tolerance test criterion for the diagnosis of diabetes. J Gen Intern Med 15:551, 2000.

45. Zimmet P, Whitehouse S: The effect of age on glucose tolerance: Studies in a Micronesian population with a high prevalence of diabetes. Diabetes 28:617, 1979.

46. McCance D, Hanson RL, Charles MA et al: Comparison of tests for glycated haemoglobin and fasting and two hour plasma glucose concentrations as diagnostic methods for diabetes. BMJ 308:1323, 1994.

47. Gordon T: Glucose tolerance of adults, United States, 1960-1962: Diabetes prevalence and results of glucose tolerance test, by age and sex. Vital and Health Statistics, Washington D.C., U.S. Government Printing Office, 1964, Series 11, No. 2.

48. Hayner NS, Kjelsberg MD, Epstein FH et al: Carbohydrate tolerance and diabetes in a total community, Tecumseh, Michigan. I. Effects of age, sex, and test conditions on one-hour glucose tolerance in adults. Diabetes 14:413, 1965.

49. The DCCT Research Group: The effect of intensive diabetes treatment on the development and progression of long-term complications in insulin-dependent diabetes mellitus. N Engl J Med 329:977, 1993.

50. The DCCT Research Group: The relationship of glycemic exposure (HbA1c) to the risk of development and progression of retinopathy in the diabetes control and complications trial. Diabetes 44:968, 1995.

51. I. Ohkubo Y, Kishikawa H, Araki E et al: Intensive insulin therapy prevents the progression of diabetic microvascular complications in Japanese patients with non-insulin-dependent diabetes mellitus: A randomized prospective 6-year study. Diabetes Res Clin Pract 28:3, 1995.

52. Krolewski AS, Laffel LMB, Krolewski M et al: Glycosylated hemoglobin and the risk of microalbuminuria in patients with insulin-dependent diabetes mellitus. N Engl J Med 332:1251, 1995.

53. Tanaka Y, Atsumi Y, Matsuoka K et al: Role of glycemic control and blood pressure in the development and progression of nephropathy in elderly Japanese NIDDM patients. Diabetes Care 21:116, 1998.

54. Warram JH, Scott LJ, Hanna LS et al: Progression of microalbuminuria to proteinuria in type 1 diabetes: Nonlinear relationship with hyperglycemia. Diabetes 49:94, 2000.

55. Bucala R, Cerami A, Vlassara H: Advanced glycosylation end products in diabetic complications. Diabetes Rev 3:258, 1995.

56. Cohen MP, Sharma K, Jin Y et al: Prevention of diabetic nephropathy in db/db mice with glycated albumin antagonists. J Clin Invest 95:2338, 1995.

57. Nakamura S, Makita Z, Ishikawa S et al: Progression of nephropathy in spontaneous diabetic rats is prevented by OPB-9195, a novel inhibitor of advanced glycation. Diabetes 46:895, 1997.

58. Clements RS Jr, Robsion WG Jr, Cohen MP: Anti-glycated albumin therapy ameliorates early retinal microvascular pathology in db/db mice. J Diabetes Comp 12:28, 1998.

59. Tattersall RB, Jackson JGL: Social and emotional complications of diabetes. In Keen H, Jarrett J, (eds): Complications of Diabetes. Year Book Medical Publishers, Chicago, 1982, p. 271.

60. Knowler WC: Screening for NIDDM: Opportunities for detection, treatment and prevention. Diabetes Care 17:445, 1994.

61. Harris MI, Cowie CC, Eastman R: Health-insurance coverage for adults with diabetes in the U.S. population. Diabetes Care 17:585, 1994.

62. Ballard DJ, Humphrey LL, Melton J III et al: Epidemiology of persistent proteinuria in type II diabetes. Diabetes 37:405, 1988.

63. Harris MI: Undiagnosed NIDDM: Public health issues. Diabetes Care 16:642, 1993.

64. Bjornholt JV, Erikssen G, Aaser E et al: Fasting blood glucose: An underestimated risk factor for cardiovascular death. Results from a 22-year follow-up of healthy nondiabetic men. Diabetes Care 22:45, 1999.

65. Coutinho M, Gerstein HC, Wang Y et al: The relationship between glucose and incident cardiovascular events: A metaregression analysis of published data from 20 studies of 95,783 individuals followed for 12.4 years. Diabetes Care 22:233, 1999.

66. Balkau B, Bertrais S, Ducimetiere P et al: Is there a glycemic threshold for mortality risk? Diabetes Care 22:696, 1999.

67. Khaw KT, Wareham N, Bingham S et al: Glycated haemoglobin, diabetes, and mortality in men in Norfolk cohort of European Prospective Investigation of Cancer and Nutrition (EPIC-Norfolk). BMJ 322:15, 2001.

68. Wild SH, Dunn CJ, McKeigue PM et al: Glycemic control and cardiovascular disease in type 2 diabetes: A review. Diabetes Metab Res Rev 15:197, 1999.

69. Lerman-Garber I, Zamora-Gonzalez J, Ono AH et al: Effect of the new diagnostic criteria for diabetes in the Mexico City study. Endocr Pract 5:179, 1999.

70. Rohlfing CL, Little RP, Wiedmeyer HM et al: Use of Ghb (Hgb A_{1c}) in screening for undiagnosed diabetes in the U.S. population. Diabetes Care 23:187, 2000.

71. Coutinho M, Gerstein HC, Wang Y et al: The relationship between glucose and incident cardiovascular events: A metaregression analysis of published data from 20 studies of 95,783 individuals followed for 12.4 years. Diabetes Care 22:233, 1999.

72. Lim S, Tai ES, Tan BY et al: Cardiovascular risk profile in individuals with borderline glycemia. The effect of the 1997 American Diabetes Association diagnostic criteria and the 1998 World Health Organization provisional report. Diabetes Care 23:278, 2000.

73. Perry RC, Baron AD: Impaired glucose tolerance. Why is it not a disease? Diabetes Care 22:883, 1999.

74. Folsom AR, Szklom M, Stevens J et al: A prospective study of coronary heart disease in relation to fasting insulin, glucose and diabetes. The Atherosclerosis Risk in Communities (ARIC) study. Diabetes Care 20:935, 1997.

75. Meigs JB, Nathan DM, Wilson PW: Metabolic risk factors worsen continuously across the spectrum of nondiabetic glucose tolerance. Ann Intern Med 128:524, 1998.
76. Tominaga M, Eguchi H, Manaka H et al: Impaired glucose tolerance is a risk factor for cardiovascular disease, but not impaired fasting glucose: The Funagata Diabetes Study. Diabetes Care 22:920, 1999.
77. Lowe LP, Liu K, Greenland P et al: Diabetes, asymptomatic hyperglycemia, and 22-year mortality in black and white men: The Chicago Heart Association Detection Project in Industry Study. Diabetes Care 20:163, 1997.
78. Barrett-Connor E, Ferara A: Isolated postchallenge hyperglycemia and the risk of fatal cardiovascular disease in older women and men: The Rancho Bernardo Study. Diabetes Care 21;1236, 1998.
79. Saydah SH, Loria CM, Eberhardt MS et al: Subclinical states of glucose intolerance and the risk of death in the US. Diabetes Care 24:447, 2001.
80. Khat KT, Wareham N, Luben R et al: Glycated haemoglobin, diabetes, and mortality in men in Norfolk cohort of European prospective investigation of cancer and nutrition (EPIC-Norfolk). BMJ 322:15, 2001.
81. Engelgau MM, Aubert RE, Thompson TJ et al: Screening for NIDDM in non-pregnant adults. Diabetes Care 18:1606, 1995.
82. Knowler WC: Screening for NIDDM. Opportunities for detection, treatment, and prevention Diabetes Care 17:445, 1994.
83. Stewart-Brown S, Farmer A: Screening could seriously damage your health. BMJ 314:533, 1997.
84. Andersson DK, Lundblad E, Svardsudd K: A model of early diagnosis in type 2 diabetes mellitus in primary health care. Diabetic Med 10:167, 1993.
85. Centers for Disease Control and Prevention: Diabetes Cost-Effectiveness Study group: The cost-effectiveness of screening for type 2 diabetes. JAMA 280:1757, 1998.
86. World Health Organization: Diabetes Mellitus: Report of a WHO Study Group (WHO Tech Rep Series 727). WHO, Geneva, 1985.
87. World Health Organization: Diabetes mellitus (WHO Tech Rep Series). WHO, Geneva, 1997.
88. Classen JB: The timing of immunization affects the development of diabetes in rodents. Autoimmunity 24:137, 1996.
89. Classen DC, Classen JB: The timing of pediatric immunization and the risk of insulin-dependent diabetes mellitus. Infect Dis Clin Pract 6:449-545, 1997.
90. Classen JB, Classen DC: Public should be told that vaccines may have long term adverse effects (Letter). BMJ 318:193, 1999.
91. Graves PM, Barriga KJ, Norris, JM et al: Lack of association between early childhood immunization and beta-cell autoimmunity. Diabetes Care 22:1694, 1999.
92. Winter WE, Maclaren NK, Riley WJ et al: Maturity-onset diabetes of youth in black Americans. N Engl J Med 316:285, 1987.
93. Banerji MA, Lebovitz HE: Remission in non-insulin-dependent diabetes mellitus: Clinical characteristics of remission and relapse in black patients. Medicine 69:176, 1990.
94. Umpierrez GE, Casals MMC, Gebhar SSP et al: Diabetic ketoacidosis in obese African-Americans. Diabetes 44:790, 1995.
95. Banerji MA, Chaiken RL, Lebovitz HE: Long-term normoglycemic remission in black newly diagnosed NIDDM subjects. Diabetes 45:337, 1996.
96. Imagawa A, Hanafusa T, Miyagawa J et al: A novel subtype of type 1 diabetes mellitus characterized by a rapid onset and an absence of diabetes related antibodies. N Engl J Med 342:301, 2000.
97. Irvine WJ, McCallum CJ, Gray RS et al: Clinical and pathogenic significance of pancreatic-islet-cell antibodies in diabetics treated with oral hypoglycemic agents. Lancet 1:1025, 1977.
98. Pozzilli P, DiMario U: Autoimmune diabetes not requiring insulin at diagnosis (latent autoimmune diabetes of the adult): Definition, characterization, and potential prevention. Diabetes Care 24:1460, 2001.
99. Carlsson A, Sundkvist G, Groop L et al: Insulin and glucagon secretion in patients with slowly progressing autoimmune diabetes (LADA). J Clin Endocrinol Metab 85:76, 2000.
100. National Diabetes Data Group: Classification and diagnosis of diabetes mellitus and other categories of glucose intolerance. Diabetes 28:1039, 1979.
101. Harris MI, Klein R, Welborn TA et al: Onset of NIDDM occurs at least 4-7 yr before clinical diagnosis. Diabetes Care 15:815, 1992.
102. Yki-Jarvinen H: Glucose toxicity. Endocr Rev 13:415, 1992.
103. Carter JS, Pugh JA, Monterrosa A: Non-insulin-dependent diabetes mellitus in minorities in the United States. Ann Intern Med 125:221, 1996.
104. Fujimoto WY, Leonetti DL, Kinyoun J et al: Prevalence of diabetes mellitus and impaired glucose tolerance among second-generation Japanese-American men. Diabetes 36:721, 1987.
105. O'Sullivan JB: Body weight and subsequent diabetes mellitus. JAMA 248:949, 1982.
106. Gerbitz KD, Gempel K, Brdiczka D: Genetic, biochemical and clinical implications of the cellular energy circuit. Diabetes 45:113, 1996.
107. Maassen JA, Kadowaki T: Maternally inherited diabetes and deafness: A new diabetes subtype. Diabetologia 39:375, 1996.
108. Karasik A, O'Hara C, Srikanta S et al: Genetically programmed selective islet cell loss in diabetes mellitus of Wolfram syndrome. Diabetes Care 12:135, 1989.
109. Fajans SS: Scope and heterogeneous nature of MODY. Diabetes Care 13:49, 1990.
110. Herman WH, Fajans SS, Ortiz FJ et al: Abnormal insulin secretion, not insulin resistance, is the

genetic or primary defect of MODY in the RW pedigree. Diabetes 43:40, 1994.

111. Wajngot A, Alvarsson M, Glaser A et al: Glucose potentiation of arginine-induced secretion is impaired in subjects with a glucokinase Glu256Lys mutation. Diabetes 43:1402, 1994.

112. Pueyo ME, Clement K, Vaxillaire M et al: Arginine-induced insulin release in glucokinase-deficient subjects. Diabetes Care 17:1015, 1994.

113. Hattersley AT, Turner RC, Permutt MA et al: Linkage of type 2 diabetes to the glucokinase gene. Lancet 339:1307, 1992.

114. Froguel P, Zouali H, Vionnet N et al: Familial hyperglycemia due to mutations in glucokinase. N Engl J Med 328:697, 1993.

115. Bell GI, Xian KS, Newman MV et al: Gene for non-insulin-dependent diabetes mellitus (maturity-onset diabetes of the young subtype) is linked to DNA polymorphism on human chromosome 20q. Proc Natl Acad Sci USA 88:1484, 1991.

116. Bowden DW, Gravius TC, Akots G et al: Identification of genetic markers flanking the locus for maturity-onset diabetes of the young on human chromosome 20. Diabetes 41:88, 1992.

117. Vaxillaire M, Boccio V, Philippi A et al: A gene for maturity onset diabetes of the young (MODY) maps to chromosome 12q. Nature Genet 9:418, 1995.

118. Menzel S, Yamagat K, Trabb JB et al: Localization of MODY3 to a 5-cM region of human chromosome 12. Diabetes 44:1408, 1995.

119. Taylor SI: Molecular mechanisms of insulin resistance: Lessons from patients with mutations in the insulin-receptor gene. Diabetes 41:1473, 1992.

120. Kahn CR, Flier JS, Bar RS et al: The syndromes of insulin resistance and acanthosis nigricans. N Engl J Med 294:739, 1976.

121. Yoshimasa Y, Seino S, Whittaker J et al: Insulin-resistant diabetes due to a point mutation that prevents insulin proreceptor processing. Science 240:784, 1988.

122. Kadowaki T, Bevins CL, Cama A et al: Two mutant alleles of the insulin receptor gene in a patient with extreme insulin resistance. Science 240:787, 1988.

123. Muller-Wieland D, van der Vorm ER, Streicher R et al: An in-frame insertion in exon 3 and a nonsense mutation in exon 2 of the insulin receptor gene associated with severe insulin resistance in a patient with Rabson-Mendenhall syndrome. Diabetologia 36:1168, 1993.

124. Senior B, Gellis SS: The syndromes of total lipodystrophy and of partial lipodystrophy. Pediatrics 33:593, 1964.

125. Davidson MB, Young RT: Metabolic studies in familial partial lipodystrophy of the lower trunk and extremities. Diabetologia 11:561, 1975.

126. van der Vorm ER, Kuipers A, Bonenkamp JW et al: Patients with lipodystrophic diabetes mellitus of the Seip-Berardineli type express normal insulin receptors. Diabetologia 36:172, 1993.

127. Desbois-Mouthon C, Magre J, Amselem S et al: Lipoatrophic diabetes: Genetic exclusion of the insulin receptor gene. J Clin Endocrinol Metab 80:314, 1995.

128. Sjoberg RJ, Kidd GS: Pancreatic diabetes mellitus. Diabetes Care 12:715, 1989.

129. Report of the Expert Committee on the Diagnosis and Classification of Diabetes Mellitus. Diabetes Care 20:1183, 1997.

130. Hoet JJ, Tripathy BB, Rao RH et al: Malnutrition and diabetes in the tropics. Diabetes Care 19:1014, 1996.

131. Mohan V, Premalatha G, Padma A et al: Fibrocalculous pancreatic diabetes. Diabetes Care 11:1274, 1996.

132. World Health Organization: Diabetes mellitus (WHO Tech Rep Series). WHO, Geneva, December 1997.

133. Handwerger S, Roth J, Gorden P et al: Glucose intolerance in cystic fibrosis. N Engl J Med 281:451, 1969.

134. Phelps G, Chapman I, Hall P et al: Prevalence of genetic haemochromatosis among diabetic patients. Lancet 2:925, 1989.

135. Morris DV, Nabarro JDN: Pancreatic cancer and diabetes mellitus. Diabetes Med 1:119, 1984.

136. Gullo L, Pezzilli R, Morselli-Labate AM et al: Diabetes and the risk of pancreatic cancer. N Engl J Med 331:81, 1994.

137. Berelowitz M, Eugene HG: Non-insulin dependent diabetes mellitus secondary to other endocrine disorders. In LeRoith D, Taylor S, Olefsky JM (eds): Diabetes Mellitus. A Fundamental and Clinical Text. Lippincott-Raven, 1996, p. 496.

138. Shen DC, Davidson MB, Kuo SW et al: Peripheral and hepatic insulin antagonism in hyperthyroidism. J Clin Endocrinol Metab 66:565, 1988.

139. Konomi K, Chijiiwa K, Katsuta T et al: Pancreatic somatostatinoma: A case report and review of the literature. J Surg Oncol 43:259, 1990.

140. Conn JW: Hypertension, the potassium ion and impaired carbohydrate tolerance. N Engl J Med 273:1135, 1965.

141. Pandit MK, Burke J, Gustafson AB et al: Drug-induced disorders of glucose tolerance. Ann Intern Med 118:529, 1993.

142. Bressler P, DeFronzo RA: Drugs and diabetes. Diabetes Rev 2:53, 1994.

143. Bouchard P, Sai P, Reach G et al: Diabetes mellitus following pentamidine-induced hypoglycemia in humans. Diabetes 31:40, 1982.

144. Gallanosa AG, Spyker DA, Curnow RT: Diabetes mellitus associated with autonomic and peripheral neuropathy after Vacor poisoning: A review. Clin Toxicol 18:441, 1981.

145. Fabris P, Betterle C, Floreani A et al: Development of type I diabetes mellitus during interferon alpha therapy for chronic HCV hepatitis. Lancet 340:548, 1992.

146. Shiba T, Morino Y, Tagawa K et al: Onset of diabetes with high titer anti-GAD antibody after

IFN therapy for chronic hepatitis. Diabetes Res Clin Pract 30:237, 1996.

147. Yoon JW: A new look at viruses in type 1 diabetes. Diabetes Metab Rev 11:83, 1995.

148. Yoon JW, Austin M, Onodera T et al: Virus-induced diabetes mellitus: Isolation of a virus from the pancreas of a child with diabetic ketoacidosis. N Engl J Med 300:1173, 1979.

149. Champsaur H, Bottazzo G, Bertrams J et al: Virologic, immunologic, and genetic factors in insulin-dependent diabetes mellitus. J Pediatr 100:15, 1982.

150. Foulis AK, McGill M, Farquharson MA et al: A search for evidence of viral infection in pancreases of newly diagnosed patients with IDDM. Diabetologia 40:53, 1997.

151. Solimena M, Folli F, Aparisi R et al: Autoantibodies to GABA-nergic neurons and pancreatic beta cells in stiff-man syndrome. N Engl J Med 41:347, 1992.

152. Taylor SI, Barbetti F, Accili D et al: Syndrome of autoimmunity and hypoglycemia. Endocrinol Metab Clin North Am 18:123, 1989.

153. Kahn CR, Flier JS, Bar RS et al: The syndromes of insulin resistance and acanthosis nigricans. N Engl J Med 294:739, 1976.

154. Raffel LJ, Scheuner MT, Rotter JI: Genetics of diabetes. In Porte D, Sherwin RS (eds): Diabetes Mellitus, 5th ed. Appleton & Lange, Norwalk, Conn, 1997, p. 401.

155. Coustan DR: Diagnosis of gestational diabetes. Diabetes Rev 3:614, 1995.

TREATMENT: GENERAL PRINCIPLES

We now have clear evidence that near-normalization of blood glucose levels in patients with type 1[1] and type 2 diabetes[2] can significantly delay the onset and retard the progression of microvascular complications associated with diabetes. Although significant morbidity and mortality results from these complications, the leading cause of death in diabetes continues to be macrovascular, namely cardiovascular (which is not as directly related to levels of glycemia). Based on the emerging knowledge of the relationship between metabolic control and the development of microvascular as well as macrovascular disease, optimal therapy becomes more important than ever. This chapter discusses the underlying metabolic abnormalities seen in diabetes, and attempts to address how these conditions intertwine to produce clinical disease. The remainder of this chapter focuses on the evidence supporting glycemic control and its impact on complications.

METABOLIC PRINCIPLES

In the postabsorptive state (usually 4 or more hours after eating), the plasma glucose concentration remains relatively constant and reflects the balance between glucose production by the liver and glucose utilization by peripheral tissues. The sources of hepatic glucose production are glycogenolysis (the breakdown of glycogen, the storage form of glucose) and gluconeogenesis (the synthesis of new glucose from noncarbohydrate precursors). After 8 to 12 hours without food intake, hepatic glycogenolysis decreases markedly, and gluconeogenesis by the liver is the main source of circulating glucose. At this time, glucose is utilized mainly by the brain and red blood cells, whereas the rest of the tissues use free fatty acids (FFA). The role of basal insulin levels in the fasting state is to oppose the effect of glucagon (a hormone that increases glycemia and increases glycogenolysis) on the liver and to restrain hepatic glucose production. Insulin does not affect glucose utilization by the brain or red blood cells.

In the 4-hour period after an oral glucose challenge, approximately 70% of glucose is taken up by peripheral tissues (primarily muscle) and the remainder is used by splanchnic tissues (probably mostly by the liver). Insulin is secreted in response to the carbohydrate and protein contents of a meal. It increases the amount of glucose transported into muscle. Its effects on hepatic carbohydrate metabolism are complex. Essentially, insulin stimulates glucose utilization by enhancing its storage as glycogen or by increasing glycolysis. The latter can lead to the conversion of hepatic glucose into adipose tissue triglycerides through a complicated series of reactions. Insulin also inhibits gluconeogenesis and glycogenolysis. The overall results of insulin action on the liver are an increase in glucose utilization after meals and a restraint on glucose production in the postabsorptive state, the period after which meal nutrients have been stored.

Insulin also has a profound influence on fat metabolism. Ingested fat is stored as triglycerides in adipose tissue. Excess carbohydrate calories also form part of the triglyceride molecule. Insulin promotes triglyceride synthesis by helping the dietary fat gain access into the fat cell and by stimulating the conversion of glucose to glycerol, the backbone of the triglyceride molecule. Most importantly, once adipose tissue triglycerides are formed, insulin has a critical role in inhibiting their breakdown. This effect is extremely critical because the FFA released as a result of triglyceride hydrolysis (lipoly-

sis) can be converted to ketone bodies in the liver. In fact, the most important determinant of the rate of formation of ketone bodies is the amount of FFA delivered to the liver. If excess FFAs are released from adipose tissue, increased production of ketone bodies by the liver follows. Although these ketone bodies can be utilized to some extent by peripheral tissues, they soon start to accumulate in the circulation and spill over into the urine.

The quantitative relation among the effects of insulin on selected aspects of carbohydrate and fat metabolism is depicted in Figure 2-1. In a nonresistant state, approximately 25 to 50 μU of insulin per milliliter is necessary to affect glucose metabolism by liver and muscle; 10 μU/ml is required to stimulate glucose uptake into fat. However, the inhibition of lipolysis requires only 1 to 2 μU of active insulin per milliliter. Therefore, as the amount of effective insulin diminishes from normal levels, the first bio-

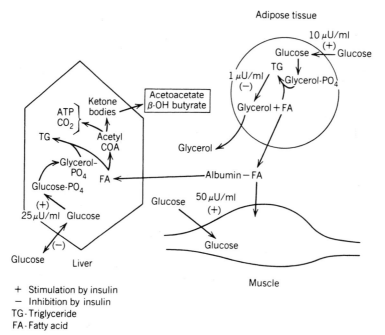

FIGURE 2-1. Pathophysiology of ketosis. (+), stimulation by insulin; (−), inhibition by insulin; ATP, adenosine triphosphate; β-OH, beta-hydroxy; CO_2, carbon dioxide; COA, coenzyme A; FA, fatty acid; PO_4, phosphate; μU, microunit; TG, triglyceride;.

chemical abnormality to develop is post-prandial hyperglycemia. Enough insulin remains to maintain normal fasting glucose concentrations and to prevent ketosis. As the process continues, fasting hyper-glycemia develops, but the patient still does not become ketotic. Only when virtually no effective insulin is available does ketosis occur. In other words, if an untreated diabetic patient does not manifest ketonuria, the pancreatic β-cells of that patient are still able to secrete some insulin. Alternatively, if a diabetic patient has ketonuria, very little if any effective insulin remains at that time.

▼
DISTINGUISHING CLINICAL AND PATHOGENETIC FEATURES OF TYPES 1 AND 2 DIABETES MELLITUS

CLINICAL DIFFERENCES:

The distinction between ketosis-resistant and ketosis-prone diabetes has important implications for therapy Because ketosis-prone (type 1) diabetic patients have virtu-ally no effective endogenous insulin, they require exogenous insulin. Although the need for insulin is not as imperative in ketosis-resistant (type 2) diabetic patients (because without it they do not become ketotic and slip into acidosis), these patients may require insulin because diet and oral med-ications fail to control their hyperglycemia. Approximately 40% of ketosis-resistant dia-betic patients take insulin either alone or in combination with other agents (see Chapter 5), 40% use oral agents as monotherapy or in combination therapy (see Chapter 4), and the remaining 20% are treated by diet (see Chapter 3) alone.[3] Patients with latent autoimmune diabetes of the adult (LADA) may initially behave as though ketosis-resist-ant and respond to oral agents, but over time they become ketosis-prone, as their β-cell function declines.[4]

Other differences between patients who are ketosis-prone (type 1) and ketosis-resist-ant (type 2) are summarized in Table 2-1. Type 1 diabetes has historically been called *juvenile-onset diabetes*. This term is not accu-rate, however, because some diabetic patients whose disease starts in adulthood may have type 1 diabetes. Furthermore, an increasing number of patients in their teens or at the end of the first decade of life have been found to have type 2 diabetes, espe-cially in African American, Native American, and Hispanic populations. Children who have type 1 diabetes usually present with a short history of the symptoms of hyper-glycemia (polyuria, polydipsia, lethargy, and weight loss), and if their condition is not rec-ognized quickly, it may develop into ketoaci-dosis. Adults tend to develop the disease more gradually.

Pathogenesis of Type 1 Diabetes

The events leading up to destruction of the pancreatic β-cell in type 1 diabetes can be divided into five stages. These are depicted in Figure 2-2, in which the hypothetical pan-creatic β-cell mass is plotted against time. Genetic, immunologic, and probably envi-ronmental (e.g., possibly viral) influences are involved, and these eventually lead to total exhaustion of the β-cell. The major genetic risk factor for the development of type 1 diabetes is the human leukocyte anti-gen (HLA) genes located on the short arm of the sixth chromosome. Their identifica-tion requires testing of white blood cells, which accounts for their name. These genes determine which surface antigens are pro-duced by nucleated cells. The surface anti-gens are involved in a host of cell-to-cell interactions, one of which includes the rejection process (i.e., the reaction when tis-sue from one host is transplanted into another). Because many different surface antigens are possible in a population, a large number of separate genes are responsible for them. Two HLA types, DR3 and/or DR4,

TABLE 2-1 METABOLIC AND CLINICAL CHARACTERISTICS OF THE TWO MAJOR TYPES OF DIABETES MELLITUS

Characteristic	Ketosis-Prone (Type 1)	Ketosis-Resistant (Type 2)
Synonyms	Juvenile-onset diabetes, growth-onset diabetes, IDDM	Adult-onset diabetes, maturity-onset diabetes, NIDDM
Age of onset	Usually during childhood (growth) but sometimes occurs in adults	Usually during adulthood (maturity) but occasionally diagnosed in children and adolescents[*]
Precipitating factors	Altered immune response; environmental "stresses"	Age, obesity
Pancreatic insulin	Very low to absent	Present
Insulin responses to glucose	Little or none	Decreased when weight and glucose levels taken into account
Insulin responses to meals	Little or none	Normal in absolute terms, but nondiabetic persons with this degree of hyperglycemia would have higher levels
Insulin resistance	Present only when diabetes is out of control	Present (independent of obesity and control)
Response to prolonged fast	Hyperglycemia, ketoacidosis	Glucose returns toward normal
Response to stress	Ketoacidosis	Hyperglycemia without ketosis
Associated obesity	Usually absent	Commonly present (~80%)
Sensitivity to insulin	Usually sensitive	Relatively resistant

IDDM, insulin-dependent diabetes mellitus; NIDDM, non-insulin-dependent diabetes mellitus.
[*]Especially in African American, Native American, and Hispanic populations.

are present in 95% of Caucasian patients with type 1 diabetes, in contrast to approximately 50% of the general population without type 1 diabetes. This means that certain genes, the ones whose expression produces these HLA types, are also common in these patients and provide a marker for the genetic background that increases susceptibility to type 1 diabetes.

The HLA system in humans is the analogue of the major histocompatibility system that occurs in all animals. This chromosomal region consists of loci that not only control the synthesis of transplantation (surface) antigens but also have fundamental roles in the immune process. Indeed,

strong evidence suggests that an immune process is active at the onset of type 1 diabetes. Lymphocytic infiltrates are seen in the islets of Langerhans of patients on whom an autopsy is performed soon after the diagnosis. Autoantibodies against islet cells are present in the sera of more than 80% of type 1 patients if they are tested near the onset of their disease; a gradual reduction in antibody titers occurs during the ensuing year in most patients. Autoantibodies against other antigens are also present.[5] Many patients have autoantibodies against the insulin molecule at the time of diagnosis. (Although it is common for patients treated with insulin to develop antibodies against the hormone

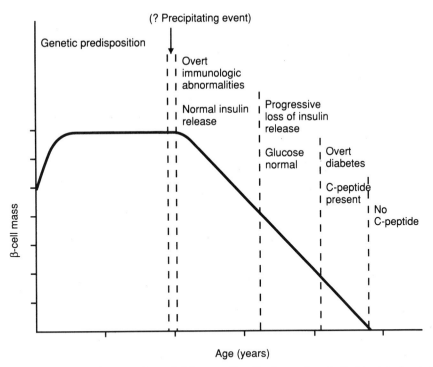

FIGURE 2-2. Stages in the development of type 1 diabetes mellitus. β-cell mass (hypothetical) is plotted against time. *(From Eisenbarth GS: Type 1 diabetes mellitus: A chronic autoimmune disease. Triangle 23:111, 1984.)*

[see Chapter 5], new-onset type 1 diabetic patients have not been exposed to exogenous insulin, and their antibodies have been generated against their own insulin.) A third autoantibody that has received much attention in recent years is one produced against glutamic acid decarboxylase (GAD), also known as the 64K antigen until it was correctly identified. This enzyme is located in the β-cell of the pancreas. Autoantibodies against antigens between 37,000 and 40,000 molecular weight (commonly called the 37K antigen) have also been found. Some or all of these autoantibodies precede the clinical appearance of type 1 diabetes, sometimes for a period of years. The higher the titer of these autoantibodies (Figure 2-3) and the more of them present (Figure 2-4), the more likely the individual is to develop type 1 diabetes.

During this preceding period before the development of diabetes in which high titers of these autoantibodies are often present, oral glucose tolerance is normal, and the insulin response to oral glucose is either normal or subtle changes only can be detected. However, the insulin response to intravenous glucose may show a progressive decline. After a bolus of glucose is injected, a rapid (within 1 to 2 minutes) rise of insulin is noted. This acute phase of insulin release falls below 5% of the response in a normal population in those individuals destined to develop type 1 diabetes (even though they still maintain relatively normal glucose and insulin responses to oral glucose). Type 1 diabetes can appear soon afterward (within weeks to months). Even with overt diabetes, these patients initially retain some insulin secretion (as assessed by measurement of C-peptide, a polypeptide packaged with insulin in β-cell granules and secreted along with insulin). Within a few years, however, the β-cell is completely

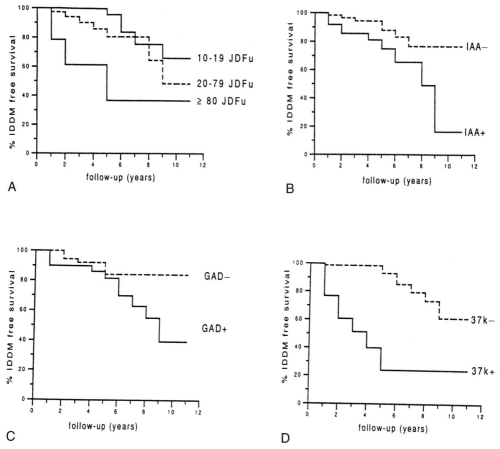

FIGURE 2-3. The cumulative risk of type 1 diabetes at 10 years in 101 unaffected first-degree relatives of children with type 1 diabetes by *(A)* level of islet cell autoantibodies measured in Juvenile Diabetes Foundation units (JDFu), *(B)* insulin autoantibodies (IAA), *(C)* autoantibodies to glutamic acid decarboxylase (GAD), and *(D)* autoantibodies to the 37K antigen. IDDM, insulin-dependent diabetes mellitus. *(From Bingley PJ for the Icarus Group: Interactions of age, islet cell antibodies, insulin autoantibodies, and first-phase insulin response in predicting risk of progression to IDDM in ICA+ relatives: The Icarus data set. Diabetes 45:1720, 1996.)*

exhausted and incapable of secreting any C-peptide or insulin.

Controversy surrounds the possible environmental "stresses" that may trigger the events leading to type 1 diabetes. Although viral infections may have a role, the evidence that viruses precipitate the *acute* clinical onset of type 1 diabetes is much weaker than the case for the importance of an appropriate genetic background and the involvement of immunologic factors. However, evidence suggests that exposure to certain enteroviruses, most commonly Coxsackie B4, may initiate the β-cell destruction starting in the months to years preceding the clinical onset of type 1 diabetes.[6] The mechanism may involve immunologic cross-reactivity between viral and β-cell antigens. Specifically, one part of the GAD molecule is structurally very similar to a portion of the Coxsackie B4 virus. It seems certain, however, that whatever initiates the chronic autoimmune process, be it viral agent, toxin, or random immunologic event, it occurs because of genetic susceptibility.

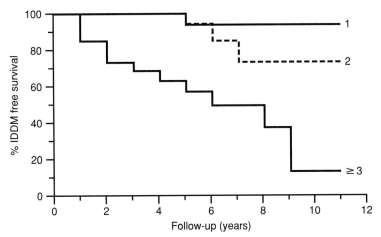

FIGURE 2-4. The cumulative risk of type 1 diabetes after 10 years in 101 unaffected first-degree relatives of a child with type 1 diabetes by the number of autoantibodies detected. IDDM, insulin-dependent diabetes mellitus. *(From Bingley PJ for the Icarus Group: Interactions of age, islet cell antibodies, insulin autoantibodies, and first-phase insulin response in predicting risk of progression to IDDM in ICA+ relatives: The Icarus data set. Diabetes 45:1720, 1996.)*

Pathogenesis of Type 2 Diabetes

Type 2 or ketosis-resistant diabetes was often called *maturity-onset* or *adult-onset* diabetes. As was stated previously, however, type 1 diabetes can start in adulthood, and type 2 diabetes (rarely progressing to ketosis) occurs in children and adolescents. The latter is much more common in African American, Native American, and Hispanic populations. Nevertheless, the majority of cases of type 2 diabetes do begin after the age of 40 years. Aging and obesity have been recognized as two associated factors. Diabetes is diagnosed in approximately 75% of type 2 patients on either a routine physical examination or during the work-up for another medical problem. Only 25% present to their physicians with symptoms.[7]

The pathogenesis of type 2 diabetes involves both relative insulin deficiency and impairment of insulin action. The insulin response to intravenous and oral glucose is decreased, although insulin concentrations after meals are normal or only slightly decreased. Because postprandial glucose levels are elevated, one might expect higher insulin concentrations, and hence a relative

insulin deficiency exists. On the other hand, the combination of normal insulin concentrations and hyperglycemia implies the presence of insulin resistance. (The term *insulin resistance* is used here, but this relatively minor degree of insulin ineffectiveness must be distinguished from the clinical syndrome of insulin resistance, in which patients require more than 200 U of insulin per day [see Chapter 5]). Indeed, sophisticated methods of evaluating insulin action have directly shown that insulin works ineffectively in the target tissues (muscle and liver) in patients with type 2 diabetes mellitus. Studies of insulin action in a large number of normal (nondiabetic) subjects have revealed a wide range of sensitivity to insulin. Some normal individuals have as much insulin resistance as those with type 2 diabetes. The former, however, are able to secrete more insulin than the latter.

The following temporal relationship between insulin secretion and sensitivity to insulin is now accepted by most investigators.[8] Insulin resistance occurs in those patients who may develop type 2 diabetes mellitus. In those in whom pancreatic β-cell reserve is sufficient, normal glucose levels are preserved at the expense of hyperinsulinemia. In those in whom the β-cell reserve is inadequate to maintain normal glucose levels, impaired glucose tolerance (IGT) appears. Hyperinsulinemia initially continues. However, as the β-cell starts to fail, glucose concentrations increase to values consistent with diabetes, and insulin concentrations decline to "normal" levels or below. Presumably, those individuals who progress from hyperinsulinemia and normal glucose tolerance through hyperinsulinemia and IGT to overt diabetes have a genetic susceptibility for a decreased β-cell reserve. Those with an adequate reserve for insulin secretion maintain normal tolerance or IGT at the expense of continued hyperinsulinemia. This scenario is supported by considering two groups of individuals who are at an increased risk for type 2 diabetes, the obese and the elderly. Not only have insulin resistance and hyperinsulinemia been documented in both groups, but IGT is also more common. If enhanced insulin secretion were unable to continue to overcome their insulin resistance, diabetes would ensue, thus accounting for the fact that 80% of type 2 patients are obese, and the prevalence of diabetes in people older than 65 years of age may be as high as 15% to 20%.

Why β-cell reserve is not maintained in those individuals developing type 2 diabetes is completely unknown. The mechanism of the insulin resistance is almost as enigmatic. The critical first step of insulin action is binding to receptors located on the cell surface. This triggers a signal (or signals) within the cell that enables insulin to carry out a myriad of effects. However, insulin binding is normal in type 2 diabetic patients. Therefore the site of the insulin resistance must be at a postbinding step. At the moment, that is all that can be said with certainty for the great majority (probably >95%) of type 2 diabetic patients. Many studies have pinpointed the lesion at the glucose transport/phosphorylation step

with evidence that glucose transport is affected.[9] Hormone regulation of glucose transport is an important action of insulin. Several mammalian glucose transporter (GLUT) genes have been identified by complementary deoxyribonucleic acid (cDNA) cloning and sequencing.[10] Four of these transporters (GLUT 1 to 4) are involved in the sodium independent facilitative diffusion of glucose into cells. GLUT 4 is the principal insulin-regulated GLUT, and changes in GLUT 4 in response to insulin are as important determinant of overall glucose uptake and plasma concentrations.[11]

However, in a small number of type 2 diabetic patients, the cause of their diabetes has been pinpointed. These fall into two general groups, maturity-onset diabetes of the young and syndromes of extreme insulin resistance. As discussed in Chapter 1, type 2 diabetes can occur in families in an autosomal dominant pattern of inheritance (i.e., it will be present in three successive generations). In many (but not all) of these families, various abnormalities occur in the gene coding for glucokinase, an enzyme important for glucose-induced insulin secretion.[8] In the rare cases of extreme insulin resistance (e.g., babies with leprechaunism, women with hyperandrogenism and acanthosis nigricans), genetic mutations of the insulin receptor have been found.[12]

In contrast to the situation in ketosis-prone diabetes, decreased food intake in the absence of drugs (insulin or sulfonylurea agents) results in improved carbohydrate metabolism in ketosis-resistant patients, especially patients who are obese. Similarly, with rare exceptions, the response to stress is hyperglycemia without ketosis or ketoacidosis. If insulin is required, relatively large amounts are needed by patients who are obese, but usually not by patients who are lean. Patients who are ketosis-resistant always respond to some extent either to dietary therapy alone or to dietary therapy supplemented with sulfonylurea agents or metformin (see Chapter 4). Thus the functional distinction between patients who are ketosis-prone and patients who are ketosis-resistant delineates certain metabolic characteristics with important clinical ramifications. Furthermore, the pathogenesis of each is completely different.

Type 1 diabetes is much less common than type 2 diabetes, occurring in 5% to 10% of patients with diabetes. Many of these with type 1 diabetes will have been diagnosed iin childhood. However, a growing number of younger individuals (<20 years of age) are being diagnosed with type 2 or ketosis-resistant diabetes. The majority of individuals with type 2 diabetes will have diabetes with onset in adulthood, mostly after the age of 40. Of these patients, most are obese and ketosis-resistant. Adults of normal weight with diabetes can have either type 1 or type 2 diabetes.

RELATION OF DIABETIC CONTROL TO DIABETIC COMPLICATIONS

The causes of death in the diabetic population changed drastically after the introduction of insulin therapy by Banting and Best in 1922. Today the vast majority of diabetic patients die of one of the vascular complications. These complications usually do not develop until many years after the onset of diabetes mellitus. Thus there is ample time in which to prevent or at least ameliorate these complications. The complications of diabetes mellitus can be divided into three general categories: macroangiopathy (coronary artery, cerebrovascular, and peripheral vascular disease), microangiopathy (retinopathy, nephropathy), and neuropathy (peripheral and autonomic neuropathy).

The morphologic hallmark of diabetic microangiopathy is increased thickness of the basement membrane surrounding capillaries, not only in the eyes and kidneys but in most other tissues throughout the body. This increase in basement membrane thick-ness is seen in all of these animal models of diabetes as well. Near euglycemia, whether accomplished by intensive insulin injection regimens or by transplantation of pancreatic β-cells in genetically identical animals, mostly prevented these complications.

Based on this body of data, large scale multicenter prospective trials were carried out in both type 1 and type 2 diabetes to determine the effects of glycemic control on the development of complications in patients with diabetes. The results of the Diabetes Control and Complications Trial (DCCT),[1] announced in June of 1993, confirmed that near-normalization of blood glucose levels in patients with type 1 diabetes can significantly delay the onset and slow the progression of complications associated with this disease. Since that time, these results have been echoed in patients with type 2 diabetes. Ohkubo et al[13] showed that intensive therapy prevented the progression of diabetic microvascular complications in a population of Japanese patients with type 2 diabetes (The Kumamoto Study), and the United Kingdom Prospective Diabetes Study (UKPDS)[2] confirmed these findings in 1998. Although these landmark trials warrant a thorough discussion (which will proceed in the following text) it is important to mention the investigative work done by individuals on a smaller scale that paved the way for these large definitive trials. In particular, work by Miki et al[14] and Pirart et al[15] helped to define the relationship between retinopathy and glycemic control. Takazakura et al[16] through biopsy specimens and Reichard et al[17] through clinical trials helped define the association between glycemic control and renal disease. The Pirart study[15] also evaluated diabetic control and the development of neuropathy. These studies are referenced at the end of this chapter, and are mentioned to remind the reader of the long and detailed process behind the research mentioned in the following text, which intuitively may be taken for granted.

Type 1 Diabetes and Microvascular Complications: Benefits of Optimal Glycemic Control

The DCCT was a multicenter randomized prospective trial sponsored by the National Institutes of Health involving 1441 patients with type 1 diabetes in Canada and the United States. The goal of this study was to address whether intensive diabetes management could prevent complications in individuals who had no complications at randomization (primary prevention), and whether intensive management could influence the course of complications in those who had diabetes for 1 to 15 years and showed early end organ involvement. Patients were randomized to receive either intensive control or standard management. The group of patients undergoing the intensive regimen did have a greater number of hypoglycemic episodes compared to the group treated with standard care. The DCCT was stopped 1 year early because the beneficial effect of intensive control was noted to far outweigh conventional control. Compared with the conventionally treated group, the intensively treated patients did achieve highly statistically significant decreases in glucose levels (averaging both preprandial and postprandial) concentrations (155 mg/dl versus 231 mg/dl) and hemoglobin A_{1c} (A1C) levels (7.2% versus 9.0%). However, the rate of severe hypoglycemic episodes increased 3-fold in the intensively treated group.

Retinopathy

Of the 1441 type 1 diabetic patients enrolled in the DCCT, 726 had no diabetic retinopathy (by seven-field stereoscopic fundus photographs), whereas 715 had mild to moderate nonproliferative (also called *background*—see Chapter 7) retinopathy at baseline. Half of the patients were randomly assigned to intensive treatment (goals—premeal blood glucose concentrations of 70 to 120 mg/dl, postprandial blood glucose con-

centrations of <180 mg/dl, and normal A1C levels [A1C < 6.05%]), and the other half remained on their conventional treatment. The fundus photographs, repeated every 6 months, were evaluated for severity of retinopathy over a 25-step scale. Clinically important changes were defined as a change of at least 3 steps that was sustained for at least 6 months. The patients were monitored for a mean of 6.5 years (range, 3 to 9). The development of retinopathy in the patients without it at baseline (called the *primary prevention cohort*) is shown in Figure 2-5A. The incidence curves begin to separate after 3 years—that is, it took that long for effects of near euglycemia to begin to show benefit. Overall, intensive treatment reduced the risk of developing clinically important (≥3-step change) diabetic retinopathy by 76% over the mean 6.5 years that these patients were studied. The progression of established nonproliferative retinopathy at baseline (called the *secondary intervention cohort*) is shown in Figure 2-5B. The intensively treated group had a higher cumulative incidence during the first year (it has been repeatedly demonstrated that bringing a patient from poor control to near euglycemia may cause transient worsening of retinopathy), but a lower cumulative incidence of clinically important retinopathy beginning again at 3 years. Overall, intensive treatment reduced the risk of progression of nonproliferative retinopathy by 54% for the duration of the DCCT. The early worsening of diabetic retinopathy during the first year (which occurred in 22% of the intensively treated patients and 13% of the conventionally treated ones) should not deter physicians from instituting tight control. These changes often disappeared by 18 months in the DCCT. Furthermore, analyzing just those patients with transient worsening, intensive treatment caused a 74% reduction in subsequent progression compared with conventional therapy. After the trial, patients returned to their usual site of care and were followed in the Epidemiology of

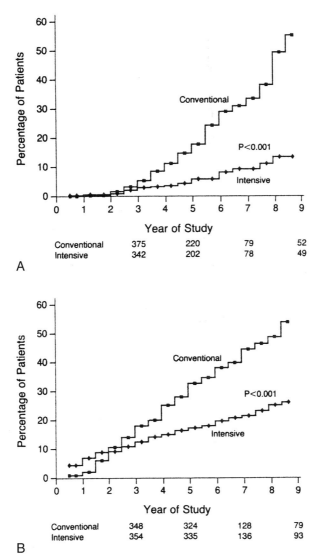

FIGURE 2-5. *A:* Cumulative incidence of developing diabetic retinopathy in the primary prevention cohort (no retinopathy at baseline). Change in retinopathy status defined as a change of at least three steps in seven-field stereoscopic fundus photographs that was sustained for at least 6 months. The numbers of patients in each therapy group who were evaluated at years 3, 5, 7, and 9 are shown below the graph. *B:* Cumulative incidence of progression of diabetic retinopathy in the secondary intervention cohort (nonproliferative retinopathy present at baseline). Change in retinopathy status defined as a change of at least three steps in seven-field stereoscopic fundus photographs that was sustained for at least 6 months. The numbers of patients in each therapy group who were evaluated at years 3, 5, 7, and 9 are shown below the graph. *(From The Diabetes Control and Complications Trial Research Group: The effect of intensive treatment of diabetes on the development and progression of long-term complications in insulin-dependent diabetes mellitus. N Engl J Med 329:977, 1993.)*

Diabetes Interventions and Complications (EDIC) study[18] to see if any benefits persisted. Despite a worsening of glycemic control off the study (both groups averaged a post-study A1C of approximately 8%), follow-up through 7 years showed that the cumulative incidence of further 3-step progression in retinopathy remained less in the former intensive treatment group than in the former conventional treatment group.

Thus it seems that the reduction in the risk of progressive retinopathy resulting from intensive therapy in patients with type 1 diabetes persists for at least 7 years, even in the face of higher A1C levels.[18]

Nephropathy

In the primary prevention cohort 726 subjects and 715 subjects in the secondary intervention cohort were followed to determine the relationship between development of nephropathy and glycemic control. Albumin excretion rates correlated positively with A1C values in both cohorts and with the duration of diabetes in the secondary cohort.[19] Thus even early in the development of nephropathy, there is a correlation with the degree of metabolic control. At the end of the DCCT, nephropathy was evaluated on the basis of urine specimens in patients 7 years after the trial. The proportion of patients with an increase in urinary albumin excretion remained significantly lower in the ex-intensive group.[18] Thus, using an aggregate endpoint of serum creatinine (2 mg/dL), chronic dialysis, or renal transplantation, only 6 of the original intensive treatment group versus 17 of the original conventional treatment group have reached that outcome. Authors of the study concluded that the reduction in the risk of progressive nephropathy resulting from intensive therapy in patients with type 1 diabetes persists for at least 7 years, despite worsening glycemic control.

Neuropathy

In the DCCT,[20] neuropathy was assessed at 5 years. Abnormal results of neurologic examinations (P <0.001), nerve conduction studies (P <0.001), and autonomic nerve studies (P <0.04) all were significantly higher in the conventionally treated group. More specifically, intensive therapy reduced the appearance of neuropathy in the primary prevention cohort by 69% and in the secondary intervention cohort by 57%.

Type 2 Diabetes and Microvascular Complications: Benefits of Optimal Glycemic Control

In the UKPDS, 5102 patients newly diagnosed as having type 2 diabetes, aged 25 to 65 years inclusive, were recruited between 1977 and 1991. All patients were prescribed a diet for 3 months and then stratified into groups based on their mean fasting plasma glucose (FPG) concentrations and weight. The first group had FPG concentrations >270 mg/dl (15 mmol/L) and were randomized to receive either sulfonylurea therapy or insulin. If obese, they were also randomized to metformin. The second group included those with FPG concentrations of 108 to 270 mg/dl (6 to 15 mmol/L). This group was randomized to either diet alone or the therapies mentioned previously. The third group had FPG concentrations of less than 108 mg/dl (6 mmol/L) and were maintained on diet therapy. Patients were followed every 3 months with the aim of achieving an FPG of less than 108 mg/dl (6 mmol/L) When protocol-defined marked hyperglycemia occurred, despite maximal doses of single therapy, additional therapy was added. Patients were followed for 3, 6, and 9 years after enrollment. The main outcome measures were FPG and A1C levels, and the proportion of patients who achieved target levels below 7% A1C or FPG levels of less than 140 mg/dl (7.8 mmol/L). After 9 years of monotherapy with diet, insulin, or sulfonylurea, 8%, 42%, and 24% respectively, achieved goal levels of FPG, and 9%, 28%, and 24% achieved goal levels of A1C (Figure 2-6A, B, C). The majority of patients needed multiple therapies to attain their target levels over the long term.[21]

Retinopathy

The risk factors related to the incidence and progression of diabetic retinopathy over 6 years from the diagnosis of diabetes was determined by the UKPDS study group.[22]

This report looked at 1919 patients who had retinal photos taken at the time of diagnosis and at 6 years later. Of these 1919 patients, 1216 (63%) had no retinopathy as defined by a modified Early Treatment of Diabetic Retinopathy Study scale. By 6 years, 22% of these patients had developed retinopathy. In the 703 subjects who had baseline eye disease, 29% progressed significantly. The development of retinopathy was strongly associated with baseline glycemic control, and subsequent control over the 6 years studied. The Kumamoto study,[13] also done in subjects with type 2 diabetes, had similar

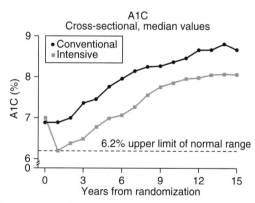

FIGURE 2-6. *A:* United Kingdom Prospective Diabetes Study (UKPDS). *B:* This slide represents the overall A1C levels maintained in the conventional and intensive therapy groups in the UKPDS.

Continued

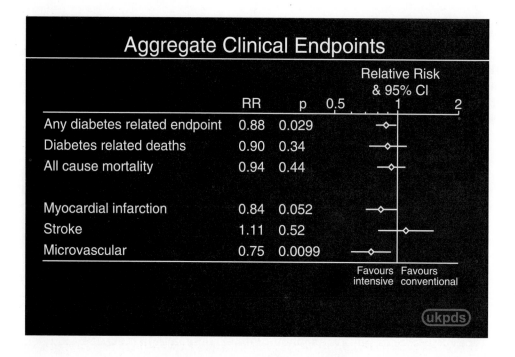

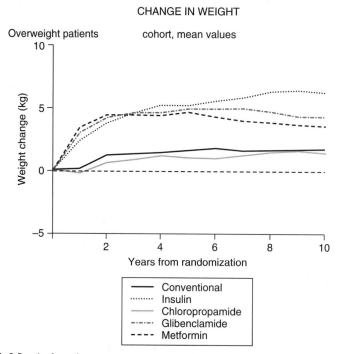

FIGURE 2-6. cont'd *C:* Results from the primary comparison in the UKPDS trial—conventional therapy versus intensive therapy using insulin and/or sulfonylurea agents. *D:* Results in patients who are overweight, comparing weight gain of patients taking metformin versus the other therapies. There were no differences in glycemic control among the intensively treated groups.

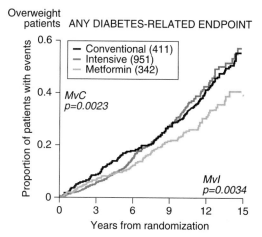

FIGURE 2-6. cont'd *E:* Metformin was associated with a statistically significant risk of myocardial infarction when compared against conventional therapy. *(Used with permission from the UKPDS Clinical Trials group.)*

findings. In this study, the primary prevention cohort had no diabetic retinopathy, whereas the secondary prevention cohort had mild background retinopathy. Development (in the primary prevention group) or progression (in the secondary prevention group) of diabetic retinopathy was defined as at least a 2-step change in a 19-step scale when the eyes were reevaluated after 6 years. Compared with the conventionally treated cohort, the intensively treated group had significantly lower fasting blood glucose concentrations (126 mg/dl versus 164 mg/dl), mean blood glucose concentrations throughout the day (157 mg/dl versus 221 mg/dl), and A1C levels (7.1% versus 9.4%). Each of the four groups maintained 25 or 26 patients at the end of the study. In the primary prevention cohort, intensive treatment resulted in a significant decrease in the development of diabetic retinopathy (7.7% versus 32.0%). Likewise, in the secondary prevention cohort, intensive treatment resulted in a significant decrease in the progression of diabetic retinopathy (19.2% versus 44.0%). Overall, repeated injections of insulin and the resultant near euglycemia reduced the risk of worsening of diabetic retinopathy by 69% over 6 years in these lean type 2 diabetic subjects.

Nephropathy

The UKPDS echoed the results of the DCCT and showed lowering of blood glucose levels prevents the progression of kidney disease. In addition, controlling hypertension plays an important role in reducing the risk of microvascular and macrovascular disease.[23] Although the role of angiotensin-converting enzyme inhibitors has long been known as beneficial in diabetic kidney disease,[24] recent data regarding hypertension control have shown that, regardless of agents used, blood pressure lowering results in effective reduction of diabetic complications.[25]

Neuropathy

Data specifically on neuropathy and diabetes control in patients with type 2 diabetes is hard to find. Observational analysis of the relationship between glycemic exposure and general microvascular complications shows that for every decrease in A1C level of 1%, a risk reduction of 37% is seen[26] (Figure 2-7). The Pirart study[15] also evaluated diabetic control and the development of neuropathy concurrently. A diagnosis of diabetic neuropathy was made if Achilles and/or patellar reflexes were lost in conjunction with a clear decrease in vibratory sensation. The prevalence of this complication lies between that

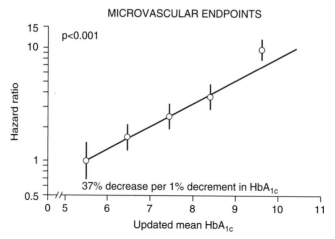

FIGURE 2-7. Epidemiologic analysis of the United Kingdom Prospective Diabetes Study data shows that there is a 37% risk reduction for the development of diabetic microvascular complications for every 1% reduction in A1C level.

of retinopathy and nephropathy. Once again, a similar relation holds between diabetic control and neuropathy. The initial low prevalence of neuropathy (Figure 2-8) did not change much as the duration of diabetes increased in the fairly well-controlled group. In sharp contrast, the prevalence increased considerably over time in the other two groups, with the most poorly controlled patients experiencing a faster deterioration of peripheral neurologic function than did the intermediate group.

Reversal of Early Changes

The most recent evidence linking strict diabetic control with a favorable effect on diabetic retinopathy, nephropathy, and neuropathy indicates that the *early* lesions are reversible if near euglycemia can be achieved with either repeated injections of insulin or insulin infusion pumps. As mentioned previously, increased capillary basement membrane thickness is the morphologic characteristic of the microvascular changes in diabetes mellitus. Because this occurs in all tissues, muscle biopsies afford an opportunity to monitor the effect of improving diabetic control. Capillary basement membrane thickness decreases considerably, almost to normal (Figure 2-9), after near euglycemia is achieved by repeated insulin injection[27] or insulin pump therapy.[28,29]

The earliest ocular abnormality in diabetes is increased leakage of the retinal vessels, which can be measured by vitreous fluorophotometry following injection of a fluorescein dye. These changes are evident years before retinal changes can be seen by ophthalmoscopic examination. In many patients, near euglycemia decreased the leakage of the fluorescein dye to normal.[30-32] Abnormal macular recovery time and oscillatory potential, two parameters of retinal function, have been shown in prospective studies[33,34] to have a highly predictive value for the eventual development of proliferative retinopathy. These two retinal functions improved significantly when strict diabetic control was implemented.[31,32] The situation in regard to retinal morphology (i.e., the result of photographic or ophthalmoscopic evaluation of the retina) was more complex. An initial worsening can occur during the first year of near euglycemia,[31,32,35-39] with subsequent stabilization or improvement such that at 2 years or beyond, diabetic retinopathy is less advanced than in control patients who had remained on their usual (suboptimal) insulin therapy.[28,31,40,41]

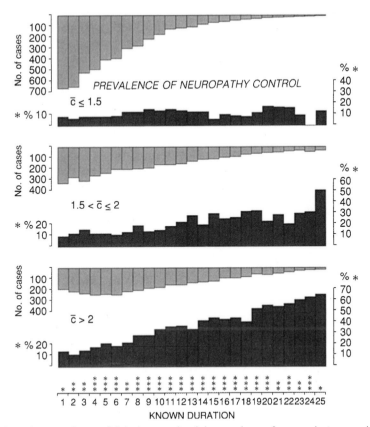

FIGURE 2-8. Relation between degree of diabetic control and the prevalence of neuropathy in a population of 4398 diabetic patients monitored by one group of physicians for up to 25 years. Light-colored bars represent the number of patients who were evaluated at each interval and who fall into the respective categories of control. Dark bars show the cumulative frequency (%) of a complication at each year of duration. Cumulative scores indicating degree of diabetic control. Based on the following scale: 1 = good control, 2 = fair control, 3 = poor control. Bottom graph therefore represents worse control. *(From Pirart J: Diabetes mellitus and its degenerative complications: A prospective study of 4,400 patients observed between 1947 and 1973. Diabetes Care 1:168, 1978.)*

Microalbuminuria and its ability to predict the eventual development of overt diabetic nephropathy was discussed earlier. Strict diabetic control decreases and in some patients entirely reverses microalbuminuria,[42–44] suggesting (but certainly not proving) that future development of diabetic nephropathy may be delayed or possibly even avoided.

In regard to neuropathy, near euglycemia diminished pain,[45] decreased the vibratory perception threshold[35,45,46] (i.e., patients were able to appreciate less intense vibrations), and increased motor nerve conduction velocities.[38,44-48] However, once morphologic changes have occurred in the eyes (i.e., retinopathy can be discerned with the ophthalmoscope) or clinical proteinuria is present, strict diabetic control does not prevent the continued deterioration of the retina[32,35,36,49,50] or kidneys.[49,51] These latter data emphasize the importance of instituting strict control at the onset of diabetes in an attempt to prevent these devastating complications.

The debate concerning the impact of hyperglycemia and diabetic complications

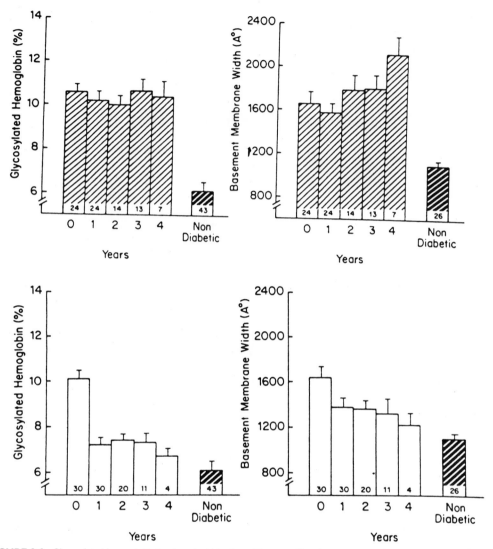

FIGURE 2-9. Glycosylated hemoglobin levels and width of quadriceps capillary basement membrane in patients with type I diabetes under conventional insulin therapy (top) or intensive therapy with insulin pumps (bottom). *(From Rosenstock J, Challis P, Stowig S, et al: Improved diabetes control reduces skeletal muscle capillary basement membrane width in insulin-dependent diabetes mellitus. Diabetes Res Clin Pract 4:167, 1988.)*

has been raging for more than half a century. With the advent of glucose self-monitoring to help achieve near euglycemia and the availability of measuring A1C levels to document it, reports clearly indicate that tight diabetic control has a major role in forestalling diabetic retinopathy, nephropathy, and neuropathy. The only serious objection raised to this conclusion is that genetic

influences may also be important in the development of these complications.[52] It is true that in diabetic patients with poor control for 25 years, 20% will not develop retinopathy, 80% will not develop nephropathy, and 35% will not develop neuropathy (Table 2-2). Perhaps genetic factors are protecting these patients. However, the overriding importance of hyperglycemia in the

TABLE 2-2	IMPACT OF DIABETIC CONTROL ON THE PREVALENCE (%) OF DIABETIC RETINOPATHY, NEPHROPATHY, AND NEUROPATHY AFTER 25 YEARS OF DIABETES MELLITUS		
Condition	**Overall**	**Good Control***	**Poor Control***
Retinopathy	60	10	80
(proliferative)		(<1)	(20)
Nephropathy	20	<1	20
Neuropathy	50	10	65

*See text for definitions.

Adapted from Gerich JE: Insulin-dependent diabetes mellitus: pathophysiology. Mayo Clin Proc 61:787, 1986.

interplay between metabolic and genetic influences is evident in that (1) renal basement membrane thickness is normal at the onset of diabetes[53]; (2) patients with secondary diabetes have the same prevalence of diabetic complications as those with "genetic" diabetes[54,55]; (3) normal kidneys transplanted into diabetic patients develop nephropathy[55]; and, conversely, (4) morphologic changes of diabetic nephropathy are reversible after transplantation into nondiabetic individuals.[56] Regardless of the genetic background, diabetic retinopathy, nephropathy, or neuropathy does not occur in the absence of hyperglycemia. Furthermore, in those who are unlikely to have a genetic background for diabetes (patients with secondary diabetes and the nondiabetic recipients of diabetic kidneys), these complications occur in a high percentage.

Clinically, it is critical to recognize that one cannot predict whether or not patients may be protected from diabetic retinopathy, nephropathy, or neuropathy. Therefore it behooves us to control their diabetes as tightly as possible without causing serious disruptions in their life styles. Which level of control to aim for and how to achieve it are discussed in detail in Chapter 9.

This chapter has reviewed the overwhelming evidence concerning the impact of near euglycemia on the development and progression of diabetic retinopathy, nephropathy, and neuropathy. This is because physicians need to be convinced of the importance of tight control so that they vigorously pursue near euglycemia. This entails not only convincing patients but taking the time and exerting the effort in working with patients to achieve it. This is not an easy task. Because most patients are asymptomatic, motivating them to do the necessary work and to continue doing it can be difficult. Physician time and motivation can also be a factor, especially because the rewards are not immediate and accrue only years later in the continued health of patients. Certain patients are not candidates for strict control—for example, the elderly, those with hypoglycemia unawareness, those with advanced microvascular and neuropathic complications, or those with severe cardiovascular disease. Some physicians believe that many other patients with type 2 diabetes should not be tightly controlled because of the theoretic risk of hyperinsulinemia.[57] Compensatory hyperinsulinemia, as a response to insulin resistance, is one of a cluster of risk factors (in which glucose intolerance or, in some cases, type 2 diabetes can also occur) for coronary artery disease (CAD). This cluster of risk factors, known as either *syndrome X* or the *insulin resistance syndrome*, should not preclude a patient from being considered for tight control.[58] In fact, new evidence that insulin may be beneficial by encouraging coronary artery vasodilation has been published.[59]

GLYCEMIC CONTROL AND MACROVASCULAR DISEASE

The relationship between glycemic control and macrovascular disease has been elusive until recently. It has long been known that CAD is the major cause of mortality in patients with type 2 diabetes mellitus, however the role of glycemic control in the prevention of mortality and morbidity related to CAD is only now being defined. This topic is discussed in more detail in Chapter 8. Initially, there was much controversy about the relationship between CAD and hyperglycemia, with a number of articles questioning an increased risk of CAD with hyperglycemia[60] and a number of articles supporting the increased risk with poor glycemic control.[61,62] Some of this dispute may have been the result of analysis techniques, patient populations used, and population sizes that were studied. Recently, it seems the debate as been resolved. Briefly, the UKPDS data showed patients without evidence of atherosclerosis when diagnosed with diabetes had an increased standardized mortality ratio compared with the normal population.[63] After 8 years of follow-up, 11% of these patients developed angina. The potentially modifiable risk factors in this group of patients included not just glycemic control, but increased concentrations of low-density lipoprotein, decreased concentrations of high-density lipoprotein, hypertension, and smoking. In fact, control of hypertension has been shown to reduce macrovascular endpoints in diabetes independent of glycemic control.[64,65] Not surprisingly, these modifiable risk factors are the same as those seen in the general population. Subsequent analysis showed that stratifying patients by A1C levels provided further proof of the relationship between glycemic control and cardiovascular risk.[66] In fact, an increase of A1C by 1% conferred an 11% increased risk of CAD. This data was similar to that reported in 1995.[67] More important, however, is the possibility that a reduction in A1C is associated with reduction in this risk score. For example, a 1% reduction in updated mean Hgb A1C levels was associated with a reduction in risk of 21% for any end point related to diabetes, 21% for deaths related to diabetes, 14% for myocardial infarction, 12% for stroke, 43% for peripheral vascular disease, and 37% for microvascular disease.[66] There was no threshold of risk observed for any end point, and the lowest risk was in those whose A1C levels fell within the normal range of less than 6.0%. This brings up some interesting questions: Is there less CAD risk if a normal person's A1C is less than 5.0% instead of simply less than 6.0%? And by association, is a lower fasting glucose in the normal range more beneficial than a fasting glucose in the upper range of normal? These questions are explored in detail in Chapter 8.

Data from the EDIC study in type 1 diabetes reveals the increased risk for atherosclerosis found in individuals with type 1 diabetes.[67a] Subjects were found to have an increase in carotid intima-media thickness (a marker for atherosclerotic plaque) compared to age- and sex-matched controls. At 6 years post-DCCT the mean progression of the intima-media thickness was significantly less in those who had been intensively treated in the DCCT compared to those who were conventionally treated. Therefore, intensive glycemic control in type 1 diabetes may reduce ratios of both micro- and macrovascular complications.[67a]

Although the previous data remind us that diabetes is really a syndrome with multiple components that need to be treated to ensure the best possible patient outcome, they also stress that glycemic control itself is an important modifiable risk factor.

THE ROLE OF POSTPRANDIAL GLUCOSE LEVELS

Until recently, most outcomes in clinical studies have been based either on A1C levels and/or fasting glucose levels. With the advent of the concept of IGT, we know that postprandial hyperglycemia occurs with great frequency before the actual diagnosis of diabetes is made. The question of how postprandial glucose relates to the complications of diabetes, and whether (either as an entity in IGT or in overt diabetes) it warrants specific therapy, are important issues of management. It is now known that men with IGT have an increased risk of ischemic heart disease[68,69] and that early intervention and lifestyle changes may be successful in resulting in lower than expected overall mortality.[70] Recent studies in diabetic patients have shown that good control of postprandial blood glucose is associated with a lower incidence of coronary heart disease and death.[71,72] In addition, therapy focusing on lowering postprandial glucose may be helpful for lowering A1C values.[73] Because of this new body of literature, the treatment of postprandial hyperglycemia has moved to the forefront of diabetes (and prediabetes) care. For this reason, postprandial hyperglycemia is covered in great detail throughout this book in the sections concerning specific complications and management issues.

▼
THE COST BENEFIT OF GLYCEMIC CONTROL

Although in an ideal world improving the quality and quantity of life would be adequate justification for spending dollars on health care, increasingly cost considerations have come into play. Patients with diabetes consume a disproportionately high percentage of healthcare resources, which has been estimated to be almost four times as high as expenditures for people without diabetes.[74] Although intensive therapy lowers the development and progression of the complications of diabetes, the costs of intensive treatment can be high. In the DCCT study the annual additional per patient cost was $4000 to $5800 per participant.[75]

Models have been developed for estimating the costs and benefits of diabetes care. One such model is based on reductions in long-term diabetic complications through intensive blood glucose control.[76] It suggests that life-long intensive treatment strategies for diabetes are economically acceptable, with a cost per quality-adjusted life-year gained of approximately $16,000 (similar to the cost of treating other chronic diseases, such as hypertension). This model does not take into account benefits that could occur through use of statin therapy and antihypertensive agents, which can lower the cost associated with cardiovascular complications in patients with diabetes.

Another approach to assessing the cost-effectiveness of diabetes care is to look at the association between A1C levels and the cost of care. Gilmer et al[77] were the first to show a relationship between A1C levels and the costs of medical care.[77] In another retrospective study[78] patients with diabetes were assigned to one of three groups: good control (A1C <8%), fair control (8% to 10%), and poor control (>10%). Inpatient admissions were tracked over 4 years, and better glycemic control was associated with a reduction in admission rates for short-term complications and a corresponding reduction in costs. However, finding an association between higher A1C levels and increased costs does not prove that lowering A1C levels will lower costs.

Data from diabetes disease management programs are beginning to provide prospective data for cost improvements.[79] A recent meta-analysis of 17 interventions for treating diabetes concluded that clearly cost-saving interventions included eye care and preconception care.[80] Cost-effective interventions included nephropathy prevention and improved glycemic control in patients with type 1 diabetes.

The Diabetes Treatment Centers of America developed a comprehensive diabetes management program. This was implemented and data were analyzed on more than 7000 patients from seven managed care plans.[81] Analysis of costs showed a gross economic savings of $44 per diabetic member per month (10.9%), with the majority of the savings coming from acute hospitalizations. However, patients followed in the program had improvements in A1C levels and other measures of diabetic control, which may eventually translate into reductions in rates of chronic complications, as well. In the UKPDS trial, a cost savings in inpatient hospitalization was seen in the intensively treated group; however, this savings was equaled by the increase in medication costs required for intensive therapy.[82]

Patients with diabetes have a considerable reduction in net earning potential, although the magnitude of the loss depends on individual characteristics.[83] Overall, the loss was approximately a one-third reduction in earnings, with a range of $3700 to $8700 per annum. Improving blood glucose control may help reduce the disability associated with diabetes, in addition to improving quality of life.[84] In this study, treatment of type 2 diabetes was associated with a greater productive capacity, less absenteeism, fewer bed-days, and fewer restrictive-activity days. Therefore improving glycemic control may have measurable benefits both in terms of the acute and chronic complications of diabetes, and it may also help improve the functional quality of the lives of patients who live with the disease.

REFERENCES

1. The Diabetes Control and Complications Trial Research Group: The effect of intensive treatment of diabetes on the development and progression of long-term complications in insulin-dependent diabetes mellitus. N Engl J Med 329:977, 1993.
2. UK Prospective Diabetes Study (UKPDS) Group: Intensive blood-glucose control with sulphonylureas or insulin compared with conventional treatment and risk of complications in patients with type 2 diabetes (UKPDS 33). Lancet 352:839, 1998.
3. Peters AL, Thompson R, Ryan D: Glycohemoglobin assessment program (GAP): What is the level of diabetes management in primary care? Diabetes 48(Suppl 1):A194, 1999.
4. Paolo P, Umberto DM: Autoimmune diabetes not requiring insulin at diagnosis (latent autoimmune diabetes of the adult): Definition, characterization, and potential prevention. Diabetes Care 24:1460, 2001.
5. Atkinson MA, Maclaren NK: Islet cell autoantigens insulin-dependent diabetes. J Clin Invest 92:1608, 1993.
6. Hyoty H, Hiltunen MK, Laakkonen M et al: A prospective study of the role of Coxsackie B and other enterovirus infections in the pathogenesis of IDDM. Diabetes 44:652, 1995.
7. Pfizer Laboratories: A study among type 2 diabetics. Survey conducted by the Gallup Organization, 1983.
8. Matschinsky F, Liang Y, Kesavan P et al: Glucokinase as pancreatic beta cell glucose sensor and diabetes gene. J Clin Invest 92:2092, 1993.
9. Cline GW, Petersen KF, Krssak M et al: Impaired glucose transport as a cause of decreased insulin-stimulated muscle glycogen synthesis in type 2 diabetes. N Engl J Med. 341:240, 1999.
10. Hayes N, Biswas C, Strout HV et al: Activation by protein synthesis inhibitors of glucose transport into L6 muscle cells. Biochem Biophys Res Commun 190:881, 1993.
11. James DE, Brown R, Navarro J et al: Insulin-regulatable tissues express a unique inslin-sensitive glucose transport protein. Nature 333:183, 1988.
12. Taylor SI: Lilly lecture: Molecular mechanisms of insulin resistance. Lessons from patients with mutations in the insulin-receptor gene. Diabetes 41:1473, 1992.
13. Ohkubo Y, Kishikawa H, Araki E et al: Intensive insulin therapy prevents the progression of diabetic microvascular complications in Japanese patients with non-insulin-dependent diabetes mellitus: A randomized prospective 6-year study. Diabetes Res Clin Pract 28:103, 1995.
14. Miki E, Fukuda M, Kuzuya T et al: Relation of the course of retinopathy to control of diabetes, age, and therapeutic agents in diabetic Japanese patients. Diabetes 18:773, 1969.
15. Pirart J: Diabetes mellitus and its degenerative complications: A prospective study of 4,400 patients observed between 1947 and 1973. Diabetes Care 1:168, 1978.
16. Takazakura E, Nakamoto Y, Hayakawa H et al: Onset and progression of diabetic glomerulosclerosis. A prospective study based on serial renal biopsies. Diabetes 24:1, 1975.
17. Reichard P, Nilsson BY, Rosenqvist U: The effect of long-term intensified insulin treatment on the development of microvascular complications of diabetes mellitus. N Engl J Med 329:304, 1993.
18. The Writing Team for the Diabetes Control and Complications Trial/Epidemiology of Diabetes Interventions and Complications Research Group. Effect of intensive therapy on the microvascular complications of type 1 diabetes mellitus. JAMA 287(19):2563-2569, 2002.
19. Molitch ME, Steffes MW, Cleay PA et al: Baseline analysis of renal function in the Diabetes Control and Complications Trial. The Diabetes Control

and Complications Trial Research Group. Kidney Int 43:668, 1993.

20. Barbosa J, Steffes MW, Sutherland DER et al: Effect of glycemic control on early diabetic renal lesions: A 5-year randomized controlled clinical trial of insulin-dependent diabetic kidney transplant recipients. JAMA 272:600, 1994.

21. Turner RC, Cull CA, Frighi V et al: Glycemic control with diet, sulfonylurea, metformin or insulin in patients with type 2 diabetes mellitus: Progressive requirement for multiple therapies (UKPDS 49). JAMA 281:2005, 1999.

22. Stratton IM, Kohner EM, aldington SJ et al: UKPDS 50: Risk factors for incidence and progression of retinopathy in type 2 diabetes over 6 years from diagnosis. Diabetologia 44:156, 2001.

23. Anonymous: Tight blood pressure control and the risk of macrovascular and microvascular complication in type 2 diabetes. UKPDS 38. BMJ 317:703, 1998.

24. Parving HH, Hovind P, Rossing K, et al: Evolving strategies for renoprotection: Diabetic nephropathy. Curr Opin Nephrol Hypertens 10:515, 2001.

25. Anonymous: Efficacy of atenolol and captopril in reducing risk of macrovascular complications in type 2 diabetes. UKPDS 39. BMJ 317:713, 1998.

26. Stratton IM, Adler AI, Neil HA et al: Association of glycaemia with macrovascular and microvascular complications of type 2 diabetes (UKPDS 35). Prospective observational study. BMJ 321:405, 2000.

27. Peterson CM, Jones RL, Esterly JS et al: Changes in basement membrane thickening and pulse volume concomitant with improved glucose control and exercise in patients with insulin-dependent diabetes mellitus. Diabetes Care 3:586, 1980.

28. Rosenstock J, Friberg T, Raskin P: Effect of glycemic control on microvascular complications in patients with type 1 diabetes mellitus. Am J Med 81:1012, 1986.

29. Rosenstock J, Challis P, Stowig S et al: Improved diabetes control reduces skeletal muscle capillary basement membrane width in insulin-dependent diabetes mellitus. Diabetes Res Clin Pract 4:167, 1988.

30. White NH, Waltman SR, Krupin T et al: Reversal of abnormalities in ocular fluorophotometry in insulin-dependent diabetes after five to nine months of improved metabolic control. Diabetes 31:30, 1982.

31. Steno Study Group: Effect of 6 months of strict metabolic control on eye and kidney function in insulin-dependent diabetics with background retinopathy. Lancet 1:121, 1982.

32. Lauritzen R, Larsen HW, Frost-Larsen K et al: Effect of 1 year of near-normal blood glucose levels on retinopathy in insulin-dependent diabetics. Lancet 1:200, 1983.

33. Simonsen SE: The value of the oscillatory potential in selecting juvenile diabetics at risk of developing proliferative retinopathy. Acta Ophthalmol 58:865, 1980.

34. Frost-Larsen K, Larsen HW, Simonsen SE: Oscillatory potential and nyctometry in insulin-dependent diabetics. Acta Ophthalmol 58:879, 1980.

35. Holman RR, Mayon-White V, Orde-Peckar C et al: Prevention of deterioration of renal and sensory-nerve function by more intensive management of insulin-dependent diabetic patients. A two-year randomised prospective study. Lancet 1:204, 1983.

36. The Kroc Collaborative Study Group: Blood glucose control and the evolution of diabetic retinopathy and albuminuria. A preliminary multicenter trial. N Engl J Med 311:365, 1984.

37. Beck-Neilsen H, Richelsen B, Mogensen CE et al: Effect of insulin pump treatment for one year on renal function and retinal morphology in patients with IDDM. Diabetes Care 8:585, 1985.

38. Dahl-Jorgensen K, Brinchmann-Hansen O, Hanssen KF et al: Effect of near normoglycaemia for two years on progression of early diabetic retinopathy, nephropathy, and neuropathy: The Oslo study. BMJ 293:1195, 1986.

39. Helve E, Laatikainen L, Merenmies L et al: Continuous insulin infusion therapy and retinopathy in patients with type 1 diabetes. Acta Endocrinol (Copenh) 115:313, 1987.

40. Lauritzen T, Frost-Larsen K, Larsen HW et al: Two-year experience with continuous subcutaneous insulin infusion in relation to retinopathy and neuropathy. Diabetes 34(suppl 3):74, 1985.

41. The Kroc Collaborative Study Group: Diabetic retinopathy after two years of intensified insulin treatment: Follow-up of the Kroc Collaborative Study. JAMA 260:37, 1988.

42. Viberti GC, Pickup JC, Bilous RW et al: Correction of exercise-induced microalbuminuria in insulin-dependent diabetics after 3 weeks of subcutaneous insulin infusion. Diabetes 30:818, 1981.

43. Feldt-Rasmussen B, Mathiesen ER, Deckert T: Effect of two years of strict metabolic control on progression of incipient nephropathy in insulin-dependent diabetes. Lancet 2:1300, 1986.

44. Pietri A, Ehle AL, Raskin P: Changes in nerve conduction velocity after six weeks of glucoregulation with portable insulin infusion pumps. Diabetes 29:668, 1980.

45. Boulton AJM, Drury J, Clarke B: Continuous subcutaneous insulin infusion in the management of painful diabetic neuropathy. Diabetes Care 5:386, 1982.

46. Service FJ, Rizza RA, Danube JR: Near normoglycaemia improved nerve conduction and vibration sensation in diabetic neuropathy. Diabetologia 28:722, 1985.

47. Chiasson JL, Ducros F, Poliquin-Hamet M et al: Continuous subcutaneous insulin infusion (Mill-Hill Infuser) versus multiple injections (Medi-Jector) in the treatment of insulin-dependent diabetes mellitus and the effect of metabolic control on microangiopathy. Diabetes Care 7:331, 1984.

48. Fedele D, Negrin P, Cardone C et al: Influence of continuous subcutaneous insulin infusion (CSII) treatment on diabetic somatic and autonomic neuropathy. J Endocrinol Invest 7:623, 1984.

49. Tamborlane WV, Puklin JE, Bergman M et al: Long-term improvement of metabolic control with the insulin pump does not reverse diabetic microangiopathy. Diabetes Care 5:58, 1982.

50. Lawson PM, Champion MC, Canny C et al: Continuous subcutaneous insulin infusion (CSII) does not prevent progression of proliferative and preproliferative retinopathy. Br J Ophthalmol 66:762, 1982.

51. Viberti GC, Bilous RW, Mackintosh D et al: Long-term correction of hyperglycaemia and progression of renal failure in insulin dependent diabetes. BMJ 286:598, 1983.

52. Raskin P, Rosenstock J: Blood glucose control and diabetic complications. Ann Intern Med 105:254, 1986.

53. Osterby R: Morphometric studies of the peripheral glomerular basement membrane in early juvenile diabetes—1. Development of initial basement membrane thickening. Diabetologia 8:84, 1972.

54. Couet C, Genton P, Pointel JP et al: The prevalence of retinopathy is similar in diabetes mellitus secondary to chronic pancreatitis with or without pancreatectomy and in idiopathic diabetes mellitus. Diabetes Care 8:323, 1985.

55. Davidson MB: The case for control in diabetes mellitus. West J Med 129:193, 1978.

56. Arouna GM, Kremer GD, Daddah SK et al: Reversal of diabetic nephropathy in human cadaveric kidneys after transplantation into nondiabetic recipients. Lancet 2:1274, 1983.

57. Nathan DM: Inferences and implications. Diabetes Care 18:251, 1995.

58. Davidson MB: Why the DCCT applies to NIDDM patients. Clin Diabetes 12:141, 1994.

59. Floras JS, Meneilly G: Insulin-mediated blood flow and glucose uptake. Can J Cardiol 17:7A, 2001.

60. Fontbonne A, Eschwege e, Cambien F et al: Hypertriglyceridemia as a risk factor of coronary heart disease mortality in subjects with impaired glucose tolerance or diabetes. Results from the 11-year follow-up of the Paris Prospective Study. Diabetologia 32:300, 1989.

61. Lehto S, Ronnemaa T, Haffner SM et al: Dyslipidemia and hyperglycemic predict coronary heart disease events in middle-aged patients with NIDDM. Diabetes 46:1354, 1997.

62. Walters DP, Gatling W, Houston AC et al: Mortality in diabetic subjects: an eleven-year follow-up of a community-based population. Diabetic Med 11:968, 1994.

63. Turner RC, Millns H, Neil HA et al: Risk factors for coronary artery disease in non-insulin dependent diabetes mellitus: United Kingdom prospective diabetes study (UKPDS:23). BMJ 316:823, 1998.

64. UK Prospective Diabetes Study Group: Tight blood pressure control and risk of macrovascular and microvascular complications in type 2 diabetes: UKPDS 38. BMJ 317:703, 1998.

65. UK Prospective Diabetes Study Group: Efficacy of atenolol and captopril in reducing risk of macrovascular and microvascular complications in type 2 diabetes: UKPDS 39. BMJ 317:713, 1998.

66. Stratton IM, Adler AI, Neil HA et al: Association of glycemia with macrovascular and microvascular complications of type 2 diabetes (UKPDS:35) prospective observational study. BMJ 321:405, 2000

67. Klein R: Hyperglycemia and microvascular and macrovascular disease in diabetes. Diabetes Care 18:258, 1995.

67a.Nathan DM, Lachin J, Cleary P et al— Epidemiology of Diabetes Interventions and Complications Research Group: Intensive diabetes therapy and carotid intima-media thickness in type 1 diabetes mellitus. N Engl J Med 348(23):2294-2303, 2003.

68. Jarret RJ: The cardiovascular risk associated with impaired glucose tolerance. Diabet Med 13:s15, 1996.

69. Knowler WC, Sartor G, Melander A et al: Glucose tolerance and mortality, including a substudy of tolbutamide treatment. Diabetologia, 40:680, 1997.

70. Eriksson KF, Lindgarde F: No excess 12 year mortality in men with impaired glucose tolerance who participated in the Malmo Preventive Trial with diet and exercise. Diabetologia 41:1010, 1998.

71. Hanefeld M, Fischer S, Julius U et al: Risk factors for myocardial infarction and death in newly detected NIDDM: The diabetes Intervention Study. 11-year follow-up. Diabetologia 39:1577, 1996.

72. Barrett-Connor E, Ferrara A: Isolated postchallenge hyperglycemia and the risk of fatal cardiovascular disease in older women and men: The Rancho Bernardo Study. Diabetes Care 21:1236, 1998.

73. Bastyr EJ, Sutart CA, Brodows RG et al: Therapy focused on lowering postprandial glucose, not fasting glucose, may be superior for lowering HbA1c. Diabetes Care 23:1236, 2000.

74. Rubin RJ, Altman WM, Mendelson DN: Health care expenditures for people with diabetes mellitus. J Clin Endo Metab 78:809A, 1992.

75. Diabetes Control and Complications Trial Research Group: Resource utilization and costs of care in the Diabetes Control and Complications Trial. Diabetes Care 18:1468, 1995.

76. Eastman RC, Javitt JC, Herman WH et al: Model of complications of NIDDM. II: Analysis of the health benefits and cost-effectiveness of treating NIDDM with the goal of normoglycemia. Diabetes Care 20:735, 1997.

77. Gilmer TP, O'Connor PJ, Manning WG, et al: The cost to health plans of poor glycemic control. Diabetes Care 20:1847, 1997.

78. Menzin J, Langley-Hawthorne C, Friedman M, et al: Potential short-term economic benefits of improved glycemic control. Diabetes Care 24:51, 2001.

79. Peters AL: Diabetes disease management: Past, present, and future. Endocrinologist 11:86, 2001.

80. Klonoff DC, Schwartz DM: An economic analysis of interventions for diabetes. Diabetes Care 23:390, 2000.

81. Rubin RJ, Dietrick KA, Hawk AD: Clinical and economic impact of implementing a comprehensive diabetes management program in managed care. J Clin Endo Metab 83:2635, 1998.

82. Gray A, Raikou M, McGuire A et al: Cost effectiveness of an intensive blood glucose control policy in patients with type 2 diabetes: Economic analysis alongside randomised controlled trial (UKPDS 41). United Kingdom Prospective Diabetes Study Group. BMJ 320:1373, 2000.

83. Chu Y, Jacobs P, Johnson JA: Productivity losses associated with diabetes in the US. Diabetes Care 24:257, 2001.

84. Testa MA, Simonson DC: Health economic benefits and quality of life during improved glycemic control in patients with type 2 diabetes mellitus. JAMA 280:1490, 1998.

NUTRITION AND PHYSICAL ACTIVITY IN DIABETES

• CHRISTINE A. BEEBE

Medical nutrition therapy (MNT) and physical activity have been considered the cornerstones of metabolic control in both type 1 and type 2 diabetes for decades. More recently, these lifestyle components have proven valuable in preventing type 2 diabetes.[1] Whereas traditional exercise recommendations have focused on vigorous activity and MNT interventions on specific percentages of macro and micro nutrients, people with diabetes generally obtain their physical activity as moderate exercise and their nutrients as food. Successful outcomes resulting from these interventions are then measured as metabolic control. Metabolic control in turn has expanded beyond a glucocentric approach to include cardiovascular and microvascular risk factor control (lipid, blood pressure, and coagulation factors) to prevent long-term complications of diabetes while maintaining an optimal quality of life.

Because diabetes spans the entire life cycle from infancy to old age, includes culturally diverse populations, and is heterogeneous for underlying defects, the behavior modification principles and strategies to implement nutritional modifications and physical activity are unique to each person. Recommendations and goals for the nutritional management of diabetes have been established by the American Diabetes Association (ADA) (Table 3-1).[2,3] Achieving these goals requires recognition of the person with diabetes as an individual and appreciating the fact that the process takes place over several months, if not years. Furthermore, not every component of a person's life style requires changing to improve metabolic control. The challenge for health professionals in implementing MNT and exercise guidelines is recognizing that the person with diabetes is responsible for 99% of the day-to-day management of diabetes, and ultimately makes the choice of what, when, and how much to eat and exercise. Helping patients prioritize strategies and develop critical thinking to problem solve around day-to-day hassles of diabetes is crucial to achieving metabolic control.

HEALTHY EATING

Regardless of the type of diabetes or stage in the life cycle, the first priority in all patients is promoting a healthy diet by implementing basic guidelines of the US Food and Drug Administration (FDA) Food Guide Pyramid (Figure 3-1). Assessing servings of fruits and

TABLE 3-1	GOALS OF MEDICAL NUTRITION THERAPY IN DIABETES

1. Attain and maintain optimal metabolic control:
   - Blood glucose levels as near normal as safely possible to reduce/prevent diabetes complications
   - Lipid and lipid profile that reduces risk for cardiovascular disease
   - Blood pressure levels that reduce risk for vascular disease
2. Prevent and treat common complications:
   - Obesity
   - Dyslipidemia
   - Cardiovascular disease
   - Hypertension
   - Nephropathy
3. Improve overall health.
4. Address individual nutritional needs considering personal, cultural, and lifestyle preferences:
   - Provide adequate energy for normal growth and development in *children with type 1 diabetes.*
   - Promote healthy eating and physical activity to reduce insulin resistance in *children with type 2 diabetes.*
   - Provide adequate energy and nutrients to support a successful pregnancy in *women of child-bearing age.*
   - Consider nutritional and psychosocial needs of the *older adult.*
   - Provide self-management training to treat and prevent hypoglycemia, illness, and exercise-related glucose excursions in *individuals treated with insulin or insulin secretagogues.*
   - Promote healthy eating and physical activity in *individuals at high risk for developing type 2 diabetes.*

MNT AND EXERCISE STRATEGIES IN DIABETES

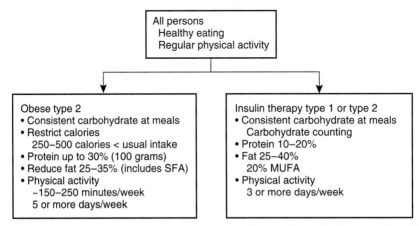

FIGURE 3-1. Approach for lifestyle recommendations for obese individuals with type 2 diabetes and in individuals taking insulin with either type 1 or type 2 diabetes. MNT, medical nutrition therapy; SFA, saturated fatty acid; MUFA, monounsaturated fat.

vegetables and promoting adherence to this one dietary modification can be valuable for overall health in the individual with diabetes. The majority of individuals do not consume the basic number of servings suggested by the Healthy Eating Guidelines (Table 3-2) and should be guided to do so.[4] This first-step approach achieves several purposes: (1) by promoting fruit and vegetable consumption, promotes consumption of micronutrients such as antioxidants that are proving to be valuable in metabolic pathways related to carbohydrate, lipid, and homocysteine metabolism, as well as reducing cardiovascular risk factors including blood pressure[5] and endothelial dysfunction; (2) promotes consumption of whole-grained cereals, breads, and other grain products that contain fiber for cholesterol regulation and gastrointestinal function,

magnesium that is involved in carbohydrate metabolism and blood pressure control, and generally yield a lower glycemic response that processed grains; (3) guides protein consumption by promoting 5 to 7 ounces of lean, protein-rich foods daily (35 to 49 grams protein); (4) initiates the concept of reduced saturated fat. Finally, starting an intervention with the Healthy Eating Guidelines focuses on a positive note of what "can" be consumed rather than what "cannot."

GLYCEMIC CONTROL

Blood glucose control, as measured by hemoglobin A_{1c} (A1C), reflects the combined effect of fasting blood glucose levels, postprandial blood glucose excursions, and

TABLE 3-2	NUTRITION INTERVENTIONS IN DIABETES
Guidelines: In Stepwise Priority	**Daily Implementation**

1. FDA Food Guide Pyramid for overall health	2–3 servings fruit
	3–4 servings vegetables
	Whole grains
	Sugar in context of healthy diet
	Salt in moderation
	    <2400 mg/day if hypertensive
	Limit alcohol
	    1 drink/day for women
	    2 drinks/day for men

2. Carbohydrate counting to reduce glucose excursions	Total carbohydrate goals/meal and
	    snacks determine insulin:CHO doses
	Evaluate individual food glycemic
	    response
	Alternative sweeteners

3. Fat modification to reduce CVD risk	Restrict SFA to ≤10% total calories ≤7% if LDL >100 mg/dl Restrict PUFA to ≤10% calories Fish at least 2×/wk Preferred fat MUFA Total fat ≤25% of calories for weight loss

5. Vitamin/mineral supplementation	Women—folic acid: 400 μg if of child-
	    bearing age
	Calcium: to intake of
	    1000–2000 mg/day

FDA, Food and Drug Administration; CHO, carbohydrate; CVD, cardiovascular disease; SFA, saturated fatty acid; LDL, low-density lipoprotein; PUFA, polyunsaturated fat; MUFA, monounsaturated fat.

mean blood glucose values throughout the day. Nutrition interventions and physical activity can affect both fasting and postprandial values. Fasting blood glucose level is determined by hepatic glucose production through the night and influenced by degree of insulin resistance and available insulin. Weight loss, calorie or nutrient restriction, and physical activity can reduce insulin resistance and decrease hepatic glucose production in type 2 diabetes.[6,7] Because all individuals with type 1 diabetes, and some individuals with type 2 diabetes, are largely insulin deficient, the amount and type of insulin provided during nighttime hours affects fasting glucose levels. Physical activity enhances insulin sensitivity, increases peripheral glucose uptake, and subsequently may result in nighttime hypoglycemia, whereas bedtime food intake in excess of insulin coverage can increase nighttime blood glucose levels.

In contrast, the postprandial blood glucose period, defined as up to 6 hours after a meal, is predominantly the result of food intake, particularly the carbohydrate load, and the availability of either endogenous or exogenous insulin to compensate for insulin resistance and cover the carbohydrate challenge.[8] Insulin secretion is influenced directly by both carbohydrate load and protein consumption, whereas insulin resistance is influenced largely by body fat, which in turn is influenced by caloric intake.

BODY WEIGHT

Energy intake is generally episodic, varying in carbohydrate, protein, and fat intake from meal to meal and day to day. Daily caloric or energy requirement is determined by daily energy expenditure. This is represented by the sum of calories required to meet the needs for resting metabolic rate (RMR), the thermic effect of food (TEF), and the thermic effect of exercise. RMR comprises 60% to 75% of daily caloric needs

and depends on age, gender, body composition, and genetics.[9] Approximately a 2% to 3% drop in RMR occurs for every decade of life, accounting for the greater caloric needs per kilogram body weight in infants, children, and adolescents. Men have a higher RMR and require more calories than women because of their larger size and greater muscle mass. The TEF (i.e., the amount of calories required to absorb, metabolize, and store nutrients) is fairly stable at 10% of daily need. Physical activity, however, varies considerably from individual to individual and from day to day and can influence caloric needs in the range of 150 to 3000 kcal/day. A very active athletic 16-year-old could require up to 6000 kcal/day, whereas his or her sedentary counterpart may need less than the recommended caloric level, which is based on light to moderate physical activity.

Estimating caloric requirements is not easy or precise, yet guidelines have been recommended based on World Health Organization (WHO) calculations and modified for U.S. populations (Table 3-3).[9] These should be used only as guidelines and are subject to variability resulting from genetic and ethnic differences as well as concurrent medical conditions. The recommendations for adults, for example, are the same for all individuals older than 51 years of age, despite the fact that a 51-year-old is very different than an 85-year-old with or without a medical condition such as heart failure.

MINIMIZING WEIGHT GAIN

A dietary assessment to evaluate usual intake can be combined with the Caloric Recommendations to arrive at a personalized caloric plan if needed. The meal plan is then evaluated by monitoring desired outcomes in terms of blood glucose and lipid levels, and also growth and body weight. Infants and small children may need specific caloric prescriptions to achieve normal

TABLE 3-3 DIETARY REFERENCE INTAKE VALUES FOR ENERGY BY ACTIVE INDIVIDUALS BY LIFE STAGE GROUP A*		
Life Stage Group	**Active PAL[†] EER (kcal/day)**	
	Male	**Female**
0–6 mo	570	520
7–12 mo	743	676
1–2 yr	1046	992
3–8 yr	1742	1642
9–13 yr	2279	2071
14–18 yr	3152	2368
>18 yr	3067	2403
Pregnancy		
14–18 yr		
First trimester		2368
Second trimester		2708
Third trimester		2820
19–50 yr		
First trimester		2403
Second trimester		2743
Third trimester		2855
Lactation (single gestation)[‡]		
14–18 yr		
First 6 months		2698
Second 6 months		2768
19–50 yr		
First 6 months		2733
Second 6 months		2803

*For healthy, moderately active Americans and Canadians.

[†]PAL, physical activity level; EER, estimated energy requirement

[‡]For multiple gestation it may be necessary to increase caloric intake by 500 calories per additional child.

Adapted from National Academies' Institute of Medicine, 2002.

growth and development; however, in general, most adult individuals with type 1 diabetes inherently adjust their food intake to meet energy needs. As a result, carbohydrate, not calories, may be the only nutrient requiring modification and monitoring.

Unfortunately, the increasing incidence of obesity in children and adults in the United States, coupled with the definite tendency to experience weight gain with intensive glucose management, may require greater attention to caloric intake. An analysis of weight gain in Diabetes Control and Complications Trial (DCCT) subjects identified that, on average, adult subjects achieving a mean A1C of 7.2% gained 4.8 kg more during a 6-year follow-up than their conventionally controlled counterparts.[10] The rate of increase was greatest in the first year of intensive therapy and slowed thereafter, and only age was consistently associated with major weight gain. Individuals with type 2 diabetes are not immune to weight gain with intensive therapy; studies identify 4 to 6 kg gains in 2- to 18-month trials using insulin or oral agents.[11,12] Despite the benefits of improved glycemic control, care should be taken to reduce weight gain and maintain a healthy weight because the physical and health consequences of excessive weight gain remain to be quantified. Daily self-monitoring of food intake and physical activity and focusing on caloric intake as well as glycemic control is a useful tool to minimize weight gain in patients on diabetes medications.

CALORIE RESTRICTION AND WEIGHT

The United Kingdom Prospective Diabetes Study (UKPDS) report of the initial 3044 patients treated with diet therapy prior to randomization expanded our understanding of the benefits of nutrition intervention early in type 2 diabetes.[13] Subjects consumed an energy restricted diet (mean 1672 cal/day) for 3 months, during which time fasting plasma glucose levels fell considerably and mean A1C levels decreased 2%. This was, in fact, the largest A1C reduction achieved throughout the 20-year trial. The presence of dietitians was directly correlated to improved outcomes, suggesting that diet therapy was key to successful management.

More than 90% of persons with type 2 diabetes are obese (body mass index [BMI] > 27), overweight (BMI > 25), or have an upper body fat distribution (waist circumference > 102 cm in men and 85 cm in women) associated with insulin resistance. Thus weight loss and/or caloric restriction are considered first-line therapy in overweight type 2 diabetes. Losing as little as 10 to 20 pounds of body weight improves blood glucose control, serum total, and low-density lipoprotein (LDL) cholesterol, corrects dyslipidemia, and reduces blood pressure.[3,14] A meta-analysis of 89 studies illustrated that weight loss in type 2 diabetes improved A1C by as much as 2.7%, which is clearly as beneficial as most pharmacologic therapies.[15]

The UKPDS also illustrated the limitations of weight loss in type 2 diabetes because only 10% of those who had a fasting plasma glucose higher than 16 mmol/L (288 mg/dl) were able to achieve a normal blood glucose with weight loss. In contrast, 50% of those who had a blood glucose level lower than 8 mmol/L (145 mg/dl) achieved normal blood glucose with weight loss. This illustrates the point that weight loss is most effective early in the course of type 2 diabetes when insulin resistance is the primary defect and insulin secretion is at least partially capable of covering the demand.

In the UKPDS diet study, blood glucose levels improved in the first month of the 500 to 1000 daily calorie reduction; however, glycemic control failed to significantly improve during the subsequent 2 months. Those individuals who resumed eating a less calorically restrictive diet after 3 months actually experienced a worsening of glycemic control despite continued weight loss. Henry et al[6] and Williams et al[16] have shown that blood glucose control generally improves within 24 hours of caloric restriction and more than 80% of the total fasting blood glucose drop occurs within the first 10 days of a diet.

Decreased hepatic glucose production and increased glucose uptake in the periphery, both indicative of increased insulin sensitivity, appear responsible for early improvements in glycemic control. Thus caloric restriction independent of weight loss has been shown to have its own unique benefits in type 2 diabetes.[17,18] Even the authors of the UKPDS concluded that the dietary improvements seen in this study were actually the result of caloric or food restriction rather than weight loss.[13]

Intermittent caloric restriction using a modified liquid fast or very low-calorie diet 1 or 2 days per week or 1 week out of every 5 has shown some benefit in regards to weight loss success and glucose control compared against a standard 1500 to 1800 kcal diet in type 2 diabetes.[16] Restricting calories by 250 to 500 kcal/day using restricted servings or meal replacements (e.g., liquid, bar, or ready-made portions) is generally preferred by most individuals and found to be efficacious in clinical trials. These diets should be attempted only under medical supervision.

NUTRIENT COMPOSITION AND WEIGHT

Few studies have examined the ideal nutrient composition for a hypocaloric weight loss diet in diabetes. Despite the popularity of high protein/low carbohydrate diets, short-term studies as to their efficacy have been published only recently. In a one-year study a high-protein diet produced more weight loss at 6 months than a more balanced weight reduction diet, but this difference was not present at one year.[18a] The few studies available have looked at the satiety effect of protein with mixed results. Hypoenergetic diets using either 12% to 15% protein or 25% to 30% protein in individuals without diabetes,[19] including one with hyperinsulinemic individuals,[20] have shown slightly more weight loss at the higher protein level. A recent study in type 2 diabetes[21] showed no added benefit of a high protein diet on weight loss, although more abdominal weight loss was observed in women than men. Such diets generally promote weight loss by limiting food choices and, as a result, limiting calories. The concern is the long-term effect on lipids and other processes; however, the study in type 2 diabetes showed no harmful effects on lipids over 6 months.[22]

Several epidemiologic studies in individuals without diabetes support the theory that dietary fat contributes to a greater body weight.[23,24] Clinical intervention studies using either ad lib food intake, weight maintenance diets, or hypocaloric diets are less conclusive, illustrating that low-calorie diets ranging from low to high dietary fat intake result in the same amount of weight loss provided that calorie values are equal.[25] This demonstration that a calorie is a calorie is relatively easy to accomplish in research studies of short duration and in controlled environments. Free-living situations in which individuals are allowed to eat ad lib, low-fat diets (25% to 30% of total calories) are related to better weight loss and weight maintenance over time.[26,27]

Perhaps the best information currently available regarding strategies associated with successful long-term weight loss comes from information obtained in the National Weight Loss Registry.[28] This program follows individuals successful at losing and keeping off at least 30 pounds for more than 1 year. Most of them have been followed for up to 6 years and have kept off approximately 60 pounds. Characteristics of success include a diet of approximately 24% fat, a reported caloric intake of approximately 1400 kcal/day, and a reported physical activity expenditure of approximately 2800 kcal/wk. Although it is a fact that obese individuals tend to under-report food intake and over-report physical activity, this does not diminish the fact that caloric intake must be less than caloric expenditure for weight loss to occur. Clinicians must assist overweight patients in making conscious changes to reduce daily caloric intake modestly (250 to 500 kcal) most likely, but not exclusively, with a low-fat diet (<30% total calories) and an increase in energy expenditure to greater than 150 to 200 min/wk or approximately 2000 cal/wk.

EXERCISE AND WEIGHT

Individuals in weight-loss programs who report the highest level of physical activity over time are most likely to maintain weight loss.[28-30] This fact holds true whether or not an individual has type 2 diabetes. Studies estimating the amount of physical activity required to lose and maintain body weight typically encourage subjects to expend 1000 to 1500 kcal/wk. The weight loss registry data suggests higher levels of physical activity are required and is supported by a randomized trial of exercise and weight control. Jakicic[29] found that after 18 months, weight loss was significantly greater in the highest quartile of subjects who reported expending a mean of 2500 kcal/wk.

Most individuals do not exercise regularly, and individuals with type 2 diabetes generally exercise less than the general population. Furthermore, minority populations who are at greatest risk for type 2 diabetes exercise even less. As a result, studies addressing how to promote physical activity are overdue. Exercising at home may be more likely associated with long-term adherence than group sessions because home exercising allows more flexibility in choosing when activity is performed.[30] In addition, most studies using home activities utilize walking, which is easily performed by most individuals and is not expensive.

Adherence may be further enhanced by encouraging activity in frequent short bouts rather than long single bouts. Four 10-minute bouts of activity per day using a personal treadmill in the home increased adherence to an activity regimen, increased expenditure, and was associated with greater weight loss over 18 months compared to single 40 minute bouts per day.[29] Exercising 200 min/wk was related to significantly better weight loss than 150 min/wk. This illustrates that patients need to be given realistic goals that are simple and flexible. Prescribing physical activity in terms of min/wk is a nonthreatening flexible approach to encouraging activity for weight loss. A good rule of thumb for obese individuals is to consider 200 minutes as expending approximately 2000 kcal, remembering that most individuals must start with a much lower goal and increase minutes gradually.

CARBOHYDRATES

The DCCT documented the importance of nutrition intervention for optimizing glycemic control in type 1 diabetes.[10] Adjusting insulin doses to food/carbohydrate intake and following a nutrition plan was associated with lowest A1C values.[31] Later, the UKPDS expanded our understanding of the progressive nature of type 2 diabetes, illustrating that gradual loss of

β-cell function and subsequent loss of insulin secretory capacity in relationship to the level of glycemia is the norm.[32,33] Weight loss and physical activity are extremely effective therapeutic tools in the early stages of type 2 diabetes because each plays a role in reducing insulin resistance. However, once β-cell function diminishes to a point at which glucose levels are consistently elevated above 140 to 180 mg/dl, therapy should move focus away from weight loss and toward modifying carbohydrate intake to work synergistically with medication, either oral agents, insulin, or a combination, to maintain near normal metabolic control. The need for antidiabetic medication does not imply that diet and exercise efforts have failed or that the patient has failed. In reality the β-cell fails to keep up with the growing need for insulin such that diet and exercise alone can no longer maintain metabolic control.

QUANTITY OF CARBOHYDRATE

Individuals with normal glucose tolerance experience a dose-related rise in postprandial blood glucose when consuming up to 60 to 75 g of carbohydrate.[34] Consuming more carbohydrate does not increase blood glucose further because insulin secretion keeps up with entry of glucose into the blood. As a result, blood glucose rarely rises higher than 140 mg/dl. In contrast, in type 2 diabetes where insulin secretion is less than adequate, or in type 1 diabetes where insulin secretion is absent or negligible, the higher the dose of carbohydrate, the greater the blood glucose response.

The optimal amount of carbohydrate to consume differs with each individual and should be based on preference and desired metabolic outcome. Carbohydrate foods such as fruits, vegetables, and whole grains and cereals provide necessary vitamins, minerals, fiber, and phytonutrients, all considered essential to health. As a result, the ADA recommends 60% to 70% of total caloric intake be derived from a combination of carbohydrate and unsaturated fat; in other words, approximately 50% of the diet should come from carbohydrate. Decreasing carbohydrate intake to a level less than 40% in an effort to attenuate postprandial blood glucose levels often results in a diet that is too high in fat and protein. Studies in individuals with type 1 diabetes show a strong relationship between the premeal short- or rapid-acting insulin dose and postprandial blood glucose response when dose is based on total carbohydrate content of the meal.[35,36] Thus a carbohydrate intake greater than 50% can be accommodated by adjusting insulin dose to carbohydrate intake. Learning to calculate and adjust insulin dose to total carbohydrate intake is the primary nutritional strategy used to optimize glycemic control in type 1 diabetes.

In contrast, studies in persons with type 2 diabetes and insulin resistance raise concern that high carbohydrate intakes (>50%) may worsen metabolic control, including serum glucose and triglyceride levels. Insulin resistance and the resultant hyperinsulinemia accentuated by a high carbohydrate intake increase hepatic synthesis of very-low-density lipoproteins-triglyceride. For this reason, the carbohydrate and fat recommendations for persons with type 2 diabetes are linked and broadly defined. Diets containing as much as 35% to 40% fat and 40% to 45% carbohydrate have shown improved metabolic control in insulin-resistant type 2 diabetes, provided that the major fatty acids consumed are of the monounsaturated variety.[37] If fat intake is highly saturated from red meats and whole-fat dairy products, then LDL cholesterol, a major risk factor for cardiovascular disease, generally increases.

TYPE OF CARBOHYDRATE/ GLYCEMIC INDEX

Despite the strong relationship between total carbohydrate intake and insulin requirement, postprandial blood glucose response to a mixed meal is not always predictable. In a classic study[38] illustrating this point, subjects with type 1 diabetes experienced a larger and longer postprandial blood glucose response when consuming a pizza meal as when consuming a standard meal, despite equivalent amounts of carbohydrate, protein, and fat It is now well accepted that the magnitude and nature of the postprandial blood glucose rise is proportional to the rate of digestion and absorption of carbohydrate in the meal. Several factors can influence the rate of digestion and absorption to a carbohydrate challenge, including premeal blood glucose values. Hyperglycemia before eating slows gastric emptying and results in a more prolonged glycemic response,[39] whereas hypoglycemia speeds emptying and results in a faster, higher, and earlier peak response.[40] The presence of some organic acids in foods, such as in sourdough bread or tannic acid in tea and wine, appears to slow gastric emptying and flatten the blood glucose response.[40a]

The optimal type of carbohydrate is considered to be one that yields a relatively flat postprandial blood glucose response. The Glycemic Index (GI) of foods is a classification of carbohydrate-rich foods based on their postprandial blood glucose and insulin response.[41] It is expressed as the percentage of blood glucose rise over 2 to 3 hours from 50 g of carbohydrate from a particular food compared with the blood glucose response to 50 g of glucose. Foods are ranked from a GI of 20 to more than 100 (pure glucose).

Research in this area has done much to dispel the myth that sugar or sucrose raises blood glucose more than starch,[42] and has provided evidence that carbohydrate foods can yield variable blood glucose and insulin responses both between and within food groups such as fruits, vegetables, and cereal grains.[43] Because blood glucose response of a carbohydrate food is directly related to the rate of glucose digestion and absorption from the gastrointestinal tract and is not a function of simple or complex carbohydrate, the terms *simple* and *complex* have been discouraged by the WHO.[44]

The molecular nature of a starch is one factor that alters the rate of digestion. Amylose, composed of straight chains of glucose molecules, is a form of starch that is slowly digested and absorbed compared with amylopectin, which is made up of branched chains. Both amylose and amylopectin are present in various amounts in all starch-containing foods. Wheat starch, containing a greater percentage of amylopectin, yields a greater glucose response than oat starch, which is higher in amylose and viscous fibers. The ratio of amylopectin to amylose is about 70:30 in most starches and accounts for the rapid blood glucose effect of most starches.[45]

Cooking, as with potatoes, and processing, as in grinding apples for applesauce, softens the starch granule and exposes it for easier enzymatic breakdown, raising blood glucose levels higher and faster.[46] This concept supports the principle that starches should be used in their whole-grain, unprocessed form such as whole wheat breads and whole grain cereals whenever possible.

Although research has provided valuable explanations for varying blood glucose responses to individual foods and mixed meals, the clinical significance of the GI remains controversial. Indeed, clinical intervention trials in type 1 diabetes have yielded inconclusive results in that, although post-meal blood glucose levels may be lower overall, blood glucose control as measured by A1C is not improved.[47,48] Adding the GI requirement to total carbohydrate counting adds another level of complexity to an already regimented diet. Studies in children found that choosing carbohydrate portions from a list of low-GI foods reduced A1C by 0.3% and improved quality of life after 12 months when compared with a carbohydrate counting exchange-type regimen.[49,50]

With the advent of rapid-acting insulin analogs, postprandial elevations with meals can be covered with insulin injections such that the greatest benefit to using low-GI foods may be between meals and as snacks when insulin concentration is waning.

Clinical intervention trials in type 2 diabetes and the GI have yielded slightly more favorable results. Postprandial values are improved and slight improvements in overall glucose control have been observed.[51,52] Lower insulin, triglyceride, and plasminogen activator inhibitor-1 levels, may prove to be the real benefit of a low-GI diet.[53] Indeed, choosing low-GI foods may be most beneficial during the prediabetes and early diabetes state when insulin resistance is high and β-cell response is limited in comparison to the glycemic load. Using the GI adds another level of complexity to an already difficult diet regimen of counting total carbohydrate. This may be helpful for some people, but is not warranted as a general recommendation for all persons with diabetes. Nonetheless, consuming whole-grain, high-fiber, unprocessed foods with the potential for producing a flatter blood glucose response is recommended as the first step in nutrition therapy for diabetes.

Fiber and Resistant Starch

Some foods such as raw cornstarch contain naturally existing resistant starches that are higher in amylose, producing a flatter glycemic response.[54] This attribute has spurred the development of designer foods such as snack bars that contain a combination of sucrose and raw cornstarch that can be used with the intent to prevent hypoglycemia.[55] There is no evidence at present that the use of resistant starch has long-term benefit in type 1 diabetes; however, the clinical value in individuals at high risk for nighttime hypoglycemia may prove beneficial.

Fiber such as that found in grains, beans, nuts, seeds, fruits, and vegetables is a form of carbohydrate that is indigestible and therefore does not contribute to the postprandial blood glucose rise. Furthermore, viscous soluble fibers found in oats and pectin limit enzyme access to other digestible carbohydrates in the gut, limiting postprandial glucose levels.[56] Early studies demonstrated a beneficial effect of fiber on glycemic control in type 1 diabetes, but were complicated by the poor glycemic control of individuals and the small number of subjects.[57] More recent studies illustrate that large amounts of fiber may be required to effect long-term glycemic control and the effects are not consistent and modest at best. A diet containing 50 g of fiber with a GI of 70% resulted in a 24% drop in mean daily blood glucose concentrations and a A1C improvement of 0.5% after 6 months in persons with type 1 diabetes, compared against a diet containing 15 g of fiber with a GI of 90%.[58] In contrast, 56 g of fiber did not have an affect in another recent study in type 1 diabetes.[59]

The best support for fiber in type 2 diabetes comes from a study comparing daily consumption of 50 g to 24 g from actual food for 6 months.[60] Glycemic control, hyperinsulinemia, and plasma lipid levels all improved. The palatability and digestibility of such large amounts of fiber may be problematic for many individuals, but should not be discouraged in those who wish to use a high-fiber diet. Because the average American consumes approximately 13 g of dietary fiber per day, progression to a high-fiber intake needs to be gradual and requires a good deal of motivation. Fiber supplements such as guar gums, psyllium, and β-glucan have had a positive short-term effect on postprandial blood glucose levels in type 2 diabetes.[3]

Persons who adjust their insulin-to-carbohydrate intake may need to subtract the grams of fiber from their total carbohydrate consumption at a particular meal if 5 or more grams of fiber are available per serving. Benefits of fiber in diabetes also include optimal overall gastrointestinal function and the LDL-cholesterol lowering effect validated in individuals without diabetes and recommended in the National Cholesterol Education Program Guidelines.[61]

Sweeteners

Sugar or sucrose (glucose + fructose) does not elevate blood glucose to a greater extent than starch.[62] Glucose is rapidly and easily absorbed, but represents only half of the sucrose molecule. As fructose passes through the liver after absorption, it is metabolized and does not immediately or directly contribute to blood glucose elevation. Ingestion of as much as 10% to 17% of total calories as sugar, consistent with typical U.S. intake, has shown no detrimental effect on blood glucose control in type 1 or type 2 diabetes.[63-65] Consumption of sugar-rich foods is recommended in moderation and in the context of a healthy diet (potentially one serving daily) while counting gram for gram as carbohydrate.

Alternative sweeteners are available for the purpose of reducing calories and carbohydrate intake. Fructose is used as an alternative sweetener and is particularly abundant in soft drinks and fruit beverages, which account for two thirds of fructose intake in the United States. Although blood glucose response is slightly flatter, concern has been raised that in large quantities fructose (20% of calories) elevates serum cholesterol levels.[66] Sugar alcohols such as sorbitol and mannitol provide fewer calories (2 to 3 cal/g) than sucrose, glucose, or fructose, and raise blood glucose to a lesser extent.[67] Yet there are no published studies illustrating a long-term benefit in glycemic control or body weight to their regular use. Because sugar alcohols have a laxative effect when consumed in more than 20-g portions or 50 g/day, they should be used with caution in small children to avoid causing diarrhea.[68]

Nonnutritive sweeteners currently approved as safe by the FDA are aspartame, saccharine, acesulfame K, and sucralose. Because of their intense sweetening capacity, they do not contribute calories or carbohydrate to the meal plan and can be used freely in the diet. However, rarely are alternative sweeteners used alone in a food except in diet drinks and some candies or gelatins. Other sources of carbohydrate may be present in combination with nonnutritive sweeteners in foods such as ice creams or deserts, requiring that total carbohydrate content per serving be calculated.

Treating hypoglycemia correctly is crucial to effectively managing diabetes. Although any form of carbohydrate raises blood glucose, sugar in the form of glucose tablets, candy, soda, juice, or milk are traditionally used. Pure glucose or sucrose in tablets or a solution elevate blood glucose equally well when treating hypoglycemia, providing a response within 10 minutes and alleviating symptoms within 15 minutes.[69] Approximately 15- to 20-g portions of these carbohydrates elevate blood glucose levels approximately 50 mg/dl when hypoglycemia is in the range of 50 to 70 mg/dl.[70] Levels less than this may require 30 g to bring the glucose level back to normal within 15 to 30 minutes. Traditional treatments such as orange juice and milk can require more than 40-g portions of carbohydrate to be as effective.[71]

CARBOHYDRATE COUNTING

Carbohydrate counting is a technique commonly used to quantify the total amount of carbohydrate consumed at a meal or snack.[72] Two basic techniques can be employed: One counts grams of carbohydrate using food labels and written sources to provide information on the grams of carbohydrate per serving in a food, whereas the second uses a modified exchange system in which carbohydrate-containing foods are classified in 15-g servings. One "carb" is equivalent to 15 g of carbohydrate. An individual's usual carbohydrate intake at meals and snacks can be assessed and used to establish carbohydrate goals for each meal and snack (Table 3-4).

The availability of rapid-acting insulin provides a means to establish an insulin/carbohydrate ratio for each meal. The ratio is determined by body weight and trial and error (e.g., one unit insulin:15 g of carbohydrate is a good place to start in the average adult). On the other hand, the ratio for a 7-year-old child may be 1:30. The insulin/carbohydrate ratio can then be adjusted until postprandial blood glucose goals are achieved.

In the DCCT, reduction in A1C was related to self-reported adherence to the diet regimen.[31] Individual dietary compo-

TABLE 3-4	SAMPLE DAILY CARBOHYDRATE DISTRIBUTION BASED ON 2000 KCAL MEAL PLAN[A]		
	Amount		
Meal		**Grams**	**Servings**
Breakfast		45	3
Snack		15	1
Lunch		60	4
Snack		30	2
Dinner		75	5
Snack		15	1
		—	—
Total		240	16

[a]50% carbohydrate.

nents identified were adjusting insulin dose to food intake and blood glucose fluctuations, and not deviating from the snack schedule. If an individual chooses to maintain a fixed dose of insulin at meals from day to day, then carbohydrate intake must be consistent or fixed as well. Deviations of more than 5 to 10 g could produce deviations in postprandial blood glucose levels. Most individuals with type 1 diabetes should, and generally prefer, to adjust their insulin dose to total carbohydrate intake. Adjusting insulin dose to carbohydrate intake allows for more flexibility in the timing and quantity of food eaten at meals. If more or less carbohydrate is desired at a meal, insulin dose can be adjusted accordingly. Rapid acting insulin, because of its quick absorption time (5 to 15 min) is effective whether taken immediately before or immediately after a meal.[73] This attribute allows for tremendous flexibility in eating and a subsequent improved quality of life. For example, a small child can be allowed to eat a meal, carbohydrate consumption can be observed, and the appropriate insulin dose provided. This has obvious advantages over predetermining and injecting an insulin dose based on potential carbohydrate intake only to discover that the child doesn't wish to eat.

The best way to evaluate the optimal amount and type of carbohydrate in meals and snacks is to use self-monitoring of blood glucose. Measuring blood glucose levels before meals estimates the previous meal's effect on blood glucose because glucose levels should return to baseline within 4 hours. Testing before and 1 to 2 hours after a meal allows fine tuning regarding the type and quantity of carbohydrate. For example, testing before and after substituting sugar-rich foods such as ice cream (15 g carbohydrate per scoop) for one slice of bread (15 g per slice) provides information for making decisions about how much of each food can be eaten. Any food can be used in the diet in type 2 diabetes; the key is portion size.

Ultimately the goal of diet therapy is to keep blood glucose values in the target range of 80 to 120 mg/dl before meals and less than 140 to 180 mg/dl after meals. As a rule, a 50 to 60 mg/dl postprandial rise is considered optimal. Records of daily food intake, physical activity, and blood glucose test results for 3 to 5 days are indispensable tools for evaluating blood glucose response to diet modification.

Traditionally diet regimens included strict attention to equal distribution of carbohydrate, protein, and fat at meals, and adhering to a rigid eating schedule. Meal frequency (three to nine meals per day) has little effect on overall metabolic control in type 2 diabetes; therefore individuals should be encouraged to consume their food in a pattern that fits their life style, matches their medication schedule, and produces optimal blood glucose levels.[74]

PHYSICAL ACTIVITY AND GLYCEMIC CONTROL

A sedentary lifestyle increases risk for type 2 diabetes. Major research trials have found that changing diet and increasing physical activity can reduce this risk by as much as 58%.[1,75] Physical activity is extraordinarily important in the medical management of type 2 diabetes. Whereas exercise has little impact on blood glucose in nondiabetic individuals, it generally lowers blood glucose in type 2 diabetes. During physical activity, glucose levels fall as a result of insulin-stimulated glucose uptake by the exercising muscle cell. This acute fall in glucose concentration is potentiated by the presence of insulin as glucose transporter 4 transport proteins are stimulated within muscle cells.[76] Repeated bouts of exercise results in both improved fasting and postprandial insulin and glucose levels.[77] This exercise-induced improvement in insulin sensitivity is the result of enhanced glycogen storage in muscle and reduced insulin resistance from mobilizing intramuscular fat. Reduced insulin resistance is by far the most important benefit of physical activity in terms of glucose tolerance and metabolic control and is thought to be responsible for the strong relationship between regular physical activity and reduced risk for developing type 2 diabetes. Furthermore, physical activity, including moderate walking, has been shown to reduce cardiovascular events in persons with type 2 diabetes.[78]

Unfortunately, improved insulin sensitivity associated with physical conditioning is short-lived, lasting approximately 24 to 72 hours. This accounts for the recommended frequency for performing physical activity of minimally 3 to 4 days each week. Both aerobic and strength-building activities such as weight lifting reduce insulin resistance and enhance glucose uptake by the muscle. However, physical activities of daily living such as gardening, house cleaning, or golfing have been associated with reduced risk of diabetes and cardiovascular disease and should be encouraged in an effort to minimize the negative association between "exercise" and rigorous activities such as running. Incorporating both structured exercise and daily physical activity require emphases in individuals with diabetes and those at risk for diabetes.

PROTEIN

GLYCEMIC EFFECTS OF PROTEIN

Protein is absorbed as amino acids and transported directly into the portal blood system. Some amino acids are metabolized immediately in the liver, but most enter the plasma as free amino acids and are transported to muscle and other tissue. Protein is not converted immediately into glucose and as a result does not immediately raise postprandial blood glucose levels. Consuming as much as 9 ounces of protein in a mixed meal elevated postprandial blood glucose levels only slightly at 3 to 5 hours after eating in persons with type 1 diabetes when compared with a standard meal with 3 to 4 ounces of protein.[79] Plasma glucagon levels appear to be stimulated by protein consumption in type 1 diabetes and mirror the delayed glucose elevation.[80] Thus increased hepatic glucose output, secondary to elevations in glucagon, during the latter half of the postprandial period appears responsible for the effect of protein when consumed along with carbohydrate. This attribute has led to the assumption that protein is required at every meal and in bedtime snacks to prolong the blood glucose response and prevent nighttime hypoglycemia. Little evidence exists to support or refute this practice. Adding 2 ounces of turkey protein to an evening carbohydrate snack (15 g) in a crossover study resulted in slightly fewer hypoglycemic episodes and an insignificant rise in fasting blood glucose the following day.[81] Adding protein to carbohydrate when treating hypoglycemia does not appear to provide benefit. One study in type 1 diabetes illustrated that 15 g of carbohydrate with or without 1 ounce of turkey produced identical blood glucose elevations over 180 minutes when treating hypoglycemia.[82]

Protein is a potent stimulator of insulin secretion in type 2 diabetes.[83,84] This increased insulin can produce a lower postprandial glucose response that returns to baseline faster. The amounts of protein studied, however, have used 50-g dose or the equivalent of 7 ounces of meat, fish, or poultry.

PROTEIN AND RENAL FUNCTION

Persons with diabetes may attempt to substitute protein for carbohydrate to attenuate postprandial glucose response. A large cross-sectional study in type 1 diabetes found that protein intakes of 20% or more of total energy intake were associated with higher albumin excretions than protein intakes of less than 20% of total energy intake.[85] Concern over the role protein intake plays in renal function suggests that consuming more than 20% protein in the diet is unwise. Furthermore, it is difficult to control total fat and saturated fat intake on a high-protein diet because saturated fat and cholesterol predominate in animal foods. Average protein consumption for most individuals is approximately 10% to 20% of total calories and consistently averaging 100 g/day. Attempts to reduce albuminuria with protein restriction have shown that even small reductions in protein intake reduce the rate of decline of glomerular filtration rate and albuminuria in persons with type 1 diabetes.[86] Most studies find that it is not feasible to reduce intake to less than 0.7 g/kg body weight. The FDA Food Guide Pyramid recommendation of 5 to 7 ounces of animal protein per day is adequate for most individuals with diabetes This level can be reduced to 0.8 to 1.0 g/kg once microalbuminuria is present and 0.8 g/kg in overt nephropathy.

FAT AND CARDIOVASCULAR RISK

Clearly, optimizing blood glucose levels is paramount to preventing the microvascular and macrovascular complications of diabetes, yet the risk of cardiovascular disease in diabetes is great. In addition to glucose intolerance, diabetic dyslipidemia characterized by elevated triglycerides and low high-density lipoprotein (HDL)-cholesterol levels, hypertension, and a prothrombotic state are common and important metabolic risk factors for cardiovascular disease in insulin-resistant type 2 diabetes. Generally LDL-cholesterol levels are normal or only slightly elevated in type 2 diabetes, but are made up of a larger proportion of small, dense, more atherosclerotic particles.[87] Thus optimizing LDL, triglyceride, and HDL levels is a primary goal of therapy in type 2 diabetes. Elevated triglycerides, low HDL levels, and elevated LDL levels are also common in untreated type 1 diabetes but

normalize with intensive glucose control. Normal LDL concentrations generally characterize treated type 1 diabetes; however, the DCCT demonstrated that intensive control can improve atherogenic risk by producing a shift in LDL particle size from small, dense to less large buoyant particles.[87]

QUANTITY OF DIETARY FAT

Dietary fatty acids can have either a positive or negative effect on lipid levels. Saturated fatty acid (SFA) is the principal determinant of serum cholesterol in diabetes as in the general population. Even on a weight loss diet containing only 31% total fat, serum LDL concentration increased in subjects with type 2 diabetes when SFA intake was high.[88] Trans fatty acids, produced during partial hydrogenation of unsaturated fat, are considered metabolically equivalent to saturated fats.[89] Few studies have been performed in type 1 diabetes; therefore any effects of dietary fat must be extrapolated from studies in the general population. The ADA and the National Cholesterol Education Program recommend that the combination of SFA and trans fatty acids not exceed 10% of calories.

If fat intake is to be reduced, the question remains as to which macronutrient should replace the 10% to 20% of calories? Substituting carbohydrate for saturated fat reduces total and LDL cholesterol levels in persons with type 2 diabetes, yet has mixed effects on HDL cholesterol and glycemic control.[90] Some studies show no negative effect of a high-carbohydrate/low fat-diet, whereas others show increased triglycerides, decreased HDL, and higher blood glucose levels.[91]

Type of Dietary Fat

Replacing SFA with polyunsaturated fat (PUFA) of the omega-6 variety (safflower, corn, soy oils) reduces total and LDL cholesterol in type 2 diabetes but may have little effect on serum triglycerides or HDL cholesterol.[92] Nor is there epidemiologic data to suggest that omega-6 PUFAs have a direct effect on reducing cardiovascular risk in individuals with or without diabetes. In contrast, omega-3 fatty acids, a form of PUFA found in cold-water fish oils, offer risk-reducing benefits by lowering triglycerides and decreasing thrombogenic factors.[93-95] Two to three 4-ounce servings of fish each week is recommended to provide beneficial effects. Fish oil supplementation can have a negative effect on serum LDL cholesterol and is therefore restricted to severe hypertriglyceridemia (>2000 mg/dl) with LDL monitoring.

Studies in the general population support that substituting monounsaturated fat (MUFA) for saturated fat is equally as effective as substituting carbohydrate for lowering total LDL levels.[96] An additional benefit of a slightly higher MUFA intake is that HDL levels are consistently maintained in type 2 diabetes and not reduced because they are on a low-fat/high-carbohydrate diet.[97] Several studies support that substituting MUFA for saturated fat improves triglyceride and HDL levels, increases LDL particle size without increasing total LDL levels, and improves glycemia.[97-100] A diet high in carbohydrate and low in fat (<30%) or a diet containing 30% to 40% total fat, if primarily MUFA, can be beneficial in insulin-resistant persons with type 2 diabetes.[101] Although it is tempting to imply benefits in type 1 diabetes when insulin is replaced physiologically and control is optimal, there are no studies specifically examining the effect of MUFA in type 1 diabetes. Because there is

no negative effect to increasing MUFA consumption within the normal range of fat intake, these fats can be encouraged. Cultural differences and food preferences may make this easier in some individuals than others (Table 3-5).

FAT REPLACERS

Fat replacers or substitutes derived from modified protein or carbohydrate were introduced into the market to assist in efforts to decrease total fat intake. Although this is theoretically possible, few studies have documented a health benefit in type 2 diabetes. Most have been behavioral studies identifying that total fat, saturated fat, and dietary cholesterol intake can be reduced with the use of these products.[102] However, little change in energy intake or body weight has been reported. Persons with diabetes using large amounts of carbohydrate-based fat substitutes (salad dressings), must consider that fat has been replaced by carbohydrate and count the carbohydrate if amounts are above 5 g per serving.

PHYSICAL ACTIVITY AND CARDIOVASCULAR RISK

Physical activity improves serum lipids indirectly by reducing insulin resistance and by promoting weight loss. Although unclear, it is thought that improved insulin sensitivity contributes to improved triglyceride levels by decreasing VLDL production and increasing

TABLE 3-5	DIETARY FAT GUIDELINES AND SOURCES BASED ON DAILY 2000 CALORIE MEAL PLAN[a]		
Type	**Source**	**% of calories**	**Amount**
Saturated/trans fats	Meats, high-fat dairy, stick margarines	<10%	2 g
Polyunsaturated omega 3	Soy, corn, safflower, fish	<10%	22 g 8 oz/wk
Monounsaturated	Olive, canola, nuts, avocados	10–20%	22–44 g
TOTAL		30%–40%	66–90 g

[a]American Diabetes Association, Nutrition Guidelines, 2002.

lipoprotein lipase activity in the muscle.[103] HDL cholesterol increases with regular physical activity as well. Effects on serum lipids require a minimum amount of activity equivalent to 10 to 12 miles of running or walking per week. A dose-response effect was observed in the Nurses Health Study.[104] Age-adjusted relative risk decreased as walking increased from less than 1 hr/wk to more than 7 hr/wk. Risk for cardiovascular events decreased and serum lipid and A1C levels improved as amount of walking and vigorousness of walking increased. Daily activity of moderate intensity for more than 200 min/wk is required for optimal outcomes.

ALCOHOL

Alcohol need not be restricted in individuals with diabetes as long as it is limited to no more than one daily serving for women and two for men. Alcohol in these amounts has little effect on glycemic control, but does potentiate the glucose lowering effect of insulin by reducing hepatic glucose production. Patients taking insulin or an insulin secretagogue should take care to consume alcohol with food to prevent hypoglycemia. Moderate consumption has been associated with reduced cardiovascular disease risk,[105] increased insulin sensitivity, and decreased risk of developing type 2 diabetes.[106] For these reasons, alcohol may in fact be beneficial to some individuals with type 2 diabetes. Although serum triglycerides can worsen with alcohol intake, small to moderate consumption is not problematic. Alcohol has been shown to increase HDL levels in the general population, which could be beneficial in insulin resistant type 2 diabetes.

SUMMARY

There is no one "diabetic diet" or exercise plan. Diabetes is heterogeneous in nature and the lifestyle, cultures, and age groups of persons with diabetes are equally heterogeneous. Physical activity and a healthy diet are part of a lifestyle that is thought to prevent type 2 diabetes and clearly plays a role in managing diabetes. A variety of strategies exist to achieve desired medical outcomes of optimal blood glucose levels, serum lipids, and blood pressure. Changing lifestyle behaviors is a gradual process that is achieved through small steps facilitated by health professionals, but is ultimately "chosen" by the person with diabetes.

REFERENCES

1. Diabetes Prevention Research Group: Reduction in the evidence of type 2 diabetes with life-style intervention or metformin. N Engl J Med 346:393, 2002.
2. American Diabetes Association: Evidence-based nutrition principles and recommendations for the treatment and prevention of diabetes and related complications. Diabetes Care 25:S50, 2002.
3. Franz MJ, Bantle JP, Beebe CA et al: Evidence-based nutrition principles and recommendations for the treatment and prevention of diabetes and related complications. (Technical Review). Diabetes Care 25:S136, 2002.
4. United States Food and Drug Administration: Major trends in U.S. food supply, 1909-99. Food Review 23:8, 2002.
5. Appel LJ, Moore TJ, Obarzanek E et al: A clinical trial of the effects of dietary patterns on blood pressure. N Eng J Med 336:1117, 1997.
6. Henry RR, Wallace P, Olefsky JM: Effects of weight loss on mechanisms of hyperglycemia in obese noninsulin-dependent diabetes mellitus. Diabetes 35:990, 1986.
7. Olefsky JM, Kolterman OG, Scarlett JA: Insulin action and resistance in obesity and noninsulin-dependent type II diabetes mellitus. Am J Physiology 243:E15, 1982.
8. American Diabetes Association. Postprandial blood glucose, consensus statement. Diabetes Care 24:775, 2001.
9. World Health Organization: Energy and protein requirements (Tech Report Ser #724). World Health Organization, Geneva, 1985.
10. The DCCT Research Group. Influence of intensive diabetes treatment on body weight and composition of adults with type 1 diabetes in the Diabetes Control and Complications Trial. Diabetes Care 24:1711, 2001.
11. Laville M, Andreelli F: Mechanisms for weight gain during blood glucose normalization. Diabetes and Metabolism 26(Suppl 3):42, 2000.
12. Rigalleau V, Delafaye C, Baillet L et al: Composition of insulin-induced body weight gain

in diabetic patients: A bio-impedence study. Diabetes Metab 25:321, 1999.

13. United Kingdom Prospective Diabetes Study Group: Response of fasting plasma glucose to diet therapy in newly presenting type II diabetic patients (UKPDS 7). Metabolism 39:905, 1990.

14. Executive Summary of the Third Report of the National Cholesterol Education Program (NCEP) Expert Panel on Detection, Evaluation, and Treatment of High Blood Cholesterol in Adults (Adult Treatment Panel III). JAMA 285:2486, 2001.

15. Brown S, Upchurch S, Anding R et al: Promoting weight loss in type 2 diabetes. Diabetes Care 19:613, 1996.

16. Williams K, Mullen M, Kelley D et al: The effect of short periods of caloric restriction on weight loss and glycemic control in type 2 diabetes. Diabetes Care 21:2, 1998.

17. Markovic T, Jenkins A, Campbell L et al: The determinants of glycemic responses to diet restriction and weight loss in obesity and NIDDM. Diabetes Care 21:687, 1998.

18. Wing R, Blair E, Bononi P et al: Caloric restriction per se is a significant factor in improvements in glycemic control and insulin sensitivity during weight loss in obese NIDDM patients. Diabetes Care 17:30, 1994.

18a.Foster GD, Wyatt HR, Hill JO et al: A randomized trial of a low-carbohydrate diet for obesity. N Engl J Med 348(21):2082-2090, 2003.

19. Skov AR, Toubro S, Ronn B et al: Randomized trial on protein vs carbohydrate in ad libitum fat reduced diet for the treatment of obesity. Int. J Obes 23:528, 1999.

20. Baba NH, Sawaya S, Torbay N et al: High protein vs high carbohydrate hypoenergetic diet for the treatment of obese hyperinsulinemic subjects. Int J Obes 23:1202, 1999.

21. Luscombe ND, Clifton PM, Noakes M et al: Effects of energy-restricted diets containing increased protein on weight loss, resting energy expenditure, and the thermic effect of feeding in type 2 diabetes. Diabetes Care 25:652, 2002.

22. Parker B, Noakes M, Luscombe N et al: Effect of a high-protein high-monounsaturated fat weight loss diet on glycemic control and lipid levels in type 2 diabetes. Diabetes Care 25:425, 2002.

23. Astrup A, Ryan L, Grunwald GK et al: The role of dietary fat in body fatness: Evidence from a preliminary meta-analysis of ad libitum low-fat dietary intervention study. Br J Nutr 83:S25, 2000.

24. Carmichael HE, Swinburn BA, Wilson MR: Lower fat intake as a predictor of initial and sustained weight loss in obese subjects consuming an otherwise adlibitum diet. J Am Diet Assoc 98:35, 1998.

25. Golay A, Allaz AF, Morel Y et al: Similar weight loss with low- or high-carbohydrate diets. Am J Clin Nutr 63:174-178, 1996.

26. Swinburn BA, Metcalf P, Lezotte DC: Long-term (5-year) effects of a reduced fat diet in individuals with glucose intolerance. Diabetes Care 24:619, 2001.

27. Prewitt TE, Schmeisser D, Bowen PE et al: Changes in body weight, body composition, and energy intake in women fed high and low fat diets. Am J Clin Nutr 54:304, 1991.

28. Klem M, Wing R, McGuire M et al: A descriptive study of individuals successful at long-term maintenance of substantial weight loss. Am J Clin Nutr 66:239, 1997.

29. Jakicic J, Wing R, Winters C: Effects of intermittent exercise and use of home exercise equipment on adherence, weight loss, and fitness in overweight women. JAMA 282:1554, 1999.

30. Perri MG, Martin AD, Leermakers EA at al: Effects of group versus home-based exercise in the treatment of obesity. J Consult Clin Psychol 65:278, 1997.

31. Delahanty LM, Halford BN: The role of diet behaviors in achieving improved glycemic control in intensively treated patients in the Diabetes Control and Complications Trial. Diabetes Care 16:1453, 1993.

32. United Kingdom Prospective Diabetes Study (UKPDS) Group: Tight blood pressure control and risk of macrovascular and microvascular complications in type 2 diabetes (UKPDS 38). BMJ 317:713, 1998.

33. United Kingdom Prospective Diabetes Study (UKPDS) Group: Intensive blood-glucose control with sulphonylureas or insulin compared with conventional treatment and risk of complications in patients with type 2 diabetes (UKPDS 33). Lancet 352:837, 1998.

34. Nuttall FQ, Gannon MC: Plasma glucose and insulin response to macronutrients in nondiabetic and NIDDM patients. Diabetes Care 14:824, 1991.

35. Rabasa-Lhoret R, Garon J, Langelier H et al: The effects of meal carbohydrate content on insulin requirements in type 1 diabetic patients treated intensively with the basal bolus (ultralent-regular) insulin regimen. Diabetes Care 22:667, 1999.

36. Heinemann L, Heise T, Wahl LCH et al: Prandial glycemia after a carbohydrate-rich meal in type 1 diabetic patients: Using the rapid acting insulin analogue [Lys(B28), Pro(B29)] human insulin. Diabetic Medicine 13:625, 1996.

37. Parillo M, Rivellese AA, Ciardullo AV et al: A high-monounsaturated-fat/low-carbohydrate diet improves peripheral insulin sensitivity in non–insulin-dependent diabetic patients. Metabolism: Clinical and Experimental 41(12):1373-1378, 1992.

38. Ahren JA, Gatcomb PM, Held NA et al: Exaggerated hyperglycemia after a pizza meal in well-controlled diabetes. Diabetes Care 16:578, 1993.

39. Fraser RJ, Horowitz M, Maddox AF et al: Hyperglycaemia slows gastric emptying rate in type 1 (insulin-dependent) diabetes mellitus. Diabetologia 33:675, 1990.

40. Schvarcz E, Palmer M, Aman J et al: Hypoglycemia increases the gastric emptying rate in healthy subjects. Diabetes Care 18:674, 1995.

40a.Liljberg H, Bjorck ME: Delayed gastric emptying rate as a potential mechanism for lowered glycemia after eating sourdough bread: Studies in humans and rats using test products with added organic acids or an organic salt. Am J Clin Nutr 64:886, 1996.

41. Jenkins DJA, Wolever TMS, Buckley G et al: Low glycemic index starchy foods in the diabetic diet. Am J Clin Nutr 48:248, 1998.

42. Venhaus A, Chanteleau E: Self-selected unrefined and refined carbohydrate diets do not affect metabolic control in pump-treated diabetic patients. Diabetologia 31:153, 1998.

43. Hughes TA, Atchison J, Hazewlrig JB et al: Glycemic responses in insulin-dependent diabetic patients: Effect of food composition. Am, J Clin Nutr 49:658, 1989.

44. Report of a Joint Food and Agriculture Organisation (FAO)/World Health Organization (WHO) Expert Consultation: Carbohydrates in Human Nutrition. FAO and WHO, Rome, 1998.

45. Behall KM, Howe JC: Effect of long-term amylose vs amylopectin starch on metabolic variables in human subjects. Am J Clin Nutr 61:334, 1995.

46. Jarvi A, Karlstrom B, Granfeldt Y et al: The influence of food structure on postprandial metabolism in patients with NIDDM. Am J Clin Nutr 61:837, 1995.

47. Calle-Pascual AL, Gomez V, Leon E et al: Foods with a low glycemic index do not improve glycemic control of both type 1 and type 2 diabetic patients after one month of therapy. Diabetic Metab 14:629, 1988.

48. Fontvieille AM, Acosta M, Rizkalla SW et al: A moderate switch from high to low glycaemic index foods for 3 weeks improves the metabolic control of type 1 (IDDM) diabetic subjects. Diab Nutr Metab 1:139, 1988.

49. Collier GR, Giudici S, Kalmusky J et al: Low glycaemic index starchy foods improve glucose control and lower serum cholesterol in diabetic children. Diab Nutr Metab 1:11, 1988.

50. Gilbertson H, Brand-Miller J, Thorburn A et al: The effect of flexible low glycemic index dietary advice versus measured carbohydrate exchange diets on glycemic control in children with type 1 diabetes. Diabetes Care 24:1137, 2001.

51. Wolever TMS, Jenkins DJA, Vuksan V et al: Beneficial effect of low glycemic index diet in type 2 diabetes. Diabetic Medicine 9:451, 1992.

52. Brand JC, Colagiuri S, Crossman S et al: Low glycemic index foods improve long term glycemic control in NIDDM. Diabetes Care 14:95, 1991.

53. Jarvi A, Karlstrom B, Granfeldt Y et al: Improved glycemic control and lipid profile and normalized fibrinolytic activity on a low glycemic index diet in type 2 diabetic patients. Diabetes Care 22:10, 1999.

54. Raben A, Tagliabue A, Christensen NJ et al: Resistant starch: The effect on postprandial glycemia, hormonal response, and satiety. Am J Clin Nutr 60:544, 1994.

55. Kaufman FR, Halvorson M, Kaufman ND: A randomized blinded trial of uncooked cornstarch to diminish nocturnal hypoglycemia at diabetes camp. Diabetes Res Clin Pract 30:205, 1995.

56. Vaaler S, Hanssen KF, Aagenaes O: Effect of different kinds of fiber on postprandial blood glucose in insulin-dependent diabetics. Acta Med Scand 15:972, 1980.

57. Riccardi G, Rivellese A, Pacioni D et al: Separate influence of dietary carbohydrate and fibre on the metabolic control in diabetes. Diabetologia 26:116, 1984.

58. Giacco R, Parillo M, Rivellese A et al: Long-term dietary treatment with increased amounts of fiber-rich low-glycemic index natural foods improves blood glucose control and reduces the number of hypoglycemic events in type 1 diabetic patients. Diabetes Care 23:1461, 2000.

59. Lafrance L, Rabasa-Lhoret R, Poisson D et al: The effects of different glycemic index foods and dietary fibre intake on glycaemic control in type 1 diabetic patients on intensive insulin therapy. Diabetic Med 15:972, 1998.

60. Chandalia M, Garg A, Luthohann D et al: Beneficial effects of a high dietary fiber intake in patients with type 2 diabetes. N Eng J Med 342:1392, 2000.

61. Expert Panel on Detection, Evaluation, and Treatment of High Blood Cholesterol in Adults: Executive summary of the Third Report of the National Cholesterol Education Program (NCEP) Expert Panel on Detection, Evaluation, and Treatment of High Blood Cholesterol in Adults (Adult Treatment Panel III). JAMA 285:2486, 2001.

62. Bantle JP, Laine DC, Castle GW et al: Postprandial glucose and insulin responses to meals containing different carbohydrates in normal and diabetic subjects. N Eng J Med 309:7, 1983.

63. Nuttall FQ, Gannon MC: Sucrose and disease. Diabetes Care 4:305, 1981.

64. Abraira C, Derler J: Large variations of sucrose in constant carbohydrate diets in type II diabetes. Am J Med 84:193, 1988.

65. Bantle JP, Swanson JE, Thomas W et al: Metabolic effects of dietary sucrose in type II diabetic subjects. Diabetes Care 16:1301, 1993.

66. Bantle JP, Raatz SK, Thomas W et al: Effects of dietary fructose on plasma lipids in healthy subjects. Am J Clin Nutr 72:1128, 2000.

67. Akgun S, Ertel NH: A comparison of carbohydrate metabolism after sucrose, sorbitol, and fructose meals in normal and diabetic subjects. Diabetes Care 3:582, 1980.

68. Payne ML, Craig WJ, Williams AC: Sorbitol is a possible risk factor for diarrhea in young children. J Am Diet Assoc 97:532, 1997.

69. Cryer PE, Fisher JN, Shamoon H: Hypoglycemia (technical review). Diabetes Care 17:734, 1995.

70. Slama G, Traynard PY, Desplanque N et al: The search for the optimized treatment of hypoglycemia: Carbohydrates in tablets, solution, or gel in the correction of insulin reactions. Arch Intern Med 150:589, 1990.

71. Brodows RG, Williams C, Amatruda JM: Treatment of insulin reactions in diabetics. JAMA 252:3378, 1984.

72. Gillespie S, Kulkarni K, Daly A: Using carbohydrate counting in diabetes clinical practice. J Am Diet Assoc 98:897-899, 1998.

73. Strachan MWJ, Frier BM: Optimal time of administration of insulin lispro. Diabetes Care 21:26, 1998.

74. Beebe CA, Van Cauter E, Shapiro T et al: Effect of temporal distribution of nutrients on diurnal patterns of glucose and insulin secretion in NIDDM. Diabetes Care 13:748, 1990.

75. Tuomilehto J, Lindstrom J, Eriksson J et al for the Finnish Diabetes Prevention Study Group: Prevention of type 2 diabetes mellitus by changes in lifestyle among subjects with impaired glucose tolerance. N Engl J Med 344:1343, 2001.

76. Mayer-Davis EJ, D'Agostino R, Karter AJ et al: Intensity and amount of physical activity in relation to insulin sensitivity: The insulin resistance Atherosclerosis Study. JAMA 279:669, 1998.

77. Goodyear LJ, Hirshman MF, Horton E: The glucose transport system in skeletal muscle effects of exercise and insulin. Med Sport Sci 37:201, 1992.

78. Hu F, Stampfer M, Solomon C et al: Physical activity and risk for cardiovascular events in diabetic women. Ann Intern Med 134:96, 2001.

79. Peters AL, Davidson MB: Protein and fat effects on glucose responses and insulin requirements in subjects with insulin-dependent diabetes. Am J Clin Nutr 58:555, 1993.

80. Nordt TK, Besenthal I, Eggstein M et al: Influence of breakfasts with different nutrient contents on glucose, C peptide, insulin, glucagon, triglycerides, and GIP in non-insulin-dependent diabetics. Am J Clin Nutr 53:155, 1991.

81. Beebe CA, Hess A: Glycemic effect of protein added to an evening snack in type 1 diabetes. (In press.).

82. Gray RO, Butler PC, Beers TR et al: Comparison of the ability of bread versus bread plus meat to treat and prevent subsequent hypoglycemia in patients with insulin-dependent diabetes. J Clin Endocrinol Metab 81:1508, 1996.

83. Nuttall F, Gannon MC: Plasma glucose and insulin response to macronutrients in nondiabetic and NIDDM subjects. Diabetes Care 145:824, 1991.

84. Gannon MC, Nuttall FQ, Neil BJ et al: The insulin and glucose responses to meals of glucose plus various proteins in type 2 diabetic subjects. Metabolism 37:1081, 1988.

85. Toeller M, Buyken A, Heitkamp G et al and the EURODIAB IDDM Complications Study: Protein intake and urinary albumin excretion rates in the EURODIAB IDDM Complications study. Diabetologia 40:1219, 1997.

86. Pedrini MT, Levey AS, Lau J et al: The effect of dietary protein restriction on the progression of diabetic and nondiabetic renal diseases: a meta analysis. Ann Intern Med 124:627, 1996.

87. American Diabetes Association Position Statement: Management of dyslipidemia in adults with diabetes. Diabetes Care 24:S58, 2001.

88. Storm H, Thomsen C, Pedersen E et al: Comparison of a carbohydrate-rich diet and diets rich in stearic or palmitic acid in NIDDM patients. Diabetes Care 20:1807, 1997.

89. Ascherio A, Katan MB, Zock PL et al: Trans fatty acids and coronary heart disease. N Engl J Med 340:1994, 1999.

90. Abbott WGH, Boyce VL, Grundy SM et al: Effects of replacing saturated fat with complex carbohydrate in diets of subjects with NIDDM. Diabetes Care 12:102, 1989.

91. Garg A, Bantle JP, Henry RR et al: Effects of varying carbohydrate content of diet in patients with non-insulin-dependent diabetes. JAMA 271:1421, 1994.

92. Sarkkinen E, Schwab U, Niskanen L et al: The effects of monounsaturated-fat enriched diet and polyunsaturated-fat diet enriched diet on lipid and glucose metabolism in subjects with impaired glucose tolerance. Eur J Clin Nutr 50:592, 1996.

93. Montori VM, Farmer A, Wollan PC et al: Fish oil supplementation in type 2 diabetes: A quantitative systematic review. Diabetes Care 223:1407, 2000.

94. Philipson BE, Rothrock DW, Conner WE et al: Reduction of plasma lipids, lipoproteins, and apoproteins by dietary fish oils in patients with hypertriglyceridemia. N Engl J Med 312:1210, 1985.

95. Leaf A, Weber PC: Cardiovascular effects of n-3 fatty acids. N Engl J Med 318:549, 1988.

96. Mensink RP, Katan MB: Effect of monounsaturated fatty acids vs. complex carbohydrates on high-density lipoproteins in healthy men and women. Lancet 1:122, 1987.

97. Garg A: High-monounsaturated fat diets for patients with diabetes mellitus: A meta-analysis. Am J Clin Nutr 67:577S, 1998.

98. Mattson FH, Grundy SM: Comparison of effects of dietary saturated, monounsaturated and polyunsaturated fatty acids on plasma lipids and lipoproteins in man. J Lipid Res 26:194, 1985.

99. Mensink RP, Katan MB: Effect of dietary fatty acids on serum lipids and lipoproteins—A meta analysis of 27 trials. Arterioscler Thromb 12:911, 1992.

100. Campbell LV, Marmot PE, Dyer JA et al: The high-monounsaturated fat diet as a practical alternative for NIDDM. Diabetes Care 17:177, 1994.

101. Rodriguez LM, Castellanos VH: Use of low-fat foods by people with diabetes decreases fat, saturated fat, and cholesterol intakes. J Am Diet Assoc 100:531, 2000.

102. Warshaw H, Franz M, Powers MA et al: Fat replacers: Their use in foods and role in diabetes medical nutrition therapy (technical review). Diabetes Care 19:1294, 1996.

103. Schneider SH, Ruderman NB: Exercise and NIDDM (technical review). Diabetes Care 13:785, 1990.

104. Kiens B, Lithell H: Lipoprotein metabolism influenced by training induced changes in

human skeletal muscle. J Clin Invest 83:558, 1989.

105. Ajani UA, Gaziano M, Lotufo PA et al: Alcohol consumption and risk of coronary heart disease by diabetes status. Circulation 102:500, 2000.

106. Wei M, Gibbon LW, Mitchell TL et al: Alcohol intake and incidence of type 2 diabetes in men. Diabetes Care 23:18, 2000.

CHAPTER 4

ORAL ANTIDIABETIC AGENTS

In recent years, the number of oral agents available with which to treat diabetes has expanded considerably. In addition to monotherapy, combination therapy has become an accepted approach for treating diabetes. Because many of these drugs function at different sites (targeting not only pancreatic production of insulin, but also muscle sensitivity and hepatic glucose regulation), combining agents produces a greater effect than any one drug in isolation. This chapter is divided into three parts. The first section describes a general approach for using oral agents in patients with type 2 diabetes. The second section deals with each class of available oral agents, and discusses in detail their background, mechanisms of action and pharmacology, appropriate usage, dosage, side effects, and contraindications. These agents are classified overall as insulin secretagogues and noninsulin secretagogues. The third section deals with combination therapy and provides strategies for managing specific patients with multiple oral medications. Case examples are included.

OVERALL STRATEGY

Previously it was fairly easy to provide an algorithm for the treatment of diabetes. A patient with new-onset diabetes who was either asymptomatic or mildly symptomatic was started on diet and exercise. Those with moderate to severe symptoms were started on a sulfonylurea agent or insulin to quickly control their hyperglycemia. Patients generally progressed from diet alone to a sulfonylurea agent to insulin. There were multiple drawbacks to this approach. The first, and most overriding problem, was that it generally did not work. The average hemoglobin A_{1c} (A1C) level in the United States in the early 1990s was 9.5%,[1] well above the goal of an A1C level of less than 7%. Second, with the exception of weight loss and exercise, this approach only treated the problem of insulin deficiency. This misses treatment of insulin resistance, which is an important component of the hyperglycemia found in many patients with type 2 diabetes.

In recent years the addition of metformin (a biguanide) and the thiazolidinediones (TZDs; troglitazone, rosiglitazone, and pioglitazone) to the arsenal of drugs available for the treatment of type 2 diabetes has allowed us to pharmacologically reduce insulin resistance and lower hepatic glucose problem.[2] Short acting insulin secretagogues (repaglinide and nateglinide), α-glucosidase inhibitors (acarbose and miglitol) and insulin analogs (Lispro,

71

aspart, glargine) have all helped further enhance our ability to treat type 2 diabetes (Tables 4-1 and 4-2 list all available oral agents with a summary of their actions). The key in using these agents is to try to individualize therapy based on a patient's needs and metabolic responses. For some individuals it is easier to comply with lifestyle recommendations when they take metformin, a TZD, or a short-acting insulin secretagogue compared with taking a sulfonylurea agent that might produce late-afternoon hyperglycemia. Others may not be able to afford the more expensive newer agents, or may prefer taking pills only once per day, so a different regimen is preferable to these individuals.

Separate from patient preferences, it is helpful if patients are divided into a more insulin-resistant group and a more insulin-deficient group. The former are started on metformin or a TZD, the latter are started on an insulin secretagogue. As a rule of thumb, patients with more insulin resistance tend to have central obesity, a strong family history of diabetes, the diabetic dyslipidemia (high triglyceride levels and low high-density lipoprotein [HDL] cholesterol levels) and/or hypertension. Patients who are more insulin-deficient are often leaner and more symptomatic. Obviously, there are individuals who do not fit these profiles, but it can be helpful to try and clinically assess the patient's diabetic metabolic profile.

Figure 4-1 provides a general schema for treating patients with new-onset type 2 diabetes. It is important to keep in mind that what medication patients are taking at one point in time is not necessarily what they will be taking later. Monotherapy loses its effectiveness in the treatment of type 2 diabetes in many patients, and it is better to add a second or even third oral agent quickly, before the patient's A1C level rises much above 8%.[3] Furthermore, although insulin is dreaded by many patients, adding insulin to the diabetes regimen should occur as soon as it is indicated and with reinforcement of

the benefits of good glycemic control for the patient.

Even as therapies change in their effectiveness, patients may also change in their need for treatment. Some older patients may present with new-onset type 2 diabetes, only to evolve into latent autoimmune diabetes of the adult (see Chapter 1) and insulin dependence. Younger individuals, particularly of Latino or African-American heritage, may present in diabetic ketoacidosis (DKA); however, once it is resolved, it may be possible to treat them for their type 2 diabetes with oral agents. Therefore it is important to react to a patient's status at the time, adding oral agents or insulin based on the clinical situation and the response to prior therapy, with a goal of keeping the patient's A1C level at or below target for most of the duration of their lifetime.

INSULIN SECRETAGOGUES

THE SULFONYLUREA AGENTS

Background

During World War II, French scientists studying the antibiotic potential of modified sulfonamides noted that the patients used in their experiments were unexpectedly dying, especially those who were malnourished. Further investigation revealed that hypoglycemia was the cause of death. The first sulfonylurea agent, carbutamide, was introduced into clinical practice for the treatment of diabetes mellitus in 1955 in Germany. Tolbutamide (Orinase) was introduced in the United States the following year, and chlorpropamide (Diabinese) became available a year later. In the 1960s, two more sulfonylurea agents, acetohexamide (Dymelor) and tolazamide (Tolinase), were introduced into clinical practice in the United States. These four agents are known as are known as *first-generation agents*. The sulfonylurea component of these compounds, which is responsible for their hypoglycemic effects, gives each

TABLE 4-1 TYPES OF DRUGS

Parameter	SUs	Non-SU Secreatagogues	Biguanides	α-Glucosidase Inhibitors	Thiazolidinediones
Primary Mechanism of Action*	Increased pancreatic insulin secretion	Increased pancreatic insulin secretion	Decreased hepatic glucose production	Decreased gut carbohydrate absorption	Increased peripheral glucose disposal
AIC Lowering in Monotherapy Trials	0.9%–2.5%	0.6%–1.9%	0.8%–3.0%	0.4%–1.3%	1.1%–2.6%
Advantages	Well established Decreases microvascular risk Daily dosing available Rapid onset	Targets postprandial glycemia Possibly less hypoglycemia and weight gain than with SUs	Well-established Weight loss (or no change) No hypoglycemia Decreases microvascular risk Decreases macrovascular risk (UKPDS) Nonglycemic benefits (decreased lipid levels, increased fibrinolysis) Daily dosing available	Targets postprandial glycemia No hypoglycemia Nonsystemic	No hypoglycemia Nonglycemic benefits (improved lipid levels [pioglitazone > rosiglitazone], increased fibrinolysis, improved endothelial function, slight lowering of blood pressure) Possible β-cell preservation Daily dosing
Disadvantages	Hypoglycemia Weight gain	More complex (three times daily) dosing schedule Hypoglycemia Weight gain No long-term data	Adverse gastrointestinal effects Many contraindications Lactic acidosis (rare)	More complex (three times daily) dosing schedule Adverse gastrointestinal side effects	Liver function test monitoring Wait gain Edema Slow onset of action

SU, sulfonylurea; UKPDS, United Kingdom Prospective Diabetes Study.

*AIC lowering greatest in drug-naïve patients. Greatest lowering often seen with highest initial AIC levels. Data provided as adjusted means the difference in AIC compared to placebo.

From Inzucchi SE: Oral antihyperglycemia therapy for type 2 diabetes. JAMA 287:360, 2002.

TABLE 4-2   SELECTED CHARACTERISTICS OF ORAL ANTIDIABETES MEDICATIONS

Generic Name	Trade Name (Manufacturer)	Tablet Size	Usual Daily Dose (mg)	Maximal Dose (mg)	Major Contraindications
Glyburide	Micronase (Pharmacia & Upjohn) Diabeta (Aventis) Glynase (micronized) (Pharmacia & Upjohn)	1.25, 2.5, 5 1.25, 2.5, 5 1.5, 3, 6	2.5–10 (single or divided) 1.5–6 (single or divided)	20 12	Severe allergy to sulfa drugs
Glipizide	Glucotrol (Pfizer) Glucotrol XL (long acting) (Pfizer)	5, 10 2.5, 5, 10	5–20 (single or divided) 5–10 (single)	40 20	Severe allergy to sulfa drugs
Glimepiride	Amaryl (Aventis)	1, 2, 4	2–4 (single)	8	Severe allergy to sulfa drugs
Repaglinide	Prandin (NovoNordisk)	0.5, 1, 2	1–2 mg three times a day before meals	16 mg per day	
Nateglinide	Starlix (Novartis)	60, 120	120 mg three times a day before meals	360 mg per day	
Metformin	Glucophage (Bristol Myers Squibb) Glucophage XR (long-acting) (Bristol Myers Squibb)	500, 850, 1000 500	1000–2000 given two to three times per day with food or once a day (if Glucophage XR)	2500 (although maximal clinical benefit seen at 2000 mg per day)	Do not use in presence of renal insufficiency, CHF, hypoxia, hepatic dysfunction
Acarbose	Precose (Bayer)	25, 50, 100	50–100 mg three times a day (with the first bite of food)	Patient ≤60 kg maximal dose is 50 mg three times a day Patient >60 kg maximal dose is 100 mg three times a day	Do not use if creatinine level >2 or patient has bowel condition (e.g., ulceration, obstruction)
Miglitol	Glyset (Pharmacia & Upjohn)	25, 50, 100	50 mg three times a day	100 mg three times a day	Do not use if creatinine level >2 or patient has bowel condition (e.g.,

Pioglitazone	Actos (*Lilly/Takeda*)	15, 30, 45	30 mg once daily	45 mg once daily	ulceration, obstruction) ALT ≥2, 5 times the upper limit of normal, NYHA class III, IV CHF
Rosiglitazone	Avandia (*GlaxoSmithKline*)	2, 4, 8	4 mg daily	4 mg twice a day	ALT ≥ 2, 5 times the upper limit of normal, NYHA class III, IV CHF
Metformin + glyburide*	Glucovance (*Bristol Myers Squibb*)	1.25/250 (glyburide/ metformin), 2.5/500, 5/500	5/500 twice a day	20 mg glyburide/ 2000 mg metformin	Contraindications for metformin and glyburide

ALT, alanine transferase; CHF, congestive heart failure; NYHA, New York Heart Association

*Additional fixed combinations increasingly available; check manufacturers' web sites for new combinations.

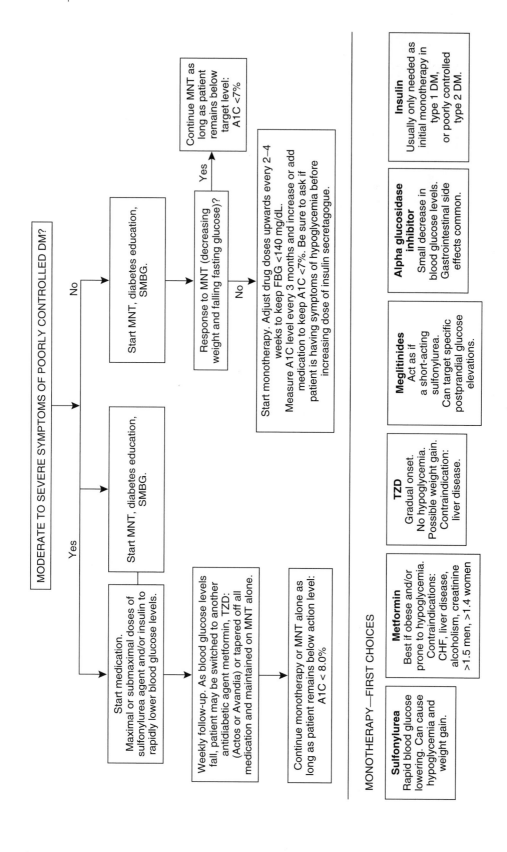

MODERATE TO SEVERE SYMPTOMS OF POORLY CONTROLLED DM?

Yes

Start medication.
Maximal or submaximal doses of sulfonylurea agent and/or insulin to rapidly lower blood glucose levels.

Weekly follow-up. As blood glucose levels fall, patient may be switched to another antidiabetic agent metformin, TZD: (Actos or Avandia) or tapered off all medication and maintained on MNT alone.

Continue monotherapy or MNT alone as long as patient remains below action level: A1C < 8.0%

Start MNT, diabetes education, SMBG.

No

Start MNT, diabetes education, SMBG.

Response to MNT (decreasing weight and falling fasting glucose)?

Yes — Continue MNT as long as patient remains below target level: A1C <7%

No

Start monotherapy. Adjust drug doses upwards every 2–4 weeks to keep FBG <140 mg/dL. Measure A1C level every 3 months and increase or add medication to keep A1C <7%. Be sure to ask if patient is having symptoms of hypoglycemia before increasing dose of insulin secretagogue.

MONOTHERAPY—FIRST CHOICES

Sulfonylurea
Rapid blood glucose lowering. Can cause hypoglycemia and weight gain.

Metformin
Best if obese and/or prone to hypoglycemia. Contraindications: CHF, liver disease, alcoholism, creatinine >1.5 men, >1.4 women

TZD
Gradual onset. No hypoglycemia. Possible weight gain. Contraindication: liver disease.

Meglitinides
Act as if a short-acting sulfonylurea. Can target specific postprandial glucose elevations.

Alpha glucosidase inhibitor
Small decrease in blood glucose levels. Gastrointestinal side effects common.

Insulin
Usually only needed as initial monotherapy in type 1 DM, or poorly controlled type 2 DM.

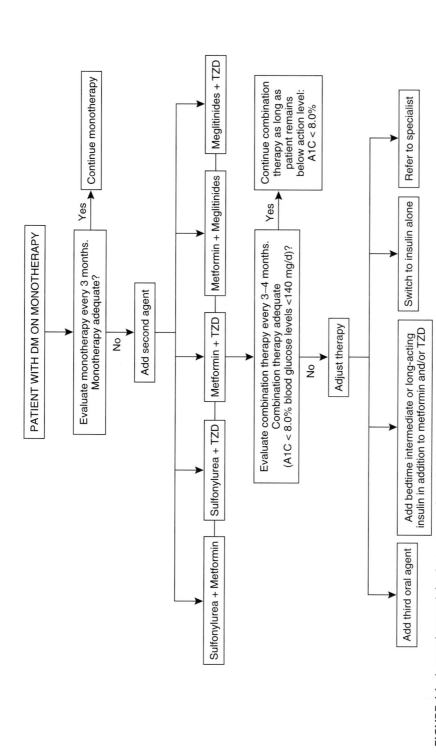

FIGURE 4-1. A general approach for the treatment of type 2 diabetes.

CHF, congestive heart failure; DM, diabetes mellitus; FBG, fasting blood glucose; A1C, hemoglobin A_{1c}; MNT, medical nutrition therapy; SMBG, self-monitoring of blood glucose; TZD, thiazolidinedione.

compound unique pharmacokinetic properties. In 1984 two sulfonylurea compounds that had been used in Europe for many years were introduced into the United States. These second-generation agents are glyburide (Micronase, DiaBeta, Glynase) and glipizide (Glucotrol, Glucotrol XL) (Figure 4-2). In 1996 another sulfonylurea agent, glimepiride (Amaryl), was approved by the Food and Drug Administration (FDA) for use in this country.

Mechanism of Action and Pharmacology

Sulfonylureas require a functioning pancreas to be effective. An increase in insulin levels in both peripheral and portal veins occurs after the *acute* administration of these compounds. These data strongly suggest that the hypoglycemic effect of the sulfonylurea agents is due to stimulation of insulin secretion. However, the situation after long-term administration of sulfonylurea agents is more complex. Glucose concentrations are lower, and insulin levels are either unchanged,[4-6] or, more likely, increased.[6] A number of studies have demonstrated that sulfonylurea agents sensitize the pancreatic β-cells to glucose and other secretagogues.[7,8]

The β-cell response, however, depends on the prevailing glucose levels, and thus interpretation of the insulin response is complicated. If the glucose concentrations are artificially raised before treatment, insulin secretion in patients on therapy is markedly enhanced compared with their initial responses.[9] Therefore the unchanged insulin levels[4-6] occurring in the presence of lowered glucose concentrations are consistent with a stimulation of insulin secretion by sulfonylurea agents.

The mechanism by which sulfonylurea agents enhance the β-cell response has been delineated in recent years.[7,8] Insulin secretion follows depolarization of the β-cell membrane, which leads to opening of voltage-dependent calcium channels and an influx of calcium ions. The increase in intracellular calcium triggers the release of insulin by a mechanism that is not clearly understood. Glucose-stimulated insulin secretion occurs after the entry and subsequent metabolism of glucose by the β-cells. This leads to increased adenosine triphosphate (ATP) synthesis, which in turn blocks an ATP-sensitive potassium channel (Figure 4-3). The closure of these ATP-sensitive potassium channels depolarizes the β-cell membrane, and the pathways of insulin

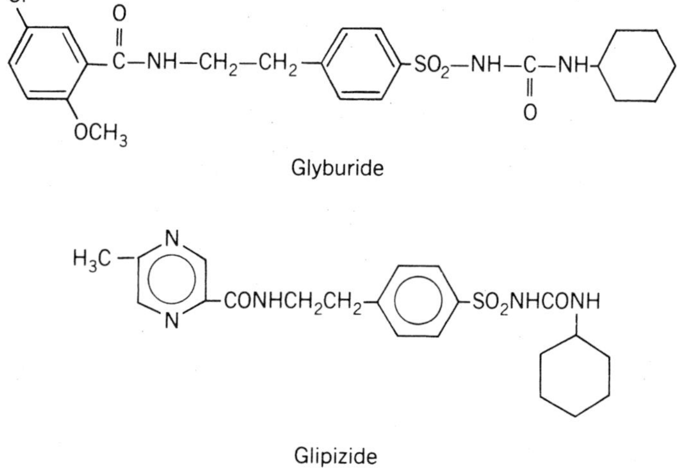

FIGURE 4-2. Chemical structure of the two second-generation sulfonylurea agents available for use in the United States.

Glyburide

Glipizide

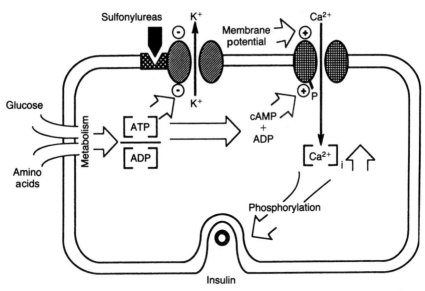

FIGURE 4-3. Proposed mechanism by which sulfonylurea agents stimulate insulin secretion. ATP, adenosine triphosphate; ADP, adenosine diphosphate; cAMP, cyclic adenosine monophosphate; P, phosphate; K^+, potassium ion; Ca^{2+}, calcium ion. *(From Gerich JE: Oral hypoglycemic agents. N Engl J Med 321:1231, 1989.)*

secretion are stimulated as just described. Sulfonylurea agents bind to a receptor that is either closely linked to or possibly part of this ATP-sensitive potassium channel and in this manner enhance both glucose-induced insulin secretion and the insulin response to nonglucose stimuli. Although non–β-cell effects have been proposed[7,8] for these agents, their role in lowering glucose levels is clinically small.

Sulfonylurea agents are rapidly absorbed from the gastrointestinal (GI) tract. The time course of their absorption does not vary with age,[10] but may be reduced by hyperglycemia in both normal[11] and diabetic[12] subjects, possibly secondary to decreased gastric motility. Appreciable concentrations in plasma can be measured by 1 hour after ingestion. The compounds are transported in the blood bound to serum proteins, mostly albumin. Plasma levels of drug vary widely for reasons that are not entirely clear. In the case of tolbutamide, rates of disappearance vary over a 10-fold range among individuals. This variation is due to genetic differences in the

enzyme of the rate-limiting degradative step.[13] Thus, although generalizations are made about the pharmacology of these drugs, the data cited may not strictly apply to individual patients.

Glyburide is metabolized in the liver. Two of its degradative products have been shown to have considerable hypoglycemic activity.[14] The metabolites are excreted roughly equally by the kidneys, appearing in the urine, and by the biliary tract, appearing in the feces. The serum half-life is approximately 10 hours, and the drug has a duration of action up to 24 hours. It is given once or twice a day, depending on the dose. A micronized formulation of glyburide, Glynase, is absorbed more completely than the nonmicronized forms DiaBeta or Micronase. This increased bioavailability simply means that lower doses are used. Otherwise, there is no difference between the micronized and nonmicronized preparations of glyburide.

Glipizide is almost completely inactivated in the liver, and the degradative products are excreted in the urine. The serum half-life of the parent compound is approximately 3 to 4 hours. Its therapeutic effect has been reported to range between 10 and 24 hours. Glucotrol is given once or twice a day, depending on the dose. A long-acting form of glipizide (Glucotrol XL) is available. Once-a-day dosing is appropriate for this formulation.

Glimepiride is metabolized in the liver to products that have no more than one-third of the biologic activity of the parent compound. Like the metabolites of glyburide, they are excreted about equally by the liver and kidneys.

Side Effects and Contraindications (Table 4-3)

Sulfonylurea agents have been taken by millions of people with diabetes over many years and are well tolerated by most patients. The prevalence of side effects is less than 5%; use of the drugs must be discontinued in only 1% to 2% of patients. Hypoglycemia, although considered to be an adverse effect, is actually an extension of the pharmacologic effect of the sulfonylurea agents. The

incidence of hypoglycemia varies among agents, but can occur with any of them. Glipizide gastrointestinal therapeutic system and glimepiride have less hypoglycemia associated with use than glyburide.

The most common side effects of the sulfonylurea agents are GI and cutaneous. The GI effects are dose-related and may disappear when the dose is reduced. These reactions often abate within several weeks even if the dose is not reduced. The GI symptoms include anorexia, heartburn, nausea with occasional vomiting, feelings of abdominal fullness, and flatulence. The common adverse cutaneous effects are morbilliform, maculopapular, or urticarial rashes, which are often characterized by erythema and pruritus. Some cross-reactivity may occur among the sulfonylurea agents. Disulfiram-like reactions have been reported to occur with chlorpropamide therapy. Disulfiram (Antabuse) is a drug used in the treatment of alcoholism. The first degradative product of ethanol is acetaldehyde, which is further metabolized to acetyl coenzyme A. Disulfiram inhibits the enzyme for the latter reaction, which causes an accumulation of acetaldehyde that can be associated with feelings of warmth, flushing,

TABLE 4-3	SIDE EFFECTS OF AND CONTRAINDICATIONS TO SULFONYLUREA AGENTS	
More Common	**Rare**
Gastrointestinal	*Skin Lesions*
Anorexia	Photosensitivity
Heartburn	Lichenoid eruptions
Nausea with occasional vomiting	Erythema multiforme
Abdominal distention	Exfoliative dermatitis
Flatulence	
Rash	*Hematologic Disorders*
Morbiliform	Leukopenia
Maculopapular	Agranulocytosis
Urticarial	Aplastic anemia
	Hemolytic anemia
Other (Chlorpropamide Only)	*Hepatic Disorders*
Alcohol flushing syndrome	Intrahepatic cholestasis (chlorpropamide usually, but others also)
Hyponatremia (syndrome of inappropriate antidiuretic hormone secretion)	Hepatitis (glyburide)

headache, nausea, vomiting, sweating, and thirst. More severe reactions occur occasionally, including respiratory difficulty, chest pain, hypotension, orthostatic syncope, confusion, and vertigo. Reactions can last from 30 minutes to several hours. Chlorpropamide also inhibits this enzyme, but much less completely. The prevalence of these reactions is unclear; various reports have cited prevalences from less than 1% to 33% among patients taking chlorpropamide.

The other side effects of the sulfonylurea agents are uncommon (<1%) or rare (isolated case reports). Other skin reactions include photosensitivity, lichenoid eruptions, erythema multiforme, and exfoliative dermatitis. Adverse hematologic effects include leukopenia, agranulocytosis, thrombocytopenia, hemolytic or aplastic anemia, or pancytopenia. Intrahepatic cholestatic jaundice, most commonly with chlorpropamide therapy, has been reported; this condition is usually reversed by discontinuation of the drug. Glyburide-induced hepatitis has been reported.[15,16] Fevers, eosinophilia, nonspecific proctocolitis, hepatic porphyria, and porphyria cutanea tarda have also been reported. Chlorpropamide[17,18] and rarely tolbutamide may cause the syndrome of inappropriate antidiuretic hormone (SIADH) secretion. The drugs cause this condition not only by stimulating the release of the hormone by the hypothalamus, but also by potentiating its inhibitory effect on free water excretion by the distal renal tubule. Older adult patients are much more susceptible to this effect, especially if they are also taking a diuretic. The other sulfonylurea agents do not cause SIADH. Some of them even appear to have a mild diuretic effect, which is not of any clinical significance. It is also important to remember that, as the name implies, sulfonylureas are sulfa-containing compounds, and should be used with caution—or not at all—in patients with documented sulfa allergies.

Finally, much has been made of the link between insulin and heart disease. Sulfonylurea compounds, which promote insulin secretion, have also been included in this debate. There is some evidence that insulin vasodilates, and may be coronary protective, whereas other authors have concluded that insulin promotes coronary artery disease. The pros and cons as they relate to sulfonylurea therapy are beyond the scope of this chapter; however, the United Kingdom Prospective Diabetes Study (UKPDS) showed that insulin and sulfonylurea therapy were not associated with an increase in cardiovascular risk in the population of patients with type 2 diabetes that were studied. The improvement in glycemic control through the use of sulfonylurea drugs and exogenous insulin actually conferred a moderate benefit in terms of myocardial risk in the UKPDS 33.[19]

Drug Interactions

Other drugs can affect the hypoglycemic action of sulfonylurea agents in two general ways. First, drugs that either impair glucose tolerance or cause hypoglycemia are expected to influence the effect of sulfonylurea agents in diabetic patients. This interaction is *indirect,* because the interfering drugs act by the same mechanisms as in nondiabetic subjects. Potassium-losing diuretics, glucocorticoids, estrogen compounds, and phenytoin (Dilantin) can impair the action of sulfonylurea agents. Conversely, salicylates, propranolol, monoamine oxidase inhibitors (of the hydrazine type), disopyramide, pentamidine, quinine, and ethanol (although not a prescribed drug) might indirectly potentiate the hypoglycemic effect of sulfonylurea agents.

Second, drugs may have a *direct* effect on the action of the sulfonylurea agents—that is, an interaction occurs in which the interfering drug affects the absorption, distribution, metabolism, or excretion of the sulfonylurea agents themselves.

Sulfonamides are the most important class of drugs that potentiate the effect of sulfonylurea agents by displacing them from their albumin binding sites.[20-23] Older drugs that have also caused hypoglycemia in patients taking sulfonylurea agents, probably by the same mechanism.

Clinical Comments

Sulfonylurea agents have been used since the 1940s and are available in low-cost generic formulations. Many patients can take them once or twice a day, with a prompt glucose lowering effect. In fact, no other agent can lower glucose levels as rapidly. In one study[23] a maximal dose of a sulfonylurea agent was given to patients with new-onset, symptomatic diabetes and blood glucose levels in the 400 mg/dl range. Within 3 days patients felt better, within a week the glucose levels had fallen to the 200 mg/dl range (Figure 4-4) and by 4 months the majority of patients were well controlled on diet therapy or on submaximal sulfonylurea agent therapy. None of the other oral agents can lower blood glucose levels as rapidly. However, it is not just bringing blood glucose levels down quickly that matters, but rather keeping them controlled over time. Sulfonylurea agents often gradually cease to be effective and combination therapy is required.

Starting doses of various sulfonylurea agents are listed in Table 4-4, designed to lower the risk of initial hypoglycemia. Additionally, patients should be warned of the risk of developing hypoglycemia, for which they are at particular risk if they decrease caloric intake, delay meals, and/or increase their aerobic exercise. The symptoms should be described and treatment suggestions given (see Chapter 7). Patients should be encouraged to eat regular meals and may need a snack in the middle of the day. However, because many patients are attempting to lose weight, the calories for the snack should be shifted from either lunch or dinner, rather than added to the meal plan. Patients should be queried about symptoms of hypoglycemia at each visit and

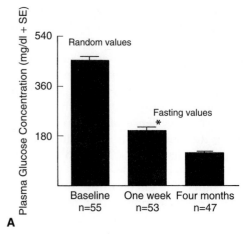

A

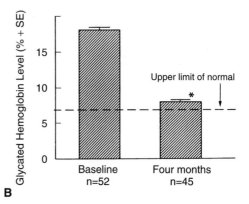

B

FIGURE 4-4. Response of markedly symptomatic patients with type 2 diabetes to maximal dose of sulfonylurea agents (or half of maximal dose in patients ≥65 years old). SE, standard error of the mean. A: Glucose concentrations. *, P <0.001 versus baseline and 4 months. B: Glycated hemoglobin levels. *, P <0.001 versus baseline.

the dose of the sulfonylurea agent decreased if these symptoms occur.

MEGLITINIDES

Background

In the early 1990s a new oral hypoglycemic agent A-4166 was shown to have stimulatory effects on insulin secretion.[24] This compound eventually became known as nateglinide (a phenylalanine derivative), with the brand name Starlix. About the same time, another compound was under

TABLE 4-4	RECOMMENDED INITIAL DOSES OF SULFONYLUREA AGENTS FOR PATIENTS WITH TYPE 2 DIABETES		
	Initial Dose (mg)		
	Asymptomatic Diet Failures[a] or Patients with Mild Symptoms with Indicated FPG		
Agent	*<180 mg/dl*	*≥180 mg/dl[b]*	*Markedly Symptomatic Patients[c]*
			—
			—
			1000 (500)
Chlorpropamide[d] (Diabinese)	100	250	750 (250)
Glyburide (DiaBeta, Micronase)	1.25	2.5	20 (7.5)
Glipizide (Glucotrol)	2.5	5.0	40 (15)
Glyburide (Glynase)	0.075	1.5	12 (6)
Glipizide (Glucotrol XL)	2.5	5.0	20 (10)
Glimepiride (Amaryl)	1.0	2.0	8 (4)

FPG, fasting plasma glucose concentration.

[a]Relatively asymptomatic patients should be treated with diet alone initially (see text for full discussion).

[b]For patients >65 years old, use dose for younger patient with FPG <180 mg/dl.

[c]Dose in parentheses indicates starting dose for patients >65 years of age. Increase quickly after 1 week if no response seen.

[d]Chlorpropamide should not be a first-line agent in patients >65 years of age.

investigation boasting similar properties and mechanisms of action with a few major differences. This compound was marketed first, as repaglinide (a benzoic acid derivative), with a trade name of Prandin. Subsequently nateglinide was released (Figure 4-5). Both of these mediations are indicated for use in the management of type 2 diabetes as monotherapy or in combination with other oral agents when diet and exercise alone are not successful.

Mechanism of Action and Pharmacology

Meglitinides are short-acting glucose lowering drugs indicated for the treatment of type 2 diabetes either alone or in combination with other agents. They require a functioning pancreas to be effective. Repaglinide and nateglinide are chemically unrelated to the oral sulfonylureas. Like sulfonylureas, both drugs work by stimulating the pancreas to release insulin by closing the ATP-dependent potassium channels in the β-cell membrane by binding at specific sites.[25] This potassium channel blockade then depolarizes the β-cell, which leads to an opening of calcium channels. The resulting influx of calcium induces insulin secretion. This action is very tissue selective and has a low affinity for heart and skeletal muscle. The insulin release is glucose dependent, unlike with sulfonylureas, and the lower the glucose level, the less insulin is released. This

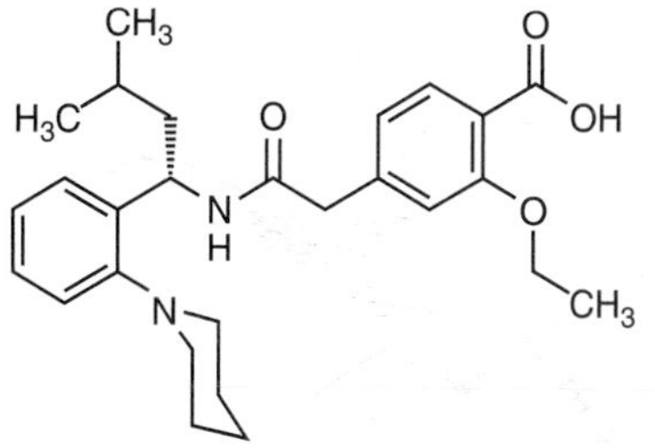

FIGURE 4-5. Structural formulae of the meglitinides.

specificity of action is particularly seen with nateglinide. Nateglinide imparts a three times more rapid and five times less persistent inhibition of β-cell potassium ATP channels than repaglinide.[26] This may result in lower meal-related glucose excursions.[27] Figure 4-6 shows the clinical effect of these agents on insulin secretion.

Repaglinide and nateglinide are rapidly and completely absorbed from the GI tract. Plasma levels peak similarly at 1 hour. Both drugs are eliminated rapidly with the half life of repaglinide being approximately 1

hour and that of nateglinide slightly longer. These drugs are metabolized by the cytochrome P-450 system to inactive metabolites. The duration of action for both of these preparations is approximately 3 to 4 hours. Nateglinide does not require dosing adjustment in patients with mild to severe renal disease, although the repaglinide dose may need to be adjusted downward if hypoglycemia occurs. In hepatic insufficiency, no change in nateglinide is needed if impairment is mild, but should be used with caution if impairment is significant. Similarly,

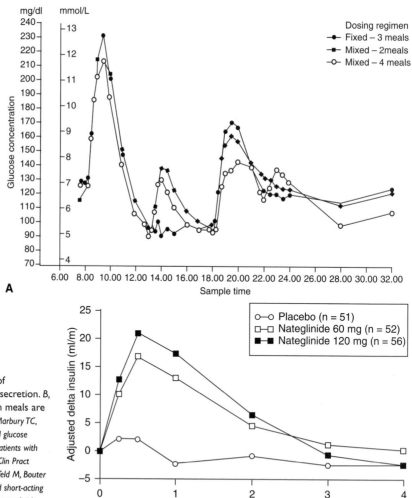

FIGURE 4-6. *A,* Effect of repaglinide *(A)* on insulin secretion. *B,* Effect of repaglinide when meals are missed. *(A, From Damsbo P, Marbury TC, Hatorp V, et al: Flexible prandial glucose regulation with repaglinide in patients with type 2 diabetes. Diabetes Res Clin Pract 45(1):31, 1999. B, From Hanefeld M, Bouter KP, Dickinson S et al: Rapid and short-acting mealtime insulin secretion with nateglinide controls both prandial and mean glycemia. Diabetes Care 23:202, 2000.)*

repaglinide should also be used with caution in patients with liver disease.

A major difference in these two medications is dosing. For patients not previously treated or whose A1C is less than 8%, the staring dose of repaglinide is 0.5 mg with each meal. If A1C levels are less than 8%, it is recommended that initial dosing begin at 2 mg with each meal. Medication is then titrated, based on glycemic response, to a total of 4 mg with each meal to a maximal dose of 16 mg per day. Patients actively involved in their own care may be taught to increase their dose of repaglinide based on the anticipated carbohydrate content of their meals. For example, if a patient usually does not eat dessert with supper, 2 mg of repaglinide may be sufficient. But if they are going to splurge and add a piece of cake and ice cream to their meal, a dose of 4 mg may be required to keep the postprandial glucose in the normal range. Dosing for nateglinide is 120 mg with each meal, with no further titration needed, aside from the liver indications noted previously. Occasionally, patients are started with 60 mg with each meal if their A1C values are close to normal.

Side Effects and Contraindications

The meglitinides listed previously are contraindicated in patients with any known hypersensitivity to their formulations, patients in current DKA (in which insulin is the only appropriate treatment), those with type 1 diabetes, and those who do not respond to sulfonylureas. In addition, the combination of sulfonylureas and meglitinides is not thought to be effective and should not be used. These medications have not been proven safe in pregnancy or breast feeding. The side effects associated with nateglinide and repaglinide therapy are essentially the same as placebo, although there is an increased incidence of hypoglycemia (a therapeutic effect rather than a side effect per se). Patients taking nateglinide were found to have a slight increase in uric acid levels, which was of no clinical consequence during the clinical trials.

Drug Interactions

Repaglinide is metabolized by the P-450 system. A decrease in its effect may be seen with drugs that induce cytochrome P-450 3A4. Nateglinide is also metabolized by the P-450 system, and includes substrate 3A4 and CYP 2C9. These following drugs may increase the metabolism of repaglinide and nateglinide: rifampin, barbiturates, and carbamazepine. Certain drugs, such as thiazides, diuretics, steroids, phenothiazines, thyroid hormones, estrogens, birth control pills, phenytoin, nicotinic acid, calcium channel blockers, and isoniazids tend to produce hyperglycemia (*indirectly,* as discussed previously for sulfonylurea agents) and may lead to loss of glycemic control. Agents that inhibit cytochrome P-450 3A4 (ketoconazole, miconazole, and erythromycin, for example) may increase repaglinide and nateglinide concentrations. Because both agents are highly protein bound, its toxic potential is increased when given with other highly protein bound drugs (such as oral anticoagulants, salicylates, nonsteroidal anti-inflammatory drugs, sulfonamides, and hydantoins), which, in theory, may increase its hypoglycemic effect. However, to date these theoretical considerations have not been clinically documented.

Clinical Comments

Short-acting insulin secretagogues are effective, but require that patients be willing to take an oral agent immediately before meals. Patients need to learn to couple taking the drug to eating their meals—if they do not eat, they should not take the drug, and they should not take the drug after the meal if they forget to take it beforehand. Although perhaps lower, the risk of hypoglycemia still exists.[28] However, the short action of these drugs allows for patients to tailor them to their meal plan with their medication (Figure 4-6, *A,* shows the results from the "Skip a Meal" Study). Patients can test their 2-hour postprandial glucose levels and determine what their postprandial glucose responses are. Some may find that very low carbohydrate meals may require a decrease in repaglinide or omission of the nateglinide dose (nateglinide is primarily used in one 120-mg dose strength). Patients taking repaglinide can increase their dose (e.g., from 2 mg to 4 mg) if they splurge and eat extra carbohydrates.

In patients taking premeal short-acting insulin secretagogues, fasting plasma glucose (FPG) levels may be higher than in patients on a longer-acting sulfonylurea agent. Therefore combination therapy with a second agent, such as metformin or a TZD, which has a synergistic mechanism of action should be considered if the FPG level increases. Although not FDA approved, some patients on bedtime NPH (neutral protein hagedorn) or glargine insulin may derive benefit from the use of premeal short-acting insulin secretagogues.

FIGURE 4-7. Structural formulae of the biguanide drugs. *(From Damsbro P, Marbury TC, Hatorp V, et al: Flexible prandial glucose regulation with repaglinide in patients with type 2 diabetes. Diabetes Clin Pract 45(1): 31–39, 1999.)*

NONSECRETAGOGUES

THE BIGUANIDES

Background

The history of biguanides can be traced back to medieval times, when, in Europe, the use of French lilac *(Galega officinalis)* in the treatment of diabetes was documented.[29] The active component of this plant is guanidine, and in the 1920s, this compound was isolated and used to synthesize several antidiabetic compounds; however, their clinical potential was not pursued. Chlorguanide hydrochloride, introduced as an antimalarial agent in the 1940s, was known to have a weak hypoglycemic effect. Phenformin and metformin (Figure 4-7) were introduced in the late 1950s as a response to the introduction of sulfonylureas.[30] In the 1970s phenformin was taken off the market in a number of countries because of its association with lac-

tic acidosis in individuals without risk factors for acidosis (see the following text)[31] Metformin is still widely available and has become a popular drug for the treatment of type 2 diabetes, both as a single agent and in combination therapy.

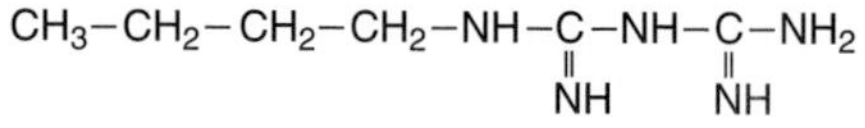

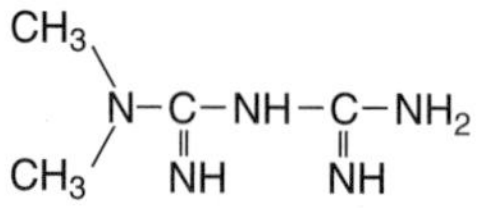

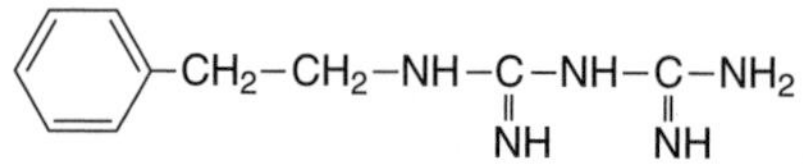

Mechanism of Action and Pharmacology

Biguanides are more accurately described as antihyperglycemics rather than hypoglycemic agents. Unlike sulfonylureas, they do not cause hypoglycemia in most cases, when used as a single agent.[32,33] Metformin does not increase insulin levels but rather improves insulin sensitivity as shown by a reduction in FPG and insulin levels[34] (Table 4-5). It is not effective in the absence of insulin.[35] In patients with type 2 diabetes, the glucose lowering effect is mainly attributed to a decrease in hepatic glucose output and a more minor effect on enhancing insulin-stimulated peripheral glucose uptake.[34] Other actions such as decreased intestinal absorption of glucose and decreased fatty acid oxidation may also contribute to its antihyperglycemic effect. Metformin decreases basal hepatic glucose output in type 2 diabetes, which is why therapy results in a lower FPG level.[36] The

TABLE 4-5	POSSIBLE SITES AND MECHANISMS OF ACTION OF METFORMIN

Gastrointestinal
Decreased or delayed absorption of glucose
Increased conversion of glucose to lactate by intestinal cells
Inducing anorexia

Hepatic (Decreased Glucose Output Secondary to Inhibition of Gluconeogenesis)
Direct effect
Potentiating insulin effect

Peripheral Tissues (Muscle and Fat)
Direct effect[a]
Potentiating insulin effect
   Increased insulin receptor binding
   Postbinding mechanism(s)[*]

[*]One of the mechanisms may be increased translocation of glucose transporters to the plasma membrane.

mechanism of this action is an enhanced suppression of gluconeogenesis by insulin and a reduction in glucagon-stimulated gluconeogenesis. Metformin also results in increased glucose disposal of muscle by enhancing insulin-stimulated uptake of glucose, resulting in increased glycogen formation and glucose oxidation.[34] There is an increase in uptake and oxidation of glucose by fat cells associated with metformin use.[37]

The pharmacokinetics of metformin reveal a bioavailability of 50% to 60% with an estimated plasma half life of 1.5 to 4.9 hours. The maximal plasma concentration is achieved 1 to 2 hours after dosing. Approximately 90% of the drug is eliminated in the urine by 12 hours, and the drug is not measurably metabolized.

Metformin offers the same metabolic control as sulfonylureas (Figures 4-8 and 4-9), without an associated weight gain.[38] Metformin actually has an anorexic effect in some patients which may be beneficial in weight loss. Metformin has modest insulin sensitizing actions, and as a result, has been used in conditions where insulin resistance is a significant pathologic condition. The classic condition is polycystic ovarian syndrome (PCOS). With the addition of metformin, patients noted more frequent and

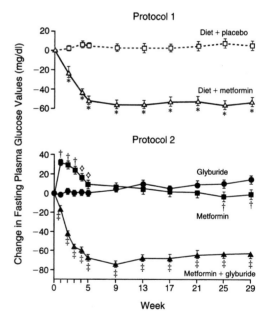

FIGURE 4-8. Mean ± standard error of changes in fasting plasma glucose concentrations in type 2 diabetic patients enrolled in two large multicenter studies in the United States. See text for description of protocols 1 and 2. [*]P < 0.001 between the placebo and metformin groups in protocol 1; [†]P < 0.001 between metformin and glyburide groups in protocol 2; [◊]P < 0.01 between metformin and glyburide groups in protocol 2; [‡]P < 0.001 between combination therapy (metformin + glyburide) and glyburide groups in protocol 2. *(From DeFronzo RA, Goodman AM, and the Multicenter Metformin Study Group: Efficacy of metformin in patients with non-insulin-dependent diabetes mellitus. N Engl J Med 333:541, 1995.)*

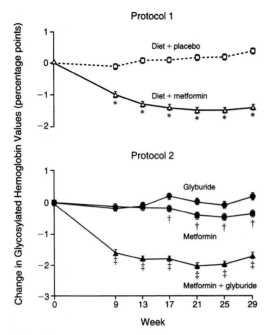

FIGURE 4-9. Mean ± standard error of changes in glycated hemoglobin levels in type 2 diabetic patients enrolled in two large multicenter studies in the United States. See text for description of protocols 1 and 2. *P <0.001 between the placebo and metformin groups in protocol 1—†P < 0.01 between metformin and glyburide groups in protocol 2; ‡P <0.001 between the combination therapy (metformin + glyburide) and glyburide groups in protocol 2. *(From DeFronzo RA, Goodman AM, and the Multicenter Metformin Study Group: Efficacy of metformin in patients with non-insulin-dependent diabetes mellitus. N Engl J Med 333:541, 1995.)*

more regular menstruation, a reduction in circulating insulin levels, and an increase in insulin sensitivity.[39] Although not an approved indication, many physicians treating PCOS have confirmed these findings, and it is quite common to see metformin used off label for this indication. When used in premenopausal women with PCOS, many have ovulated and some have become pregnant.

Metformin has generally been shown to have the added benefit of lowering triglycerides and total and low-density lipoprotein (LDL) cholesterol levels (Table 4-6). This lipid-lowering effect appears to be dose-dependent.[40] This effect suggests that metformin, particularly in higher doses, may have a beneficial effect on cardiovascular risk factors, even if adequate blood glucose levels have been achieved.[41] In UKPDS 34,[42] metformin had a greater beneficial effect on the incidence of coronary heart disease than did sulfonylureas or exogenous insulin in a cohort of overweight patients, suggesting a possible role for insulin-sensitizing drugs, but the interpretation of the data was complicated. Clearly, the issue of the relative pros and cons of insulin-sensitizing drugs versus the pros and cons of drugs that stimulate insulin secretion on macrovascular dis-

TABLE 4-6	EFFECTS OF METFORMIN ON LIPID PARAMETERS FROM INITIAL CLINICAL MONOTHERAPY TRIAL	
Lipid Parameter (change from baseline)	**Metformin (up to 2500 mg/day)[a]**
Triglycerides	placebo: +1.0% metformin: −16.0%
Total cholesterol	placebo: +1.0% metformin: −5.0%
LDL cholesterol	placebo: +1.0% metformin: −8.0%
HDL cholesterol	placebo: −1.0% metformin: +2.0%

HDL, high-density lipoprotein; LDL, low-density lipoprotein.
[a]Values from the package insert.

ease in patients with type 2 diabetes remains unresolved, and needs to be studied in new clinical trials.

Side Effects and Contraindications

Patients starting metformin therapy may experience minor side effects, mostly involving the GI tract. These side effects include diarrhea, abdominal discomfort, anorexia, nausea and rarely a metallic taste in the mouth.[43] Symptoms are dose-related and can improve if the dose is reduced. Some patients experience fewer GI side effects on long-acting metformin (Glucophage XR) than on regular metformin. Gradual increase in dosing tends to be less associated with discomfort. Approximately 5% of patients cannot tolerate even low doses of metformin therapy.

The more serious side effect of metformin is lactic acidosis. Although rare, it can occur in patients who have renal or hepatic insufficiency. Therefore states that lead to the excess accumulation of met-

formin (which is cleared exclusively by the kidney) or lactic acid (such as liver or respiratory failure) are contraindications to use of the drug. The listed exclusion criteria are renal impairment with a serum creatinine level value of 1.5 mg/dl or higher in men and 1.4 mg/dl or higher in women (or an abnormal creatinine clearance, which may be helpful in evaluating the risk for developing metformin-related lactic acidosis in the elderly), cardiac disease or respiratory disease that may result in a reduced peripheral perfusion, severe infection that may lead to decreased tissue perfusion, liver disease as documented by elevated transaminase levels, alcohol abuse with binges, and use of radiographic contrast dyes[44] (Table 4-7) The latter contraindication is particularly important in management, because outpatients often undergo procedures such as magnetic resonance imaging or intravenous pyelograms. The metformin should be stopped 24 hours before the procedure and continued after the procedure once normal renal function is demonstrated. This reduces the

---

TABLE 4-7 METFORMIN: CONTRAINDICATIONS/MONITORING

Contraindications	Monitoring
Renal disease or dysfunction (as suggested by serum creatinine level $\geq$1.5 mg in males, $\geq$1.4 mg/dl in females, or an abnormal creatinine clearance)	Liver and renal function measured yearly; more often if abnormal
Congestive heart failure requiring pharmacologic therapy	If patient older than 80 years of age, documentation of a normal creatinine clearance before use of metformin with regular monitoring of renal function
Acute or chronic metabolic acidosis	CBC count at baseline and yearly (metformin can lower vitamin B_{12} levels)
States of hypoxemia	
Chronic alcoholism or binge drinking	Stopped 24 hours prior to the start of a radiographic procedure or significant surgery and restarted after 48 hours, after re-evaluation reveals normal renal function
Impaired hepatic function	
Use of iodinated radiographic dye or other condition that could precipitate acute renal dysfunction	
Surgery or acute medical condition requiring hospitalization	

CBC, complete blood cell.
Adapted from Metformin package insert, 2002.

risk of having metformin cause problems in the event of renal impairment from the contrast dye. The major risk of metformin is lactic acidosis, and this is rare, with an incidence of 0.03 per 1000 patients per year.[44] In the majority of patients, this complication is related to use in the presence of contraindications. The mortality reported in these cases is approximately 50%. It is important to remember when looking at these data that these patients often had other causes for lactate accumulation such as hypoperfusion and sepsis; thus metformin accumulation as a causal factor may be overestimated.[45]

Drug Interactions

Cationic drugs (e.g., amiloride, digoxin, morphine, procainamide, quinidine, quinine, ranitidine, triamterene, trimethoprim, or vancomycin) that are eliminated by renal tubular excretion have the theoretical potential for competing with metformin for renal tubular transport systems.[46] In studies with metformin and cimetidine, elimination of metformin (but not cimetidine) was impaired. The clinical significance of this is not known and other drug interactions have not been reported.

Clinical Comments

Metformin has been used worldwide since 1957. A great deal of information is known about its risks and benefits, although interestingly its mode of action has not been clearly elucidated. Metformin can be used safely, as long as compliance with clinical prescribing guidelines are followed. Although there are specific prescribing instructions for the use of metformin, physicians do not always follow them, leading to an increased risk for the development of lactic acidosis in patients erroneously prescribed the drug.[47] The most common error in prescribing is to give the drug to patients with an elevated serum creatinine level. Metformin is 100% excreted by the kidneys, so renal insufficiency can easily lead to the accumulation of metformin and the subsequent development of lactic acidosis.

Patients should be told of the risk for lactic acidosis and that kidney and liver function need to be normal for them to stay on the drug. Patients should be warned to stop the metformin if they are undergoing a contrast study or an acute hospitalization (any state that could compromise renal function) and not restart the drug until normal kidney function is documented. Excessive use of alcohol is also a contraindication to the use of metformin and should be discussed with the patient.

Patients should also be warned of the risk of the less serious (but more common) GI side effects. They should be instructed to take the metformin with meals, to decrease the risk for GI side effects, and should have the drug increased gradually. These side effects should be discussed with patients in advance and checked for at follow-up visits. All too often, patients undergo extensive GI work-ups for symptoms such as diarrhea that end up being the result of the metformin and would have been relieved by a decrease in dose and/or cessation of the drug.

ALPHA GLUCOSIDASE INHIBITORS

Background

Acarbose (Precose) (Figure 4-10) was introduced in the United States in the mid 1990s, followed shortly by the introduction of miglitol (Glyset). Both of these agents are α-glucosidase inhibitors, and function similarly. The concept behind these medications is to attempt to slow the absorption of carbohydrates to lower postprandial blood glucose levels. The slower rise in postprandial glucose levels is potentially beneficial in both type 1 and type 2 diabetes.

Mechanism of Action and Pharmacology

In the brush border of the intestine, starch is broken down to oligosaccharides by amylase and further digested into monosaccharides by membrane-bound α-glucosidases

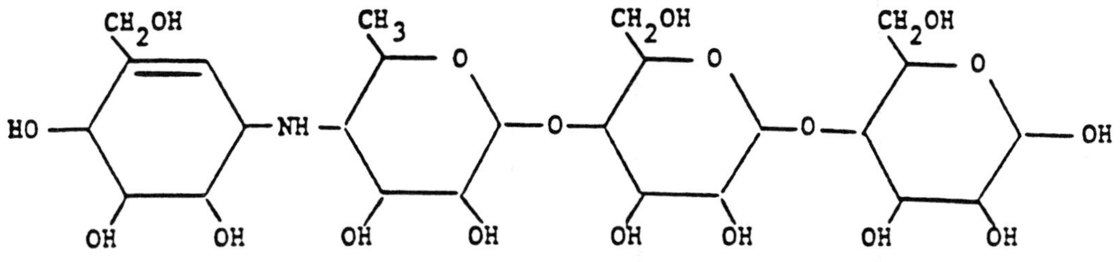

FIGURE 4-10. Structural formula of acarbose.

(isomaltase, maltase, and glucomaltase). Sucrose is broken down by membrane-bound sucrase, also an α-glucosidase enzyme. The α-glucosidase inhibitor drugs competitively inhibit the ability of amylase (acarbose only) and the membrane-bound alpha glucosidases (acarbose and miglitol) to function[48] in the proximal small bowel (Figure 4-11). The inhibitory effect on lactase (a β-glucosidase), which breaks down lactose, is minimal. Because the digestion of carbohydrates is delayed, absorption occurs more slowly. The undigested carbohydrate eventually reaches the ileum, where there is little native α-glucosidase activity. However, use of these drugs (particularly a gradual period of dose titration) will cause induction of α-glucosidase in the ileum, so that carbohydrate can be absorbed before it reaches the colon, where it can cause flatulence and diarrhea. At therapeutic doses, the α-glucosidase inhibitors do not cause malabsorption because the colon has a large capacity to absorb undigested carbohydrate.

As monotherapy, acarbose decreases FPG by 25 to 30 mg/dl and A1C values are reduced by 0.5% to 1% (Figure 4-12). The greatest benefit is seen in postprandial glucose levels, which may drop by 40 to 50 mg/dl.[49] Given its postprandial benefit, the drug is being studied in people with impaired glucose tolerance (where an early defect is isolated postprandial hyperglycemia) and is useful in patients who have diabetes with mildly elevated FPG levels but high excursions after meals.

Miglitol appears to have similar efficacy based on studies in which it was given alone,

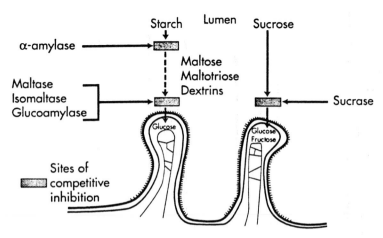

FIGURE 4-11. Sites of action of acarbose in the gastrointestinal tract. In normal digestion, pancreatic α-amylase hydrolyzes complex starches into oligosaccharides, which are further hydrolyzed by α-glucosidases located in the intestinal brush border to glucose and other monosaccharides, which are then absorbed. Acarbose competitively inhibits both of these enzymatic steps.

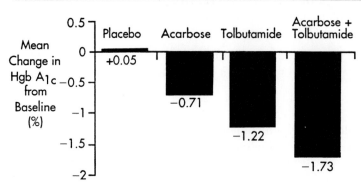

FIGURE 4-12. Mean changes in glycated hemoglobin levels in type 2 diabetic patients receiving either placebo, acarbose, tolbutamide, or acarbose + tolbutamide. A1C, hemoglobin A_{1c}. *(From Coniff RF, Shapiro JA, Seaton TB: Multicenter, placebo-controlled trial comparing acarbose [BAY g 5421] with placebo, tolbutamide, and tolbutamide-plus-acarbose in non-insulin-dependent diabetes mellitus. Am J Med 98:443, 1995.)*

combined with insulin or a sulfonylurea as compared to placebo. There are no head to head studies with miglitol and acarbose, but they appear to be comparable. Miglitol and acarbose are also effective when combined with metformin, although GI tolerance may be an issue. Some studies have reported a modest decrease in plasma triglyceride levels without a change in LDL and HDL in patients on acarbose.[50]

Onset and Duration of Action

α-Glucosidase inhibitors work locally, within the GI tract. In healthy subjects, less than 2% of an oral dose is absorbed systemically. When studies of absorption have been done, the peak plasma concentrations of active drug are seen at 1 hour. An average of 51% of an oral dose is excreted in the feces within 96 hours of ingestion.[51]

These drugs are metabolized within the GI tract by intestinal bacteria as well as by digestive enzymes. The absorbed drug is excreted almost entirely by the kidneys, and in renal insufficiency levels that can cause liver toxicity can be reached, which is why the drug is contraindicated in patients with

a serum creatinine level higher than 2 mg/dl.

Side Effects and Contraindications

GI side effects, including bloating, abdominal discomfort, diarrhea, and flatulence, occur in up to 30% of patients, and diminish with use. Slow titration upward, starting at a low dose, helps build tolerance. With very high doses of acarbose (200 to 300 mg per day) liver toxicity has been reported particularly in patients with renal dysfunction.[52] Abnormal liver function testing resolves with discontinuation of the drug. Hypoglycemia does not usually occur on these agents, unless they are used in combination with other agents that increase insulin levels. If hypoglycemia does occur in a patient using miglitol or acarbose, only pure glucose (which can be absorbed without enzymatic degradation) or milk (lactase not inhibited) will be absorbed quickly enough to aid in treating the patient. Patients on these agents must be advised that standard hypoglycemia therapy such as juice is not appropriate in their case. These agents are contraindicated in patients with inflammatory bowel disease, those with elevated creatinine (>2.0 mg/dl) or cirrhosis. Bowel or intestinal disease (such as irritable bowel syndrome), liver disease, and/or a history of intestinal obstruction are also contraindications (Table 4-8).

Drug Interactions

Most drugs are not affected by coadministration with α-glucosidase inhibitors, although digoxin bioavailability may be affected and levels should be followed when the drugs are used concurrently.

Clinical Comments

Use of α-glucosidase inhibitors is often limited by GI side effects. These can be reduced if patients start at the lowest possible dose of the drugs, sometimes starting with it only once a day, gradually increasing to three times per day with the first bite of each major meal. After a patient tolerates a low dose of the drug three times a day, it is increased at 4- to 8-week intervals. It is best to monitor changes in 1-hour postprandial glucose levels to judge the response to the drug. The overall fall in A1C level may be relatively small (see Figure 4-12), but the postprandial values should become markedly lower.

The maximal dose of acarbose is based on the patient's weight. In a patient weighing 60 kg or less, the maximal dose is 50 mg three times a day. In patients who weigh more than 60 kg, the maximal dose is 100 mg three times a day.

THIAZOLIDINEDIONES

Background

TZDs are a new class of compounds for use in the treatment of type 2 diabetes (Figure 4-13). The effectiveness of these agents in decreasing glycemic control is well documented[53] troglitazone (Rezulin), the first member of this class to be approved for use by the FDA in the United States, was taken off the market because of the occurrence of severe hepatic toxicity and failure associated with its use. Two related compounds, rosiglitazone (Avandia) and pioglitazone (Actos) are currently available in the United States after approval by the FDA in 1999. Although they are sister compounds to troglitazone, they do not seem to be associated with the same liver toxicity. Although there is a baseline rate of liver function abnormality in

TABLE 4-8	α-GLUCOSIDASE INHIBITORS: CONTRAINDICATIONS/ MONITORING	
Contraindications	**Monitoring**
Serum creatinine >2 mg/dl	Serum transaminases every 3 months for
Cirrhosis	the first year and periodically
Inflammatory bowel disease	thereafter (for acarbose)
Colonic ulceration	Annual serum creatinine level
Partial intestinal obstruction	
Predisposition to intestinal obstruction	
Disorders of digestion or absorption that may deteriorate as a result of increased gas formation	
Diabetic ketoacidosis	
Known hypersensitivity to the drug	

Adapted from acarbose and miglitol package inserts, 2002.

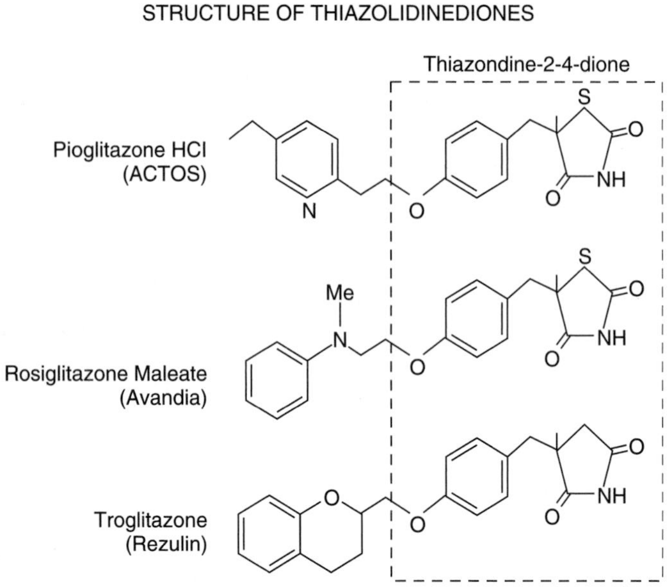

STRUCTURE OF THIAZOLIDINEDIONES

Thiazondine-2-4-dione

Pioglitazone HCl
(ACTOS)

Rosiglitazone Maleate
(Avandia)

Troglitazone
(Rezulin)

FIGURE 4-13. Chemical structures of the thiazolidinediones.

patients with diabetes, both during clinical trials and in postmarketing surveillance, rosiglitazone and pioglitazone appear to be much less hepatotoxic than troglitazone. Severe liver toxicity has been reported,[54] but it is often ultimately found to be caused by something other than the TZD.[55] For the time being, however, the FDA recommends every-other-month liver monitoring for patients started on these agents (see the following text) and these guidelines should be followed.

Mechanism of Action and Pharmacology

Both rosiglitazone and pioglitazone act by enhancing the effect of insulin in muscle, adipose tissue, and liver. They are commonly known as *insulin sensitizers,* which work by decreasing insulin resistance. Circulating insulin must be present for these drugs to be effective. They increase glucose uptake in muscle and fat, probably by stimulating glucose transport through a reduction in circulating free fatty acid lev-

els. There is a modest decrease in hepatic glucose production as well.[56] These drugs have been effective in lowering blood glucose levels in patients with type 2 diabetes, and because they do not exert effect on the pancreas, circulating insulin levels do not increase. Their hallmark is a decrease in insulin levels because as they decrease insulin resistance, glucose falls and the pancreas needs to secrete less insulin. These agents are highly selective agonists for the peroxisome proliferator-activated receptor-gamma (PPAR-gamma) (Figure 4-14). These receptors are found in tissues important for insulin action such as adipose tissue, skeletal muscle, and liver. Activation of PPAR-gamma nuclear receptors modulates the transcription of a number of insulin responsive genes in the control of glucose and lipid metabolism.

TZDs decrease plasma concentrations of free fatty acids, which improves insulin sensitivity.[57] They may also activate other members of the PPAR family (such as PPAR-alpha and PPAR-delta), and the resulting effects

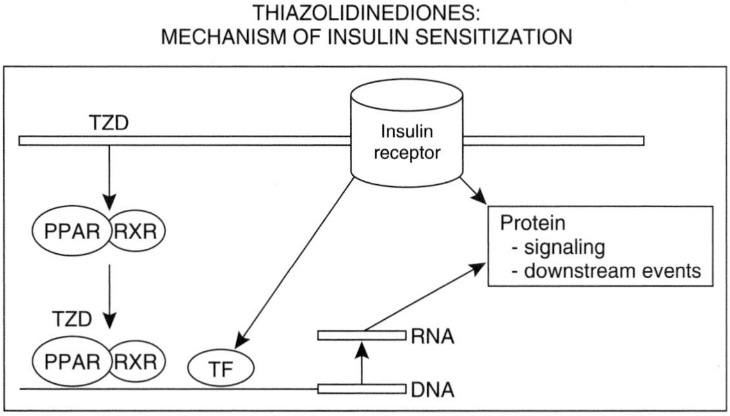

THIAZOLIDINEDIONES:
MECHANISM OF INSULIN SENSITIZATION

FIGURE 4-14. Potential effects of thiazolidinediones on the PPAR-gamma receptor with resultant impact on insulin resistance. PPAR, peroxisome proliferator-activated receptor; RXR, retinoid x receptor; TF, transcription factors; TZD, thiazolidinedione.

are currently being elucidated.[58] As an aside, this class of agents is being extensively studied for its potential benefits on the cardiovascular system. There is mounting evidence that this class of agents decreases blood pressure and peripheral vascular resistance,[59] improves HDL cholesterol and decrease triglyceride levels,[60] exerts a beneficial effect on vascular smooth muscle cell proliferation,[61] and reduces carotid intimal-medial thickness.[62] The reduction in insulin resistance is being explored as a therapeutic option in other disease states, such as PCOS.[63] There is also evidence that this class of compounds has an anti-inflammatory effect that may be beneficial in other diseases as well.[64]

The effects on the lipid profile appear to differ between rosiglitazone and pioglitazone (Table 4-9).[65-67] The major difference is that pioglitazone tends to lower triglyceride levels, whereas rosiglitazone generally does not.[67a] Both drugs have a positive effect on HDL cholesterol concentrations (they both increase it) and both increase LDL particle size. Because patients with type 2 diabetes

are at such high risk for cardiovascular disease (see Chapter 8), it is important that lipid targets are reached and maintained. Therefore particularly when starting a patient with an elevated LDL cholesterol and/or triglyceride level on rosiglitazone, it is important to remeasure the lipids after 3 months on the drug to ensure that patients stay within recommended lipid targets. Conversely, patients with elevated triglyceride levels started on pioglitazone may experience a decrease in their levels, and occasionally patients who are on a fibric acid derivative may no longer need the additional drug.

Pioglitazone and rosiglitazone act within 1 to 2 hours of administration and are dosed daily. At the highest dose, rosiglitazone is maximally effective when given as 4 mg twice a day. It is important to note that it takes up to 4 weeks to see a drop in blood glucose levels on these agents and up to 12 weeks to see a maximum benefit. Steady-state serum concentrations are achieved within 7 days. Pioglitazone and rosiglitazone have been approved as first-line therapy in

| TABLE 4-9 | THIAZOLIDINEDIONES: EFFECTS ON LIPID PARAMETERS LIPID CHANGES ASSOCIATED WITH THE USE OF ROSIGLITAZONE AND PIOGLITAZONE |

A. Rosiglitazone

Study	HDL change (%)	LDL change (%)	TG change (%)
Study 1[a]			
Placebo	5.0	0	20.6
4 mg	5.8	7.5	9.4
8 mg	13.6	15.5	2.0
Study 2[b]			
Placebo	8.0	4.8	Not reported
4 mg	11.4	14.1	Not reported
8 mg	14.2	18.6	Not reported
Study 3[c]			
Placebo	4.3	−0.9	Not reported
8 mg	14.0	11.9	Not reported
Study 4[d]			
Placebo	5.3	3.0	0.4
4 mg	11.9	15.4	3.1
8 mg	13.3	18.6	0.4

B. Pioglitazone

Study	HDL change (%)	LDL change (%)	TG change (%)
Study 1[e]			
Placebo	6.2	2.2	−3.8
15 mg	12.4	4.8	−20.4
30 mg	10.3	2.8	−13.7
45 mg	17.4	6.9	−15.7
Study 2[f]			
Placebo	−4.7	5.6	3.1
15 mg	7.3	3.2	−15.4
30 mg	9.5	2.4	−23.8
Study 3[g]			
Placebo	8.1	4.8	4.8
15 mg	14.1	7.2	−9.0
30 mg	12.2	5.2	−9.6
45 mg	19.1	6	−9.3

[a]Raskin P, Rendell M, Riddle MC et al: A randomized trial of rosiglitazone therapy in patients with inadequately controlled insulin-treated type 2 diabetes. Diabetes Care 24:1226, 2001.

[b]Rosiglitazone package insert—monotherapy data.

[c]Rosiglitazone package insert—combination with SA.

[d]Fonseca V, Rosenstock J, Patwardhan R, Salzman A: Effect of metformin and rosiglitazone combination therapy in patients with type 2 diabetes mellitus: A randomized controlled trial. JAMA 283:1695, 2000.

[e]Arnoff S, Rosenblatt S, Braithwaite S et al: Pioglitazone hydrochloride monotherapy improves glycemic control in the treatment of patients with type 2 diabetes: A 6 month randomized placebo-controlled dose-response study. Diabetes Care 23:1605, 2000.

[f]Kipnes MS, Krosnick A, Rendell MS et al: Pioglitazone hydrochloride in combination with sulfonylurea therapy improves glycemic control in patients with type 2 diabetes mellitus: A randomized, placebo-controlled study. Am J Med 111:10, 2001.

[g]Pioglitazone package insert monotherapy data.

diabetes, and for use in combination with other oral agents. Pioglitazone and rosiglitazone are FDA approved for use in conjunction with insulin in patients with type 2 diabetes.[68,69] It should be noted that both drugs cause an increase in plasma volume and it is possible that a patient with underlying cardiac dysfunction can be tipped into congestive failure on these agents. This may occur more frequently in patients with a longer duration of diabetes, who are taking insulin and who are on higher doses.

Side Effects and Contraindications (Table 4-10)

Therapy with rosiglitazone and pioglitazone should not be initiated in patients with clinical evidence of active liver disease or increased serum transaminases of greater than 2.5 times normal. There are no clinically relevant differences in the metabolism of these agents in patients with mild to moderate renal impairment or in those on dialysis. No dose adjustment is required in renal failure.

The FDA recommends that liver function be measured at baseline and then every other month for the first year of therapy. After that point, the frequency of monitoring may be decreased. The most significant contraindications to these medications include any type of liver disease, and heart failure. These medications may cause a significant increase in fluid retention along with weight gain, particularly when used in combination with other agents. There is debate as to how much of this change is actually true weight gain versus fluid retention. Most likely, in the majority of patients, it is a combination. There is an association with a reduction in A1C levels and an increase in weight in patients on these agents. Although the reports of weight gain are generally 3 to 8 pounds, clinical experience shows that a large amount of weight gain can sometimes occur. The weight gain seems to be more common with higher doses of the drug. In patients with mild to moderate edema, the resulting ankle swelling and puffiness can be controlled with the addition of a diuretic such as furosemide, or by reducing the dose of pioglitazone or rosiglitazone. On occasion, patients may have such excessive weight gain (30 to 40 pounds) or such severe edema or even shortness of breath that this class of drug must be discontinued altogether.

Other side effects include a decrease in hemoglobin and hematocrit, which is likely related to an increase in plasma volume, and ovulation in premenopausal anovulatory women, which may result in increased risk for pregnancy. Premenopausal women on these agents should be counseled on birth control.

Drug Interactions

No clinically significant drug interactions have been reported for rosiglitazone or pioglitazone. Initially, there was some concern that pioglitazone would have some drug interactions resulting from its possible induction of hepatic cytochrome P450 isoform CYP3A4, but this has been found to be clinically insignificant.[70] Therefore drug interactions are not a concern with either drug. However, women who are anovulatory may resume ovulation when treated for their insulin resistance, and pregnancy can ensue. Therefore women of childbearing age should be told of the risk for pregnancy during treatment with these agents.

Clinical Comments

The TZDs work to lower glucose levels in patients with insulin resistance (Figures 4-15 and 4-16). They work gradually, with the peak effect occurring 12 to 16 weeks after the maximal dose is reached. Some practitioners start at higher doses from the first (4 mg twice a day of rosiglitazone or 45 mg of pioglitazone), whereas others find few side effects when lower doses are smaller and increased gradually. The TZDs cause an increase in plasma volume, and the most common side effect is edema, which is usually not clinically significant. However, occasionally patients develop severe edema and, even more rarely, the increase in fluid volume can precipitate congestive heart failure. Therefore these drugs should not be used in patients with a tenuous volume status (such as class III or IV congestive heart failure). Some patients with mild to moderate edema may benefit from concomitant use of a diuretic.

TABLE 4-10	CONTRAINDICATIONS/MONITORING FOR THIAZOLIDINEDIONES	
Contraindications	**Monitoring**	
• ALT >2.5 times the upper limit of normal at baseline • Stop drug if ALT becomes greater than 3 times the upper limit of normal • NYHA class III or IV congestive heart failure • Edema (relative contraindication) • Concomitant use of insulin (rosiglitazone only)	• Measure ALT at baseline and then every other month for the first year; periodically therafter • Ovulation may occur in premenopausal women and adequate contraception while on these drugs should be recommended	

ALT, alanine transferase; NYHA, New York Heart Association.

Adapted from rosiglitazone and pioglitazone package inserts.

Patients who are taking insulin or an insulin secretagogue with a TZD may notice a further fall in their blood glucose levels, even hypoglycemia, as the insulin resistance diminishes. The drug that can cause hypoglycemia, either the insulin or the insulin secretagogue, should be decreased as a response is noted. It is not recommended that an anticipatory decrease in the drug should be made, in case the patient does not respond to the TZD.

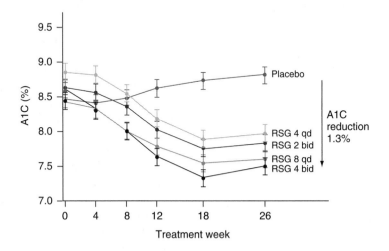

ROSIGLITAZONE THERAPY
Mean A1C (drug-naïve subset*)

*Efficacy-evaluable population (n = 225)

FIGURE 4-15. The effect of rosiglitazone on A1C levels when used as monotherapy in patients with type 2 diabetes. RSG, rosiglitazone.

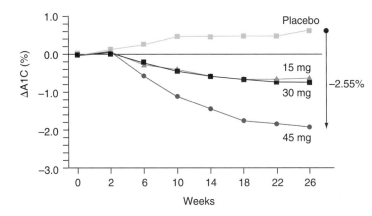

PIOGLITAZONE MONOTHERAPY
Change in Hgb A_1 from baseline—treatment naïve patients

FIGURE 4-16. The effect of pioglitazone on AIC levels when used as monotherapy in patients with type 2 diabetes. *(Courtesy Glaxo SmithKline)*

Because rosiglitazone and pioglitazone are of the same class as troglitazone, and troglitazone was associated with rare episodes of severe hepatic toxicity, liver monitoring is required when using the newer agents. Liver function tests should be measured at baseline and then every 2 months of the first year of use of rosiglitazone or pioglitazone and periodically thereafter (every 3 to 6 months). Patients with abnormal liver function or active liver disease at baseline should not be started on a TZD. These newer agents do not seem to have the same liver toxicity as does troglitazone, but the liver monitoring guidelines should be followed. Additionally, because of potential negative effects on the lipid profile, patients should have their lipids remeasured 2 to 3 months after starting on rosiglitazone and lipid medication adjusted (if needed) to maintain lipids at target levels.

THE USE OF ORAL AGENTS IN COMBINATION

Currently, sulfonylurea agents are the most prescribed class of oral agents in the United States, but metformin is increasingly being used as initial monotherapy in obese patients with type 2 diabetes (and it is now available as a cheaper generic, as well as the sulfonylurea agents). Sulfonylurea therapy is inexpensive and reliably effective in early type 2 diabetes. Aside from the tendency to cause hypoglycemia and weight gain, the chief draw back of sulfonylurea therapy is the secondary failure rate. For patients who respond to therapy, treatment fails at a rate of 5% or more per year.[71] Some have theorized that this is due to "burn out" of the β-cells through years of hyperstimulation, but the secondary failure rate with metformin is similar,[72] so the progressive hyperglycemia seen may be due to the progressive nature of the disease. However, only limited long-term data on the TZDs is available, and in certain individuals these drugs may help prevent β-cell failure. On a purely practical level, it is sometimes easier to work with a patient on weight loss and exercise when they are taking an agent that does not cause an increase in insulin secretion and hypoglycemia. Regardless of the choice of monotherapy, many patients require combination therapy and the important goal is to maintain good glycemic control throughout the patient's diabetes treatment.

In this day and age, the role of combination therapy for the treatment of diabetes is a valuable option for treatment because we are equipped with a growing list of drugs that have specific sites of action. The thought process to treating diabetes has changed in recent years. Instead of simply stopping a medication and starting another, the possibility of an additive effect of the medications in combination has prompted clinicians to use combination therapy as state-of-the-art care (Table 4-11). Whereas much of medicine is pure science, combination therapy for the treatment of diabetes— although based in sound scientific principals—is really the art of medicine. Medical professionals must use their powers of reasoning to derive the best combination of medications and take into account lifestyle, patient preferences, other comorbid conditions, compliance issues, cost, and a host of other factors to ensure the best possible outcomes for both short-term and long-term care.

Metformin plus a sulfonylurea agent is the most commonly used combination.[73] Using these agents together gives an additive effect on glucose lowering.[74] Whether one agent is started before the other does not seem to affect the ultimate fasting blood glucose values obtained on combination therapy as shown in a study by Hermann et al.[75] In another large study of combination therapy,[76] patients of glyburide received either addition of metformin or placebo. In the placebo group, A1C values increased by 0.2% and FPG values increased by 14 mg/dl, whereas in the metformin-added group, A1C values decreased by 1.7% and FPG values dropped by 63 mg/dl. The combination of metformin and sulfonylurea therapy has become so popular that a fixed-dose combination pill called Glucovance has been approved for use in the United States. Although this medication allows for greater compliance because the medications are combined, it may not be clinically beneficial. First, the weight-sparing relative effect of the metformin is lost with the combination pill because the weight gain with Glucovance is equal to that with glyburide alone and more than metformin alone. Second, the plasma levels of sulfonylurea (in this case, glyburide) peak earlier, and the hypoglycemic effect may be more pronounced. Third, glyburide causes more hypoglycemia and weight gain than some of the other sulfonylureas (such as glimepiride). The side effect and safety profile is similar to that of each drug used separately. Whether to use a combination pill is really a matter of personal preference. The major drawback is

TABLE 4-11   BENEFITS OF COMBINATION THERAPIES

Combination Therapy for Type 2 Diabetes *Effect on A1C*		
Current Rx	Therapy Added	Change in A1C
Sulfonylurea	Metformin	↓ 1.6%
	Glitazone	↓ 0.9–1.9%
Metformin	Glitazone	↓ 0.8–1.5%
Glitazone	Sulfonylurea	↓ up to 2.0%

DM Kendall. Data adapted from multiple references.

the inability to titrate each agent without adjusting the other, and the metformin (which does not increase insulin secretion) cannot be increased separately from the glyburide. For this reason, physicians may choose to adjust each medication individually until a therapeutic dose of each has been found, and then switch to the equivalent dose of Glucovance for compliance.

Studies have also shown an additive benefit with acarbose in combination with both metformin[77] and sulfonylurea agents.[78,79] GI side effects may preclude the use of metformin with acarbose and need to be followed. The use of all three agents in combination is also acceptable if tolerated, because once again, all three agents work at different sites and their effects may be additive.

Meglitinides are short-acting agents that are particularly beneficial in reducing mealtime glucose excursions. As a result, the combination of these agents with metformin is particularly effective, providing both a mechanism to control hepatic glucose output in the fasting state, and insulin secretion in the post prandial state.[80] There is no demonstrable benefit of combining meglitinides with sulfonylurea agents.

Much of the work done on combination therapy with TZDs has been done with troglitazone. Studies are currently underway to determine the effects of currently available agents such as rosiglitazone and pioglitazone in combination with other oral agents. In one combination study,[81] 560 patients with type 2 diabetes on a sulfonylurea, either alone or in combination with another antidiabetic agent, were randomly assigned to receive 15 mg or 30 mg of pioglitazone or placebo. The addition of pioglitazone to a sulfonylurea agent significantly reduced the mean A1C by 0.9% and 1.3% in the 15-mg and 30-mg treated groups, respectively. Compared with placebo, the FPG decreased by 39 mg/dl and 58 mg/dl in the 15-mg and 30-mg treated groups. In a sec-

ond combination study,[82] 328 patients with type 2 diabetes on metformin either alone or in combination with another agent were randomized to received 30 mg pioglitazone or placebo in addition to metformin, while the other antidiabetic agents were withdrawn. Compared with placebo, the addition of pioglitazone to metformin significantly reduced the mean A1C by 0.8%. Both of these studies observed benefit regardless of the dose of sulfonylurea or biguanides. In the case of rosiglitazone, a study[83] of 348 poorly controlled patients with type 2 diabetes showed a significant improvement on the combination of rosiglitazone and metformin over metformin and placebo over a 26-week period. This improvement over placebo was seen in both A1C levels and FPG levels. Similarly, rosiglitazone in combination with a sulfonylurea in patients with inadequately controlled type 2 diabetes showed a significant reduction in FPG and A1C levels.[84] Triple combination therapy (TZD plus metformin plus a sulfonylurea agent) has also been shown to be effective[85] (Figure 4-17).

WHEN SHOULD COMBINATION THERAPY BE CONSIDERED?

Given the high failure rate of monotherapy and what we know about the importance of achieving glycemic control in reducing the complications of diabetes, the authors feel that combination therapy should be considered early in the course of the disease process. If a single drug treatment is unable to keep A1C values under 7% (or under an individually chosen goal), a second agent should be added. Although some clinicians prefer to maximize one medication before adding another, there is some evidence that starting a second agent before maximizing the first may be beneficial in reducing both cost and side effects.[86] For many drugs, maximal therapeutic effects are seen at 50%

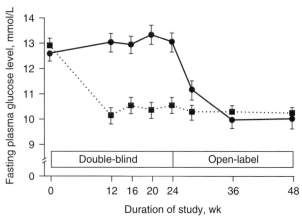

TRIPLE COMBINATION THERAPY IN THE
TREATMENT OF TYPE 2 DIABETES

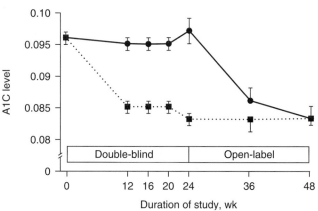

FIGURE 4-17. This figure depicts the effectiveness of triple drug therapy (sulfonylurea agent, metformin, and troglitazone) in patients poorly controlled on double agent therapy. During the double-blind phase, some patients were on placebo troglitazone instead of active troglitazone; in the open label phase, all patients were on triple active drug therapy. *(From Yale JF, Valiquett TR, Ghazzi MN et al: The effect of a thiazolidinedione drug, troglitazone, on glycemia in patients with type 2 diabetes mellitus poorly controlled with sulfonylurea and metformin: A multicenter, randomized, double-blind, placebo controlled trial. Ann Int Med 134:737, 2001.)*

maximal dosage. In the case of metformin, increasing doses beyond 2000 mg daily has no added benefit, and actually may be associated with a decline in efficacy, whereas 1000 mg daily yields approximately 65% of maximal therapeutic effect with fewer side effects.[87] A similar dose response may be seen for glimepiride. However, the other side of the issue is that all drugs have side effects, and limiting a patient to use of fewer agents may limit the risk of side effects. Therefore decisions on use of drugs should be weighed individually with the knowledge that A1C levels should be kept below 7% whenever possible.

Insulin and Oral Agent Therapy

Insulin and oral agent therapy is discussed in detail in Chapter 5. In type 2 diabetes, patients have both insulin resistance and insulin deficiency. Therefore it makes sense to treat both defects. Bedtime insulin daytime oral agent (BIDO) therapy is an effective way to treat type 2 diabetes that cannot be controlled with oral agents alone. In particular, maintaining sulfonylurea therapy after secondary failure while adding insulin at bedtime shows an advantage.[88] By using insulin (bedtime NPH or glargine insulin) to restrain hepatic glucose output during

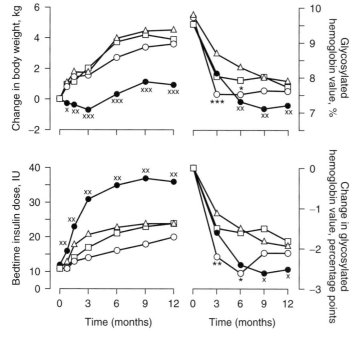

FIGURE 4-18. Effects of combination insulin plus oral agent therapy on glucose levels and body weight in patients with type 2 diabetes after 1 year of treatment. Dark circles = bedtime insulin plus metformin; white squares = bedtime insulin plus glyburide; white circles = bedtime insulin plus glyburide and metformin; white triangles = twice daily insulin. *(From Yki-Jarvinen H, Ryysi L, Nikkila K et al: Comparison of bedtime insulin regimens in patients with non-insulin–dependent diabetes mellitus. N Engl J Med 327: 1426–1433, 1992.)*

the night and early morning, fasting hyperglycemia can be better controlled. Once this is achieved, daytime administered sulfonylurea agents seem better able to maintain postprandial euglycemia. Short-acting insulin secretagogues can also be used before meals in patients who are willing to take a drug three times a day. This offers a bit more flexibility than longer-acting sulfonylurea agents because patients can skip meals (and hold the corresponding dose of the insulin secretagogue.) By using metformin in combination with insulin, glycemic control can be comparable with other insulin regimens[89] and there may be less weight gain than is seen in multiple injection regimens (Figure 4-18). If multiple injections of insulin become needed, continuation of a sulfonylurea agent may not provide added benefit.[90] TZD may also be continued with the addition of insulin. In cases in which multiple injections of insulin become needed, TZD and met-

formin may be continued after secretagogue therapy is stopped. The insulin sparing/sensitizing effects may allow for smaller doses of insulin to be required to maintain glycemic control.

CASE 1

MONOTHERAPY

TW is a 56-year-old Hispanic woman with new-onset type 2 diabetes. Her diabetes was diagnosed when she went to see her gynecologist for a recurrent vaginal yeast infection. A random blood glucose level was found to be 255 mg/dl and a FPG level was 180 mg/dl. She was referred to a primary care physician. She had no symptoms of polyuria or polydipsia. Her weight had been gradually increasing. She gave birth to four children, birth weights (from first to last) 7 pounds 2 ounces, 7 pounds 6 ounces, 8 pounds 2 ounces, and 9 pounds 3 ounces. Her mother developed "old-age diabetes" when she was 76 years of age. On examination, the patient was 5 feet 2 inches tall and weighed 195 pounds. Her blood pressure was 128/78. She had no diabetic retinopathy or neuropathy. Her laboratory test results revealed an A1C level of 8.9%, normal serum creatinine level, a urine albumin/creatinine ratio of 10, triglycerides of 210 mg/dl, total cholesterol of 198 mg/dl, HDL cholesterol of 52 mg/dl, and LDL cholesterol of 104 mg/dl.

The patient was given a preprinted 1200 kcal diabetic diet and told to lose weight and exercise. After 3 months there was no change in the patient's weight, although she had started walking for 20 minutes 2 to 3 days per week. Her fasting blood glucose level was 178 mg/dl. She was started on glyburide 5 mg per day. She started the medication and went to see a dietitian on her own. She reduced her caloric intake and increased her activity further. She began to develop symptoms of hypoglycemia in the late afternoon. She went back to see her physician who started self-monitoring of blood glucose levels and switched her glyburide to metformin 500 mg twice a day. After 1 month on the metformin her FPG had fallen to 132 mg/dl and her weight had fallen by 8 pounds. She was maintained on the metformin with a A1C level of 6.8%. The patient was encouraged to continue with her diet and exercise program.

Comment

Many patients with type 2 diabetes are relatively asymptomatic prior to diagnosis. This patient should have been screened for diabetes long before she was diagnosed. She had multiple risk factors: she is Latina (a high-risk ethnic group), overweight, has a first-degree relative with type 2 diabetes, and has a history of having a baby weighing more than 9 pounds (suggesting gestational diabetes during the pregnancy). But this individual, like many people, did not receive regular medical care. For women, their primary care physician is often their gynecologist. Based on this patient's risk factors and the presence of recurrent vaginal candidiasis (which can be a presenting symptom of diabetes in women), a blood glucose level was measured. This led to the patient receiving treatment for her diabetes.

The initial laboratory tests and evaluation were appropriate, although the patient was not sent to see a dietitian for nutritional counseling. Medical nutrition therapy and exercise are the initial treatments for patients with asymptomatic or

minimally symptomatic diabetes and should be continued throughout the patient's lifetime. Weight loss and exercise reduce insulin resistance and lower the risk for cardiovascular disease. In this patient's case, no initial change in lifestyle occurred, but when placed on a sulfonylurea agent, she began to restrict her caloric intake. The increase in insulin secretion caused by the sulfonylurea agent caused late-afternoon hypoglycemia. The patient was changed to metformin, which could have also been used as the initial choice of therapy in this obese patient with new-onset diabetes. On the metformin her symptoms of hypoglycemia resolved and she was able to lose some weight on her diet plan. Her A1C level remained below the target of 7%.

• • •

CASE 2

COMBINATION ORAL AGENTS

RW is a 52-year-old African American woman with a 5-year history of type 2 diabetes. Her past medical history is notable for hypertension (treatment was lisinopril) and endometriosis. She has a family history that is positive for type 2 diabetes in both of her sisters. She is married, works as a secretary, and denies use of alcohol or cigarettes. On micronized glyburide (Glynase) 6 mg twice a day (the maximal dose), her A1C level is 10.1%, triglyceride level is 210 mg/dl, total cholesterol is 240 mg/dl, LDL cholesterol level is 160 mg/dl, and her HDL level is 38 mg/dl. She did not adhere to any particular diet and did not exercise routinely. She had no known complications of her diabetes but did have mild polyuria and polydipsia.

The patient had normal kidney and liver function and metformin 500 mg twice a day with breakfast and dinner was added to her glyburide. After 1 month her FPG level had fallen from 240 mg/dl to 215 mg/dl. The metformin dose was increased to 1 g twice a day. This lowered her FPG level to 180 mg/dl with a fall in her A1C level to 8.4% after 3 months on maximal dose glyburide and metformin therapy. A statin was also started and adjusted, and her follow-up lipid profile was at target, with a triglyceride level of 154 mg/dl, total cholesterol level of 168 mg/dl,

HDL cholesterol level of 39 mg/dl, LDL cholesterol level of 98 mg/dl.

Rosiglitazone 4 mg per day was added to the other two agents. Over the next 3 months the dose was increased to 4 mg twice a day. Her FPG level gradually fell to 136 mg/dl and her HbA1c level fell to 7.2%. She gained 11 pounds of weight as her blood glucose levels fell. Her lipid profile improved further with an increase in her HDL cholesterol to 45 mg/dl and no change in her triglycerides or LDL cholesterol level while maintained on a statin.

Buoyed by her success (and her increase in energy) the patient began to become more adherent to her nutritional plan and exercise. Although her weight remained approximately the same, with the increase in exercise her presupper blood glucose levels fell to 70 to 80 mg/dl. Her glyburide dose was decreased gradually by 50% to 6 mg once a day.

Comment

This patient represents a fairly classic response to combination oral agent therapy, which allows some patients to remain in good control without taking insulin injections. Many patients fear taking insulin injections, and although most find the reality less burdensome than they anticipated, insulin injections often impose lifestyle changes that are unnecessary with oral agents. RW did not achieve adequate control with combination sulfonylurea agent plus metformin therapy, and a third agent was quickly added to reduce her blood glucose levels further. Rosiglitazone acts gradually, and over time brought her glucose levels near the target range. This was very encouraging for the patient and she began to become more adherent to lifestyle recommendations. As her control improved, her blood glucose levels fell. The sulfonylurea agent, which increases insulin secretion, was lowered and the patient was then able to maintain normal glucose (and lipid) levels.

• • •

CASE 3

INSULIN PLUS A THIAZOLIDINEDIONE

LH is a 60-year-old white man with a 14-year history of type 2 diabetes. Initially he was started on a sulfonylurea agent, but over time his blood glucose levels rose. Five years after diagnosis, he was started on a twice-daily insulin regimen.

When he was referred, his A1C level was 9.9% on 40 units of 70/30 insulin in the morning and 20 units before supper. He had background diabetic retinopathy, mild peripheral sensory polyneuropathy, and microalbuminuria. He monitored his blood glucose levels twice a day and was fairly regular with his dietary intake. After his initial assessment, he was seen by a diabetes educator and a nutritionist. He began to test more often and his 70/30 insulin was switched to self-mixed NPH and regular to allow for more flexibility in dosing. He improved, although his A1C level remained elevated at 8.6%.

The patient had a normal serum creatinine level, and metformin was added to his insulin regimen because he was trying hard to lose weight. On the metformin he was able to lower his insulin dose by approximately 15 units and he lost 8 pounds. His A1C level did not fall much, however, and was 8.4%. Pioglitazone was added to his insulin at a dose of 15 mg per day. He was warned of the risk of edema and instructed to call if he developed side effects or his blood glucose level fell below 100 mg/dl. After 2 weeks his glucose levels did start to respond and as his glucose levels fell, his corresponding insulin doses were lowered. After 6 months his pioglitazone dose was increased to 45 mg per day and 18 units of NPH insulin at bedtime. His A1C level fell to 7.3% and his weight increased by 12 pounds. His self-monitoring of blood glucose levels showed that his postsupper glucose levels were consistently 180 to 240 mg/dl and the remainder of his values were within target. Presupper nateglinide (Starlix) 120 mg was added with a corresponding fall in his postprandial value and a further improvement in his A1C level to 6.9%.

In addition to his glucose lowering, the patient was started on an angiotensin-converting enzyme inhibitor therapy, aspirin, and a statin to maintain his blood pressure at less than 130/80, treat his microalbuminuria, maintain his LDL cholesterol level at less than 100 mg/dl, and reduce his cardiovascular disease risk.

Comment

It is often hard to lower blood glucose levels into the normal range in patients with type 2 diabetes using insulin alone. Theoretically it is possible, but it is often difficult to do in an individual patient. LH responded well to the sequential addition of metformin, and then an insulin sensitizer. Finally, targeting pharmacology to his physiology, a high supper postprandial glucose level was identified and treated with a short-acting insulin secretagogue. Ultimately, treatment of type 2 diabetes involves global risk reduction so measures to lower risk for both microvascular and macrovascular complications were employed.

REFERENCES

1. Peters AL, Davidson MB: Quality of outpatient care provided to diabetic patients: A health maintenance organization experience. Diabetes Care 6:601, 1996.
2. Inzucchi SE: Oral antihyperglycemic therapy for type 2 diabetes. JAMA 287:360, 2002.
3. Yki-Jarvinen H: Combination therapies with insulin in type 2 diabetes. Diabetes Care 24:758, 2001.
4. Chu PC, Conway MJ, Krouse HA, Goodner CJ: The pattern of response of plasma insulin and glucose to meals and fasting during chlorpropamide therapy. Ann Intern Med 68:757, 1968.
5. Reaven G, Dray J: Effect of chlorpropamide on serum glucose and immunoreactive insulin concentrations in patients with ketosis-resistant diabetes mellitus. Diabetes 16:487, 1967.
6. Peters AL, Davidson MB: Reduction of hyperinsulinemia by glyburide—Scientific fact or advertising fiction? Diabetes Care 15:719, 1992.
7. Gerich JE: Oral hypoglycemic agents. N Engl J Med 321:1231, 1989.
8. Groop LC: Sulfonylureas in NIDDM. Diabetes Care 15:737, 1992.
9. Judzewitsch RG, Pfeifer MA, Best JD et al: Chronic chlorpropamide therapy of noninsulin-dependent diabetes augments basal and stimulated insulin secretion by increasing islet sensitivity to glucose. J Clin Endocrinol Metab 55:321, 1982.
10. Sartor G, Melander A, Schersten B et al: Influence of food and age on the single-dose kinetics and effects of tolbutamide and chlorpropamide. Eur J Clin Pharmol 17:285, 1980.
11. Groop LC, Luzi L, DeFronzo RA et al: Hyperglycaemia and absorption of sulphonylurea drugs. Lancet 2:129, 1989.
12. Esmatjes E, Vinuesa P, Navarro P et al: The effect of hyperglycemia on glipizide absorption in NIDDM patients. Diabetes Care 18:1075, 1995.
13. Scott J, Poffenbarger PL: Pharmacogenetics of tolbutamide metabolism in humans. Diabetes 28:41, 1979.
14. Rydberg T, Roder M, Jonsson A et al: Hypoglycemic activity of glyburide (glibenclamide) metabolites in humans. Diabetes Care 17:1026, 1994.
15. Goodman RC, Dean PJ, Radparvar A, Kitabchi AE: Glyburide-induced hepatitis. Ann Intern Med 106:837, 1987.
16. Meadow P, Tullio CJ: Glyburide-induced hepatitis. Clin Pharmacol 8:470, 1989.
17. Garcia M, Miller M, Moses AM: Chlorpropamide-induced water retention in patients with diabetes mellitus. Ann Intern Med 75:549, 1971.
18. Kadowaki T, Hagura R, Kajinuma H et al: Chlorpropamide-induced hyponatremia: Incidence and risk factors. Diabetes Care 6:468, 1983.
19. Intensive blood-glucose control with sulphonylureas or insulin compared with conventional treatment and risk of complications in patients with type 2 diabetes (UKPDS 33). Lancet 352:837, 1998. (Erratum, Lancet 354:602, 1999.)
20. Jackson JE, Bressler R: Clinical pharmacology of sulphonylurea hypoglycemic agents. Drugs 22:211, 1981.
21. Hansen JM, Christensen LK: Drug interactions with oral sulphonylurea hypoglycaemic drugs. Drugs 13:24, 1977.
22. Edwards TH, Braunstein GD, Davidson MB: Glyburide-induced hypoglycemia in an elderly patient: Similarity of first-generation and second-generation sulfonylurea agents. Mt Sinai J Med 52:644, 1985.
23. Peters AL, Davidson MB: Maximal dose glyburide therapy in markedly symptomatic patients with type 2 diabetes: A new use for an old friend. J Clin Endocrinol Metab 81:2423, 1996.
24. Sato Y, Nishikawa M, Shinkai H, Sukegawa E: Possibility of ideal blood glucose control by a new oral hypoglycemic agent, N-[trans-4-isopropylcyclohexyl)-carbonyl]-D-phenylalanine (A-4166) and its stimulatory effect on insulin secretion in animals. Diabetes Res Clin Pract 12:53, 1991.
25. Kikuchi M: Modulation of insulin secretion in non-insulin-dependent diabetes mellitus by two novel oral hypoglycemic agents, NN623 and A4166. Diabet Med 13:S151, 1996.
26. Hu S, Wang S, Fanelli B, et al: Pancreatic beta-cell K (ATP) channel activity and membrane binding studies with nateglinide: A comparison with sulfonylureas and repaglinide. J Pharmacol Exp Ther 293:444, 2000.
27. Kalbag JB, Walter YH, Nedelman JR, McLeod JF: Mealtime glucose regulation with nateglinide in healthy volunteers. Comparison with repaglinide and placebo. Diabetes Care 24:73, 2001.
28. Flood TM: Serious hypoglycemia associated with misuse of repaglinide. Endocrine Pract 5:137, 137–138, 1999.
29. Bailey CJ, Day C: Traditional plant medicines as treatment for diabetes. Diabetes Care 12:553, 1989.
30. Sterne J: Pharmacology and mode of action of hypoglycemic guanidine derivative. In Campbell GD (ed): Oral Hypoglycaemic Agents. Academic Press, London, 1969, pp. 193–245.
31. Nattrass M, Alberti KG: Biguanides. Diabetologia 14:71, 1978.

32. Hsia SH, Davidson MB: Established therapies for diabetes mellitus. Curr Med Res Opin 18(Suppl):13–21, 2002.

33. McLelland J: Recovery from metformin overdose. Diabetic Med 2:410, 1985.

34. Bailey CJ: Biguanides and NIDDM. Diabetes Care 15:755, 1992.

35. Hermann LS: Metformin: A review of its pharmacological properties and therapeutic use. Diabete Metab 5(3):233–245, 1979.

36. DeFronzo RA, Barzilai N, Simonson DC: Mechanism of metformin action in non-insulin-dependent diabetic subject. J Clin Endocrinol Metab 73:1294, 1991.

37. Cigolini M, Bosello O, Zancanaro C et al: Influence of metformin on metabolic effect of insulin in human adipose tissue. Diabete Metab 10:311, 1984.

38. Johansen K: Efficacy of metformin in the treatment of NIDDM. Diabetes Care 22:33, 1999.

39. Moghetti P, Castell R, Negri C et al: Metformin effects on clinical features, endocrine and metabolic profiles and insulin sensitivity in polycystic ovary syndrome: A randomized, double blind placebo controlled 6 month trial followed by open long term clinical evaluation. J Clin Endocrinol Metab 85:139, 2000.

40. Howlett HC, Bailey CJ: A risk benefit assessment of metformin in type 2 diabetes. Drug Saf 20(6):489–503, 1999.

41. Grant PJ: The effects of high- and medium-dose metformin therapy on the cardiovascular risk factors in patients with type 2 diabetes. Diabetes Care 19:64, 1996.

42. UK Prospective Diabetes Study (UKPDS) Group: Effect of intensive blood-glucose control with metformin on complications in overweight patients with type 2 diabetes (UKDPS 34). Lancet 352:854, 1998.

43. Dandona P, Fonseca V, Mier A, Beckett AG: Diarrhea and metformin in a diabetic clinic. Diabetes Care 6:472, 1983.

44. Bailey CJ, Turner RC: Metformin. N Engl J Med 334:574, 1996.

45. Lalau JD, Lacroix C, Compagnon P et al: Role of metformin accumulation in metformin-associated lactic acidosis. Diabetes Care 18:779, 1995.

46. Metformin Package Insert, 2002.

47. Calabrese AT, Coley KC, DaPos SV et al: Evaluation of prescribing practices: Risk of lactic acidosis with metformin therapy. Arch Intern Med 162:434, 2002.

48. Rosak C. The pathophysiologic basis of efficacy and clinical experience with new oral diabetic agents. J Diabetes Complications 16(1): 123–132, 2002.

49. Coniff RF, Shapiro JA, Robbins D et al: Reduction of glycosylated hemoglobin and post prandial hyperglycemia by acarbose in patients with NIDDM. A placebo controlled dose comparison study. Diabetes Care 18:817, 1995.

50. Hoffmann J, Spengler M: Efficacy of 24-week monotherapy with acarbose, metformin, or placebo in dietary treated NIDDM patients: The Essen-II study. Am J Med 103:483, 1997.

51. Acarbose Package Insert, 2002.

52. Krentz AJ, Ferner RE, Bailey CJ: Comparative tolerability profiles of oral antidiabetic agents. Drug Saf 11:223, 1994.

53. Saltiel AR, Olefsky JM: Thiazolidinediones in the treatment of insulin resistance and type 2 diabetes. Diabetes 45:1661, 1996.

54. Al-Salman J, Arjomand H, Kemp DG, Mittal M. Hepatocellular injury in a patient receiving rosiglitazone. A case report. Ann Int Med 132:121, 2000.

55. Correction: Liver injury and rosiglitazone. Ann Intern Med 133:237, 2000.

56. Maggs DG, Buchanan TA, Burant CF et al: Metabolic effects of troglitazone monotherapy in type 2 diabetes mellitus. A randomized double-blind placebo controlled trial. Ann Intern Med 128:176, 1998.

57. Santomauro AT, Boden G, Silva ME et al: Overnight lowering of free fatty acids with Acipimox improves insulin resistance and glucose tolerance in obese diabetic and nondiabetic subjects. Diabetes 48:1836, 1999.

58. Ziouzenkova O, Perrey S, Marx N et al: Peroxisome proliferator-activated receptors. Curr Atheroscler Rep 4:59–64, 2002.

59. Parulkar AA, Pendergrass ML, Granda-Ayala R et al: Nonhypoglycemic effects of thiazolidinediones. Ann Inter Med 134:61, 2001.

60. Ghazzi MN, Perex JE, Anonucci TK et al: Cardiac and glycemic benefits of troglitazone treatment in NIDDM. The Troglitazone Study Group. Diabetes 46:433, 1997.

61. Peuler JD, Phare SM, Iannucci AR et al: Differential inhibitory effects of antidiabetic drugs on arterial smooth muscle cell proliferation. Am J Hypertens 9:188, 1996.

62. Koshiyama H, Shimono D. Kuwamura N et al: Rapid communication: Inhibitory effect of pioglitazone on carotid arterial wall thickness in type 2 diabetes. J Clin Endo Metab 86:3452, 2001.

63. Ehrmann DA, Schneider DJ, Sobel BE et al: Troglitazone improves defects in insulin action, insulin secretion, ovarian steroidogenesis, and fibrinolysis in women with polycystic ovary syndrome. J Clin Endo Metab 82:2108, 1997.

64. Lewis JD, Lichtenstein GR, Stein RB et al: An open-label trial of the PPAR-gamma ligand rosiglitazone for active ulcerative colitis. Am J Gastro 96:3323, 2001.

65. King AB: A comparison in a clinical setting of the efficacy and side effects of three thiazolidinediones. Diabetes Care 23:557, 2000.

66. Gegich CG, Altheimer MD: Comparison of effects of thiazolidinediones on cardiovascular risk factors: Observations from a clinical practice. Endo Pract 7:162, 2001.

67. Sakamoto J, Kimura H, Moriyama S et al: Activation of human peroxisome proliferator-activated receptor (PPAR) subtypes by pioglitazone. Biochem Biophys Res Commun 278:704, 2000.

67a.Boyle PJ, King AB, Olansky L et al: Effects of pioglitazone and rosiglitazone on blood lipid levels and glycemic control in patients with type 2 diabetes mellitus: A retrospective review of randomly selected medical records. Clin Ther 24:378-396, 2002.

68. Pioglitazone Package Insert, 2002.

69. Rendell RP, Riddle MC, Dole JF et al: A randomized trial of rosiglitazone therapy in patients with inadequately treated type 2 diabetes. Diabetes Care 24:1226, 2001.

70. Glazer NB, Sanes-Miller C: Pharmacokinetics of coadministration of pioglitazone with ranitidine. Diabetes 50:455, 2001.

71. Groop LC, DeFronzo RA: Sulfonylureas. In Defronzo RA (ed): Current Therapy of Diabetes Mellitus. Mosby, St. Louis, 1998, pp. 96–101.

72. Turner RC, Cull CA, Frighi V et al: Glycemic control with diet, sulfonylurea, metformin, or insulin in patients with type 2 diabetes mellitus: Progressive requirement for multiple therapies (UKPDS 49). United Kingdom Prospective Diabetes Study (UKPDS) Group. JAMA 281:2005, 1999.

73. DeFronzo RA: Pharmacologic therapy for type 2 diabetes. Ann Intern Med 131:281, 1999.

74. Dunn CJ, Peters DH: Metformin. A review of its pharmacological properties and therapeutic use in non-insulin dependent diabetes mellitus. Drugs 49:721, 1995.

75. Hermann LS, Schersten B, Bitzen PO et al: Therapeutic comparison of metformin and sulfonylurea, alone and in various combination. A double-blind controlled study. Diabetes Care 17:1100, 1994.

76. DeFronzo RA, Goodman AM: Efficacy of metformin in patients with non-insulin-dependent diabetes mellitus. The Multicenter Metformin Study Group. N Engl J Med 333:541, 1995.

77. Rosenstock J, Brown A, Fischer J et al: Efficacy and safety of acarbose in metformin-treated patients with type 2 diabetes. Diabetes Care 21:2050, 1998.

78. Rodger NW, Chiasson JL, Josse RG et al: Clinical experience with acarbose: Results of a Canadian multicenter study. Clin Invest Med 18:318, 1995.

79. Coniff RF, Shapiro JA, Seaton TB et al: Multicenter placebo controlled trial comparing acarbose (BAY g 5421) with placebo, tolbutamide and tolbutamide-plus-acarbose in non-insulin dependent diabetes mellitus. Am J Med 98:443, 1995.

80. Hirschberg Y, Karara AH, Pietri AO et al: Improved control of mealtime glucose excursions with coadministration of nateglinide and metformin. Diabetes Care 23:349, 2000.

81. Kipnes MS, Krosnick A, Rendell MS et al: Pioglitazone hydrochloride in combination with sulfonylurea therapy improves glycemic control in patients with type 2 diabetes mellitus. Am J Med 111:10, 2001.

82. Einhorn D, Rendell M, Rosenzweig J et al: Pioglitazone hydrochloride in combination with metformin in the treatment of type 2 diabetes mellitus: A randomized, placebo-controlled study: The Pioglitazone 027 Study Group. Clin Ther 22:1395, 2000.

83. Fonseca V, Rosenstock J, Patwardhan R et al: Effect of metformin and rosiglitazone combination therapy in patients with type 2 diabetes mellitus. A randomized controlled trial. JAMA 283:1695, 2000.

84. Wolffenbuttel BH, Gomis R, Squatrito S et al: Addition of low-dose rosiglitazone to sulphonylurea therapy improves glycaemic control in type 2 diabetic patients. Diabetic Med 17:40, 2000.

85. Yale JF, Valiquett TR, Ghazzi MN et al: The effect of a thiazolidinedione drug, troglitazone, on glycemia in patients with type 2 diabetes mellitus poorly controlled with sulfonylurea and metformin. Ann Int Med 134:737–745, 2001.

86. Riddle M: Combining sulfonylureas and other oral agents. Am J Med 108:15S, 2000.

87. Garber AJ, Duncan TG, Goodman AM et al: Efficacy of metformin in type II diabetes: Results of a double-blind placebo controlled dose response trial. Am J Med 103:491–497, 1997.

88. Yki-Jarvinen H, Kauppila M, Kujansuu E et al: Comparison of insulin regimens in patients with non-insulin dependent diabetes mellitus. N Engl J Med 327:1426–1433, 1992.

89. Yki-Jarvinen H, Ryysy L, Nikkila K et al: Comparison of bedtime insulin regimens in patients with type 2 diabetes mellitus. A randomized, controlled trial. Ann Int Med 130:389, 1999.

90. Peters AL, Davidson MB: Insulin plus sulfonylurea agent for treating type 2 diabetes. Ann Intern Med 115:45, 1991.

INSULIN THERAPY

INSULIN PREPARATIONS

More types of insulin are becoming available, from the traditional insulins to insulin analogues (Table 5-1). This diversity of choice in terms of onset and duration of action allows use of exogenous insulin to mimic normal physiology more closely, thereby allowing for improvements in glycemic control with less hypoglycemia. However, the increasing numbers of insulin options on the market can make choosing which insulin preparations to order for a patient confusing. Once the pharmacology of each of the agents is understood, it can make the choice of insulin clearer, particularly if coupled with a knowledge of each individual's physiology. In addition to choices about the type of insulin, there are also an increasing number of insulin delivery systems available. For some patients, use of an insulin pen is preferred over the use of a syringe and vial.[1] However, because of variability in insurance coverage for insulin pens, it is best to train patients to use insulin initially with a vial and syringe, and then provide them with insulin delivery options subsequently.

Four properties characterize insulin preparations used for injection: concentra-

tion, species source, purity, and type—that is, certain physicochemical modifications that determine the time course of action. Choosing the concentrations and types of insulin to use require clinical judgment. Therefore these two aspects of insulin preparations are discussed at the beginning of this chapter. The choices concerning the species source and purity are less important than they used to be, because most insulin is now some form of human insulin. However, species source and purity are related to some of the side effects of insulin. Therefore these characteristics of insulin preparations are discussed later in conjunction with a description of the immunologic responses to insulin therapy.

CONCENTRATION

Insulin is usually marketed in 10-ml vials at a concentration of 100 U/ml (U-100). If a patient injects 0.5 ml, she or he receives 50 U of insulin. From another viewpoint, administration of 20 U of insulin requires injection of 0.2 ml of U-100 insulin. Fortunately, calculations by the patient are obviated by the use of syringes with the number of units marked directly on the barrel. In Europe, other concentrations of insulin can be obtained (such as U-40). Additionally, a more concentrated form of insulin known as U-500 can be purchased by special order in the United States for use in patients who require large amounts of insulin because of insulin resistance.

TIME COURSE OF ACTION

From a therapeutic point of view, three characteristics of the time course of action of the different types of insulin preparations are important: onset of action, time of peak activity, and duration of action. These depend on the rate of absorption after the subcutaneous injection. Table 5-1 summarizes the data on the insulin preparations currently on the market. These are general guidelines and may not pertain exactly to the clinical situation in which patients' physical activity and eating patterns differ from conditions imposed by the metabolic ward setting. These ranges are only approximations because of the great intrinsic variability among patients and because the response of an occasional patient may differ considerably from the values listed

VARIABILITY OF INSULIN

There are many reasons that insulin has a variable action in a given individual. The type of insulin influences variability, with lispro and aspart being the least variable (that is, they have the least intrasubject variability when injected in the same individual, and their activity is measured on different days) and lente and ultralente being the most variable.[2] The volume of a dose of insulin may alter its absorption, although this may be less true with the newer analogues.[3] The site of injection can influence rate of absorption of the insulin as well as the depth of injection (intramuscular versus subcutaneous versus intradermal).[4] Finally, regional blood flow can alter the absorption of insulin, with factors such as exercise, skin temperature and hydration status also affecting absorption.[5]

SPECIES/SOURCE

The initial insulins were created from actual animal pancreases. They were named from

TABLE 5-1 TIME COURSE OF ACTION OF INSULINS*

Type	Onset (h)	Peak (h)	Duration (h)	Mixability
Rapid-acting • Lispro • Aspart	0.25–0.50	1.0–2.0	3.0–5.0	Good
Short-acting • Regular	0.50–1.0	2.0–4.0	6.0–8.0	Good
Intermediate- acting • NPH • Lente	1.0–3.0	4.0–12.0	18.0–24.0	Good
Long-acting • Glargine • Ultralente	2–4 4–8	None 8–12 (variable)	~24 18–36	Never mix Avoid mixing
Mixtures • 70/30 • 75/25 • 50/50	Actions based on components of the mixture			

NPH, neutral protein hagedorn.
*Times are approximations; insulins may act differently in different individuals.

the species they came from: pork, beef, and beef/pork. In 1986 the first recombinant human insulin was released. Because it is human insulin, produced in *Escherichia coli*, it is less immunogenic than the older animal insulins. It has largely replaced use of the older animal insulins.

The very first type of insulin produced was regular insulin. It has no modifying agent and is the only one that should be administered intravenously (the analogs Lispro and Aspart are for subcutaneous injection only). To prolong the absorption of insulin, protamine was added and Neutral Protamine Hagedorn (NPH) insulin was created. In the lente series, insulin is buffered by acetate, and the size of the crystal determines the rate of absorption. Lente insulin has a time course of action that is indistinguishable from that of NPH insulin.

When regular insulin is injected there is a slight delay in its absorption as a result of self-aggregation that occurs between insulin molecules (Figure 5-1). Regular insulin forms a hexamer in subcutaneous tissue and must dissociate into a monomeric form to be absorbed. To overcome this problem insulin analogues have been created. An

analogue is regular human insulin that has been altered through an amino acid substitution, addition, deletion, or rearrangement that changes its activity.

We now have analogues that allow insulin to be absorbed more quickly (lispro [Humalog] and aspart [NovoLog])[6-8] (because they are monomeric) as well as more slowly (glargine [Lantus])[9-11] (because the isoelectric point is altered). Table 5-2 lists the amino acid alterations that have been made to these insulins. The rapid-acting insulins can be injected immediately before a meal, and glargine may only be needed once a day as a basal insulin (although in certain individuals it needs to be given twice a day).

USE OF INSULINS: GENERAL CONSIDERATIONS

The goal of insulin therapy is to provide insulin replacement in as physiologic a fashion as possible. Figure 5-2 shows the time course of action for the available times of insulin: rapid-, short-, intermediate- and long-acting. Ideally, for patients with type 1 diabetes, the most physiologic regimen

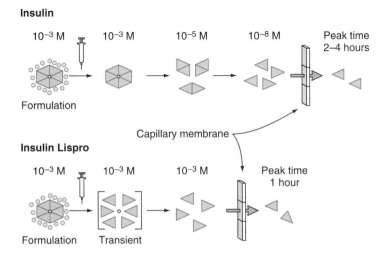

INSULIN FORMULATION
Lispro versus regular

FIGURE 5-1. Self-aggregation of regular insulin compared with the insulin analogue Lispro.

TABLE 5-2	DIFFERENCES IN AMINO ACID SEQUENCE OF DIFFERENT INSULIN ANALOGUES		
Type	**Chain**	**Alteration**	
Lispro	b-chain	Proline (b28)/lysine (b29) switched to lysine (b28)/proline (b29)	
Aspart	b-chain	Proline (b28) switched to aspartic acid (b28)	
Glargine	b-chain	Two arginines added to end (b30) of b-chain	
	a-chain	Asparagine (a21) switched to glycine (a21)	

would include use of a basal insulin combined with premeal boluses (Figure 5-3). This approach offers the most flexibility in lifestyle. However, this type of regimen requires that patients give four to six injections of insulin per day, learn how to do carbohydrate counting (for best results), and test their blood sugar levels before each insulin injection. Easier regimens, such as twice-a-day NPH and regular insulin (Figure 5-4), may require less testing by the patient, but because the patient is taking an intermediate-acting insulin (NPH) they have much less flexibility in lifestyle. The insulin will peak 6 to 12 hours after injection and the patient will need to eat at that time. Treating patients effectively with insulin requires patient education and time spent teaching patients their treatment goals. Often a patient starts with one regimen and switches to another because he or she wants to have tighter control. Overall, the goal for every patient is to keep his or her A1C level as close to normal as possible with a minimum number of hypoglycemic reactions, particularly avoiding severe reactions (that is, insulin reactions that require assistance of another for treatment).

In type 2 diabetes, in which treatment involves both reversing insulin deficiency and resistance, patients may benefit from a combination of a drug that improves insulin sensitivity (such as metformin or a glitazone) plus insulin.[12,-15] In each case, the treatment should be individualized—many patients with type 2 diabetes start with the evening addition of NPH insulin or glargine, with the goal of normalizing the fasting blood glucose level.[16-18] Some patients do well on this regimen, whereas others need the addition of premeal short- or rapid-acting insulin.

INSULIN TIME ACTION PROFILE

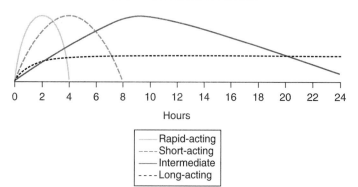

FIGURE 5-2. Time course of action of rapid-, short-, intermediate-, and long-acting insulins.

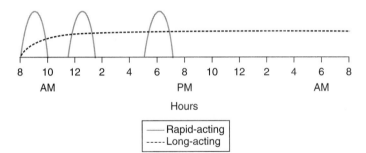

FIGURE 5-3. Use of a basal insulin with premeal insulin boluses.

Figures 5-3 and 5-4 show the usual time course of the activity of two common patterns of insulin use. To start a patient on insulin, a basal insulin should be provided. This can either be provided as NPH insulin given before breakfast and before dinner or as a morning or evening injection of glargine.[18a] Patients who are on a bedtime insulin daytime oral agent (BIDO) regimen will remain on oral agents used to control the premeal blood glucose levels. This approach is described in the following text and is a common approach for using insulin in patients with type 2 diabetes. When starting patients on an insulin-only regimen, preprandial insulin will need to be given in addition to the basal insulin. Patients can change from one type of insulin to another as their responses to insulin become apparent and their involvement in their diabetes

management evolves. The key to using insulin in the treatment of type 1 or type 2 diabetes is use of self-monitoring of blood glucose (SMBG) with assessment of a patient's response and need for the addition of (or for changes in) basal and preprandial insulin doses.

In patients on twice-a-day NPH, patients should test their blood glucose levels before meals and at bedtime. The NPH doses should bring the fasting and predinner blood glucose levels into the near normal range (80 to 140 mg/dl). If the prelunch and prebedtime blood glucose levels are high (40 mg/dl greater than the prebreakfast or predinner blood glucose level), then a short- or rapid-acting insulin should be added to the NPH. Rapid-acting insulins have the advantage of working immediately after injection, so that patients do not need

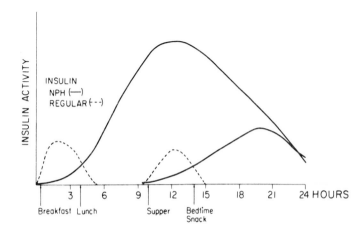

FIGURE 5-4. Time course of action of two injections of insulin. *(From Davidson MB: The case for control in diabetes mellitus. West J Med 129:193, 1978.)*

to wait between injecting the insulin and eating. They also cause less postmeal hypoglycemia because their activity tends to more closely follow the pattern of ingested carbohydrates.[7]

In general, between two thirds and three fourths of the intermediate-acting insulin is given in the morning and the remainder before supper (or before bedtime). If short- or rapid-acting insulin is also required, 4 to 8 U at each time usually suffices (in nonobese patients). Ideally, *only after the appropriate dose of intermediate-acting insulin has been established should short- or rapid-acting insulin be added.* In a patient starting on long-acting insulin, premeal rapid-acting insulin needs to be started simultaneously. In patients taking intermediate-acting insulin, short-/rapid-acting insulin is usually necessary in the morning to handle the breakfast calories because of the lag period before NPH insulin starts to work. Even though the intermediate-acting insulin administered in the morning exerts its maximal effect in the afternoon and early evening, an amount appropriate to cover the interval

before supper may be inadequate to cover the mealtime hyperglycemia. In that case, short-/rapid-acting insulin should be added to the second insulin injection if given before supper. If not, the short-/rapid-acting insulin should be given before supper and the intermediate-/long-acting insulin given at bedtime. The advantage of this approach is that each component of the insulin prescription can be regulated independently (Table 5-3). Thus, as can be deduced from the intervals of maximal action of the various insulin preparations (see Table 5-1), the blood test that best reflects the patient's response to the morning NPH insulin injection is the one before supper; the following morning's test is the best indicator of the effect of NPH insulin given before supper (or bedtime); the test before lunch best reflects the action of rapid- or short-acting insulin given before breakfast; and the test at bedtime is the most sensitive indicator of the action of rapid- or short-acting insulin received before supper. In patients who are striving to obtain nearly normal blood glucose levels, a 2-hour postpran-

TABLE 5-3	PERIOD DURING WHICH GLUCOSE IS CONTROLLED BY VARIOUS COMPONENTS OF THE INSULIN REGIMEN AND TIMING OF TESTS REFLECTING THAT ACTIVITY		
Insulin	Time Injected	Period of Activity	Test Reflecting Insulin Action
Rapid- or short-acting insulin	Before a meal	Between that meal and either the subsequent one or the bedtime snack (if insulin is taken before supper)	Two-h postprandial blood glucose level Blood glucose level prior to next meal or snack
Intermediate-acting (e.g., NPH)	Before breakfast	Generally between lunch and supper	Before supper
Intermediate-acting	Before supper or bedtime	Overnight	Before breakfast
Long-acting (e.g., glargine)	Before bedtime	Overnight (although acts throughout the next day as well)	Before breakfast

NPH, neutral protein hagedorn.

dial blood glucose level may be the most useful in terms of assessing the adequacy of the premeal insulin dose. Therefore obtaining occasional 2-hour prandial blood glucose levels, particularly after the meal containing the highest carbohydrate content, can also be helpful in guiding insulin dosing.

Because of the clear evidence that strict diabetic control is beneficial in attenuating the microvascular and neuropathic complications of diabetes, an increasing number of physicians and their patients are attempting to achieve near euglycemia. When a split/mixed (i.e., NPH and regular) insulin regimen is used with this goal in mind, patients have relatively limited flexibility in their eating patterns. Not only must their meals not be delayed, but the amount of carbohydrate in each meal must be close to the prescribed amount, or hypoglycemia is likely to occur (unless the patient does carbohydrate counting and adjusts the short- or rapid-acting insulin before breakfast and supper). In addition, extra exercise may also pose a problem because of the enhanced absorption from the large depots of injected

insulin. Patients have much more flexibility in regard to both eating and exercise with four to six injections of insulin each. With this approach, rapid-acting insulin is taken before each meal or snack, and the test after the meal or before the next one reflects the effectiveness of that dose. For instance, an injection before lunch is judged by the result of the postprandial lunch test or the presupper test. Control of glucose levels overnight is provided by glargine insulin injected before bedtime (in a separate syringe). Alternatively, patients can be managed on an insulin pump.

Five different insulin regimens are described in Table 5-4. Certain caveats should be kept in mind with each of the regimens listed. In regimens A and B (as already mentioned), patients have the least flexibility with regard to the timing and content of meals. Hypoglycemia is most likely to occur with these two regimens if meals are delayed. In regimen A, the intermediate-acting insulin taken before supper may have peak activity in the middle of the night rather than toward morning in some

TABLE 5-4 VARIOUS INSULIN REGIMENS

Regimen	Before Breakfast	Before Lunch	Before Supper	Before Bedtime
A	NPH/short- or rapid-acting insulin*	—	NPH/short- or rapid-acting insulin*	
B	NPH/short- or rapid-acting insulin*		Short- or rapid-acting insulin	NPH
C	Short- or rapid-acting insulin	Short- or rapid-acting insulin	Short- or rapid-acting insulin	Glargine†
D	Daytime oral agent(s)			Glargine or NPH
E	Insulin pump therapy with rapid-acting insulin (usually, although short-acting insulin can also be used), using both a basal rate(s) as well as premeal bolus of insulin			

NPH, neutral protein hagedorn.
*Can be given as premixed or self-mixed insulin.
†Glargine should not be mixed with any other insulins. In some individuals it can be given before breakfast or split between breakfast and bedtime.

patients. In this situation, increasing the dose may lead to hypoglycemic reactions overnight before the target level of glucose before breakfast is achieved. If this should occur, switching the intermediate-acting insulin to before bedtime (regimen B) should solve the problem. Alternatively, the NPH insulin can be changed to glargine and regimen C followed. With glargine insulin (regimen C) some patients may need to split the dose and take it twice a day. The need for this is suggested by a normal fasting glucose level combined with a high predinner blood glucose level. Occasionally, patients benefit from switching the dose of glargine from bedtime to prebreakfast, instead of splitting it. Another caveat concerning glargine insulin is that because its duration of action is so long, the effect of changing the dose may not become apparent for 2 to 3 days, until a new equilibrium is reached. Finally, with regimen D, late-morning or late-afternoon hypoglycemia may occur after the fasting glucose level is lowered by bedtime NPH or glargine insulin, even though the patient had been in poor control with maximal doses of oral agents previously. In that case, the dose of the oral agent that increases insulin secretion (a sulfonylurea agent or repaglinide or nateglinide) should be decreased.

INITIATION OF INSULIN THERAPY IN HOSPITALIZED PATIENTS

Although initiating insulin therapy in an outpatient or office setting is common, how it may be done in the hospital is described first because the general principles are the same regardless of the location. The initial dose of insulin given to a patient is to some extent empirically based. Lean individuals are given 12 to 15 U of NPH insulin: 8 to 10 U before breakfast and 4 to 5 U before supper. Obese patients (>125% of desirable body weight) receive a total of 30 U of NPH

insulin: 20 U in the morning and 10 U in the evening. A patient's response is monitored closely, and the amounts of intermediate-acting insulin are adjusted accordingly, usually by 4 or 5 U at a time initially. In extremely obese patients and in any others with plasma glucose levels exceeding 300 mg/dl, increments of 8 to 10 U may initially be advisable to achieve control faster. (An important point to remember is that these results are obtained at times of maximal action of NPH insulin and that glucose concentrations presumably are even higher at other times.) In the early stages of therapy with NPH insulin, amounts are adjusted daily.

For patients receiving intermediate-acting insulin twice a day, glucose concentrations in blood glucose measurements before breakfast and before supper determine what adjustments should be made in the amounts of NPH insulin administered. If a patient's hospital stay is to be minimized, these test results must be made available in time to change the appropriate NPH insulin dose if necessary. Because the amount of insulin given before breakfast depends on the result of the test before supper on the preceding day, this result must be communicated to the physician during the evening. By the same token, the fasting glucose concentration must be made available to the physician during the day so that the evening NPH insulin dose can be altered if necessary.

The physician should write insulin orders on a continuing basis (rather than repeated orders for one dose only) to ensure that the patient receives insulin at the proper times. Even if an appropriate change in dose is not made, at least the previous dose will automatically be given, and the orderly flow of gradually increasing amounts of insulin will not be interrupted. If the physician orders each insulin dose or each day's insulin prescription separately (with the intent of using the most recent appropriate glucose results to determine the amount of insulin given the next day), he or she may for some reason fail to write a particular order, and valuable time is lost. Even if the error is caught quickly and the patient receives insulin late, the response to that dose may not accurately reflect the efficacy of injected insulin because of the altered relation between the times of peak insulin action and meals. If the patient has been approaching reasonable control and his or her control deteriorates significantly because a dose is missed, the amount of insulin required to return to the control attained previously may exceed the requirement once control has been regained. (For reasons that are not entirely clear, diabetic patients are often less sensitive to insulin when their glucose levels are very high than when these levels are more near normal. This is termed *glucose toxicity*.) In instances such as these, hospitalization is prolonged, and with current daily hospital rates, such errors can be expensive.

Diabetic control should not be too tight in patients who are started on insulin in the hospital. Their diets, exercise, and emotional pattern will almost certainly be different when they return to the usual home environment, and these changes will certainly influence the insulin requirements. Therefore the goal while these patients are in the hospital is to achieve preprandial glucose concentrations of less than 200 mg/dl. Intermediate-acting insulin is used alone until the prebreakfast and presupper values are lowered to these levels. At this point, short-/rapid-acting insulin is added in small amounts (if necessary) to attain similar levels of glucose before lunch and before the bedtime snack. However, in today's climate of shortened hospital stays, if insulin is started in the hospital, a small, fixed amount (2 to 4 U in lean and obese patients, respectively) of short- or rapid-acting insulin is added to each injection of NPH insulin. In this manner, patients can be taught how to mix insulins while in the hospital; this may be important if outpatient education is difficult to arrange. Generally, short-/rapid-acting insulin is not added until the corre-

sponding fasting and presupper glucose concentrations are <200 mg/dl. If one starts to adjust the amounts of regular insulin immediately, more may be required when the prebreakfast or presupper glucose concentration is higher than when lower. For instance, 20 U of regular insulin before breakfast may not lead to hypoglycemia before lunch if the fasting glucose value is 250 mg/dl, but may do so after the prebreakfast value has been reduced to 150 mg/dl by increasing evening doses of NPH insulin. Sometimes, however, to achieve control more rapidly, short-/rapid-acting insulin can be added sooner, with the knowledge that the dose will be decreased as the prebreakfast and predinner blood sugar levels fall to prevent hypoglycemia. Once all preprandial and bedtime snack glucose concentrations are <200 mg/dl in the hospital, the patient is discharged and final adjustments of the insulin doses are carried out in the usual home environment. The illustrative case study that follows brings out these points.

CASE STUDY

PATIENT 1

This 48-year-old woman has had diabetes mellitus for 3 years. She is 5 feet 2 inches tall, has a medium frame, and currently weighs 165 pounds. Despite institution of an 1100-calorie diet (which, she admits, is difficult for her to follow) and treatment with 10 mg of glyburide twice per day and pioglitazone 45 mg per day (metformin was not tolerated because of gastrointestinal side effects), her fasting plasma glucose levels consistently exceed 250 mg/dl. She tests her blood glucose levels rarely. The patient has only mild symptoms of polyuria and polydipsia. Because of her failure to respond to maximal tolerated doses of oral agents, she is started on insulin therapy during a hospital admission for chest pain.

The patient agrees to test her blood sugar levels twice a day once discharged. Because the weight of the patient exceeds 125% of her desirable body weight (which is approximately

110 pounds), a 20 U–10 U split NPH regimen is initially prescribed. Her oral agents are stopped. The patient's response to insulin is summarized in the flow sheet in Table 5-5. She is discharged with a prescription for 45 U of NPH and 8 U of regular insulin before breakfast and 20 U of NPH and 8 U of regular insulin before supper.

COMMENT

A simple flow sheet like the one shown in Table 5-5 is extremely helpful in monitoring the progress of a patient. Anyone reviewing the chart can quickly and easily determine the patient's degree of diabetic control and response to insulin. Whether as an outpatient or an inpatient, the blood glucose flow log should be available for review by members of the diabetes health care team.

With regard to the patient just described, the initial morning injection of 20 U of NPH insulin was clearly suboptimal because the 1600 glucose level (i.e., at 4 PM) was 306 mg/dl. As the morning dose of NPH insulin was increased, the glucose concentration before supper gradually decreased to acceptable levels. Similarly, the initial amount of NPH insulin (10 U) given before supper was inadequate; the next morning's fasting glucose concentration was 254 mg/dl. Increases over several days to a dose of 20 U in the evening finally brought the fasting glucose level below 200 mg/dl. Note that the morning and evening insulin doses were adjusted independently of each other. For example, on 9/22 the morning dose of NPH insulin was increased, whereas the evening dose remained the same.

It is a common practice to measure glucose levels routinely before meals and the bedtime snack, especially if bedside monitoring on samples

TABLE 5-5	FLOW SHEET SHOWING RESPONSE OF PATIENT 1 TO INITIATION OF INSULIN THERAPY			
		Blood Glucose[a]	Insulin (U)	
Date	Time	(mg/dl)	NPH	Regular
9/19	0800	285		
	0920		20	
	1600	306	10	
	2200	328		
9/20	0700	254	30	
	1100	333		
	1600	278	15	
	2200	346		
9/21	0700	222	40	
	1100	280		
	1600	232	20	
	2200	302		
9/22	0700	172	45	
	1100	248		
	1600	163	20	
	2200	278		
9/23	0700	178	45	4
	1100	210		
	1600	152	20	4
	2200	223		
9/24	0700	165	45	8
	1100	183		
	1600	157	20	8
	2200	195		
9/25	0700	172	45	8

NPH, neutral protein Hagedorn.

produced by a finger stick is ordered. However, in keeping with the approach discussed earlier, the prelunch and bedtime values of 9/20 and 9/21 were ignored (i.e., no short-/rapid-acting insulin was added to the appropriate NPH insulin injections). Importantly, no extra short-/rapid-acting insulin was given for these elevated glucose levels at the time they were obtained. If that had been done, the subsequent glucose concentrations (i.e., before supper if short-/rapid-acting insulin had been given before lunch, and the next day's fasting glucose value if short-/rapid-acting insulin had been given at bedtime) would not reflect the effect of the corresponding NPH insulin alone. The action of both the short-/rapid-acting and intermediate-acting insulins would have coincided. If this had occurred, valuable information about the effect of the dose of NPH insulin would have been lost. However, once the prebreakfast and supper glucose levels fell to below 200 mg/dl on 9/22, the prelunch and bedtime snack values were taken into consideration. A gradual increase of regular insulin added to the morning and evening NPH insulin lowered these concentrations to less than 200 mg/dl.

• • •

P A T I E N T   1   (Revisited)

Let us assume that this patient is willing and capable of learning SMBG and that her physician is able to initiate insulin therapy in the office setting. She is seen in the afternoon, and it is decided to place her on a mixed/split insulin regimen (i.e., NPH and regular insulin taken before breakfast and before supper). The diabetes educator teaches her to perform SMBG, and her blood glucose is 295 mg/dl (Table 5-6). By now it is late afternoon, and the timing of the insulin injection is nearly before her usual supper time. Because she is obese, the 20 U–10 U split NPH regimen is initially prescribed. (No regular insulin is given until the prebreakfast and presupper SMBG values are lowered to <150 mg/dl.) She is taught to draw up 10 U of NPH insulin into a syringe, and with the help of the diabetes educator, it is injected subcutaneously into the abdomen. The patient is told to discontinue her oral agents. She returns the next morning before breakfast, and the diabetes educator supervises the performance of SMBG. This value is 254

mg/dl. Again under supervision by the diabetes educator, the patient draws up 20 U of NPH insulin into the syringe and injects it subcutaneously into the abdomen. She is also taught the signs, symptoms, and treatment of hypoglycemia. Because her fasting blood glucose concentration is so high, her presupper NPH insulin dose is increased to 14 U. She is asked to perform SMBG (and record the values in the glucose monitoring book given to her) before breakfast and before supper each day and to return one more time the next morning before breakfast. At that time, the patient's insulin administration and SMBG techniques are reviewed and both her prebreakfast and presupper NPH insulin doses are increased based on the corresponding glucose values obtained the evening before (252 mg/dl) and that morning (216 mg/dl) (see Table 5-6). She is instructed in the time course of action of NPH insulin and asked to call the office every 2 to 3 days for adjustment of her NPH insulin doses.

On 4/14, both doses of NPH insulin were raised because of elevated corresponding SMBG values (see Table 5-6). On 4/17, the glucose values for the previous several days before breakfast and supper were above 150 mg/dl, and therefore no further increases were made in the NPH insulin doses. The patient was told to start measuring before lunch and before the bedtime snack to ascertain the need for regular insulin. If these were above 150 mg/dl, she was to be seen in the office to learn how to mix regular insulin with NPH insulin in the same syringe. This occurred in the afternoon of 4/19, at which time 4 U of regular insulin was added to both NPH doses and she was taught the time course of action of the short-acting insulin. When she called on 4/22, the before supper dose of regular insulin was increased to 6 U because of elevated glucose values before her bedtime snack on the previous three evenings. The dose of morning regular insulin was not changed because the prelunch glucose values were approximately 150 mg/dl. A further increase to 8 U in the before supper dose of regular insulin was made on 4/25 because the prebedtime snack glucose levels were still less than 150 mg/dl. When she called on 4/27, she was told to send in her SMBG results in 1 month because almost all of the values were now less than 150 mg/dl. Final adjustments to achieve goal values of less than 120 mg/dl with minimal

TABLE 5-6 FLOW SHEET SHOWING RESPONSE OF PATIENT 1 TO INITIATION OF INSULIN THERAPY IN AN OFFICE SETTING (MIXED/SPLIT REGIMEN)

	Before Breakfast	Before Lunch	Before Supper	Before Bedtime*
4/10				
SMBG (mg/dl)			295	
Insulin dose (U)			10 NPH	
4/11				
SMBG (mg/dl)	254		252	
Insulin dose (U)	20 NPH		14 NPH	
4/12				
SMBG (mg/dl)	216		222	
Insulin dose (U)	24 NPH		18 NPH	
4/13				
SMBG (mg/dl)	183		198	
Insulin dose (U)	24 NPH		18 NPH	
4/14†				
SMBG (mg/dl)	176		202	
Insulin dose	24 NPH		20 NPH	
4/15				
SMBG (mg/dl)	142		153	
Insulin dose (U)	28 NPH		20 NPH	
416				
SMBG (mg/dl)	138		142	
Insulin dose (U)	28 NPH		20 NPH	
4/17†				
SMBG (mg/dl)	146		144	
Insulin dose (U)	28 NPH		20 NPH	
4/18				
SMBG (mg/dl)	132	213	162	247
Insulin dose (U)	28 NPH		20 NPH	
4/19				
SMBG (mg/dl)	142		146	
Insulin dose (U)	28 NPH	208	20 NPH/4 Reg	203
4/20				
SMBG (mg/dl)	129		132	
Insulin dose (U)	28 NPH/4 Reg	154	20 NPH/4 Reg	212
4/21				
SMBG (mg/dl)	135		148	
Insulin dose (U)	28 NPH/4 Reg	142	20 NPH/4 Reg	196
4/22†				
SMBG (mg/dl)	128		141	
Insulin dose (U)	28 NPH/4 Reg	139	20 NPH/6 Reg	163
4/23				
SMBG (mg/dl)	119		161	
Insulin dose (U)	28 NPH/4 Reg	145	20 NPH/6 Reg	191
4/24				
SMBG (mg/dl)	132		146	
Insulin dose (U)	28 NPH/4 Reg	151	20 NPH/6 Reg	183
4/25†				
SMBG (mg/dl)	135		138	
Insulin dose (U)	28 NPH/4 Reg	142	20 NPH/8 Reg	147

TABLE 5-6	FLOW SHEET SHOWING RESPONSE OF PATIENT 1 TO INITIATION OF INSULIN THERAPY IN AN OFFICE SETTING (MIXED/SPLIT REGIMEN)—CONT'D			
	Before Breakfast	Before Lunch	Before Supper	Before Bedtime*
4/26				
SMBG (mg/dl)	121		132	
Insulin dose (U)	28 NPH/4 Reg	148	20 NPH/8 Reg	138
4/27†				
SMBG (mg/dl)	133			
Insulin dose (U)	28 NPH/4 Reg	151		

SMBG, Self-monitoring of blood glucose.

*Glucose should be measured before snack (if eaten).

†Phone call to office during the day.

hypoglycemia should be made to analyze glucose patterns occurring over longer periods.

. . .

PATIENT 1 (Revisited Again)

An increasingly popular insulin regimen to use for patients failing to respond to maximal doses of sulfonylurea agents is BIDO (see regimen D in Table 5-4). The concept behind BIDO therapy is simple. The evening NPH or glargine insulin lowers the fasting blood glucose level to an acceptable value, and the oral agent maintains it during the day. With the use of increasing doses of bedtime NPH or glargine insulin, the fasting blood glucose level is lowered into the normal range and the oral agents maintain the daytime glucose levels. For this approach to be successful, the postprandial excursion of glucose during the day should come back to baseline (80 to 140 mg/dl) before each meal. With the use of bedtime NPH, a high presupper blood glucose level predicts a lack of efficacy of the daytime oral agents to maintain normal glucose control. In some individuals this can be overcome by switching from NPH to bedtime glargine insulin to lower both the fasting and presupper blood glucose levels.

Let us assume that patient 1 is to be placed on BIDO therapy. Her maximal dose of glyburide

and pioglitazone are continued, and on the afternoon of 4/10 the diabetes educator is able to get her to inject saline into her abdomen and shows her how to draw up insulin into the syringe. The diabetes educator supervises the patient as she draws up 14 U of NPH insulin into an insulin syringe (lean and obese patients are started on 8 to 10 U and 14 to 16 U of NPH insulin, respectively.) The patient takes the syringe home and is instructed to inject the contents subcutaneously into her abdomen at bedtime. The patient is also taught how to perform SMBG and is told to measure her fasting blood glucose value with the machine and strips to be purchased that evening. She returns the next day, at which time the diabetes educator observes both her SMBG and injection (of saline) techniques and teaches her the signs, symptoms, and treatment of hypoglycemia. Because the patient's fasting blood glucose value that morning was 243 mg/dl (Table 5-7), her NPH dose is increased to 18 U. The diabetes educator supervises the drawing up of that amount, and the patient is told to take this dose each evening, to measure her fasting blood glucose, and to call the office with the results in 2 days. Her course is summarized in Table 5-7. She is to return to the office in 1 week for a final review of her SMBG technique and ability to draw up insulin accurately. Note that at this visit (on 4/17) her fasting glucose values were low enough (although not at target) that she was instructed to wait

TABLE 5-7	FLOW SHEET SHOWING RESPONSE OF PATIENT 1 TO INITIATION OF BIDO THERAPY IN AN OFFICE SETTING					
Date	Fasting Blood Glucose (mg/dl)	Bedtime NPH Insulin (U)	Date	Blood Glucose (mg/dl)	Bedtime NPH Insulin (U)	
4/10		14	4/18	132	26	
4/11	243	18	4/19	135	26	
4/12	196	18	4/20	128	26	
4/13*	208	22	4/21	142	26	
4/14	172	22	4/22	137	26	
4/15*	163	24	4/23	131	26	
4/16	148	24	4/24*	129	28	
4/17†	144	26				

*Phone call to office.
†Office visit.

another week before calling the office. The response to that call (on 4/24) was to increase the NPH dose slightly, to begin monitoring before supper, and to send the results to the office in 1 month. To reiterate, to avoid hypoglycemia when a patient is approaching the lower target goals, the final adjustments should be made only after analysis of glucose patterns over longer periods (at least several weeks).

If a patient is capable of following a simple algorithm, it is possible to reduce the number of calls to the office. The algorithm summarized in Table 5-8 is very useful in the initial dose adjustments until the fasting blood glucose level decreases to less than 150 mg/dl. At that point, the patient is asked to send in the results each month.

BIDO therapy is particularly useful in type 2 diabetic patients who fail to respond to maximal doses of oral agents and who are reluctant to start insulin. One injection and (at least initially) one finger stick for SMBG a day is easier to sell than two or more injections and two to four fingersticks per day. Importantly, a patient's life style is less interrupted in terms of eating and exercise patterns with BIDO therapy. Several studies compared BIDO therapy (using a sulfonylurea agent) with two or more injections of insulin and found no difference in the level of diabetic control achieved after 3[19] or 6[18,20] months. In one study,[21] excellent control was maintained for a year with bedtime NPH and daytime glipizide. Patients who take an evening shot of NPH with daytime metformin tend to have improved glycemic control with less weight

TABLE 5-8	INITIATION OF BIDO THERAPY[a] IN PATIENTS ABLE TO FOLLOW SIMPLE ALGORITHM AND SELF-ADJUST NPH INSULIN DOSES OR GLARGINE DOSES		
		Lean	Obese
Initial dose		8–10 U	14–16 U
FBG >200 mg/dl for 2 days in a row		Increase by 2 U	Increase by 4 U
FBG between 150–200 mg/dl for 2 days in a row[b]		Increase by 1 U	Increase by 2 U

[a]Goal is fasting blood glucose (FBG) <150 mg/dl; to lower to <120 mg/dl, glucose pattern over a longer period of time should be analyzed.
[b]Applies if one day >200 mg/dl and the next day between 150-200 mg/dl or vice versa.

gain when compared with regimens using sulfonylurea agents or twice daily insulin.[16] Patients with type 2 diabetes on two or more injections of insulin per day may have an improvement in their A1C levels with the addition of metformin[12,13] or a glitazone.[14,15] Combination therapy with oral agents and glargine insulin is also effective. Glargine can lower glucose levels throughout 24 hours without hypoglycemia and can be an effective alternative to NPH. Glargine can also be given in the morning or evening, depending on which is easier for a patient to fit into his or her lifestyle.

• • •

PATIENT 2

A 27-year-old financial planner reports a 3-week history of increasing urination, thirst, and a 6-pound weight loss despite an increased appetite. He denies blurring of vision or a family history of diabetes. Additionally, he denies signs or symptoms of infection or a coexisting illness and is able to eat and drink normally. He is 5 feet 11 inches tall and weighs 155 pounds. A glucose value measured on a meter is 420 mg/dl, and his urine shows 2% glucose and strong ketone bodies. His breathing appears normal. It is late morning. The patient has blood drawn for serum electrolyte and acetoacetate measurement, he is given 5 U of rapid acting insulin subcutaneously, and his diabetes education is begun.

His laboratory values are as follows: Na, 135 mEq/L; K, 3.6 mEq/L; Cl, 98 mEq/L; HCO_3, 22 mEq/L; and acetoacetate trace positive in the undiluted serum. Based on these results, the patient is told he has new-onset type 1 diabetes, nearing ketoacidosis, and will require immediate initiation of insulin therapy. Mixed/split, multiple injection (rapid-acting insulin before each meal and bedtime glargine insulin) and insulin pump therapy are described to him. Because of a variable eating schedule (erratic timing of meals because of meetings with clients) as well as an inconstant exercise pattern, he chooses the multiple injection regimen with an interest in learning about the pump at a later date.

He is taught SMBG and how to draw up insulin into a syringe. The initial doses for this regimen that are as follows: for lean patients, 4 to 5 U of premeal rapid acting insulin and 8 to 10 U of bedtime glargine insulin; for obese patients, 8

to 10 U of premeal rapid acting insulin and 14 to 16 U of glargine insulin. He was started on the former regimen because he is lean. He is taught a simple correction dose algorithm for his premeal rapid acting insulin: Add 1 unit of insulin for every 50 units above 150 mg/dl. He was instructed to measure his blood glucose levels before each meal and his bedtime snack, and to return to the office the next day to review and reinforce the material that had just been taught and to be trained on the use of an insulin pen, to use for his premeal insulin. In addition, an appointment was made with the dietitian to instruct him on topics such as carbohydrate counting (a good rule of thumb to start carbohydrate counting is for patients to take 1 unit of rapid-acting insulin for every 15 g of carbohydrate they eat, in addition to their correction dose instead of giving a fixed premeal insulin dose).

His course is summarized in Table 5-9. Note that the glargine insulin dose was increased the next day at the office visit because of the elevated fasting glucose value, but that the doses of rapid-acting insulin were increased more slowly because the differences between the preprandial levels were fairly low. That is, the amount of rapid-acting insulin given before a meal was able to bring the postprandial glucose rise back to the preprandial level. This *delta response* to rapid-acting insulin is a useful index of the efficacy of the dose. If the succeeding preprandial glucose concentration (i.e., before the next meal or bedtime snack) was much higher, more rapid-acting insulin would be needed. Conversely, if the preprandial level could be lowered (e.g., by increasing the bedtime glargine insulin), an amount of rapid-acting insulin that yielded a small delta response between two meals (or between supper and the bedtime snack) would provide near euglycemia throughout the day. If preprandial glucose values are high and enough rapid-acting insulin is given to achieve satisfactory levels before the next meal, hypoglycemia will ensue once the high preprandial glucose concentrations are lowered. For this reason, doses of rapid-acting insulin should be raised cautiously when initiating insulin therapy until preprandial glucose concentrations are satisfactory. Or patients can be taught to base their preprandial doses based on carbohydrate counting and a compensatory scale for extra insulin if the blood glucose levels are

TABLE 5-9 FLOW SHEET SHOWING RESPONSE OF PATIENT 2 TO INITIATION OF INSULIN THERAPY IN AN OFFICE SETTING (PREPRANDIAL REGULAR/BEDTIME GLARGINE)

	Before Breakfast	Before Lunch	Before Supper	Before Bedtime*
5/23[b]				
SMBG (mg/dl)		420	333	286
Insulin dose (U)		4 rapid-acting insulin	4 rapid-acting insulin	8 glargine
5/24[b]				
SMBG (mg/dl)	243	268	222	193
Insulin (U)	4 rapid-acting insulin	4 rapid-acting insulin	4 rapid-acting insulin	10 glargine
5/25				
SMBG (mg/dl)	208	175	196	200
Insulin (U)	4 rapid-acting insulin	4 rapid-acting insulin	4 rapid-acting insulin	10 glargine
5/26[†]				
SMBG (mg/dl)	183	188	155	182
Insulin (U)	4 rapid-acting insulin	5 rapid-acting insulin	5 rapid-acting insulin	12 glargine
5/27				
SMBG (mg/dl)	152	163	145	175
Insulin (U)	5 rapid-acting insulin	5 rapid-acting insulin	5 rapid-acting insulin	12 glargine
5/28				
SMBG (mg/dl)	148	172	139	163
Insulin (U)	5 rapid-acting insulin	5 rapid-acting insulin	6 rapid-acting insulin	14 glargine
5/29				
SMBG (mg/dl)	135	154	128	148
Insulin (U)	6 rapid-acting insulin	5 rapid-acting insulin	6 rapid-acting insulin	14 glargine
5/30[‡]				
SMBG (mg/dl)	129	163	137	162
Insulin (U)	6 rapid-acting insulin	5 rapid-acting insulin	6 rapid-acting insulin	14 glargine
5/31				
SMBG (mg/dl)	131	172	148	182
Insulin (U)	6 rapid-acting insulin	5 rapid-acting insulin	6 rapid-acting insulin	14 glargine
6/1[‡]				

SMBG (mg/dl)	125	148	125	151
Insulin (U)	6 rapid-acting insulin	5 rapid-acting insulin	7 rapid-acting insulin	14 glargine
6/2				
SMBG (mg/dl)	133	127	119	147
Insulin (U)	7 rapid-acting insulin	5 rapid-acting insulin	7 rapid-acting insulin	14 glargine
6/3†				
SMBG (mg/dl)	121	138		
Insulin (U)	7 rapid-acting insulin	5 rapid-acting insulin		

SMBG, self-monitoring of blood glucose.

*Glucose should be measured before snack (if eaten).

†Office visit.

‡SMBG results phoned to office.

high, which allows for maximal flexibility and takes away the risk for hypoglycemia that could occur if fixed doses are used.

USE OF URINE TESTS TO INITIATE INSULIN THERAPY

Meters for glucose monitoring are now widely available and take only 5 to 15 seconds to measure the blood glucose level. However, an occasional patient may still prefer to perform urine testing for glucose. Additionally, it may be useful to have patients test their urine for glucose when they awaken to urinate in the middle of the night—it helps to differentiate between nocturia resulting from high levels of glucose in the urine and other causes. Detailed examples of how to monitor patients with urine testing can be found in earlier editions of this textbook.

PREMIXED INSULINS

Premixed insulin preparations, either commercially available containing either 70% NPH insulin and 30% regular insulin (70/30), 50% NPH insulin and 50% regular insulin (50/50), 75% neutral protamine lispro and 25% lispro (75/25), 70% neutral protamine aspart and 30% aspart (70/30) or insulins mixed by family members or diabetes educators in syringes (or bottles) with various proportions of intermediate- and short-acting insulins, are increasingly being used, especially for older patients who have difficulty mixing insulins. The relationship between each test and the individual component of the insulin prescription for both two injections (see Table 5-1) and one injection per day (discussed earlier) applies to premixed insulins as well. However, there are certain constraints on adjusting doses because the amounts of both intermediate-acting and short-/rapid-acting insulins are being changed concomitantly.

The general rule to follow is that the lowest glucose value limits the dose. For instance, in a patient taking two injections of premixed insulin, the morning dose can be increased as long as neither the prelunch or presupper glucose level is too low. If either of these declines below the target range or the patient experiences unexplained hypoglycemia between breakfast and lunch or between lunch and supper, the dose cannot be increased any further and indeed probably needs to be decreased slightly. This should occur even if one of the test results (before lunch or before supper) is too high. Similarly, the presupper injection of premixed insulin can be increased as long as the prebed and fasting test results are not too low and unexplained hypoglycemia does not occur between supper and breakfast. If either test results are too low or unexplained hypoglycemia occurs during this period, the dose of the premixed insulin must be adjusted downward accordingly. The situation is a little more complex in a patient taking a single daily injection of premixed insulin. Any test result that is too low or unexplained hypoglycemia at any time necessitates decreasing the dose even if three of the four test values are too high. Thus, although using premixed insulins may be easier for patients, their use usually leads to higher glucose levels than if the doses of NPH and regular insulin could be adjusted separately.

TREATMENT OF HOSPITALIZED PATIENTS WITH INSULIN

There is increasing literature to suggest that patients with higher blood glucose levels presenting with events such as stroke,[22] have poorer outcomes than do patients with more normal blood glucose levels. Additionally, nondiabetic and diabetic patients with conditions such as sepsis in the intensive care unit (ICU)[23] to postmyocardial infarction[24] to postcoronoray artery bypass surgery[25] have improved outcomes with the inpatient use of insulin for even mildly elevated blood glucose levels. However, insulin is often used incorrectly in hospitalized patients. This is often due to a constellation of findings including disruption of normal routines and food intake, fear of hypoglycemia, and stress of illness leading to insulin resistance. Additionally, sliding scale insulin therapy is often prescribed, even though when used inappropriately this leads to worse, not improved, outcomes.[26]

Two principles guide a physician in using insulin. First, insulin should be administered in anticipation of subsequent events so that it is available to *prevent* inordinate hyperglycemia. This can be done through the use of a basal long-acting insulin such as glargine or with doses of NPH insulin given every 12 hours. In patients receiving total parenteral nutrition, regular insulin should be given mixed in with the parenteral nutritional solution and in patients treated in an ICU, insulin drips based on standardized protocols can be very helpful at maintaining normal glucose levels.

Second, sliding scales of short- or rapid-acting insulin should be applied in a standard fashion and should be used in addition to the longer-acting insulin that is adjusted to maintain a smooth blood glucose profile. Patients already on a multiple injection regimen know what their premeal insulin requirements are, and have an idea of their own adjustment scale for high and low blood glucose levels. Patients' own knowledge of their response to insulin should never be discounted; however, while in the hospital patients may have more insulin resistance or a different routine that will require a change in their normal insulin doses.

Patients with type 1 diabetes who are not eating regularly need to have a continuous source of carbohydrate and insulin provided at all times to avoid the development of ketoacidosis. Patients with type 2 diabetes who are not eating may require very little or no insulin. Regardless, in a patient who is not eating routine meals, the longer-acting insulin should either be given every 12 hours (for NPH) or at bedtime (for glargine). Once a patient begins eating on a normal meal schedule, the insulin regimen should be adjusted to fit the new pattern, with insulin given before meals, at bedtime, or both.

SIDE EFFECTS OF INSULIN THERAPY

The side effects of insulin therapy include delayed *local* skin reactions to injected insulin, true or *systemic* insulin allergy, insulin resistance, insulin-induced lipoatrophy, and insulin-induced lipohypertrophy. Three other possible sequelae of insulin administration are considered *therapeutic* effects, not side effects. The most obvious one, of course, is hypoglycemia. The other two are associated with weight gain in patients whose diabetes was uncontrolled before the initiation or intensification of insulin therapy. These patients commonly gain weight, usually because the glucose calories that were lost in the urine in the markedly hyperglycemic state are now being stored under the influence of insulin. These formerly lost but now retained calories can account for 70% to 100% of the weight gained.[21,27] An occasional patient accumulates enough extra fluid so that localized or even generalized edema may occur.[28,29] This *insulin edema* is reversible over time (up to a month) but may be helped by a mild diuretic or in refractory cases by low-dose ephedrine.[30] Insulin normally causes sodium reabsorption in the proximal tubules of the kidneys, and it is believed that insulin edema is a very unusual manifestation of this action. It is more likely to occur in those patients whose diabetes had been markedly out of control for a long time.

Some information about the structure, biosynthesis, and purification of insulin is necessary for an understanding of the pathogenesis of these complications of insulin therapy. Insulin is a polypeptide hormone with a molecular weight of approximately 6000. As illustrated in the dark area of Figure 5-5, the insulin molecule consists of A and B chains joined by two disulfide bridges. In addition, a disulfide linkage connects amino acids 6 and 11 within the A chain. The steps by which insulin is synthesized in the pancreatic β-cells include (1) the formation of a single long-chain polypeptide; (2) the curving of this string of amino acids back on itself in a configuration that aligns the future A and B chains of insulin opposite each other; (3) the closing of the two disulfide bridges to form a larger

polypeptide (molecular weight, approximately 9000) called *proinsulin*, which is illustrated by the entire structure in Figure 5-5; and (4) the breaking of this curvilinear molecule at two points, yielding insulin (see Figure 5-5, solid circles) and the connecting peptide (C-peptide) (see Figure 5-5, open circles).

Insulin and C-peptide are packaged in equimolar amounts in the granules of the β-cells and released into the circulation together. C-peptide has no well-known biologic function, although some recent papers have defined an effect on endothelial and renal function.[31,32] It does serve as an important marker of insulin secretion in patients whose insulin levels cannot be measured directly (e.g., because of insulin-binding antibodies).

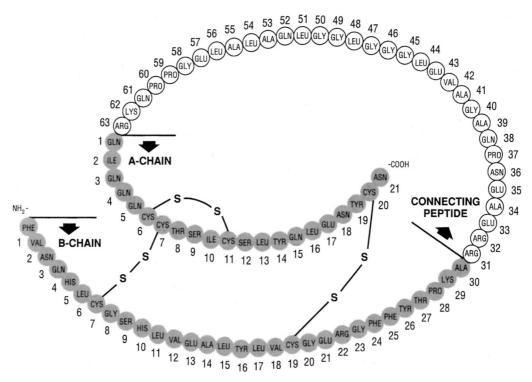

FIGURE 5-5. Structure of porcine proinsulin. Cleavage occurs at the points marked by straight lines, yielding equimolar amounts of connecting peptide and insulin. The letter *S* connected to the heavy bars represents disulfide linkages between the amino acids indicated. *(From Chance RE: Amino acid sequences of proinsulins and intermediates. Diabetes 21 [suppl 2]:461, 1972.)*

The conventional way to monitor the purity of insulin preparations is to measure the amount of proinsulin contained in them, which is expressed as parts per million (ppm). In the past 25 years, the purification of insulin preparations has improved dramatically so that now there is <10 ppm in the *impure* preparations used. The pure ones contain <1 ppm of proinsulin.

Both immunoglobulin (Ig)G and IgE antibodies to insulin are found in patients treated with insulin. Only rarely, however, do these antibodies cause clinical problems in diabetic patients. The IgE antibody seems to be directed specifically against insulin, and high titers are associated with systemic insulin allergy. The situation with regard to IgG antibodies is less clear. It was initially believed that insulin itself stimulated the formation of IgG antibodies. This antigenic response was later thought to be mainly (if not entirely) caused by the impurities (proinsulin and other larger-molecular-weight compounds) in the preparation. Although purified insulins were once thought not to be antigenic, studies clearly indicate that IgG antibodies are formed against these purer preparations.[33] Thus, although impurities enhance the IgG antibody response to insulin, insulin itself is probably mildly antigenic.

DELAYED LOCAL REACTION AT THE SITE OF INJECTION

With the earlier, more impure preparations of insulin, local skin reactions at the site of injection were common, occurring in as many as 50% of patients receiving injections for the first time. In patients who have these reactions, symptoms start within 1 month of institution of insulin therapy. A 3- to 6-hour lag period passes before the appearance of the lesions, which are characterized by pruritic, erythematous, indurated areas from 1 to 5 cm in diameter. The lesions become maximal 18 to 24 hours later and last for several days. They are often heralded by a stinging or burning sensation at the time of injection. These reactions are self-limited, invariably disappearing within 1 to 3 months. Because the prevalence and severity of these lesions had been markedly diminished by recrystallization of the older insulin preparations to rid them of contaminants, it is likely that the impurities cause these local reactions. The mechanism may involve a delayed hypersensitivity reaction.[34] In any event, use of the new, more pure preparations has alleviated this problem to a large extent.

Treatment of local delayed reactions to insulin injections should be conservative. If the symptoms are not too troublesome to a patient, no therapy is indicated because the lesions will resolve spontaneously within several months. Skin reactions to the intermediate-acting insulins seem more common than those to the short-acting insulins. Delayed local reactions may occasionally be due to the zinc in the insulin preparations; such reactions can be successfully treated with zinc-free insulin.[35] Antibodies to protamine in patients taking NPH insulin are common.[36] However, the clinical manifestation of protamine allergy is not a delayed local reaction, but either an extremely rare generalized urticarial reaction occurring spontaneously[37] or an anaphylactoid reaction. The latter occurs when protamine is given to reverse heparinization after cardiac catheterization[38] or cardiac surgery[39] in approximately 1% of diabetic patients taking NPH insulin. The treatment of protamine allergy is discussed under systemic reactions to insulin.

Switching to a different insulin preparation is often helpful for the treatment of local reactions. Skin testing by an allergist can help guide the clinician in doing this, because the component causing the allergy can often be identified. Other therapeutic approaches that have been suggested include systemic use of antihistamines or local injections of antihistamines or glucocorticoids. The adverse effects of these medications must be weighed against the possible benefits in this benign situation. If local injections of an antihistamine are tried, 1 mg of diphenhydramine (Benadryl) for each 10 U of insulin can be added to the same syringe, although antihistamines may be effective only in true or systemic insulin allergy[40] (see the following text). As long as small doses of steroids are used, adrenal suppression, insulin resistance, and other adverse effects of glucocorticoid therapy should not be a problem. Two glucocorticoid preparations, hydrocortisone and dexamethasone, have been used in the same syringe with insulin. The initial doses of hydrocortisone and dexamethasone are 2 mg and 0.1 mg per injection, respectively. These amounts are gradually increased until the desired effect is achieved. The replacement doses of hydrocortisone and dexamethasone (i.e., the amounts that suppress the hypothalamic-pituitary-adrenal axis) are 20 mg and 0.75 mg, respectively. It is important to use the smallest possible effective dose—one that preferably is considerably smaller than a full replacement dose. Another important point is that the effect of dexamethasone lasts for more than 24 hours, whereas the effect of hydrocortisone lasts for approximately 8 hours. This shorter-lived effect of hydrocortisone is a theoretic argument for its use, because adrenal suppression may be less likely. On the other hand, if the local reaction flares up after the effect of the glucocorticoid wears off, dexamethasone may be the better agent.

TRUE OR SYSTEMIC INSULIN ALLERGY

NATURE OF INSULIN ALLERGY

True allergy to insulin, also called *systemic insulin allergy*, is (fortunately) rare, occurring in approximately 0.1% of diabetic patients receiving insulin. The same sort of a reaction can occur to protamine. It is much more common in patients with a history of interrupted insulin therapy than in those whose therapy has been continuous and in those who have received protamine in large doses previously. The manifestations of insulin allergy are usually seen within 1 or 2 weeks of the resumption of interrupted insulin therapy. The hallmark of true insulin allergy is an *immediate* local reaction (within 30 to 60 minutes) that gradually increases until large areas surrounding the injection site are involved. In approximately half of patients, the reaction soon spreads into a generalized urticarial pattern and is occasionally associated with angioneurotic edema or even anaphylactic shock.[41,42] These systemic reactions are often preceded by gradual increases in the severity of the immediate local reaction, which may serve as a warning that serious difficulties lie ahead unless appropriate therapy (desensitization) is instituted (in the instance of protamine allergy, a nonprotamine form of insulin can be substituted).

These immediate reactions (both local and systemic) seem to be allergic responses to the insulin molecule itself. They are rarely alleviated by the use of extremely pure insulin preparations. The clinical similarity to penicillin allergy is striking, and indeed, the immunologic characteristics of true insulin allergy are almost identical to those of penicillin allergy. Both types of allergy involve (1) exquisite sensitivity to minute amounts of the antigen on conjunctival or intradermal testing, (2) passive transfer of an antibody (identified as IgE) that is capable of sensitizing normal skin to a subsequent challenge by the antigen (i.e., a positive result of Prausnitz-Küstner test), (3) high titers (as measured by direct assays) of IgE antibodies to the particular antigen in question, and (4) successful treatment by desensitization in almost all cases. Although true insulin allergy is mediated by the same antibody (IgE) that causes atopic disease (asthma, allergic rhinitis, urticaria), patients allergic to insulin apparently have no greater predisposition to atopy than do other patients. On the other hand, one third of patients with true insulin allergy have a history of penicillin allergy.[43]

Patients with systemic insulin allergy have high titers of IgE antibodies; these levels decline rapidly (within days) after desensitization but only gradually (over months) after discontinuation of insulin.[44-46] These antibodies also characterize the immunologic response of patients who develop persistent, immediate local reactions without systemic symptoms.[47] The IgE antibodies fix to tissue mast cells (and circulating basophils). When the IgE–mast cell combination is exposed to insulin, a complicated reaction causes the degranulation of the mast cells. The material released by the mast cells is composed of chemical inflammatory mediators, including large amounts of histamine, and is responsible for the urticaria and anaphylactic symptoms exhibited by patients with true insulin allergy.

TREATMENT OF INSULIN ALLERGY

Because pork and human insulin differ slightly in their amino acid composition, it is theoretically possible that IgE antibodies may be directed against insulin from only one of these species and that switching insulin preparations may be of value. However, this approach to true insulin allergy works only very rarely and should not be tried. On the other hand, switching to an insulin analogue (lispro, aspart, or glargine) has been useful.[48-50,50a] Until the recent availability of insulin analogues, desensitization was required in almost all cases to treat patients with an allergy to insulin, whether animal or human.[51-53]). Skin testing by an allergist can be helpful; a variety of different types and species of insulin can be tested to determine if there are any that can be tolerated by the patient.

To desensitize a patient, very small but gradually increasing amounts of insulin are injected after relatively short periods. These minute doses of the antigen bind to IgE, but the amount of histamine and other chemical mediators of inflammation released by the IgE–mast cell combination is too small to cause clinical symptoms. As the dose of injected insulin is gradually increased, the amount of insulin bound to IgE is thought to increase at a slow enough pace that the resultant mast cell degranulation causes no symptoms. Eventually, all of the IgE affixed to mast cells are bound to the increasing doses in insulin and the patient can tolerate the usual therapeutic doses of insulin.

Desensitization can be achieved by either of two methods. If the patient has received insulin within the preceding 24 hours, the dose is first decreased by 80% and then increased by 3 to 5 U per injection at daily or twice-daily intervals. In this manner, many patients can be successfully desensitized. If administration of 20% of the usual insulin dose still leads to symptoms of insulin allergy, or if the patient has not received insulin within the preceding 24 hours, enough unbound IgE antibodies (affixed to mast cells) are probably present to cause difficulties. Under these conditions, injection of more than very small amounts of insulin is extremely uncomfortable for the patient and possibly dangerous; therefore a complete desensitization program is advisable.

A reasonable schedule for complete desensitization is presented in Table 5-10. The footnote to the table describes the four diluted insulin solutions used, and the table gives details of administration. All injections may be given subcutaneously. If rapid desensitization is required (i.e., if the patient's glucose levels are markedly out of control or diabetic ketoacidosis is an imminent problem and substantial amounts of insulin are needed soon), insulin is given every 30 minutes. If subtherapeutic amounts of insulin can be tolerated for a day or two, insulin is administered every 2 hours. Regular insulin is given for the first 12 injections (until a dose of 5 U is reached). After that, the required

| TABLE 5-10 | DESENSITIZATION SCHEDULE FOR PATIENTS WITH TRUE (SYSTEMIC) INSULIN ALLERGY |

Order of Doses	Solution*	Volume Injected (ml)	Amount of Insulin Injected (U)
1	D	0.1	0.001
2	D	0.2	0.002
3	D	0.4	0.004
4	C	0.1	0.01
5	C	0.2	0.02
6	C	0.4	0.04
7	B	0.1	0.1
8	B	0.2	0.2
9	B	0.5	0.5
10	A	0.1	1
11	A	0.2	2
12	A	0.5	5†

*Solutions are designed as follows: A, 1 ml of U-100 (regular insulin) + 9 ml of normal saline (final concentration, 10.0 U/ml); B, 1 ml of solution A + 9 ml of normal saline (final concentration, 1.0 U/ml); C, 1 ml of solution B + 9 ml of normal saline (final concentration, 0.1 U/ml); and D, 1 ml of solution C + 9 ml of normal saline (final concentration, 0.01 U/ml).

†Required therapeutic dose may be tried after this point.

therapeutic dose of either intermediate-acting or fast-acting insulin (depending on the circumstances) may be tried.

If a severe local or systemic reaction occurs during the gradual increase of the amount of insulin administered, the dose should be reduced by one dilution and the schedule resumed. If the weakest dilution (0.001 U) listed in Table 5-10 elicits a positive reaction, then even weaker dilutions injected *intradermally* must be tried. Tests with gradually increasing amounts above the dilution that causes no reaction should be continued.

During the course of desensitization, adequate anaphylactic precautions must be taken. Epinephrine, diphenhydramine, methylprednisolone (Solu-Medrol), and intubation equipment must be immediately available. A physician should be immediately available for at least 30 minutes after the administration of each increasing amount of insulin. If this restriction should prove difficult (during the night, for example), the continued administration of the last dilution that was well tolerated by the patient should

be performed by an experienced nurse. In this case, injections should be given at 2-hour intervals. The presence of a physician and anaphylactic precautions are mandatory when insulin-allergic patients are receiving increasing amounts of insulin because anaphylactoid reactions can occur suddenly, even when previous smaller doses of insulin administered at 30-minute intervals have not elicited any local reactions.[54]

Desensitization is successful in approximately 95% of patients manifesting systemic insulin allergy.[43] Approximately 50% of patients with persistent local reactions of the immediate type also seem to be helped by desensitization.[43] Once desensitized, these patients should not have their insulin therapy interrupted. Because a schedule calling for at least two injections a day has the theoretic advantage of supplying insulin more constantly to the circulation (as well as usually improving diabetic control), such a regimen should probably be used for all patients who have been successfully desensitized. Indeed, treatment by continuous subcutaneous insulin infusion via an insulin pump has been successful in a patient who was not helped by desensitization to highly purified pork or human insulin.[55] However, some patients may require repeated desensitization despite continuous insulin administration.

Treatment of true insulin allergy with glucocorticoids should be avoided if possible because of the effectiveness of desensitization and the long-term adverse effects of steroid therapy. However, if repeated desensitizations are ineffective, prednisone may bring relief, probably by blocking IgE production. An initial dose of 30 to 40 mg/day should be tapered as rapidly as possible to the lowest amounts feasible, with the patient's allergic manifestations serving as the endpoint. If discontinuation of prednisone is not possible within several weeks, alternate-day therapy may be tried to minimize the adverse effects of the glucocorticoid. Alternatively, injection of dexamethasone[56] or methylprednisolone[54] via the insulin syringe has also been advocated. Because so little experience with glucocorticoid therapy for patients with true insulin allergy has been reported, it is difficult to offer firm recommendations. Fortunately, the need for glucocorticoid therapy in this situation is unusual.

Some patients develop both a delayed local reaction and a true insulin allergy (immediate reaction) concurrently.[40,55] Taking a detailed history to differentiate the symptoms and signs of this biphasic insulin allergy is important because the treatment for each component may be different.[40]

Occasionally, these patients with systemic signs of allergy are not allergic to the insulin molecule but are reacting to the zinc,[37,56-58] protamine,[37,57] or diluting medium[56-58]) of the insulin preparation. Also, allergies to substances found in insulin vials and syringes, such as latex tops, can cause allergic reactions.[59] Insulin desensitization kits obtained from two pharmaceutical companies that manufacture insulin (Lilly and Novo Nordisk) contain appropriate solu-

tions for intradermal testing that allow one to make specific diagnoses.

INSULIN RESISTANCE

Clinically severe insulin resistance is defined as a situation in which a patient requires more than 200 U of insulin daily for more than 2 days. This definition was coined more than 40 years ago, when it was erroneously believed that the human pancreas secreted approximately 200 U of insulin per day. Although it is now known that the normal pancreas secretes only 20 to 40 U of insulin per day, this clinical definition is helpful because it delineates a very small group of patients with a number of unusual underlying problems.

Use of the term *insulin resistance* in this context must be clearly differentiated from its more general use to describe situations in which any impairment of insulin action is noted. (See Chapter 8 for full details on the insulin resistance syndrome.) The broad spectrum of insulin resistance includes (1) situations in which the pancreas hypersecretes a quantity of insulin that maintains carbohydrate metabolism within normal limits; (2) mild glucose intolerance; (3) definite diabetes controlled by diet alone, by oral antidiabetes medications, or by the usual amounts of injected insulin; and (4) cases in which the insulin requirement of a patient clearly falls outside the doses required by the great majority of diabetic patients. The situations to be discussed under the clinical definition of the term *insulin resistance* represent the far end of this spectrum at which the action of insulin is markedly inhibited. For instance, although every acromegalic patient with or without diabetes mellitus manifests insulin resistance in the general sense, only those few requiring the large amounts of insulin specified in the clinical definition of this term need special therapeutic considerations.

CONDITIONS ASSOCIATED WITH INSULIN RESISTANCE

The conditions associated with the clinical definition of insulin resistance are listed in Table 5-11. Infection, regardless of the causative organism, clearly is a state in which insulin resistance exists, but the mechanisms involved are unknown. The insulin requirements of most diabetic patients with infections rise, but the requirement reaches 200 U per day in only a small minority of patients. Because the host's defenses against infections caused by bacteria and certain fungi are impaired in the setting of uncontrolled diabetes, it is important to increase the insulin dose appropriately in a vigorous attempt to lower glucose concentrations.

Although obese diabetic patients require significantly more insulin than their nonobese counterparts, relatively few obese patients could be termed insulin resistant in the clinical sense of the term. There seems to be a rough correlation between a patient's degree of obesity and the insulin requirement. The clinical approach to obese diabetic patients is considered in Chapter 3.

Glucocorticoids are potent insulin antagonists that increase hepatic gluconeogenesis and interfere with the ability of insulin to enhance glucose use by the peripheral tissues. Most cases of insulin resistance secondary to Cushing's syndrome are iatrogenic—that is, glucocorticoid therapy is prescribed for treatment of other severe problems (asthma, lupus erythematosus, myasthenia gravis, rejection of transplanted organs, and so on). In general, the increase in the insulin requirement is proportional to the amount of glucocorticoids given. Thus most patients classified as clinically insulin resistant are taking at least 50 mg of prednisone or its equivalent. (That is not to say that most patients taking 50 mg or more of prednisone are clinically insulin resistant.) Noniatrogenic cases of insulin resistance caused by excessive secretion of glucocorticoids are very unusual.

Acromegaly is the clinical syndrome caused by excessive secretion of growth hormone, usually from a pituitary tumor. One metabolic aspect of this syndrome is insulin resistance induced by growth hormone, the mechanism of which is unknown. Like obese patients and those affected by excessive doses of glucocorticoids, acromegalic patients may manifest a spectrum of conditions ranging from normal carbohydrate metabolism to diabetes of varying severity. Effective therapy exists for most patients with acromegaly, and those whose condition falls under the clinical definition of insulin resistance are few.

TABLE 5-11	CONDITIONS ASSOCIATED WITH CLINICAL INSULIN RESISTANCE
Infection	
Gross obesity	
Cushing's syndrome	
Acromegaly	
Hemochromatosis	
Lipodystrophic diabetes	
Acanthosis nigricans	
Werner's syndrome (adult form of progeria)	
Insulin degradation at injection site	
Idiopathic or immune-mediated (mediated by IgG antibody)	
Ig, immunoglobulin.	

Although the great majority of patients whose diabetes is secondary to hemochromatosis do not develop clinical insulin resistance, the number of patients with clinical insulin resistance and hemochromatosis is certainly higher than would be expected. Insulin resistance has also been reported in isolated cases of acute and chronic hepatic degeneration, hepatic infarcts, common-duct stones, fatty liver, Laënnec's cirrhosis, and hepatic failure. The mechanism involved in insulin resistance associated with hemochromatosis and other liver diseases is unknown. Although most reports of such cases originated before IgG antibodies were routinely measured, the production of such antibodies clearly cannot explain many of these cases.

Patients with lipodystrophic diabetes[60] are often unresponsive to large amounts of insulin. Total lipodystrophy, often called *lipoatrophy*, is a syndrome characterized by a complete loss of adipose tissue associated with some or all of the following: ketosis-resistant diabetes, hyperlipidemia, hepatomegaly, increased basal metabolic rates (but normal thyroid test results), and acanthosis nigricans. The genes associated with several types of congential generalized lipodystrophy have been identified.[61,62] These genetic defects appear to result in poor development of metabolically active adipose tissue.[63]

Partial lipodystrophy, in which loss of adipose tissue occurs in only parts of the body, is more common and is also associated with some or all of the features just listed. Partial lipodystrophy takes two general forms. In the cephalothoracic form, the loss of fat occurs in the upper part of the body, with normal or even excessive amounts of adipose tissue remaining in the lower half. In the second form, the loss of fat occurs in the lower half of the body and sometimes in the upper extremities, but adipose tissue remains over the face and trunk.[64-66] Lipodystrophy syndromes can occur in patients with HIV treated with protease inhibitors.[67,68]

Studies have revealed prereceptor[69] (i.e., increased insulin clearance from the circu-lation), receptor[70] (i.e., decreased binding of insulin to its receptor), and postbinding defects[71] in various patients with total lipodystrophy. These rare lipoatrophic syndromes with marked systemic effects should not be confused with insulin-induced (local) lipotrophy, one of the side effects of insulin (described later).

Insulin resistance is occasionally seen in patients who have acanthosis nigricans without lipoatrophy. Genes associated with these syndromes have also been identified.[72-74] Almost all such individuals studied have been women in whom obesity, hirsutism, amenorrhea, and/or polycystic ovaries were also noted. These individuals may tolerate thousands of units of insulin. Insulin resistance in these patients is caused by a marked defect in the binding of insulin to its receptor.[75] There are two clinical subtypes. In some patients (type A), both decreased binding of insulin to its receptor and decreased functioning of the activated receptor have been demonstrated. These abnormalities have been the result of various genetic alterations of the insulin receptor in different patients.[76] Type A patients manifest no immunologic features. In contrast, other patients with this syndrome (type B) have antibodies to the insulin receptor itself.[75,77,78] These antibodies do not affect the number of receptors available, but interfere with the affinity of insulin for its receptor. Some type B patients have intermittent hypoglycemia,[79,80] which is occasionally life threatening. The hypoglycemia is thought to be due to an insulin-like effect caused by the binding of the antireceptor antibody to the receptor. Why binding of the antireceptor antibody to the receptor only intermittently triggers postreceptor events mimicking the action of insulin is unclear. Type B patients also manifest other immunologic features, such as very high erythrocyte sedimentation rates; elevated levels of antinuclear and antideoxyribonucleic acid (DNA) antibodies; decreased complement levels; proteinuria; elevated IgG, IgM, and IgA levels; leukopenia; alopecia; and vitiligo. The type B syndrome is one of the autoimmune diseases and has been associated with lupus erythematosus,[81,82] scleroderma,[83] myositis,[81,84] and both thrombocytopenia and primary biliary cirrhosis in the same patient.[85]

Werner's syndrome, the adult form of progeria,[86] is a rare familial condition that appears in adults and is characterized by diabetes, short stature, slender extremities but a stocky trunk, premature graying of the hair, baldness, cataracts, skin ulcers, early appearance of atherosclerosis, and premature death. Although diabetes is usually mild, these patients are often unresponsive to large amounts of insulin for unknown reasons.

Destruction of subcutaneously injected insulin in a 16-year-old diabetic girl has been reported.[87] This patient's condition could not be controlled by even as much as 3000 U of injected insulin per day. Control was achieved by continuous intravenous infusion of approximately 50 to 60 U over a 24-hour period. Although a few more patients with this kind of problem have been described since the original one, this kind of insulin resistance fortunately is very rare.[88] If this cause of clinical insulin resistance can be documented, these patients respond best to continuous intravenous[89] or intraperitoneal[90] insulin.

All of the conditions listed in Table 5-11 and discussed so far can usually be easily excluded in the differential diagnosis. A patient's insulin resistance most often falls into the category described by the term *idiopathic*. In actuality, this designation is not entirely accurate because the basis for the high insulin requirement is known. Many patients receiving insulin injections develop IgG insulin-binding antibodies during the ensuing weeks or months. These antibodies are produced whether or not the patient has diabetes (e.g., they were found to be present in mentally ill patients undergoing insulin shock treatment 40 to 50 years ago). Although IgG antibody production to insulin is much less with the more pure insulin preparations used today, detectable amounts are still found in many patients. In the vast majority of diabetic patients, modest levels of IgG antibodies to insulin (<10 mU of insulin bound per milliliter) cause no difficulty. In approximately 0.1% of insulin-requiring patients, the concentration increases to very high levels (ranging from 50 to many thousands of milliunits of insulin bound per milliliter). The reason for this markedly enhanced response and the subsequent decline to normal levels is completely unknown. As with true insulin allergy, intermittent insulin therapy seems to predispose patients to insulin resistance. Indeed, both insulin allergy (IgE mediated) and insulin resistance (IgG mediated) can be found in the same patient.

TREATMENT OF INSULIN RESISTANCE

Several approaches can be effective in patients with immune-mediated (idiopathic) insulin resistance. Theoretically, it may be possible for patients to switch to another insulin preparation that the IgG antibodies either do not recognize or bind to much more weakly. This has been shown to be the case when switching a patient to lispro insulin.[91]

Interestingly, although two insulin preparations have been extremely effective in treating insulin resistance, neither is readily available to physicians in this country at present. If insulin is treated with sulfuric acid under the appropriate chemical conditions, the modified insulin molecule that emerges retains some biologic activity but shows a markedly reduced affinity for binding to IgG antibodies and very little antigenicity in patients never before treated with insulin. It is not surprising, then, that sulfated beef insulin has been used effectively in therapy of insulin resistance.[92] However, although sulfated insulin was first prepared and tested by a Canadian laboratory approximately 50 years ago, it is still not available in the United States except by direct petitioning to the Food and Drug Administration.

The (nonmammalian) fish insulins (sometimes called Bonito insulin) differ markedly from mammalian insulins in structure. For instance, cod and beef insulins differ in 24 positions on the A chain and 9 positions on the B chain. As might be anticipated, antibodies directed against beef insulin do not bind cod insulin. However, cod insulin retains its biologic activity in mammals and therefore is effective in treating insulin resistance.[93] Unfortunately, nonmammalian insulins are not available in this country.

If none of these techniques work, other avenues of therapy are usually necessary. Glitazone therapy may be useful in certain cases of insulin resistance.[94] Some physicians treat insulin resistance with high doses of glucocorticoids. Although the mechanism by which these agents decrease insulin requirements is not known with certainty, inhibition of IgG antibody production has been postulated. Even if antibody formation were immediately curtailed, however (and this is probably not the case), high insulin requirements would persist for a while because the half-life of IgG is approximately 3 to 4 weeks. Thus the clinical response to glucocorticoids is often delayed for 1 to 2 weeks, with initial responses occasionally occurring as late as a month after commencement of therapy. During the initial period of treatment, deterioration in diabetic control and even higher insulin requirements are common secondary to the insulin resistance caused by high doses of glucocorticoids. If this therapeutic approach is tried, doses equivalent to approximately 60 mg of prednisone should be used initially and maintained for at least several weeks or until insulin requirements are definitely lowered. The amount of steroid administered is then decreased rapidly, until either the patient can be taken off the medication entirely or a level is reached below which insulin requirements definitely increase

again. Patients frequently require 5 to 10 mg of prednisone for maintenance therapy. Some individuals who are in remission and either are taking low doses of steroids or have discontinued therapy completely may suffer relapse and need subsequent courses. In view of the adverse effects of long-term glucocorticoid administration, complete discontinuation of therapy should be attempted repeatedly. If it is not possible to discontinue treatment, alternate-day therapy should be tried, although there are no published results concerning its efficacy.

Immune-mediated insulin resistance is self-limited, with antibody titers and insulin requirements returning to the usual levels within several months to a year. Because of the potential hazards of long-term glucocorticoid administration, the relatively long lag period before this type of therapy becomes effective, the frequent deterioration in diabetic control after initiation of steroid therapy, and the temporary nature of the clinical course of insulin resistance, it is usually best to avoid administering glucocorticoid therapy altogether and simply use enough insulin to keep patients relatively asymptomatic and to prevent the development of ketosis.

A special preparation of highly concentrated regular insulin (U-500) is available for this purpose. The high concentration of insulin in this preparation (500 U/ml) is very convenient for these patients because the usual U-100 insulin would have to be injected in large volumes. Even though the U-500 preparation contains regular insulin, the action is prolonged because of the extremely high antibody titers. After absorption from the subcutaneous injection site, the insulin is quickly bound by the enlarged pool of circulating IgG antibodies before it can act on the insulin-sensitive tissues. Free insulin is subsequently released at a rate that clinically approximates a time course of action between those of short- and intermediate-acting insulins. Thus one or two injections per day of U-500 regular insulin in appropriate amounts usually control diabetes in a patient with immune-mediated insulin resistance. Patients seem to require much less (50% to 75%) of the U-500 preparation than the amounts of U-100 insulin for which it is substituted.[95,96] Obviously, in this temporary situation, good control is difficult to achieve and should probably not be sought. The goals should be to keep patients from developing ketosis and to lower glucose concentrations to a degree such that the symptoms of hyperglycemia (polyuria, polydipsia, nocturia, and increased susceptibility to infection) are avoided.

Several important considerations must be kept in mind during the treatment of immune-mediated insulin resistance with U-500 regular insulin. Small increments in insulin dose are usually ineffective when more insulin is needed. The increase per dose should be at least 10 U and probably close to 20 U, depending on the clinical picture. That is, if a patient's glucose levels are clearly out of control and have shown little or no response to the current insulin regimen (by definition the dose would be 200 units of insulin or more per day), increases of 20 to 25 U should be prescribed. If a patient has begun to respond to increased amounts of insulin, the additional increases in dose should be smaller, that is, 10 to 15 U each time. However, it must be emphasized again that responses to these large amounts of insulin are usually not consistent and predictable in patients with immune-mediated clinical insulin resistance. The dose of insulin may be varied considerably with little change in glucose levels, or conversely, glucose concentrations may vary considerably despite administration of a fixed amount of insulin. Thus simply keeping patients free of ketosis and symptomatic hyperglycemia is a realistic goal, but can often be quite a therapeutic challenge.

RETURN OF INSULIN SENSITIVITY

Insulin sensitivity can return relatively quickly. The reason for a marked decrease in IgG production is unknown. At this point in the clinical course, hypoglycemia can become a serious problem as the large amounts of already bound insulin are released and act on the tissues. Furthermore, the number of available binding sites for the recently injected insulin on the circulating anti-insulin IgG pool is not large. For this reason, the dose of insulin must be decreased in large decrements (20 to 40 U) once symptoms of hypoglycemia are detected. The reversal of insulin resistance is one of the few situations in which the insulin dose is lowered in *anticipation* of hypoglycemia. If the fasting and/or presupper glucose concentrations are more than 200 mg/dl, the dose of insulin should be decreased. If the degree of diabetic control remains the same, further decreases in the dose of insulin should be tried until control deteriorates. If the insulin-resistant state has finally been reversed, the decrease stops when the usual therapeutic dose of insulin is reached. If not, continued administration of larger amounts of insulin and continued close follow-up are required.

A smooth transition from insulin resistance to insulin sensitivity often does not occur, and insulin requirements may have to be juggled from day to day, depending on a patient's responses. However, at some point in the clinical course, excessive production of IgG antibodies to insulin ceases, and the return of insulin sensitivity becomes obvious. This change usually takes place over several weeks, an interval consistent with the half-life of IgG antibodies. Although the timing of the decision to return to therapy with intermediate-acting insulins varies from patient to patient, once fewer than 100 U of regular insulin is being given at each injection, intermediate- or long-acting insulin may be tried again. A short interval (2 to 4 hours) between the injection of U-500 regular insulin and a clear metabolic response (marked lowering of glucose concentrations) and/or clinical symptoms of hypoglycemia suggests that the high titers of IgG antibodies have diminished; thus a short interval of action of U-500 insulin may serve as a clue about when to resume therapy with long- or intermediate-acting insulins.

INSULIN-INDUCED LIPOATROPHY

Insulin-induced lipoatrophy (Figure 5-6) is a loss of subcutaneous fat at the sites of insulin injections. Although this condition seems to be more common in young females than in other patients, it certainly is not limited to this group of insulin-requiring diabetic patients. Even though this form of local lipoatrophy is a benign condition, the cosmetic effect can be disturbing, especially to adolescent girls and young women. Although the cause of this reaction is not known for certain, an immune response to contaminants in the administered insulin preparation may be involved. First, lipoatrophy was found to be two to three times more common in patients who had received the more impure preparations compared with the purified ones.[97,98] Second, patients with lipoatrophy often describe a local delayed reaction at the site of injection,[43] a response that may be associated with delayed hyper-

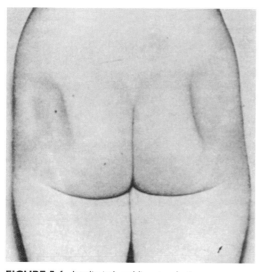

FIGURE 5-6. Insulin-induced lipoatrophy in a young woman. *(From Mazzaferi EL: Endocrinology Case Studies. Medical Examination Publishing Co, Flushing, NY, 1975, p. 161.)*

sensitivity to impurities in the insulin preparation.[34] Third, the condition of some patients improves in response to local injections of dexamethasone. Fourth, abnormal deposition of immunologic components was found in the dermal vessel walls in biopsy specimens taken from lipoatrophic sites.[99] In addition, these patients had much higher serum insulin-binding capacities (IgG titers) than insulin-requiring patients without lipoatrophy.[99] Finally, cytokine (tumor necrosis factor-α and interleukin-6) production was markedly increased by macrophages of a patient with lipoatrophy.[100]

An effective treatment is available for insulin-induced local lipoatrophy. This treatment simply (and perhaps paradoxically) involves injection of pure insulin preparations directly into the involved areas. The response is probably due to a local lipogenic effect of insulin. The technique for injection in these atrophic areas is shown in Figure 5-7, and the results 6 months later are shown in Figure 5-8. In a series of more than 300 patients,[43] more than 80% were successfully treated by injection of standard mixed beef-pork insulin, a preparation more pure than the ones used in the early 1970s. Approximately one quarter of those in whom this approach was not helpful responded to injection of a standard pork preparation. The remainder were successfully treated when a purified preparation of pork insulin was used. Human insulin was successful in a few patients in whom purified pork insulin was ineffective.[101] Thus in keeping with an allergic basis for lipoatrophy, using the least immunogenic insulin to treat it is the most effective therapy.

Several other considerations need to be kept in mind. First, patients who may still be experiencing delayed local reactions to insulin are often refractory to treatment for lipoatrophy until the skin reaction abates. Second, local injections must be given for 2 to 4 weeks before normal subcutaneous fat tissue even begins to reaccumulate. Third, areas that have filled in may lose their fatty tissue again unless they are

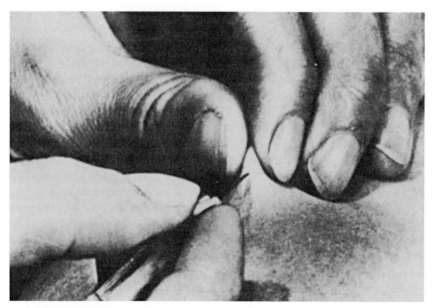

FIGURE 5-7. Injection of insulin into the affected area of a patient with lipoatrophy.

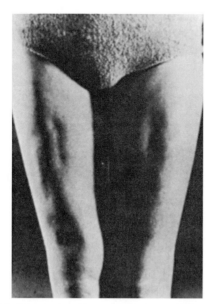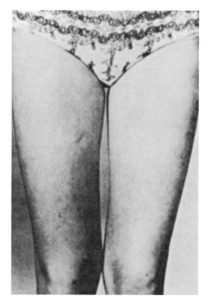

FIGURE 5-8. Insulin-induced lipoatrophy before *(left)* and after *(right)* 6 months of treatment with a purified insulin preparation.

reinjected periodically (every 2 to 4 weeks). Fourth, although the evidence implicating an immunogenic basis for lipoatrophy is substantial and injection of pure preparations of insulin into the affected sites is "virtually 100% effective,"[43] an occasional patient develops lipoatrophy in response to subcutaneous injections of human insulin,[102-104] which is a recombinant DNA–derived preparation.

INSULIN-INDUCED LIPOHYPERTROPHY

Some diabetic patients receiving insulin manifest lipohypertrophy of subcutaneous fat tissue at the site of injection (Figure 5-9). This condition is no doubt due to a

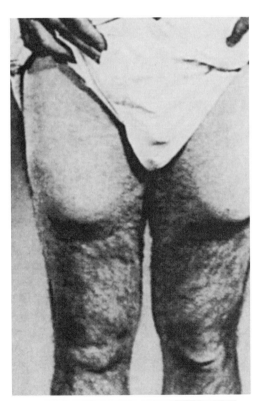

FIGURE 5-9. An extreme example of insulin-induced lipohypertrophy.

local lipogenic effect of insulin. Although patients are less likely to comment on lipohypertrophy than on atrophy, an older careful study of almost 600 patients[105] revealed some increases in subcutaneous fat at the sites of insulin injection in approximately 40% of males and 18% of females younger than 20 years old and in 20% of males and 12% of females older than 20 years. The use of more pure insulin preparations has not changed the approximately 20% prevalence of lipohypertrophy.[43,106] Lipohypertrophy is also common at the abdominal sites of needle placement in patients using insulin pumps. One factor that predisposes to this reaction is repeated injections in the same place.[106] Once lipohypertrophy develops, patients may tend to continue injecting at this site because many report less pain than at other sites. In addition to cosmetic considerations, continued injection into these areas is probably not wise because absorption of insulin from such sites is delayed[107,108] and erratic.[108] Avoidance of these lipohypertrophic areas for future insulin injection sometimes results in a gradual disappearance of this extra tissue. Severe insulin-induced lipohypertrophy has been successfully treated with liposuction.[109]

Thus, except for lipohypertrophy, the pathogenesis of the other four side effects of insulin therapy seems to be immunogenic (Figure 5-10). Stimulation of the T-lymphocyte arm of the immune system leads to delayed hypersensitivity manifested by a *delayed local reaction*. Activation of B lymphocytes leads to formation of IgE and IgG antibodies, causing *true* or *systemic insulin allergy* and *immune-mediated insulin resistance*, respectively. Finally, *lipoatrophy* may be the result of an Arthus type of reaction in which immune complexes are formed between the antigen (insulin) and circulating (IgG insulin-binding) antibodies, causing activation of complement and infiltration of inflammatory cells.[99]

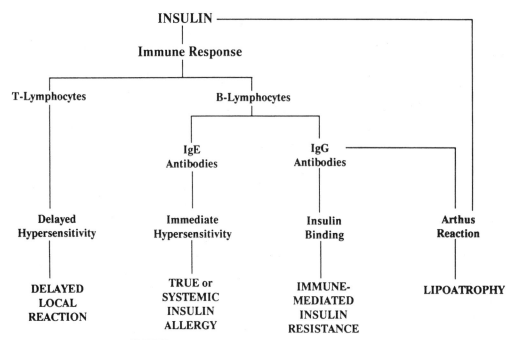

FIGURE 5-10. Immunogenic side effects of insulin therapy.

REFERENCES

1. Dunbar JM, Madden PM, Gleeson DT et al: Premixed insulin preparations in pen syringes maintain glycemic control and are preferred by patients. Diabetes Care 17:874, 1994.
2. Galloway JA, Spradlin CT, Nelson RL et al: Factors influencing the absorption, serum insulin concentration, and blood glucose responses after injections of regular insulin and various insulin mixtures. Diabetes Care 4(3):366-76, 1981.
3. Binder C, Lauritzen T, Faber O, et al: Insulin pharmacokinetics. Diabetes Care 7(2):188-99, 1984.
4. Sindelka G, Heinemann L, Berger M et al: Effect of insulin concentration, subcutaneous fat thickness and skin temperature on subcutaneous insulin absorption in healthy subjects. Diabetologia 37:377, 1994.
5. Koivisto VA, Felig P: Alterations in insulin absorption and in blood glucose control associated with varying insulin injection sites in diabetic patients. Ann Intern Med 92:59, 1980.
6. Holleman F, Van den Brand JJG, Hoven RA et al: Comparison of LysB28, ProB29 human insulin analog and regular human insulin in the correction of incidental hyperglycemia. Diabetes Care 19:1426, 1996.
7. Brunelle BL, Llewelyn J, Anderson JH Jr et al: Meta-analysis of the effect of insulin lispro on severe hypoglycemia in patients with type 1 diabetes. Diabetes Care 21:1726, 1998.
8. Raskin P, Guthrie RA, Leiter L, et al: Use of insulin aspart, a fast-acting insulin analog, as the mealtime insulin in the management of patients with type 1 diabetes. Diabetes Care 23:583, 2000.
9. Heinemann L, Linkeschova R, Rave K et al: Time-action profile of the long-acting insulin analog insulin glargine (HOE901) in comparison with those of NPH insulin and placebo Diabetes Care 23:644, 2000.
10. Yki-Järvinen H, Dressler A, Ziemen M: Less nocturnal hypoglycemia and better post-dinner glucose control with bedtime insulin glargine compared with bedtime NPH insulin during insulin combination therapy in type 2 diabetes. Diabetes Care 23:1130, 2000.
11. Rosenstock J, Park G, Zimmerman J: Basal insulin glargine (HOE 901) versus NPH insulin in patients with type 1 diabetes on multiple daily insulin regimens. U.S. Insulin Glargine (HOE 901) Type 1 Diabetes Investigator Group. Diabetes Care 23:1137, 2000.
12. Fritsche A, Schmulling RM, Haring HU et al: Intensive insulin therapy combined with metformin in obese type 2 diabetic patients. Acta Diabetol 37(1):13-18, 2000.
13. Aviles-Santa L, Sinding J, Raskin P: Effects of metformin in patients with poorly controlled, insulin-treated type 2 diabetes mellitus. A randomized, double-blind, placebo-controlled trial. Ann Intern Med 131(3):182, 1999.
14. Yu JG, Kruszynska YT, Mulford MI et al: A comparison of troglitazone and metformin on

insulin requirements in euglycemic intensively insulin-treated type 2 diabetic patients. Diabetes 48(12):2414, 1999.

15. Buse JB, Gumbiner B, Mathias NP et al: Troglitazone use in insulin-treated type 2 diabetic patients. The Troglitazone Insulin Study Group. Diabetes Care 21(9):1455, 1998.

16. Yki-Järvinen H, Ryysy L, Nikkilä K et al: Comparison of bedtime insulin regimens in patients with type 2 diabetes mellitus. A randomized controlled trial. Ann Intern Med 130:389, 1999.

17. Landstedt-Hallin L, Adamson U, Arner P et al: Comparison of bedtime NPH or preprandial regular insulin combined with glibenclamide in secondary sulfonylurea failure. Diabetes Care 18:1183, 1995.

18. Peters AL, Davidson MB: BIDS therapy for treatment of NIDDM: effectiveness and predictors (if any) of success. Diabetes Spectrum 7:152, 1994.

18a. Fritsche A, Schweitzer MA, Haring HU: Glimepiride combined with morning insulin glargine, bedtime neutral protamine hagedorn insulin, or bedtime insulin glargine patients with type 2 diabetes: A randomized controlled trial. Ann Intern Med 138(12):952-959.

19. Yki-Jarvinin H, Kauppila M, Kujansuu E et al: Comparison of insulin regimens in patients with non-insulin-dependent diabetes mellitus. N Engl J Med 327:1426, 1992.

20. Chow C-C, Tsang LWW, Sorensen JP et al: Comparison of insulin with or without continuation of oral hypoglycemic agents in the treatment of secondary failure in NIDDM patients. Diabetes Care 18:307, 1995.

21. Shank ML, Del Prato S, DeFronzo RA: Bedtime insulin/daytime glipizide: Effective therapy for sulfonylurea failures in NIDDM. Diabetes 44:165, 1995.

22. Weir CJ, Murray GD, Dyker AG et al: Is hyperglycemia an independent predictor of poor outcome after acute stroke? Results of a longterm follow-up study. BMJ 314:1303, 1997.

23. van den Berghe G, Wouters P, Weekers F et al: Intensive insulin therapy in the surgical intensive care unit. N Engl J Med 345:1359, 2001.

24. Malmberg K, Ryden L, Efendic S, Herlitz J. Randomized trial of insulin-glucose infusion followed by subcutaneous insulin treatment in diabetes patients with acute myocardial infarction (DIGAMI Study): effects on mortality at 1 year. J Am Coll Cardiol 26:57-65, 1995

25. Kalin MF, Tranbaugh RF, Salas J et al: Intensive intervention by an endocrinologist-directed diabetes team diminishes excess mortality in patients with diabetes who undergo coronary artery bypass graft. Diabetes 47(Suppl 1):A87, 1998.

26. Queale WS, Seidler AJ, Bracati FL: Glycemic control and sliding scale insulin use in medical inpatients with diabetes mellitus. Arch Int Med 157:545, 1997.

27. Carlson MG, Campbell PJ: Intensive insulin therapy and weight gain in IDDM. Diabetes 42:1700, 1993.

28. Saudek CD, Boulter PR, Knopp RH et al: Sodium retention accompanying insulin treatment of diabetes mellitus. Diabetes 23:240, 1974.

29. Wheatley T, Edwards OM: Insulin oedema and its clinical significance: Metabolic studies in three cases. Diabetic Med 2:400, 1985

30. Hopkins DFC, Cotton SJ, Williams G: Effective treatment of insulin-induced edema using ephedrine. Diabetes Care 16:1026, 1993.

31. Samnegard B, Jacobson SH, Jaremko G et al: Effects of C-peptide on glomerular and renal size and renal function in diabetic rats. Kidney Int 60(4):1258, 2001.

32. Fernqvist-Forbes E, Johansson BL, Eriksson MJ: Effects of C-peptide on forearm blood flow and brachial artery dilatation in patients with type 1 diabetes mellitus. Acta Physiol Scand 172(3):159, 2001.

33. Fineberg SE, Galloway JA, Fineberg NS et al: Immunogenicity of recombinant DNA human insulin. Diabetologia 25:465, 1983.

34. Ross JM: Allergy to insulin. Pediatr Clin North Am 31:675, 1984.

35. Feinglos MN, Jegasothy BV: "Insulin" allergy due to zinc. Lancet 1:122, 1979.

36. Nell JL, Thomas JW: Frequency and specificity of protamine antibodies in diabetic and control subjects. Diabetes 37:172, 1988.

37. Shore NR, Shelley WB, Kyle CC: Chronic urticaria from isophane insulin therapy. Arch Dermatol 111:94, 1975.

38. Levy JH, Ziadan JR, Faraj B: Prospective evaluation of risk of protamine reactions in patients with NPH insulin-dependent diabetes. Anesth Analg 65:739, 1986.

39. Levy JH, Schwieger IM, Zaidan JR et al: Evaluation of patients at risk for protamine reactions. J Thorac Cardiovasc Surg 98:200, 1989.

40. Loeb JA, Herold KC, Barton KP et al: Systematic approach to diagnosis and management of biphasic insulin allergy with local anti-inflammatory agents. Diabetes Care 12:421, 1989.

41. Hanauer L, Batson JM: Anaphylactic shock following insulin injection: Case report and review of the literature. Diabetes 10:105, 1961.

42. Scheer BG, Sitz KV: Suspected insulin anaphylaxis and literature review. J Ark Med Soc 97(9):311, 2001.

43. Galloway JA, Bressler R: Insulin treatment in diabetes. Med Clin North Am 62:663, 1978.

44. Patterson R, Mellies CJ, Roberts M: Immunologic reactions against insulin. II. IgE anti-insulin, insulin allergy and combined IgE and IgG immunologic insulin resistance. J Immunol 110:1135, 1973.

45. Mattson JR, Patterson R, Roberts M: Insulin therapy in patients with systemic insulin allergy. Arch Intern Med 135:818, 1975.

46. Bruni B, Barolo P, Blatto A et al: Treatment of allergy to heterologous monocomponent insulin with human semisynthetic insulin. Long-term study. Diabetes Care 11:59, 1988.

47. deShazo RD, Mather P, Grant W et al: Evaluation of patients with local reactions to insulin with skin

tests and in vitro techniques. Diabetes Care 10:330, 1987.

48. Abraham MR, al-Sharafi BA, Saavedra GA et al: Lispro in the treatment of insulin allergy. Diabetes Care 22(11):1916, 1999.

49. Airaghi L, Lorini M, Tedeschi A. The insulin analog aspart: A safe alternative in insulin allergy. Diabetes Care 24(11):2000, 2001.

50. Moriyama H, Nagata M, Fujihira K et al: Treatment with human analog (GlyA21, ArgB31, ArgB32) insulin glargine (HOE901) resolves a generalized allergy to human insulin in type 1 diabetes. Diabetes Care 24(2):411, 2001.

50a.Wessbecher R, Kiehn M, Stoffel E et al: Management of insulin allergy. Allergy 56:919, 2001.

51. Grammer LC, Metzger BE, Patterson R: Cutaneous allergy to human (recombinant DNA) insulin. JAMA 251:1459, 1984.

52. Child DF, Johansson GO: IgE antibody studies in a case of generalized allergic reaction to human insulin. Allergy 39:630, 1984.

53. Berke L, Owen JA, Atkinson RL: Allergies to human insulin. Diabetes Care 7:402, 1984.

54. Goldman RA, Lewis AE, Rose LI: Anaphylactoid reaction to single-component pork insulin. JAMA 236:1148, 1976.

55. Valentini U, Cimino A, Rocca L et al: CSII in management of insulin allergy. Diabetes Care 11:97, 1988.

56. Wiles PG, Guy R, Watkins SM et al: Allergy to purified bovine, porcine, and human insulins. BMJ 287:531, 1983.

57. Grant W, deShazo RD, Frentz J: Use of low-dose continuous corticosteroid infusion to facilitate insulin pump use in local insulin hypersensitivity. Diabetes Care 9:318, 1986.

58. deShazo RD, Boehm TM, Kumar D et al: Dermal hypersensitivity reactions to insulin: Correlations of three patterns to their histopathology. Allergy Clin Immunol 69:229, 1982.

59. Bruni B, Campana M, Gamba S et al: A generalized allergic reaction due to zinc in insulin preparation. Diabetes Care 8:201, 1985.

60. Garg A: Lipodystrophies. Am J Med 108:143, 2000.

61. Garg A, Wilson R, Barnes R et al: A gene for congenital generalized lipodystrophy maps to human chromosome 9q34. J Clin Endocrinol Metab 84:3390, 1999.

62. Magre J, Delepine M, Khallouf E et al: Identification of the gene altered in Berardinelli-Seip congenital lipodystrophy on chromosome 11q13. Nat Genet 28:365, 2001.

63. Garg A, Fleckenstein JL, Peshock RM, Grundy SM: Peculiar distribution of adipose tissue in patients with congenital generalized lipodystrophy. J Clin Endocrinol Metab 75:358, 1992.

64. Davidson MB, Young RT: Metabolic studies in familial partial lipodystrophy of the lower trunk and extremities. Diabetologia 11:561, 1975.

65. Garg A, Peshock RM, Fleckenstein JL: Adipose tissue distribution pattern in patients with familial partial lipodystrophy (Dunnigan variety). J Clin Endocrinol Metab 84:170, 1999.

66. Ursich MJ, Fukui RT, Galvao MS et al: Insulin resistance in limb and trunk partial lipodystrophy (type 2 Kobberling-Dunnigan syndrome). Metabolism 46:159, 1997.

67. Tsiodras S, Mantzoros C, Hammer S et al: Effects of protease inhibitors on hyperglycemia, hyperlipidemia, and lipodystrophy: A 5-year cohort study. Arch Intern Med 160:2050, 2000.

68. Martinez E, Mocroft A, Garcia-Viejo MA et al: Risk of lipodystrophy in HIV-1 infected patients treated with protease inhibitors: A prospective cohort study. Lancet 357:592, 2001.

69. Golden MP, Charles MA, Arquilla ER et al: Insulin resistance in total lipodystrophy: Evidence for a pre-receptor defect in insulin action. Metabolism 34:330, 1985.

70. Kriauciunas KM, Kahn CR, Muller-Wieland D et al: Altered expression and function of the insulin receptor in a family with lipoatrophic diabetes. J Clin Endocrinol Metab 67:1284, 1988.

71. Magre J, Reynet C, Capeau J et al: In vitro studies of insulin resistance in patients with lipoatrophic diabetes. Evidence of heterogeneous postbinding defects. Diabetes 37:421, 1988.

72. Peters JM, Barnes R, Bennett L et al: Localization of the gene for familial partial lipodystrophy (Dunnigan variety) to chromosome 1q21-22. Nat Genet 18:292, 1998.

73. Peters JM, Barnes R, Bennett L et al: Localization of the gene for familial partial lipodystrophy (Dunnigan variety) to chromosome 1q21-22. Nat Genet 18:292, 1998.

74. Cao H, Hegele RA: Nuclear lamin A/C R482Q mutation in Canadian kindreds with Dunnigan-type familial partial lipodystrophy. Hum Mol Genet 9:109, 2000.

75. Kahn CR, Flier JS, Bar RS et al: The syndromes of insulin resistance and acanthosis nigricans. Insulin-receptor disorders in man. N Engl J Med 294:739, 1976.

76. Taylor SI: Molecular mechanisms of insulin resistance: Lessons from patients with mutations in the insulin-receptor gene. Diabetes 41:1473, 1992.

77. Rodriguez O, Collier E, Arakaki et al: Characterization of purified autoantibodies to the insulin receptor from six patients with type B insulin resistance. Metabolism 41:325, 1992.

78. Freeland BS, Paglia RE, Seal DL. Clinical challenges of type B insulin resistance: A case study. Diabetes Educ 24(6):728, 1998.

79. Flier JS, Bar RS, Muggeo M et al: The evolving clinical course of patients with receptor autoantibodies: Spontaneous remission or receptor proliferation with hypoglycemia. J Clin Endocrinol Metab 47:985, 1978.

80. Taylor SI, Barbetti F, Accili D et al: Syndromes of autoimmunity and hypoglycemia: Autoantibodies directed against insulin and its receptor. Endocrinol Metab Clin North Am 18:123, 1989.

81. Tsokos GC, Gorden P, Antonovych T et al: Lupus nephritis and other autoimmune features in patients with diabetes mellitus due to autoantibody to insulin receptors. Ann Intern Med 102:176, 1985.

82. Di Paolo S, Giorgino R: Insulin resistance and hypoglycemia in a patient with systemic lupus erythematosus: Description of antiinsulin receptor antibodies that enhance insulin binding and inhibit insulin action. J Clin Endocrinol Metab 73:650, 1991.

83. Bloise W, Wajchenberg BL, Moncada VY et al: Atypical antiinsulin receptor antibodies in a patient with type B insulin resistance and scleroderma. J Clin Endocrinol Metab 68:227, 1989.

84. Fonseca V, Khokher MA, Dandona P: Insulin receptor antibodies causing steroid responsive diabetes mellitus in a patient with myositis. BMJ 288:1578, 1984.

85. Selinger S, Tsai J, Pulini M et al: Autoimmune thrombocytopenia and primary biliary cirrhosis with hypoglycemia and insulin receptor autoantibodies. A case report. Ann Intern Med 107:686, 1987.

86. Epstein CJ, Martini GM, Schultz AL, et al: Werner's syndrome: a review of its symptomatology, natural history, pathological features, genetics, and relationship to the natural aging process. Medicine 45:177, 1966.

87. Paulsen EP, Courtney JW III, Duckworth WC: Insulin resistance caused by massive degradation of subcutaneous insulin. Diabetes 28:640, 1979.

88. Schade DS, Duckworth WC: In search of the subcutaneous-insulin-resistance syndrome. N Engl J Med 315:147, 1986.

89. Paterson KR, Campbell IW, MacRury SM et al: Management of diabetes resistant to subcutaneous insulin with intravenous insulin via an implanted infusion pump. Scot Med J 33:239, 1988.

90. Riveline JP, Capeau J, Robert JJ et al: Extreme subcutaneous insulin resistance successfully treated by an implantable pump. Diabetes Care 24(12):2155, 2001.

91. Lahtela JT, Knip M, Paul R et al: Severe antibody-mediated human insulin resistance: Successful treatment with the insulin analog lispro. Diabetes Care 20:71, 1997.

92. Davidson JK, DeBra DW: Immunologic insulin resistance. Diabetes 27:307, 1978.

93. Yalow RS, Berson SA: Reaction of fish insulins with human insulin antiserums. Potential value in the treatment of insulin resistance. N Engl J Med 270:1171, 1964.

94. Arioglu E, Duncan-Morin J, Sebring N et al: Efficacy and safety of troglitazone in the treatment of lipodystrophy syndromes. Ann Intern Med 133(4):263, 2000.

95. Nathan SM, Axelrod L, Flier JS et al: U-500 insulin in the treatment of antibody-mediated insulin resistance. Ann Intern Med 94:653, 1981.

96. Baumann G, Drobny EC: Enhanced efficacy of U-500 insulin in the treatment of insulin resistance caused by target tissue insensitivity. Am J Med 76:529, 1984.

97. Deckert T, Andersen O, Poulsen JE: The clinical significance of highly purified pig-insulin preparations. Diabetologia 10:703, 1974.

98. Wilson RM, Douglas CA, Tattersall RB et al: Immunogenicity of highly purified bovine insulin: A comparison with conventional bovine and highly purified human insulins. Diabetologia 28:667, 1985.

99. Reeves WG, Allen BR, Tattersall RB: Insulin-induced lipoatrophy: Evidence for an immune pathogenesis. BMJ 1:1500, 1980.

100. Altan-Gepner C, Bongrand P, Farnarier C et al: Insulin-induced lipoatrophy in type 1 diabetes: a possible tumor necrosis factor-α-mediated dedifferentiation of adipocytes. Diabetes Care 19:1283, 1996.

101. Valenta LJ, Elias AN: Insulin-induced lipodystrophy in diabetic patients resolved by treatment with human insulin. Ann Intern Med 102:790, 1985.

102. Rosman MS: Fat atrophy in human insulin therapy. Diabetes Care 9:436, 1986.

103. Page MD, Bodansky HJ: Human insulin and lipoatrophy. Diabetic Med 9:779, 1992.

104. Jaap AJ, Horn HM, Tidman MJ et al: Lipoatrophy with human insulin. Diabetes Care 19:1289, 1996.

105. Marble A, Renold AE: Atrophy of subcutaneous fat following injections of insulin. Proc Am Diabetes Assoc 2:171, 1942.

106. Young RJ, Steel JM, Frier BM et al: Insulin injection sites in diabetes—a neglected area? BMJ 283:349, 1981.

107. Kolendorf K, Bojsen J, Deckert T: Clinical factors influencing the absorption of ^{125}I-NPH insulin in diabetic patients. Horm Metab Res 15:274, 1982.

108. Young RJ, Hannan WJ, Frier BM et al: Diabetic lipohypertrophy delays insulin absorption. Diabetes Care 7:479, 1984.

109. Hardy KJ, Gill GV, Bryson JR: Severe insulin-induced lipohypertrophy successfully treated by liposuction. Diabetes Care 16:929, 1993.

CHAPTER 6

HYPERGLYCEMIC AND HYPOGLYCEMIC EMERGENCIES

Diabetic ketoacidosis (DKA) and hyperosmolar hyperglycemic state (HHS) are profound metabolic complications of diabetes and are the among the most serious acute complications, along with severe hypoglycemia. Previously it was thought that only patients with type 1 diabetes developed DKA and those with type 2 diabetes developed HHS. This dogmatic view is incorrect; both of these disorders can occur in patients with type 1 and type 2 diabetes. As the population of type 2 patients gets younger, the overlap occurs with increasing frequency. This chapter addresses the pathophysiology, causes, signs, symptoms, and treatment of hyperglycemic emergencies, and outlines specific differences between DKA and HHS in these regards. The final section of this chapter focuses on hypoglycemia, its causes, manifestations, and management.

DIABETIC KETOACIDOSIS

PATHOPHYSIOLOGY

DKA is caused by a profound lack of effective insulin. Published studies routinely report some measurable insulin concentrations, but these low levels (usually <10 µU/ml) are clearly inadequate in the metabolic milieu of marked hyperglycemia, ketosis, and acidosis. Although levels of the counter-regulatory hormones (catecholamines, glucagon, growth hormone, and cortisol) are elevated as the result of stress,[1] such elevations do not *cause* the metabolic derangements that lead to DKA. Elevated levels of these hormones simply potentiate the effect of a lack of insulin; patients can become at least mildly ketoacidotic in the absence of high levels of these hormones.

The clinical hallmarks of DKA are acidosis, dehydration, and electrolyte depletion. The mechanisms behind these conditions are outlined in Figure 6-1. The effect of a lack of insulin on all three general areas of metabolism—carbohydrate, protein, and fat—figures prominently in the pathophysiology of DKA. In the absence of effective insulin, ingested carbohydrate is not utilized by the three insulin-sensitive tissues (liver, muscle, and adipose tissues). This impairment of glucose uptake causes hyperglycemia. Furthermore, in the late postprandial state, after the carbohydrate content of the diet has been stored, insulin is critically important in the modulation of glucose production by the liver. In the absence of effective insulin, enhanced hepatic

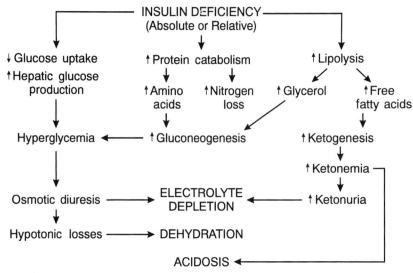

FIGURE 6-1. Pathophysiology of diabetic ketoacidosis.

glucose production further increases the already elevated glucose concentrations. In fact, more than half of the reduction in plasma glucose concentrations secondary to insulin administration in the treatment of DKA is due to decreased hepatic glucose production.[1] Hyperglycemia, in turn, causes an osmotic diuresis that results in water and electrolyte depletion. The water and electrolyte losses cause dehydration, which is clinically manifested as intravascular volume depletion. The fluid losses are hypotonic to plasma, and a hyperosmolar state therefore develops.

In protein metabolism, a lack of insulin reinforces fluid and electrolyte depletion. In the absence of effective insulin, the transport of amino acids into cells and the incorporation of these intracellular amino acids into protein are decreased. In addition, the inhibition of protein degradation by insulin is lost. Therefore the effects of a lack of insulin on amino acid transport, protein synthesis, and protein degradation all cause protein catabolism, which results in increased release of amino acids from muscle tissue. Some of these amino acids are gluconeogenic precursors and are converted to glucose by the liver. The rate of gluconeoge-

nesis is controlled by the amount of appropriate substrates delivered to the liver. Therefore the increased flux of amino acids from muscle contributes significantly to hyperglycemia, with its attendant fluid and electrolyte losses. The amino acids not utilized for gluconeogenesis are metabolized by the liver to fulfill energy demands. This increased nitrogen loss leads to a depletion of lean body mass, which is an important component of the weight loss suffered by the affected patients.

In the case of fat metabolism, the lack of effective insulin also contributes to fluid and electrolyte depletion. However, ketosis and eventual acidosis are solely attributable to the lack of an insulin effect on adipose tissue. A critical aspect of insulin action on this tissue is an inhibition of the breakdown of triglycerides, a pathway termed lipolysis (see Chapter 2). Increased lipolysis results in elevated concentrations of glycerol and free fatty acids (FFAs) in plasma. Because glycerol is a gluconeogenic precursor, its increased flux from adipose tissue enhances gluconeogenesis even further. This enhancement, of course, leads to more pronounced hyperglycemia and greater fluid and electrolyte losses. Some of the FFA can be utilized by tissues for energy purposes or reconstituted as hepatic triglycerides. However, the most important determinant of ketone body formation (ketogenesis) is the amount of FFA delivered to the liver. The ketogenic pathway is further activated by the presence of the low insulin and high glucagon concentrations that characterize DKA. The ketone bodies (acetoacetate and β-hydroxybutyrate) are weak acids that must be buffered on release by the liver into the circulation (ketonemia). As more and more ketone bodies are produced, the body bases become depleted and acidosis ensues. In addition to causing acidosis, the ketone bodies also contribute to the loss of electrolytes. Although they can be utilized to some extent by various body tissues, the capacity to metabolize ketone bodies is soon exceeded, and they are excreted into the urine (ketonuria).

This event exacerbates electrolyte depletion because cations must be excreted with the ketone bodies. These are the mechanisms, then, by which a lack of insulin affects carbohydrate, protein, and fat metabolism, and leads to the dehydration, electrolyte depletion, and acidosis that characterize DKA.

ELECTROLYTE AND FLUID SHIFTS

The usual fluid and electrolyte losses sustained by patients experiencing DKA are marked, as shown in Figure 6-2. The values in this figure are derived from two kinds of studies. In one type of study, the use of insulin was discontinued in ketosis-prone diabetic patients, and the amounts of fluid and electrolytes lost over a 24-hour period were measured. In the other type, the amounts of fluid and electrolytes needed to treat patients experiencing DKA in the first 24-hour period

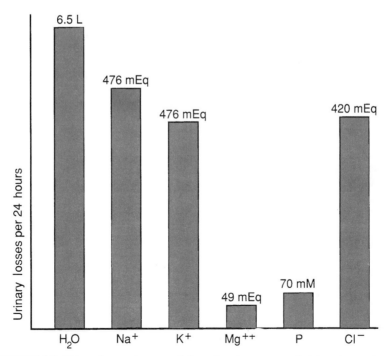

FIGURE 6-2. Urinary losses of water and electrolytes in patients with diabetic ketoacidosis.

were carefully tabulated. In a "typical" 70-kg individual, the fluid, sodium, potassium, and chloride losses depicted in Figure 6-2 are indeed impressive. Extracellular water represents 17% of body weight, or ~12 L in our reference subject. Therefore more than half of the extracellular fluid compartment was lost. The amount of exchangeable sodium in a normal individual is 41 mEq/kg. The sodium loss in these diabetic subjects represented over 15% of this total exchangeable pool. Similarly, the chloride loss was between 15% and 20% of the normal chloride pool (33 mEq/kg). Approximately 10% of total body potassium (50 to 54 mEq/kg) was excreted by these subjects. Of the total exchangeable magnesium pool (10 mEq/kg), 7% was lost under these circumstances.

The situation with regard to phosphorus is more complicated. The body of a 70-kg man, for example, contains ~712 g, or 23,000 mmol, of phosphorus. Of this amount, 80% is in bone and 9% in muscle. However, the bulk of the intracellular phosphorus is in organic form, and only a small fraction is inorganic. Thus although the amount of phosphorus lost in the urine of these diabetic subjects during a 24-hour period is a minuscule percentage of total body phosphorus, it represents a relatively substantial part of the available inorganic phosphorus pool. Balance studies performed during several weeks after recovery from DKA have demonstrated substantial retention of phosphorus (up to 400 mmol). These studies probably underestimate net phosphorus losses because they were completed before the pre-DKA weight had been regained. The problems of phosphorus homeostasis in the treatment of DKA are discussed in greater detail later.

PRECIPITATING FACTORS

The precipitating causes of DKA are listed in Table 6-1. The most common cause is infection. New onset of type 1 diabetes is the second most common cause, followed closely by omission or reduction of the current insulin dose. Various medical conditions account for the remainder of the identifiable causes. These include cerebrovascular accidents, alcohol abuse, pancreatitis, myocardial infarction, trauma, and drugs. Drugs that affect carbohydrate metabolism, such as steroids, thiazide diuretics, and sympathomimetic agents may also precipitate DKA. Eating disorders, particularly in young females, may be a contributing factor in up to 20% of recurrent DKA. In younger patients, one must think of factors relating to social issues. For example, not wanting to take insulin in a social situation, fear of weight gain associated with insulin, and age-related

TABLE 6-1 PRECIPITATING CAUSES OF DIABETIC KETOACIDOSIS

Cause	Percent
Infection	30–40
Cessation of insulin	15–20
New-onset diabetes	20–25
Myocardial infarction	
Pancreatitis	
Shock and hypovolemia	10–15
Stroke	
Other medical diseases	
No precipitating event	20–25

From DeFronzo RA, Matsuda M, Barrett EJ: Diabetic ketoacidosis: A combined metabolic-nephrologic approach to therapy. Diabetes Rev 2:209, 1994

rebellion against authority may all affect compliance. All may play a role in recurrent DKA behavior. No precipitating event can be identified in approximately one quarter of patients admitted to the hospital with DKA. It should be emphasized, however, that DKA is potentially preventable in the approximately 50% of patients in whom the precipitating cause is infection or reduced insulin doses (often a combination of the two).

SIGNS AND SYMPTOMS

The evolution of DKA in patients with type 1 and type 2 diabetes is rapid, over the course of hours or days, whereas HHS may be more insidious. The signs and symptoms of DKA are listed in Table 6-2. Low body temperatures are not generally recognized as characteristic of patients experiencing DKA. If present, it is a poor prognostic sign.[2] The depth of respiration, not the rate, characterizes Kussmaul respirations. Patients often have a normal respiratory rate but on closer inspection are noted to be breathing very deeply. The signal for this hyperventilation is acidosis, which stimulates the respiratory center in the brain. The resulting respiratory alkalosis offsets the metabolic acidosis to some extent, but cannot compensate for

it entirely in the absence of treatment. Through the pathophysiology described previously, the accumulation of ketones occurs. Acetone has a fruity odor that is often apparent on a patient's breath, although not all observers can distinguish this odor.

Although the term *dehydration* is often used to describe patients experiencing DKA, the signs really result from intravascular volume depletion. In adults, the most sensitive sign of intravascular volume depletion is a change in the way in which the neck veins fill. When normally hydrated subjects lie entirely horizontally (i.e., without a pillow), the neck veins fill from below up to one half to two thirds of the way to the angle of the jaw. This sign is essentially a clinical measurement of venous pressure, which is normally ~7 cm H_2O. To ascertain whether the jugular veins are filling from below, the vein near the clavicle should first be occluded just above the clavicle so that its course can be delineated as it fills from above. Next, the vein should be occluded near the angle of the jaw to determine how far over the clavicle it fills from below. It is helpful to empty the vein by "milking" it while it is occluded from above so that the advancing column of blood can be seen as the vein subsequently fills from below the clavicle. If the vein is not

TABLE 6-2	SYMPTOMS AND SIGNS OF DIABETIC KETOACIDOSIS
Symptoms	**Signs**
Polyuria	Hypothermia
Polydipsia	Hyperpnea (Kussmaul respirations)
Weakness	Acetone breath
Lethargy	"Dehydration" (intravascular volume depletion)
Myalgia	Hyporeflexia
Headache	Acute abdomen
Anorexia	Stupor ($\rightarrow$ coma)
Nausea	Hypotonia
Vomiting	Uncoordinated ocular movements
Abdominal pain	Fixed, dilated pupils
"Dyspnea"	

filled from below or is filled to less than half of the distance to the angle of the mandible, the intravascular volume is significantly reduced.

The only other reliable sign of intravascular depletion in adults is supine hypotension or a fall of systolic blood pressure by 20 mm Hg or greater when the patient moves from a lying to a sitting or standing position. So that equilibrium is ensured, at least 1 minute should elapse before the semivertical or vertical blood pressure is recorded. This orthostatic change in systolic blood pressure is a less sensitive measurement than decreased filling of the neck veins and thus represents a more marked deficit in intravascular volume. (It must be kept in mind, however, that diabetic patients with dysfunction of the autonomic nervous system may manifest orthostatic changes in blood pressure in the absence of any fluid loss.)

Hyporeflexia may be noted in patients experiencing DKA. If not present initially, it often develops during treatment if the potassium concentration (K) falls. (The response of potassium to therapy is discussed later.)

The abdominal examination of patients experiencing DKA can yield striking results. Abdominal tenderness to palpation and muscle guarding are usual. Bowel sounds may be diminished or even absent. Rebound tenderness is often noted. In an occasional patient, a boardlike abdomen with no bowel sounds and rebound tenderness may suggest a catastrophic intraabdominal process requiring immediate surgery. However, these signs are caused by DKA, although the mechanism underlying them is unknown. Although documentation is difficult, ketosis is probably responsible for many of the gastrointestinal symptoms. (Ketosis secondary to low carbohydrate intake—starvation ketosis—is associated with anorexia, nausea, and occasionally vomiting.) In any event, nausea, vomiting, and abdominal pain are often noted in patients with DKA. Up to 25% of patients with DKA have emesis, which may actually be hematemesis. Endoscopy of these patients often reveals hemorrhagic

gastritis. Except for the unusual patient in whom DKA may be precipitated by such an event, these signs resolve as the patient's biochemical status improves. In any event, because surgery is contraindicated in patients with DKA because of the extremely high related mortality, treatment of DKA must precede surgical intervention, and signs suggesting the need for surgery almost invariably disappear with treatment.

The mental status of patients experiencing DKA ranges from completely alert to comatose and is not related to the degree of ketosis or acidosis. In fact, a patient's mental status seems best correlated with plasma osmolarity (Figure 6-3). Various degrees of

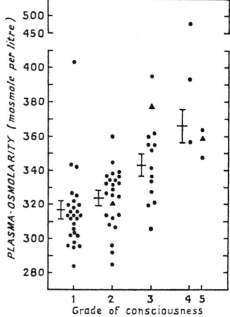

FIGURE 6-3. Relation between state of consciousness and calculated plasma osmolarity in 70 episodes of diabetic ketoacidosis. The means (horizontal line) are shown, and ± 1 SEM (standard error of the mean) is enclosed in brackets. The three triangles refer to three values reported as exceeding those shown. States of consciousness were defined as follows: (1) awake or mildly drowsy (26 episodes); (2) moderately drowsy but easily arousable and fully oriented (24 episodes); (3) very drowsy but arousable by loud questioning and then partially oriented (14 episodes); (4) stuporous, barely responsive, and then not oriented (3 episodes); and (5) comatose (4 episodes). *(From Fulop M, Tannenbaum H, Dreyer N: Hyperosmolar coma. Lancet 2:635, 1973.)*

lethargy, stupor, and coma are observed in most patients, and altered mental status is an important sign of DKA.

Hypotonia, uncoordinated ocular movements, and fixed, dilated pupils are fortunately unusual symptoms that are associated with a poor prognosis, as is very deep coma.

The symptoms of DKA are listed in Table 6-2. Polyuria and polydipsia are simply manifestations of osmotic diuresis secondary to hyperglycemia. Weakness, lethargy, headache, and myalgia are relatively nonspecific symptoms. The gastrointestinal and respiratory symptoms, however, are specifically related to DKA.

When questioned more closely, patients who complain of dyspnea (shortness of breath on exertion) are found actually to be having difficulty in catching their breath even while sitting or lying quietly. This symptom represents hyperventilation, which is the ventilatory response to metabolic acidosis originally described by Kussmaul.

DIFFERENTIAL DIAGNOSIS

The diagnosis of DKA is simple if it is considered in the differential. A urine sample showing marked glucosuria and ketonuria or an undiluted plasma sample giving a strongly positive result in the nitroprusside test for acetoacetate is sufficient for the diagnosis. However, too often these tests are not performed and the diagnosis is regrettably delayed.

Other conditions that may mimic DKA to various degrees and the clinical similarities between these conditions and DKA are listed in Table 6-3. Although coma is certainly encountered in DKA, most diabetic patients who present in coma are found to have suffered cerebral vascular accidents, simply because many more diabetic patients have strokes than have episodes of DKA.

A brainstem hemorrhage may be confused with DKA because both conditions may be associated with glucosuria and hyperventilation. The hyperventilation in brainstem hemorrhage is explained by the fact that the respiratory center is located in the brainstem. In the 19th century, Claude Bernard showed that stimulation of an area in the brainstem resulted in glucosuria, or "piqûre" diabetes.

The many features that distinguish DKA from hypoglycemia are listed in Table 6-4. Hypoglycemic signs and symptoms are listed later in this chapter.

The other conditions listed—metabolic acidosis, gastroenteritis, and pneumonia—all can be ruled out by the absence of significant ketosis. Although ketonuria may be present if carbohydrate intake has been poor, a less than strongly positive result in the nitroprusside test for ketone bodies in undiluted plasma essentially rules out DKA.

TABLE 6-3 DIFFERENTIAL DIAGNOSIS OF DIABETIC KETOACIDOSIS

Cerebrovascular accident (altered mental status)[*]
Brainstem hemorrhage (hyperventilation, glucosuria)
Hypoglycemia (altered mental status, tachycardia)
Metabolic acidosis (hyperventilation, anion gap acidosis)
  Uremia
  Salicylates
  Methanol
  Ethylene glycol
Gastroenteritis (nausea, vomiting, abdominal pain)
Pneumonia (hyperventilation)

[*]Clinical similarities to diabetic ketoacidosis are listed in parentheses.

TABLE 6-4	FEATURES DISTINGUISHING DIABETIC KETOACIDOSIS FROM HYPOGLYCEMIA		
		Condition	
Feature		**DKA**	**Hypoglycemia**
Onset		Slow	Fast
Gastrointestinal symptoms		Yes	No
Intravascular volume depletion		Yes	No
Respiration		Deep	Normal
Sympathetic nervous system signs and symptoms		Tachycardia only	Yes
Glucosuria		≥2%	±
Ketonuria		Strong	Negative

DKA, diabetic ketoacidosis.

Although ketosis helps to make the diagnosis of DKA, not all patients with ketones actually have DKA. Other causes of ketosis include starvation and alcohol excess. These conditions can be distinguished by clinical history and laboratory testing showing glucose values from hypoglycemic to slightly elevated in range. In the case of starvation, a modest acidosis may be present. The differential diagnosis of DKA should also include other causes of a high anion gap acidosis. These include ingestion of excess amounts of salicylates, methanol, ethylene glycol, and paraldehyde. The accumulation of lactate can also cause a similar picture, which should trigger questions about possible metformin use and renal insufficiency. A thorough history, drug screen, and measurements of serum methanol, lactate, and renal function can be helpful in these cases.

INITIAL LABORATORY VALUES

The results of pertinent laboratory tests in patients presenting with DKA are listed in Table 6-5. Glucose concentrations obviously can vary considerably, and a substantial number of patients experiencing DKA have initial glucose values of less than 300 mg/dl.[3] In a series of 211 episodes of DKA, 37 patients had severe acidosis—that is, HCO_3 less than 10 mEq/L—and "euglycemia."

Glucose concentrations were between 200 and 300 mg/dl in 21 patients, between 100 and 200 mg/dl in 9, and less than 100 mg/dl in 7. Thus 17.5% of patients in this report presented with glucose levels of less than 300 mg/dl although they were experiencing severe DKA.[3] Others have also found that glucose concentrations are unrelated to the severity of the acidosis.[4] In essence, this means that although there is a standard presentation we think of with DKA, nothing is absolute, and variations in degree and severity of metabolic abnormalities will be observed.

The initial laboratory investigations should be guided by clinical suspicion, and in the majority of cases should include the following: plasma glucose level, blood urea nitrogen (BUN) level, creatinine level, serum ketones, electrolyte levels, osmolality, urinalysis, urine ketones, initial arterial blood gas, complete blood cell count with differential, and electrocardiogram (ECG).[5] Serum osmolality can also be estimated by the following formula: 2 [measured Na (Meq/l)] + glucose (mg/dl)/18. Bacterial cultures of blood, urine, throat, and wound sites, along with chest x-ray examinations and abdominal films should also be considered. A hemoglobin A_{1c} (A1C) level may provide evidence for baseline control.

The nitroprusside test for ketone bodies yields strongly positive results in undiluted

TABLE 6-5	**INITIAL LABORATORY VALUES FOR PATIENTS EXPERIENCING DIABETIC KETOACIDOSIS**	

Test	Result	Remarks
Glucose	300–800 mg/dl	Concentrations not related to severity of DKA
Ketone bodies	Strong at least in undiluted plasma	Measures only acetoacetate, not β-hydroxybutyrate
HCO_3	0–15 mEq/L	
pH	6.8–7.3	
Na	Low, normal, or high	Total body depletion; concentration dependent on relative H_2O loss and amount shifted from intracellular to extracellular space
K	Low, normal, or high	Total body depletion; heart responsive to extracellular concentration
Phosphate	Usually normal or slightly elevated; occasionally slightly low	Associated with phosphaturia; marked decrease with treatment in levels of both serum and urine phosphates
Creatinine/BUN	Usually mildly increased	May be prerenal; spurious increases in creatinine by acetoacetate in some automated methods
WBC count	Usually increased	Possibility of leukemoid reaction (even in absence of infection)
Amylase	Often increased	Predominant form of salivary gland origin
Lipase	Sometimes increased	Even markedly elevated values do not necessarily mean acute pancreatitis present
Hemoglobin, hematocrit, total protein	Often increased	Secondary to contracted plasma volume
AST, ALT, LDH	Can be mildly elevated	Spurious increases in transaminases caused by acetoacetate interference in older colorimetric methods

ALT, alanine aminotransferase; AST, aspartate aminotransferase; BUN, blood urea nitrogen; DKA, diabetic ketoacidosis; HCO_3, concentration of bicarbonate; K, concentration of potassium; LDH, lactic dehydrogenase; Na, concentration of sodium; WBC, white blood cell.

plasma, and these results most often remain strongly positive through several dilutions (Figure 6-4). The result of this test does not represent the full extent of the ketosis, however, because the nitroprusside reagent measures only acetoacetate and not β-hydroxybutyrate. (Actually, acetone is also measured, but it is only 5% as active as acetoacetate on a molar basis and occurs in patients with DKA at levels that are only two to four times higher than those of acetoacetate.) The ratio of β-hydroxybutyrate to acetoacetate varies greatly in DKA, but may be as high as 3:1 to 5:1.[6-8] A rapid and specific assay for β-hydroxybutyrate that can be carried out on a drop of blood or plasma (e.g., KetoSite-ketone test card, GDS Diagnostics, Elkhart, IN) is also available. Finally, some blood glucose monitoring meters can also measure serum ketones (e.g., Precision Meter by Medisense).

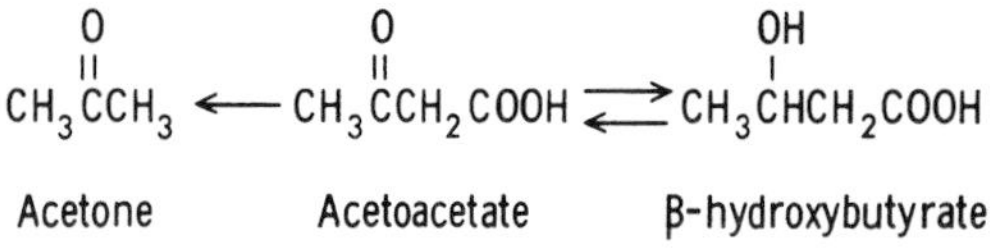

$$CH_3\overset{\overset{O}{\|}}{C}CH_3 \longleftarrow CH_3\overset{\overset{O}{\|}}{C}CH_2COOH \rightleftharpoons CH_3\overset{\overset{OH}{|}}{C}HCH_2COOH$$

Acetone   Acetoacetate   β-hydroxybutyrate

FIGURE 6-4. Structure of and relation among the ketone bodies.

The decreases in HCO_3 and pH do reflect the severity of metabolic derangement. However, if a patient is vomiting excessively, the tendency for a metabolic alkalosis blunts the decline in HCO_3 and pH.[1] In fact, patients have been reported with marked hyperglycemia and ketosis and such severe vomiting that the resulting metabolic alkalosis has more than compensated for the ketoacidosis causing initial elevations of HCO_3 and pH.[9] Severe intravascular volume depletion causes a contraction alkalosis, further limiting the reduction of HCO_3 and pH.

Although total body depletion of sodium stores occurs in DKA, the serum concentration of sodium may be low, normal, or high, and depends on water balance. If hyperlipidemia is present, the serum sodium measured is falsely low. If hyperlipidemia is absent, the serum sodium is simply a measure of the relative amounts of the cation and body water. Because urinary fluid losses are hypotonic, plasma osmolality becomes elevated, and a high serum sodium would be expected. However, polyuria leads to polydipsia and the amount of water ingested affects the Na. If an appropriate amount of water is consumed, the sodium may be normal. If an excess amount is ingested, the sodium decreases. Vomiting further complicates the relation between sodium and water. In addition, the osmolar contribution of the hyperglycemia tends to decrease sodium by drawing water from the intracellular to the extracellular space. Finally, if intravascular volume depletion is profound, antidiuretic hormone is secreted in an attempt to restore the vascular volume, even at the expense of decreasing serum osmolality and sodium.[10] (Hypertriglyceridemia can cause a pseudohyponatremia by displacing plasma water with lipid, and elevated triglyceride levels commonly occur in patients with markedly uncontrolled diabetes. The sodium is decreased by 1.6 mEq/L for each 1000 mg/dl triglyceride concentration.) At presentation, the sodium is normal in half of the patients, low in one quarter, and elevated in one quarter.[1] Although correcting the sodium to take into account the effect of hyperglycemia (i.e., by raising the value by 1.6 mg/dl for each 100 mg/dl of glucose above 100 mg/dl[11]) has been advocated to give a truer picture of water balance,[1] the corrected value does not alter the clinical dictum that patients in DKA need saline repletion to restore their vascular volume, regardless of the sodium. (The rate and osmolality of the replacement solutions are discussed later in the treatment section.)

Similar considerations pertain to the initial potassium, which may be low, normal, or high. There is a profound total body depletion of potassium regardless of the serum concentration, and affected patients must have their stores replenished with potassium salts. The clinical situation with regard to potassium homeostasis in DKA is somewhat complicated and is also discussed in greater detail later in the treatment section.

Serum phosphorus concentrations are usually normal or even slightly elevated in untreated DKA. This finding is associated with marked phosphaturia (which accompanies all forms of metabolic acidosis). The explanation given is that acidosis leads to the breakdown of intracellular organic compounds and that inorganic phosphate is thus liberated, transferred into the plasma, and subsequently excreted in the urine. Treatment of DKA results in a gradual reduction of phosphaturia (over 8 to 10 hours) and a marked decrement of serum phosphorus concentrations, which may not reach their nadir for several days. The hypophosphatemia is presumably the result of the uptake of inorganic phosphorus by cells that had been phosphorus deficient.

Creatinine and BUN levels are usually increased in DKA. This increase often represents prerenal azotemia caused by diminished perfusion of the kidneys secondary to intravascular volume depletion. An additional reason for elevated creatinine concentrations (but not BUN values) is interference by acetoacetate in some automated assays.[10] Therefore a valid assessment of renal function must await resolution of DKA. In many cases, however, BUN and creatinine values do not return to normal, a result reflecting underlying diabetic nephropathy.

Not only is leukocytosis common in DKA, but leukemoid reactions with white blood cell (WBC) counts of $20,000/mm^3$ to $40,000/mm^3$ are occasionally seen. The high WBC counts are associated with lymphopenia and eosinopenia. This leukocyte response to DKA is thought to reflect increased adrenocortical activity and dehydration. Therefore leukocytosis itself is not a reliable sign of infection in this setting. However, the WBC differential may provide an important clue. Patients with a higher percent of band neutrophils (bands) and a lower percent of segmented ones (segs) are much more likely to have a major infection.[12] Using an admission band neutrophil count of more than 10% as diagnostic of a major infection, the sensitivity was 100% and the specificity was 80%. That is, all patients with a major infection had over 10% band neutrophils (sensitivity) whereas 80% of patients with over 10% band neutrophils had a major infection (specificity).

Amylase values are elevated in more than 50% of patients with DKA.[13] However, the increase in the majority of instances is in amylase of salivary origin rather than in that of pancreatic origin.[14,15] Furthermore, the levels and origin of amylase do not correlate with signs and symptoms suggestive of pancreatitis.[14,15] Thus hyperamylasemia probably represents transient nonspecific leakage of this enzyme from its two tissues of origin and does not support a diagnosis of pancreatitis in DKA. Liver function tests are also often non-

specifically elevated. In the recent past, tests for the enzymes serum aspartate aminotransferase (AST), alanine aminotransferase (ALT), and lactic dehydrogenase (LDH) often gave falsely elevated results because of interference by acetoacetate in the colorimetric methods used. Many laboratories are now using kinetic procedures for the measurement of these enzymes; in these procedures, false-positive results are not a problem. If the level of any of these enzymes is found to be elevated in patients who are ketotic, the physician should ascertain that the method used involves direct measurements of reduced nucleotides via changes in ultraviolet absorption rather than coupling with a diazonium salt (the colorimetric method). However, levels of serum enzymes such as AST, ALT, creatine phosphokinase (CPK), and 5'-nucleotidase may truly be elevated in many patients with DKA. Severe abnormalities are usually explained by readily apparent clinical disease. Elevated levels are not related to the degree of abdominal symptoms, nor are they caused by acidosis per se. When no cause can be found, the enzyme levels usually return to normal after treatment for DKA. The transaminitis and rise in amylase are more often seen in DKA versus HHS. Lipase levels, which are considered more specific for pancreatic damage than amylase, can also be elevated in DKA, although not as frequently as amylase.[13] Although it is stated in textbooks that hyperlipasemia in DKA diagnoses pancreatitis, the published data do not substantiate that claim. Nsien and colleagues[13] reported that three patients with DKA, no abdominal symptoms, and marked elevations of lipase had negative results of computed tomography (CT) scans of the pancreas. Clinical judgment is required here. If a patient with marked hyperlipasemia can resume oral intake within a day or two, this would seem to be inconsistent with the diagnosis of acute pancreatitis. If the biochemical changes of DKA have been reversed and the patient remains unable to tolerate oral feedings for several more days, the patient may have acute pancreatitis.

The frequent increases in hemoglobin, hematocrit, and total proteins in DKA simply reflect the decreased volume of plasma. Therefore a low normal or slightly decreased hematocrit or hemoglobin value on admission indicates a probable anemia that will require further evaluation after DKA is treated.

Discerning readers have probably noticed that the anion gap ($Na-Cl-HCO_3$) has not been discussed. Because of the affect of vomiting and contraction alkalosis discussed earlier, as well as other limitations in its interpretation,[16] uncritical reliance on the anion gap in the diagnosis and treatment of DKA can be misleading.

TREATMENT

The treatment of DKA can be conveniently discussed under six separate categories: general therapeutic approaches, fluid replacement, insulin therapy, potassium replacement, phosphate replacement, and bicarbonate therapy. Obviously, all six areas must be considered in clinical decisions, but if each area is considered separately, the decisions are usually straightforward and a coherent treatment plan emerges. Some of these areas of treatment are controversial, and valid arguments can be made on both sides of the issues. Indeed, in many cases, it is difficult to be certain that one course of action is distinctly better for a given patient The modified American Diabetes Association (ADA) steps for DKA management in adults are shown in Figure 6-5.

General Considerations

The use of all deliberate speed is appropriate in the treatment of DKA. Therapy within minutes is not necessary, but a delay of treatment for several hours can be detrimental to patients. The fundamentals of care should be aimed toward correction of dehydration,

hyperglycemia, and electrolyte abnormalities, as well as toward identifying precipitating factors. Certain general principles should be followed. First, only one physician should be in charge of the patient's care and should assume full responsibility for therapeutic decisions.

Second, a DKA progress record (Figure 6-6) should be started *as soon as therapy is initiated*. Too often, this record is constructed from memory many hours after treatment has begun. An accurate and updated progress record enables any health professional involved in the care of the patient to become quickly familiar with the treatment given and the response to therapy. This progress record is extremely important in situations in which responsibility for the patient's care is transferred (e.g., when house staff coverage in teaching hospitals or evening and weekend coverage in the private sector causes a transfer of responsibility to personnel not familiar with the patient). At that juncture, it is wise for the two physicians involved to discuss the patient's progress record, what has transpired, and what is planned.

Third, and most obvious, an appropriate site for intravenous (IV) fluid administration is necessary. Because many hours of fluid administration will be necessary, reliance on a small-gauge catheter tenuously placed in a peripheral vein is not advisable.

Fourth, urine samples are necessary not only in making the diagnosis of DKA, but in monitoring a patient's response to therapy. In addition, it must be ascertained that a patient is not experiencing renal shutdown before potassium replacement is started. Therefore if a patient does not urinate spontaneously, bladder catheterization is indicated. In this instance, the initial bladder specimen should be cultured to ascertain whether the DKA is associated with or precipitated by a urinary tract infection.

Fifth, because the possibility of pulmonary aspiration is enhanced considerably

MANAGEMENT OF ADULT PATIENTS WITH DKA*

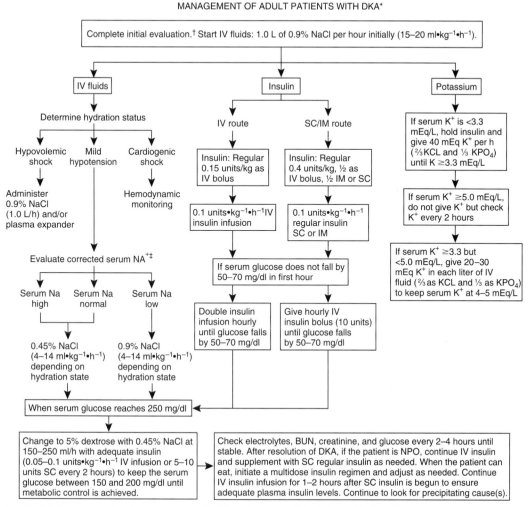

FIGURE 6-5. Protocol for the management of adult patients with diabetic ketoacidosis (DKA).

*DKA diagnostic criteria: blood glucose >250 mg/dl, arterial pH <7.3, bicarbonate <15 mEq/L, and moderate ketonuria or ketonemia.

†After history and physical examination, obtain arterial blood gases, complete blood count with differential, urinalysis, blood glucose, blood urea nitrogen (BUN), electrolytes, chemistry profile, and creatinine levels as soon as possible as well as an electrocardiogram. Obtain chest x-ray examination and cultures as needed.

‡Serum sodium should be corrected for hyperglycemia (for each 100 mg/dl glucose >100 mg/dl, add 1.6 mEq to sodium value for corrected serum sodium value). IM, intramuscular; IV, intravenous; NPO, nothing by mouth; SC, subcutaneous.

(From Hyperglycemic crises in patients with diabetes mellitus. Diabetes Care 26(suppl):S109-S117, 2003.)

in comatose patients, a nasogastric tube should be put in place and continuous suction applied until patients become more responsive. In more alert patients, this maneuver is restricted to those with signs of gastric distention.

The sixth general principle concerns the ordering of laboratory tests and the timing of samples. This discussion is limited to those tests that are concerned specifically with the diagnosis and treatment of DKA. Measurements of glucose, electrolytes,

SUGGESTED
DKA/HHS FLOWSHEET

DATE: HOUR:														
Weight (daily)														
Mental status*														
Temperature														
Pulse														
Respiration/depth**														
Blood pressure														
Serum glucose (mg/dl)														
Serum ketones														
Urine ketones														
ELECTOLYTES														
Serum Na* (mEq/L)														
Serum K* (mEq/L)														
Serum HCO$_3$ (mEq/L)														
Serum BUN (mg/dl)														
Effective osmolality														
2 [measured Na(mEq/L)]														
+Glucose (mg/dl)/18														
Anion gap														
A.B.G.														
pH Venous (V) Arterial (A)														
pO$_2$														
pCO$_2$														
O$_2$ SAT														
INSULIN														
Units past hour														
Route														
INTAKE FLUID/METABOLITES														
0.45% NaCl (ml) past hour														
0.9% NaCl (ml) past hour														
5% Dextrose (ml) past hour														
KCL (mEq) past hour														
PO$_4$ (mMOLES) past hour														
Other (e.g., HCO$_3$)														
OUTPUT														
Urine (ml)														
Other														

*A-ALERT   D-DROWSY   S-STUPOROUS   C-COMATOSE
**D-DEEP   S-SHALLOW   N-NORMAL

FIGURE 6-6. Diabetic ketoacidosis/hyperosmolar hyperglycemia state flowsheet for the documentation of clinical parameters, fluid and electrolytes, laboratory values, insulin therapy, and urinary output. *(From Hyperglycemic crises in patients with diabetes mellitus. Diabetes Care26(supp1):5109-5117, 2003.)*

phosphate, and creatinine or BUN values should be obtained and followed. Although measuring the initial pH and degree of ketosis is not necessary for either diagnosis or monitoring the response to therapy, these values will document the severity of the DKA. A serum sample for measurement of ketones should be sent to confirm the diagnosis of DKA.

After treatment is started, glucose and electrolyte concentrations should be measured every 1 to 2 hours until the HCO_3 reaches ~12 mEq/L; at this time, sampling every 4 hours becomes appropriate. Phosphate concentrations should be measured initially and every 4 to 6 hours. If phosphate levels are elevated, calcium and magnesium concentrations in serum should also be measured. The BUN or creatinine test is repeated after the patient is adequately rehydrated.

Fluid Administration

Solutions containing dextrose should not be used initially (unless the glucose concentration is <200 mg/dl) because the additional glucose cannot be utilized and would simply increase the degree of hyperglycemia. Because an occasional patient with DKA also has lactic acidosis (as described later), most diabetologists also avoid the use of solutions containing lactate. The controversy surrounding fluid administration involves the osmolality of the saline solution that should be used.

A patient experiencing DKA has two separate problems that are specifically treated by fluid administration. One is the hyperosmolar state of the circulation (secondary to hypotonic fluid losses), and the other is intravascular volume depletion. The first problem should be treated with hypo-osmolal solutions, and the second requires saline to replenish the plasma volume. The argument against using a hypo-osmolal solution (usually one-half normal or 0.45% saline) as the initial fluid replacement in DKA is that it

does not reverse intravascular volume depletion as rapidly as does normal saline, and vital organs may continue to be underperfused for a longer period. On the other hand, the argument against the use of normal or isotonic (0.9%) saline as the initial fluid is its hyperosmolality (308 mOsm/kg) compared with normal plasma osmolality (285 mOsm/kg). Proponents of the use of normal saline point out that plasma osmolality in DKA is most often above 310 mOsm/kg, and therefore a hyperosmolal solution is not really being infused. However, potassium and its anion (20 to 40 mEq of each) are often added to the first bottle (as described later) so that the osmolality is increased to 348 or 388 mOsm/kg. The need to reduce the plasma osmolality in DKA (and the possible danger of increasing it) is represented by the inverse relation between the patient's level of consciousness and plasma osmolality, as depicted in Figure 6-3. It is important to remember that the main goal of fluid therapy is mainly to expand volume and restore renal perfusion.

Given these considerations, normal saline is an appropriate choice when intravascular volume depletion is profound. The two clinical signs of intravascular volume depletion (an orthostatic decline in systolic pressure of 20 mm Hg or greater and decreased neck vein filling from below) are very helpful in making this clinical distinction. (Supine hypotension reflects an even greater degree of intravascular volume depletion than a normal supine systolic blood pressure with orthostatic changes on sitting or standing.) As long as a patient has supine hypotension or orthostatic changes, reflecting more profound dehydration, normal saline is the preferred solution. When the blood pressure can be maintained while the patient is sitting or standing but neck vein filling is still low, the administration of 0.45% saline can be begun if one chooses. Regardless of the degree of dehydration, 0.9% saline is used if the serum Na is less than 130 mEq/L, and 0.45% saline is used if the serum Na is less than 150 mEq/L. Patients with known orthostatic changes in blood pressure secondary to dysfunction of the autonomic nervous system present a problem. Other signs of dehydration may help to address fluid status, as will BUN/creatinine (Cr) ratios. In the majority of these patients, it is reasonable to use 1 L of 0.9% saline unless the serum Na dictates otherwise.

The rate of fluid administration is important. A common cause of an apparent lack of response to insulin treatment is too slow a rate of fluid replacement. (A typical situation might involve an infusion rate of 200 ml/hr and glucose concentrations that remain within 50 mg/dl of their initial level for several hours.) It has even been suggested that initially insulin has little, if any, effect on hyperglycemia and that the reduced glucose concentrations are secondary to rehydration, which results in urinary disposal of the excess glucose.[17,18] The most recent recommendations by the ADA for hydration rates are 0.9% NaCl infused at a rate of 15 to 20 ml/kg/hr or greater during the first hour.[5] These translate into approximately 1.0 to 1.5 L. Pending serum Na levels, subsequent infusion rates of 0.9% NaCl or 0.45% NaCl should be continued at 4 to 14 ml/kg/hr. It is important to remember that the average total body water deficit in DKA is 6 to 7 L, so replacement may continue for several hours. In pediatric patients, the complication of rapid hydration to be considered is that of cerebral edema. Although it has been hard to implicate any one parameter as causal for cerebral edema, in the first hour, pediatric patients should receive fluid at a rate of 10 to 20 ml/kg/hr, and total expansion should not exceed 50 ml/kg over the first 4 hours of therapy. The guidelines to choosing appropriate fluids are as mentioned previously.

Because it takes longer to correct acidosis and ketonemia than to correct hyperglycemia, it is almost always necessary to add dextrose to the fluids being administered at some point during treatment. When glucose concentrations have declined to ~250 mg/dl, 5% dextrose should be added to the infusion. (The reason for preventing glucose levels from falling rapidly to <250 mg/dl is discussed later). The average decrement in glucose concentrations is 75 to 100 mg/dl/hr. Therefore the time at which dextrose is needed can often be estimated if this rate of reduction in glucose level can be documented during the early phase of treatment. Because the osmolality of 5% dextrose in water is 277 mOsm/kg, the appropriate fluid for infusion is 5% dextrose–0.45% saline. By the time dextrose is needed, most patients have been rehydrated to the point at which 0.45% saline is appropriate. However, if intravascular volume depletion is still severe, a 5% dextrose–0.9% saline solution should be used. The hyperosmolality of the infusate decreases appreciably as glucose is metabolized or excreted and leaves the vascular space.

Insulin Treatment

In the past, most authorities recommended administration of high doses of insulin at frequent intervals for the treatment of DKA. Several studies have directly compared the efficacy and side effects of using much lower doses of insulin (2 to 10 U/hr) instead of the previously recommended approach.[19-22] The reversal of the DKA state was similar regardless of the dose of insulin given. However, patients treated with lower doses of insulin had less hypoglycemia and hypokalemia than those given the higher "conventional" amounts. No differences were found in the rate of decrement of glucose concentrations, the control of acidosis, or the time elapsed before the patient became mentally alert. Finally, mortality in DKA was similar in 113 episodes treated with infrequent large amounts of insulin (4.4%) and in 237 episodes treated with frequent or continuous small doses of insulin (4.6%).[23] Unless the episode of DKA is mild (defined as plasma glucose >250 mg/dl, pH >7.25, serum bicarbonate of >15 mEq/L and an anion gap of >10 in an alert patient), regular administration of insulin by IV infusion is the treatment of choice.

Once potassium status has been assessed, and no hypokalemia is found, insulin is started. Although the benefit of an initial bolus is debatable, and patients will recover regardless of bolus administration of insulin, it is recommended that a bolus of regular insulin be administered upon initiation of therapy at a dose of 0.15 U/kg, followed by a continuous infusion of 0.1 U/kg/hr in adult patients. In pediatric patients, the bolus is avoided and the rate of regular insulin infusion is started at 0.1 U/kg/hr. The goal in all patients is a slow and steady decrease in glucose levels between 50 and 75 mg/hr. With hourly monitoring, the infusion rate can be titrated up or down to achieve such a rate of decline. When the plasma rate of glucose reaches approximately 250 mg/dl, the infusion rate of insulin may be decreased to 0.05 to 0.1 U/kg/hr, and dextrose added to the IV solution. Frequent monitoring must continue to allow for titration with the goal of reversing acidosis, hyperosmolarity, and any mental changes without causing hypoglycemia. Although insulin is adsorbed to the glass bottle and plastic tubing, it is not necessary to add albumin to this solution. Rather, to avoid the expense and time wasted in waiting for albumin to arrive from the pharmacy, 50 to 100 ml of the insulin solution may simply be discarded into the sink (through the tubing after it is attached to the bottle). This procedure saturates the adsorption sites, and the appropriate amount of insulin is delivered to the patient.[24] The insulin is either piggy-backed onto the IV line delivering the rehydration fluid or administered via a separate vein.

Criteria for resolution of DKA includes a glucose value of less than 200 mg/dl, a serum bicarbonate value of 18 mEq/L or higher and a pH of more than 7.3 (venous sample). At this point, subcutaneous (SC) insulin may be started. Starting insulin doses and regimens in this setting can be based on body weight, total insulin requirements over the preceding 24 hours, or previous regimens. Details of types of insulins available and starting regimens are discussed elsewhere in this book. In general, because patients recovering from DKA probably are not eating the usual number of calories initially, the first dose of insulin should be approximately two thirds of the usual amount. If a patient has a documented infection, however, the prehospitalization dose of insulin may be given because the decreased caloric intake is probably offset by the insulin resistance associated with infection. A question often arises about the interval between the discontinuation of regular insulin infusions and the administration of SC insulin. If a patient is eating at the time when SC insulin is first administered, the insulin infusion is continued for 1 or 2 hours (with the interval determined by the size of the meal). This regular insulin helps dispose of the ingested calories during the 2- to 4-hour lag period before intermediate-acting insulin (which is usually the insulin of choice in this setting) starts to act. A multiple dose schedule should be started as soon as possible, and regimens are discussed elsewhere in this book. On the other hand, if SC insulin is injected when the patient has been ordered to eat nothing by mouth, the IV insulin and fluids are continued with SC regular insulin added as needed every 4 hours. In adults, a guideline is 5 units for every 50 mg/dl increase in blood glucose above 150 mg/dl up to 20 units for a blood glucose of 300 mg/dl. Once able to eat, the patient can be switched over as noted previously.

Potassium Replacement

In considering potassium therapy, one is faced with a certain dilemma. Although the total body depletion of potassium is profound (see Figure 6-2), the heart responds to extracellular concentrations, which, as shown in Table 6-5, can be high as well as normal or low. Therefore potassium replacement may be contraindicated initially. However, because all modes of therapy reduce the serum potassium, unless the patient is anuric, potassium replacement is required at some time (usually soon) after treatment is started.

Rehydration lowers the serum potassium in two ways. First, as the plasma volume is expanded, the potassium decreases simply through dilution. Second, an expanding intravascular volume improves renal perfusion. Improved perfusion increases urinary glucose excretion, and the resulting osmotic diuresis enhances urinary potassium losses.

Insulin treatment also lowers the serum potassium by two separate mechanisms. First, insulin directly stimulates the uptake of potassium by adipose tissue, muscle, and liver. Second, the entry of glucose into these tissues further enhances potassium uptake. Although it is commonly held that potassium leaves the cell and enters the extracellular fluid compartment as hydrogen ions enter the cell to be buffered, this probably does not occur in DKA.[25] Therefore correction of the acidosis (with a postulated subsequent return of potassium into the cell) does not result in lowering of potassium. The major determinants of the serum potassium on admission for DKA are the degree of ketoacidemia and hyperglycemia,[25] both of which are accounted for solely by the insulinopenia.

Although the potassium measured in the laboratory is obviously the ultimate criterion on which clinical decisions must be based, the ECG provides a reasonable alternative in the interval before laboratory results are available. The effect of potassium on the T-wave of the ECG is depicted in Figure 6-6. Hyperkalemia causes a tall, symmetrically peaked T-wave, whereas hypokalemia is associated with low or flat T-waves and the development of U-waves if the potassium is low enough. The relation between the shape of the T-wave and the serum potassium may vary among patients. Therefore the actual potassium cannot be predicted by the T-wave

configuration on the ECG. However, in a given patient, the changes in the T-waves are consistent and predict corresponding changes in potassium. That is, a serum potassium of 6.0 mEq/L may be associated with abnormally tall and peaked T-waves in one patient but with normal-appearing T-waves in another. In both patients, however, the T-wave decreases in amplitude during treatment. By the same token, a serum potassium of 2.6 mEq/L may be associated with low T-waves in one patient and flat T-waves in another. Treatment (without appropriate potassium replacement) flattens outthe T-waves in the first patient and causes the appearance of U-waves in the second. Thus no matter what the actual configuration of the T-wave at the beginning of treatment, the change from the initial serum potassium can be predicted by a corresponding change in the T-wave.

Because both hyperkalemia and hypokalemia have detrimental effects on the cardiovascular and respiratory systems, the goal of potassium replacement is to maintain the serum potassium within the normal range. If a patient presents with hyperkalemia, potassium replacement should be delayed until the serum potassium has fallen into the normal range. If the initial serum potassium is normal, the goal of potassium replacement should be to maintain this normal level. If hypokalemia is initially noted, potassium replacement should restore the serum potassium to normal relatively quickly; however, the patient's cardiovascular system must not be jeopardized by too rapid administration of potassium. At presentation, the great majority of patients have a normal or elevated potassium level.[1] A low potassium level reflects very severe potassium deficiency. If the potassium is less than 3.0 mEq/L, insulin should be withheld until potassium repletion raises the potassium above that value. Remember that initial rehydration alone is effective therapy.[17,18]

To replete potassium in a safe, timely manner, the following approach is recommended. If easily obtained, and ECG is performed as soon as is feasible, and the lead II, V_1, or V_2 tracing is either placed in the patient's chart or posted at the bedside for further comparisons. Potassium replacement is not begun if the patient is anuric or if the T-waves either are abnormally tall and peaked or have a high normal configuration consistent with excessively high extracellular concentrations, accompanied by serum levels that are consistent. Laboratory testing should be obtained first. Fluid resuscitation is started as otherwise outlined with a repeat potassium obtained within 1 hour along with a follow-up ECG. If the T-waves are normal or slightly low and serum potassium levels are low, normal or modestly elevated, 20 to 40 mEq of potassium (⅔ KCL and ⅓ KPO$_4$) is added to the first liter of replacement fluid. If the T-waves are flat, or if significant hypokalemia is present, potassium replacement should begin with fluid therapy and insulin treatment should be delayed until the potassium concentration is restored to more than 3.3 mEq/L to avoid arrhythmias and other cardiac sequelae.

Phosphate Replacement

Serum phosphate concentrations are usually slightly elevated or in the high-normal range in patients admitted in DKA, despite whole body deficits. Levels decline, during the first 24 hours of treatment without phosphate replacement.[20,26-30] Some earlier evidence showed that these low levels of phosphate might impair tissue oxygenation by inhibiting the production of red blood cell 2,3-diphosphoglycerate.[31] This compound decreases the affinity of hemoglobin for oxygen, thereby enhancing oxygen delivery to peripheral tissue. Hence, lower levels would theoretically cause oxygen to be more tightly bound to hemoglobin and less available to the tissues. However, impairment of tissue oxygenation could not be corroborated in subsequent studies.[27,29] Furthermore, phosphate replacement had no effect on the rates of (1) glucose decrement,[28-30] (2) pH rise,[27,29,30] (3) increase in bicarbonate lev-

els,[29] (4) fall in ketone bodies,[29] (5) recovery of mental status,[28,29] (6) requirements for insulin,[28,29] or (7) mortality.[28-30] In addition to the lack of demonstrable clinical efficacy for phosphate treatment in DKA, there are two other reasons to be wary of its use. First, phosphate infusions are contraindicated for patients with renal insufficiency, and initially it is difficult to ascertain whether the increased Cr and BUN levels represent prerenal azotemia, spurious increases in Cr values secondary to high acetoacetate concentrations, or true renal failure. Second, overly zealous administration of phosphate has been reported to cause symptomatic hypocalcemia,[32,33] although in general the reduction in calcium levels during phosphate replacement in DKA is modest.[27-29] Prospective data has failed to show any beneficial effect on clinical outcome in DKA[34]; however, serum phosphate concentrations can fall to extremely low levels (even to <1 mg/dl) during therapy for DKA, and the potential hazards of severe hypophosphatemia (muscle weakness, respiratory failure, hemolytic anemia, hemorrhage, rhabdomyolysis, and neurologic dysfunction) must be kept in mind.[35] In certain cases, careful phosphate replacement may be warranted if serum levels are less than 1.0 mg/dl.

The following approach for phosphate replacement may be used. Potassium is replaced with the chloride anion unless the serum phosphate concentrations are initially low or in the low-normal range. In that case, half of the potassium is given as the chloride and half as the phosphate salt. In addition, phosphate may be used for one half of the potassium replacement as soon as an initially high serum level declines into the normal range because of the likelihood of a continued decrease unless phosphate is given. In any event, continued monitoring of serum phosphate and calcium levels is important to prevent unexpected hyperphosphatemia or hypocalcemia.

Inorganic phosphate exists in serum in two valence states, HPO_4^{2-} and $H_2PO_4^-$; the proportions vary with the pH. Therefore the number of milliequivalents in 1 mmol of phosphate is not constant. In contrast, because the amount of phosphate as expressed in millimoles does not vary, phosphate replacement should be calculated in millimoles.[36] Although potassium phosphate for injection is a mixture of two salts, KH_2PO_4 and K_2HPO_4, the important consideration is the total amount of phosphate being administered. Most potassium phosphate preparations for IV use contain 4.4 mEq/ml of potassium and 3 mmol/ml of phosphate.

Bicarbonate Therapy

The use of bicarbonate is another controversial area in the treatment of DKA.[37] At a pH of above 7.0, reestablishing insulin activity adequately blocks lipolysis and resolves ketoacidosis, and no bicarbonate is needed. Most patients experiencing DKA do not require and therefore should not receive bicarbonate therapy. Although some standard texts state that a pH of <7.0 is incompatible with life (or words to that effect), two important caveats must be issued. First, this assertion applies to a chronic situation, whereas DKA is an acute acidosis. Second, and probably more important, the acid-base status of the cerebrospinal fluid (CSF), not the pH of the systemic circulation, determines brain function.[38] In contrast to respiratory acidosis, in which systemic pH and that of CSF diminish in parallel,[38] the pH of CSF is much higher than the systemic pH in DKA,[38,39] for reasons discussed later.

There are many cogent arguments against the administration of bicarbonate to patients with DKA. First, endogenous bicarbonate is generated during insulin treatment.

Second, not only is intracellular pH normally much lower than extracellular pH, it is relatively uninfluenced by the acid-base status of the surrounding interstitial fluid. Rather, the partial pressure of carbon dioxide (PCO_2) has a much greater effect. The lowered PCO_2 of DKA raises the intracellular pH.[40] Thus the intracellular pH may be normal or close to it even though a patient has a systemic acidosis.

Third, because bicarbonate administration usually reverses systemic acidosis relatively quickly, hypokalemia becomes a much greater problem. Indeed, before the relation between bicarbonate therapy and hypokalemia was recognized, a number of patients treated with alkali died of cardiac arrhythmias. More recently, hypokalemic respiratory arrest occurring during bicarbonate administration in DKA has been rediscovered.[41]

Fourth, administration of bicarbonate enhances the paradoxic acidosis of the CSF that develops during the treatment of DKA. The mechanism of enhancement can be understood by means of the following rearrangement of the Henderson-Hasselbalch equation, which expresses the relation among pH, HCO_3, and PCO_2.

$$pH \propto \frac{[HCO_3]}{PCO_2} \qquad (1)$$

Because CO_2 crosses freely from blood to CSF and vice versa, it quickly equilibrates between the two. Bicarbonate, on the other hand, diffuses much more slowly across the blood-brain barrier.[38] The difference between the rate of diffusion of CO_2 and that of bicarbonate explains both the higher pH of the CSF in DKA and the paradoxic fall of the pH of CSF during treatment. In the untreated state, as the HCO_3 falls, it is lower in the systemic circulation than in the CSF because of the delayed attainment of equilibrium. Because CO_2, on the other hand, equilibrates rapidly between the blood and CSF, CO_2 tension is the same on both sides of the blood-brain barrier. As can be appreciated from the equation just cited, the pH is higher in the CSF than in the plasma. As treatment progresses, both the PCO_2 and the HCO_3 increase in the plasma. In the CSF, the increase in the HCO_3 is delayed compared with that in the PCO_2, so that the pH actually falls. Bicarbonate therapy enhances this decrease in the pH of CSF.[39,42] Because mental status correlates with the pH of CSF rather than with systemic pH,[38] bicarbonate therapy could be deleterious.

Fifth, fatal cerebral edema is a rare cause of death in DKA that is discussed in more detail later. The histologic changes in the brain resemble those of anoxia.[40] Treatment of experimentally induced DKA in dogs with systemic bicarbonate caused a marked reduction in the partial pressure of oxygen in the CSF compared with that in dogs whose regimen did not include bicarbonate.[43]

Sixth, bicarbonate administration in patients with DKA increased hepatic ketogenesis, resulting in an initial rise in acetoacetate concentrations followed by a rebound increase in β-hydroxybutyrate levels after the alkali was discontinued.[44] There was a 6-hour delay in the improvement of ketosis compared with the control group in DKA not receiving bicarbonate.[44]

Seventh, a retrospective analysis[45] of 73 cases of severe DKA treated with bicarbonate compared with 22 episodes of DKA treated without bicarbonate revealed no differences between the two groups in rates of (1) decrease in plasma glucose levels, (2) increase in plasma bicarbonate concentrations, (3) arterial pH, and (4) neurologic recovery. This study is representative of several other retrospective studies that could not document improved outcome in patients treated with bicarbonate.

Eighth, a prospective study[46] of patients with severe DKA (pH 6.9 to 7.14), half of whom received bicarbonate, also showed no difference in the rates of (1) decrease in plasma glucose levels, (2) decrease in concentrations of plasma ketone bodies, (3) increase in arterial pH, (4) increase in plasma bicarbonate levels, and (5) increase in CSF pH and bicarbonate concentrations. Thus in the absence of any advantages to bicarbonate therapy in DKA, why expose patients routinely to the potential hazards of this treatment?

In several situations, however, bicarbonate therapy should be considered. First, patients with life-threatening hyperkalemia should be given bicarbonate. A second circumstance in which bicarbonate therapy might be considered is in severe acidosis with shock that is unresponsive to intravascular volume repletion. If rehydration with saline (which is distributed throughout the entire extracellular fluid compartment) is initially ineffective, the intravascular volume should be expanded with plasma, albumin, or even whole blood (all of which are contained within the vascular volume). If these measures do not restore the blood pressure, bicarbonate therapy is indicated. The rationale for the use of alkali under these circumstances is that severe, prolonged acidosis may impair left ventricular contractility, whereas a more rapid reversal of acidosis may improve cardiac output.

Finally, a patient with a maximal ventilatory response (PCO_2 ≤10 mm Hg) and an HCO_3 of 5 mEq/L or higher has a very small buffer reserve. Any further reduction in HCO_3 would theoretically have a profound effect on the pH. Although patients with these values have been successfully treated without bicarbonate administration, alkali treatment is often used under these circumstances. To avoid alkalosis overshoot (i.e., posttreatment alkalosis), it is recommended to infuse only that amount of bicarbonate that raises the HCO_3 to 10 to 12 mEq/L.[1] Other sources of an alkalosis overshoot are bicarbonate generated from the metabolism of ketone bodies and the 24- to 36-hour persistence of hyperventilation after the acidosis is corrected.[47] Because these two are beyond the control of the physician, it makes sense to limit the amount of exogenous bicarbonate to minimize the possibility of an alkalosis overshoot.

If bicarbonate therapy is to be used to treat DKA, it should *never* be given in the form of an IV bolus. Death secondary to hypokalemia has occurred under these circumstances, even when the K was elevated at the time of administration. Although every case must be reviewed on an individual basis, the ADA position statement[5] advocates that for adult patients with a pH of <6.9, 100 mmol sodium bicarbonate should be added to 400 ml of sterile water and given at a rate of 200 ml/hr. In patients with a pH of 6.9 to 7.0, 50 mmol of sodium bicarbonate should be diluted in 200 ml of sterile water and infused at a rate of 200 ml/hr. They note that if the pH is 7.0 or greater, no bicarbonate is needed in regular circumstances without the previously noted complications.

In pediatric patients there are no studies done in situations in which pH levels are less than 6.9. It may be appropriate to consider bicarbonate therapy if the pH after an hour of fluid resuscitation does not climb above 7.0. The ADA recommends 1 to 2 mEq/kg sodium bicarbonate be given as added to NaCl over the course of an hour.

RESPONSE TO THERAPY

Glucose concentrations decline at a rate of 75 to 100 mg/dl/hr in patients receiving low-dose insulin infusions for the treatment of DKA. In general, glucose levels reach 200 to 300 mg/dl within 4 to 5 hours. At this time, because of the continued need for insulin to treat the still uncorrected ketosis and acidosis, dextrose must be added to the infusion to avoid hypoglycemia. The insulin infusion rate can be decreased to 2 to 3 U/hr unless the addition of dextrose to the rehydration fluid (usually as 5% dextrose in one-half normal saline) increases plasma glucose concentrations.

Ketosis is reversed in ~12 to 24 hours, although some patients may have detectable ketone bodies for several days. This may be due to the generation of acetone by the spontaneous decarboxylation of acetoacetate. As mentioned earlier, acetone is weakly reactive to nitroprusside. Its concentration in DKA exceeds that of acetoacetate.[48] Because of its solubility in fat and slow excretion via the lungs and kidneys, the

half-life of plasma acetone in treated patients with DKA ranged from 8 to 15 hours.[48] These factors probably account for the persistence of ketonuria and the smell of acetone on the breath 24 to 48 hours after the correction of acidosis. As shown in Figure 6-7, levels of β-hydroxybutyrate and acetoacetate (which initially favors the former by a ratio of 3:1 to 5:1) shifts so that the concentration of the latter falls less rapidly (and may even increase early in treatment) than that of the former. This has important clinical ramifications if the patient's course is being monitored by the nitroprusside test for plasma ketone bodies. Because only acetoacetate is measured by this method, it may appear that the ketosis is not responding to treatment or even that it is worsening, although the total amount of ketone bodies is actually decreasing (hours 2 through 8 in Figure 6-7). Direct measurement of β-hydroxybutyrate concentrations, which is becoming more common, avoids the uncertainties of interpretation surrounding the assessment of ketosis by nitroprusside.

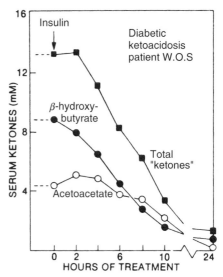

FIGURE 6-7. Response of serum ketone bodies to treatment in diabetic ketoacidosis. *(From Upjohn Co: Current Concepts. Coma in the Diabetic. The Upjohn Co, Kalamazoo, MI, 1974, p. 16.)*

Monitoring of the reversal of acidosis strictly on the basis of changes in the HCO_3 may also be somewhat misleading. Frequently, the HCO_3 seems to remain low (between 12 and 18 mEq/L) after most other signs, symptoms, and biochemical abnormalities associated with DKA have markedly improved. If the pH is measured at this time, it is frequently above 7.3, whereas both the HCO_3 and the PCO_2 are low.[49,50] Thus the metabolic acidosis has been almost compensated at this point by a respiratory alkalosis (see Equation 1). Indeed, if patients are observed closely, deep respirations are noted even though tachypnea is frequently absent. This explains the discrepancy between the time when the pH returns to more than 7.3 (~8 to 9 hours) and that when the HCO_3 returns to normal (14 to 24 hours).

During this period of recovery from DKA, the acid-base status is labeled as a hyperchloremic acidosis. The anion gap has returned to normal, and increased chloride levels replace the ketone bodies. The mechanism of these changes is thought to be the following. The conversion of ketone bodies to bicarbonate is the major source of the regenerated alkali. However, ketone bodies are lost in the urine before treatment and during rehydration, and therefore an insufficient amount of bicarbonate is formed to replace totally the acidic ketone bodies in the extracellular space.[51,52] The chloride ion makes up the deficit during this period until more bicarbonate ion is generated from other sources. The important clinical lesson to keep in mind is that decreased HCO_3 after approximately 8 hours of treatment probably does not mean that the patient's pH is still low and requires further therapy for an acidosis. The increase in HCO_3 and decline in serum chloride levels to normal values should occur spontaneously in the next 12 to 24 hours.

Full replacement of total body water may require 1 or 2 days and obviously can be completed by the oral route. Full repletion of intracellular electrolytes can take up to 10 days. Nitrogen balance may require several weeks to return to normal.

Life-threatening complications associated with DKA are listed in Table 6-6. The most common complications are hypoglycemia and hypokalemia. Hyperglycemia also occurs with frequency if therapy is interrupted or insufficient. Transient hyperchloremia is often seen as a result of choice of fluid replacement, and is usually self-limited. Mortality in DKA has been reported to be between 3% and 30%, although the more recent figures have been between 5% and 10%. No single factor seems to predict which patients will fare poorly. The presence of a complicating condition is often associated with a poor outcome. Age and the duration and degree of unconsciousness have also been cited as relevant factors. For instance, in 317 episodes of DKA in adults admitted to a hospital in England, 43% of those of older than 50 years of age died, whereas the mortality rate was only 3.4% in patients younger

TABLE 6-6	LIFE-THREATENING COMPLICATIONS ASSOCIATED WITH DIABETIC KETOACIDOSIS
Cerebral edema	*Disseminated intravascular coagulation*
Serious infection	Adult respiratory distress syndrome (smokers)
Unrelenting shock	Aspiration
Cardiac arrest (hyperkalemia)	Pulmonary embolus
Respiratory arrest (hypokalemia)	Rhabdomyolysis
Arterial thrombosis	Pneumomediastinum and subcutaneous emphysema

than 50 years.[53] In 128 episodes of DKA in adults admitted to a hospital in the United States, 18% of those older than 50 years of age died, compared with 6% of those younger than 50.[54] The severity of hyperglycemia or acidosis does not seem to be of prognostic importance. Deaths are usually a result of infections, arterial thrombosis, or unrelenting shock.[18] Because infection leads to death in only 2% of patients with DKA, routine antibiotic coverage is not indicated. On the other hand, a thorough evaluation for a source of infection is mandatory in every patient with DKA. Adult respiratory distress syndrome (almost always in smokers) is as an important cause of death in DKA.[55]

Death secondary to arterial thrombosis has been reported to be relatively common in all published studies of patients with DKA. The site may be ubiquitous and can involve any of the following arteries: coronary, carotid, mesenteric, iliac, renal, splenic, or pancreaticoduodenal. The clinical manifestations usually become apparent late in the course of treatment or even after recovery from DKA. It has been suggested that the treatment itself may trigger a number of phenomena that increase the propensity of patients with DKA to develop vascular thromboses.

Hypotension, azotemia, and oliguria leading to anuria as a result of severe intravascular volume depletion in combination with hyperosmolality are often associated with a poor prognosis.[56] Like vascular thrombosis, irreversible shock may develop during the course of treatment. Thus vigorous rehydration at the beginning of treatment may be helpful. Decreased cardiac output secondary to severe prolonged acidosis may also contribute to a poor outcome through impairment of left ventricular function. If acidosis does not improve in this situation, treatment with bicarbonate may be helpful. However, preexisting heart disease may also be a major and untreatable factor.

Rhabdomyolysis is a common complication of DKA and is related to the degree of hyperosmolality.[57,58] Pneumomediastinal

emphysema secondary to the 20 to 30 mm Hg increase in alveolar pressure caused by Kussmaul respirations is probably much more common than realized.[59] Fortunately, neither of these seems to make a major contribution to mortality.

Although cerebral edema is an unusual cause of death in the entire population of patients with DKA, 95% of cases occur in patients less than 20 years of age and 33% in children less than 5 years old.[60] The usual clinical setting is one in which the patient is showing marked clinical and biochemical improvement but then lapses back into a fatal coma while the metabolic abnormalities return completely to normal. At autopsy, cerebral edema is found. Although clinically evident cerebral edema is often fatal, rapid recognition and treatment with mannitol is helpful. If treatment is administered soon after signs of neurologic deterioration, approximately half of patients (most often children) are left with mild or no disability.[61,62]

It was once thought that cerebral edema was solely a manifestation of treatment. In fact, several studies documented that most patients undergoing treatment for DKA probably go through a stage of mild cerebral edema. In one study,[63] CSF pressures were monitored continuously in five adult patients during the first 10 hours of therapy. In four of the five patients, the CSF pressure was normal before initiation of treatment, but became elevated during the course of therapy. In the fifth patient, the CSF pressure was elevated initially and increased even further during treatment. The highest pressure recorded was 600 mm H_2O, and four of the five patients had sustained elevations in pressure for at least 2 hours. All of these patients were alert on admission but became drowsy during the interval when CSF pressure was greater than normal. One patient developed slurred speech and became semistuporous 3 hours after treatment was begun. Another patient became incoherent and agitated at 4 hours and semistuporous at 6 hours.

Cerebral edema during the treatment of DKA with low-dose insulin infusions was evaluated by means of serial repeat echoencephalograms.[64] A decrease in the width of the lateral ventricles was taken as an indication of cerebral edema. Of 11 patients, 9 showed significant decreases in lateral ventricle size at some time during the 15-hour period after treatment was started. Seven of the nine patients who had diminished lateral ventricle width also showed "hash marks," which are characteristic of cerebral edema by this technique. By 20 hours, the size of the lateral ventricle had returned to normal in all patients. In this study, no patient exhibited clinical evidence of cerebral edema. More recently, cerebral edema was evaluated by performing cranial CT scans in six children being treated for DKA.[65] The scans were performed as soon as possible after the blood glucose level had fallen to less than 250 mg/dl and 3 to 6 days after admission, just before discharge from the hospital. Two patients were lethargic at the time of the first scan, but no patient had any other abnormal neurologic sign during treatment. All of the initial scans showed a statistically significant narrowing of the third and lateral ventricles compared with the subsequent one. Although the results on the early scan did not permit an unequivocal diagnosis of cerebral edema, comparison of the two scans showed an alteration in brain volume compatible with mild brain swelling during treatment for DKA in these children who showed no clinical signs of abnormal neurologic function (except for lethargy).

It now seems clear that cerebral edema is also present before treatment. Not only is it evident on CT scans before therapy is initiated,[66,67] but fatal cerebral edema has been reported either before treatment was begun[68] or 1.5 hours after it was started, with only minimal changes in pH, glucose, and electrolytes values.[69] The degree of cerebral edema before therapy was proportional to the glucose concentration and inversely proportional to the bicarbonate level.[67] The

recognition that cerebral edema is present before treatment may help lessen the emotional and legal consequences that can attend this unfortunate outcome.

Why an occasional, usually young patient develops fatal cerebral edema and how this devastating outcome can be prevented are unknown. Three observations, however, suggest a therapeutic approach that may limit the possibility of developing clinical cerebral edema during therapy. First, changes of cerebral edema on CT scan during treatment correlated very highly with changes in calculated plasma osmolality[67]—that is, the more rapid the fall, the more brain swelling.

Second, although Rosenbloom[61] could find no correlation between clinical cerebral edema and rates of hydration, tonicity of administered fluid, or rates of correction of glucose (or bicarbonate) concentrations, others have noted that clinical cerebral edema occurred in patients whose Na failed to rise as glucose concentrations fell[70] and did not if [Na] remained stable or increased.[70,71] Because Na would be expected to increase as glucose levels declined (all other things being equal),[11] the failure to rise implies overhydration with free water.

Third, experiments in animals have demonstrated that a rapid decline of the plasma glucose concentration after a 4-hour period of marked hyperglycemia causes cerebral edema. The mechanism involved may be the delay in attainment of equilibrium between glucose levels in CSF and those in plasma. Glucose concentrations decrease more rapidly in the blood than in the CSF during treatment. This discrepancy results in a less marked decrease in CSF osmolality than in plasma osmolality, so that fluid enters the CSF compartment. Because expansion of this compartment is limited by the cranium, increased pressure and cerebral edema develop. Greater decrements in glucose concentrations and osmolalities in plasma than in CSF have been documented in patients undergoing treatment with high-dose insulin regimens.[39,42]

These observations suggest that the development of clinical cerebral edema during treatment may be associated with a rapid decline in plasma osmolality. This could occur if glucose concentrations are lowered too quickly and/or hypotonic solutions are given too rapidly. Thus it seems wise to lower glucose levels gradually (75 to 100 mg/dl/hr) and to support the glucose concentration by adding dextrose to the infusate when it reaches ~250 mg/dl. In children, avoiding rapid rates of rehydration to less than 4 L/m² during the first 24 hours[72] and ensuring that Na does not decline during treatment by adjusting the tonicity of the infusate[70,71] may also be beneficial.

HHS

Although HHS was first described before 1900 and sporadic cases were reported in the first half of this century, this syndrome has received ever-increasing attention since 1957. The "pure" syndrome has been defined[73] variously as glucose concentrations of 500 to 800 mg/dl, hyperosmolality above 320 to 350 mOsm/kg, and profound intravascular volume depletion in the absence of "significant" ketosis (usually defined as a nitroprusside reaction of 2 or less in a 1:1 dilution of plasma). The serum bicarbonate concentration is above 15 mEq/L, and by definition, the serum pH is above 7.3. The plasma glucose values often are even higher (ranging to >2000 mg/dl), as is the hyperosmolality (sometimes >400 mOsm/kg). A depressed sensorium is frequently encountered, especially if the plasma osmolality is above 350 mOsm/kg. Affected patients are usually older than those presenting with DKA. In practice, patients who have these characteristics of HHS are often also mildly ketotic and acidotic. Indeed, DKA and HHS represent two ends of a continuous spectrum, and many patients have various aspects of each syndrome (Table 6-7).[74] As might be expected, the pathogenesis, clinical presentation, and treatment of HHS are similar to those of DKA in most respects. Several exceptions are important, however. The following discussion briefly mentions the similarities between the two conditions, but emphasizes the differences.

PATHOPHYSIOLOGY

As outlined in Figure 6-1, a lack of effective insulin in carbohydrate and protein metabolism leads to intravascular volume deple-

TABLE 6-7	DIAGNOSTIC CRITERIAL FOR DKA AND HHS			
	DKA			
	Mild	**Moderate**	**Severe**	**HHS**
Plasma glucose (mg/dl)	>250	>250	>250	>600
Arterial pH	7.25–7.30	7.00–7.24	<7.00	>7.30
Serum bicarbonate (mEq/L)	15-18	10 to <15	<10	>15
Urine ketones*	Positive	Positive	Positive	Small
Serum ketones*	Positive	Positive	Positive	Small
Effective serum osmolality (mOsm/kg)†	Variable 0	Variable	Variable	>320
Anion gap‡	>10	>12	>12	<12
Alteration in sensoria or mental obtundation	Alert	Alert/drowsy	Stupor/coma	Stupor/coma

DKA, diabetic ketoacidosis; HHS, hyperosmolar hypoglycemia state.
*Nitroprusside reaction method; †calculation: 2[measured Na (mEq/l)] + glucose (mg/dl)/18; ‡calculation: (Na⁺) − (Cl⁻ + HCO₃⁻) (mEq/L).
See text for details.

tion ("dehydration") and electrolyte depletion. The unregulated lipolysis that results from a lack of effective insulin on fat metabolism causes ketosis and the resultant acidosis. If lipolysis were not increased, ketosis and acidosis would not ensue and patients would manifest only depletion of intravascular volume and electrolytes. Because, in fact, only the latter two manifestations characterize patients in HHS, the relatively normal lipolysis in this setting must be explained.

Two explanations have been offered. Because the regulation of lipolysis is so sensitive to insulin, the levels of insulin in patients in HHS may be sufficient to control this pathway but not to prevent catabolism in the carbohydrate and protein pathways. In general, however, plasma insulin concentrations have been similar in DKA and in HHS when measured. On the other hand, FFA levels are generally lower in HHS than in DKA, a finding that reinforces the view that lipolysis is better controlled in HHS. In vitro data suggest that hyperosmolality itself inhibits lipolysis.[75] Thus the combination of some effective insulin acting in an environment of greatly increased osmolality may account for the lack of ketosis and subsequent acidosis. This is not an entirely satisfactory explanation, however, because the marked increase in serum osmolality occurs later in the evolution of HHS and would not account for the restrained lipolysis early on.

LOSSES

The losses sustained in DKA and depicted in Figure 6-2 are often exceeded in patients in HHS (Table 6-8). In the absence of ketosis and acidosis, which cause severe gastrointestinal symptoms in patients with DKA and force them to seek medical attention within 1 or 2 days, many patients tolerate polyuria and polydipsia for weeks, thus losing great quantities of fluid and electrolytes.

CAUSES

Conditions associated with the onset of HHS are listed in Table 6-9. The mechanism by which these conditions induce HHS is evident in most but not all cases. HHS can be the initial manifestation of diabetes mellitus in older patients. In most other cases, the onset of HHS is associated with a condition that is known to impair insulin action or insulin secretion or both, especially if ready access to fluids is not available. The patient usually is ill, although the mechanistic relationship to HHS is not always clear. *The important point to keep in mind, however, is that patients with HHS are very likely to have a*

TABLE 6-8	TYPICAL TOTAL BODY DEFICITS OF WATER AND ELECTROLYTES IN DKA AND HHS	
	DKA	HHS
Total water (L)	6	9
Water (ml/kg)*	100	100–200
Na^+ (mEq/kg)	7–10	5–13
Cl^- (mEq/kg)	3–5	5–15
K^+ (mEq/kg)	3–5	4–6
PO_4 (mmol/kg)	5–7	3–7
Mg^{2+} (mEq/kg)	1–2	1–2
Ca^{2+} (mEq/kg)	1–2	1–2

DKA, diabetic ketoacidosis; HHS, hyperosmolar hypoglycemia state.

*Per kilogram of body weight.
‡From Ennis et al. (20) and Kreisberg (24).

TABLE 6-9	PREDISPOSING OR PRECIPITATING FACTORS OF HYPEROMOLAR NONKETOTIC SYNDROME	
Acute Illness	**Drugs/Therapy**	
Previously undiagnosed diabetes mellitus	Calcium channel blockers	
	Chlorpromazine	
Acute infection (32% to 60%)	Chlorthalidone	
Pneumonia	Cimetidine	
Urinary tract infection	Diazoxide	
Sepsis	Encainide	
Cerebrovascular accident	Ethacrynic acid	
Myocardial infarction	Immunosuppressive agents	
Acute pancreatitis	L-Asparaginase	
Acute pulmonary embolus	Loxapine	
Intestinal obstruction	Phenytoin	
Dialysis, peritoneal	Propranolol	
Mesenteric thrombosis	Steroids	
Renal failure	Thiazide diuretics	
Heat stroke	Total parenteral nutrition	
Hypothermia		
Subdural hematoma		
Severe burns		
Endocrine		
Acromegaly		
Thyrotoxicosis		
Cushing's syndrome		

precipitating cause that requires a diligent search unless it is obvious. Even patients in whom HHS is the initial manifestation of diabetes may have an underlying condition that precipitated it.

Infection, occurring commonly in patients with HHS, is well known to cause insulin resistance. Inflammation or tumors of the pancreas probably reduce insulin secretion. The potent insulin resistance of growth hormone and glucocorticoids explains the association of HHS with acromegaly and Cushing's syndrome, respectively.

Several of the miscellaneous conditions listed in Table 6-9 would be expected to cause stress-related secretion of growth hormone, catecholamines, cortisol, and glucagon. These conditions include extensive burns, hypothermia, and heat stroke. HHS in patients who have been burned is often associated with high carbohydrate intake, either orally or intravenously. It may also develop in hospitalized patients given large amounts of carbohydrate in tube feedings or via total parenteral nutrition without enough free water and/or insulin. Dialysis patients have usually received hypertonic solutions in the dialysate. Secretion of the stress hormones would also be expected if a patient were ill enough with any of the other conditions listed in Table 6-9.

The mechanisms by which the drugs listed in Table 6-9 cause HHS are clear. Diazoxide and phenytoin (Dilantin) directly inhibit insulin secretion, as does hypokalemia. Propranolol, a β-adrenergic blocker, inhibits lipolysis. As was just mentioned, glucocorticoids cause insulin resistance. Finally, HHS was found to occur in patients treated for cardiac arrest with 7.5% $NaHCO_3$ (although it is no longer routinely used). The injection of a hypertonic solution in a situation of overwhelming stress (in which levels of all of the counterregulatory hormones were no doubt extremely elevated) would explain this association. Because older patients take many drugs, it is possible that some of the ones listed in Table 6-10 are not related to the onset of HHS despite the fact that in some cases a clear temporal relationship was found between starting the drug and the onset of the syndrome.

SIGNS AND SYMPTOMS

Except for dyspnea, all of the symptoms of DKA listed in Table 6-2 also apply to HHS. Polyuria and polydipsia are very intense for 3 to 7 days before treatment and have often been present for several weeks. Although less prevalent than in DKA, abdominal pain, nausea, and vomiting do occur in HHS. However, rather than the gastrointestinal symptoms that often motivate patients with DKA to seek medical attention, the usual reason for which patients in HHS are brought to a medical facility is their lack of normal responsiveness. Many also present with focal neurologic symptoms, which are discussed in more detail in the next section.

Many of the signs of DKA (see Table 6-2) do not apply to HHS. Patients in HHS often have an elevated temperature, which is usually caused by an infection.[76] Because marked ketosis and acidosis are not present, hyperpnea, acetone breath, and signs of an acute abdomen are lacking. Intravascular volume depletion is usually profound, and the related signs are therefore uniformly present.

The neurologic picture in HHS differs dramatically from that in DKA in many patients. Coma resulting from the altered

| TABLE 6-10 | COMPARISONS OF SOME SALIENT FEATURES OF DIABETIC KETOACIDOSIS AND HYPEROSMOLAR NONKETOTIC SYNDROME |

	Conditions	
Feature	Diabetic Ketoacidosis	Hyperosmolar Nonketotic Syndrome
Age of patient	Usually <40 years	Usually >40 years
Duration of symptoms	Usually <2 days	Usually >5 days
Glucose	Usually <800 mg/dl	Usually >800 mg/dl
Na	More likely to be normal or low	More likely to be normal or high
K	High, normal, or low	High, normal, or low
HCO$_3$	Low	Normal
Ketone bodies	At least 4 + in 1:1 dilution	<2 + in 1:1 dilution
pH	Low	Normal
Serum osmolality	Usually <350 mOsm/kg	Usually >350 mOsm/kg
Cerebral edema	Often subclinical; occasionally clinical	Not evaluated if subclinical; rarely clinical
Prognosis	3% to 10% mortality	10% to 20% mortality
Subsequent course	Insulin therapy required in virtually all cases	Insulin therapy not required in many cases

Glucose, serum concentration of glucose; HCO$_3$, serum concentration of bicarbonate; K, serum concentration of potassium; Na, serum concentration of sodium.

metabolic conditions per se is not noted when the serum osmolality is <340 to 350 mOsm/kg.[73] Thus it is more likely in patients with HHS, occurring in 10% to 20% of episodes.[73,76,77] Although a depressed sensorium (albeit not coma) is common to both syndromes, focal neurologic signs and symptoms are frequently noted in patients in HHS.[78-80] Seizures, often resistant to anticonvulsant therapy, are frequent (occurring in 10% to 15% of patients), and hallucinations and psychic disturbances are not uncommon. Focal dysfunctions include aphasia, homonymous hemianopsia, hemiparesis, hemisensory defects, unilateral hyperreflexia, and unilateral Babinski signs; all of these focal dysfunctions may be postictal, but may also occur independently of seizures. Abnormal muscle tone, tonic eye deviations, and nystagmus are less frequent. Hyperpnea (in the absence of acidosis) is common and probably reflects stimulation of the medullary centers by non–acid-base parameters. In contrast to the Kussmaul respirations of DKA, in which both inspiratory and expiratory phases are increased, the hyperpnea of HHS is reported to affect the expiratory phase only. Hyperthermia is a terminal event. Signs of nuchal rigidity have been reported in patients in HHS, even though meningitis was found to be absent by means of appropriate tests. Abnormalities in electroencephalograms are seen and are unaffected by treatment with anticonvulsant agents. These abnormalities disappear when hypotonic fluids are given, although it may take several days for a complete return to normal.

DIFFERENTIAL DIAGNOSIS

As with DKA, the diagnosis of HHS is easily made once it is considered. The usual difficulty is that only various neurologic possibilities are considered initially. Patients in HHS are commonly admitted to the neurology or neurosurgical service, and the diagnosis of HHS is made only when the results of routine urine and blood tests are known. This delay in the institution of appropriate treatment is partially responsible for the much poorer prognosis in HHS than in DKA.

INITIAL LABORATORY VALUES

The similarities and differences between the initial laboratory values in DKA and those in HHS should be apparent from the foregoing discussion (see Tables 6-7 and 6-8). Glucose concentrations are generally higher in HHS. Although the sodium and potassium can be low, normal, or high in both syndromes, the sodium in HHS is more likely to be higher than in DKA. As discussed earlier, an artificial reduction of the sodium caused by hypertriglyceridemia must be kept in mind, especially because patients in HHS have a longer prodrome than those in DKA and consequently are more likely to develop elevated triglyceride levels. (During therapy, as glycemia is lowered and serum osmolality decreases, the sodium rises because water is drawn back into the intracellular space, the reverse of what occurs as HHS developed.) Serum osmolality is also higher in HHS than in DKA. The *total* serum osmolality can be calculated as follows.

$$\text{Osmolality} = 2\,[\text{Na} + \text{K}] + \frac{[\text{glucose}]}{18} + \frac{[\text{BUN}]}{2.8} \quad (2)$$

To determine the *effective* serum osmolality, the final term is dropped from Equation 2 because urea is freely distributed between the extracellular and intracellular compartments. However, the calculated *total* osmolality corresponds better with the measured serum osmolality values. Changes in serum phosphate levels are similar to those in DKA. Both HCO_3 and pH values are normal in the pure syndrome of HHS. The biochemical indices of plasma volume contraction (BUN, creatinine, hematocrit, hemoglobin, and total protein) are generally higher in HHS because intravascular volume depletion is usually greater. Phosphate concentration, amylase levels, WBC counts, and serum enzyme changes have not been systematically reported in HHS. The latter two values depend on the presence of associated conditions. CPK levels may be elevated, sometimes to extremely high values, secondary to the rhabdomyolysis caused by the marked hyperosmolality.[76]

TREATMENT

The points discussed in the earlier section on general considerations in the treatment of DKA apply for the most part in HHS, with several modifications. The ADA suggestions for treatment are provided in Figure 6-8. With regard to laboratory tests, if significant ketosis is absent, an initial measurement of pH is unnecessary. In the unusual event that the HCO_3 is low (<15 mEq/L), pH can be measured. Because most patients in HHS are older and many have preexisting heart disease, monitoring of their cardiovascular status during fluid replacement is critically important. For this reason, placement of a central venous pressure line or, if possible, a right-sided heart catheter that measures pulmonary capillary wedge pressure should be considered in patients with a history of congestive heart failure.

The same controversy surrounding fluid administration in DKA exists in relation to HHS. Because the correlation between plasma osmolarity and depression of sensorium is even higher in HHS (Figure 6-9) than in DKA (see Figure 6-3), some investigators argue that hypotonic solutions should be used and plasma osmolality reduced fairly rapidly. Others point out that patients in HHS are even more vulnerable to the effects of intravascular volume depletion than are those with DKA and thus that rehydration with 0.9% saline should take precedence. If normal saline is used as the initial fluid in resuscitation, fluid administration may be switched to 0.45% saline when volume status normalizes. As was just men-

tioned, precipitation of congestive heart failure during saline administration is all too common in patients in HHS. Frequent monitoring of their cardiovascular status by physical examination and hemodynamic methods (if available) is extremely important to a successful outcome. The one exception to the previous discussion on fluid replacement involves patients who have advanced renal failure and who develop HHS. Under these conditions, glucosuria leading to an osmotic diuresis may be markedly impaired[81] so that the hyperglycemia-induced shift of water from the intracellular to the extracellular space is retained. These patients differ from the typical presentation of HHS in that the prodrome of polyuria and polydipsia is absent and the initial Na is low. In this situation, little or no fluid may be required—only insulin to lower glucose concentrations so that water shifts back from the extracellular to the intracellular space. Dialysis may be necessary in some instances.

Insulin is given to patients in HHS in the same manner as to those with DKA. When the glucose concentration declines to ~250 mg/dl, the rate of insulin infusion is decreased to 2 to 3 U/hr and dextrose is added to the administered fluid. Cerebral edema is much less common in HHS than in DKA. In the few reported cases, the symptoms began when the glucose concentration was well below 250 mg/dl,[79,82] and almost all occurred in children,[82] similar to the situation in DKA.

Because patients in HHS are not experiencing ketosis or acidosis, the glucose level is the sole biochemical endpoint. However, it often is many hours or even a few days before these patients are able to tolerate oral intake because of their mental status and/or associated conditions. Under these circumstances, 50 g of dextrose should be administered every 8 hours, and the dose of insulin infused should be decreased appropriately (1 to 3 U/hr) on the basis of plasma glucose determinations every 4 hours. The

MANAGEMENT OF ADULT PATIENTS WITH HHS*

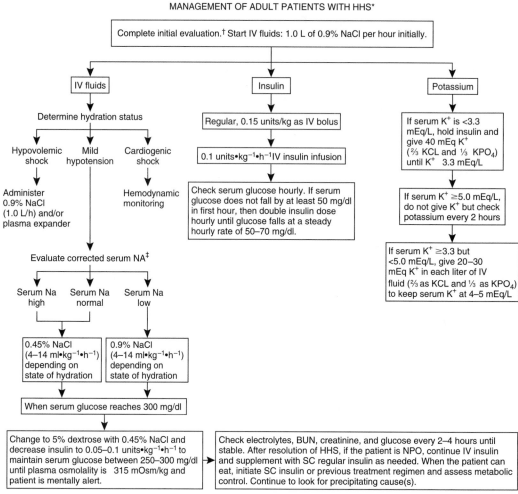

FIGURE 6-8. Protocol for the management of adult patients with hyperosmolar hyperglycemia state (HHS). *Diagnostic criteria: blood glucose >600 mg/dl, arterial pH >7.3, bicarbonate >15 mEq/L, mild ketonuria or ketonemia, and effective serum osmolality >320 mOsm/kg H_2O. This protocol is for patients admitted with mental status change or severe dehydration who require admission to an intensive care unit. Effective serum osmolality calculation: 2 [measured Na (mEq/L)] + glucose (mg/dl)/18. †After history and physical examination, obtain arterial blood gases, complete blood count with differential, urinalysis, plasma glucose, blood urea nitrogen (BUN), electrolytes, chemistry profile, and creatinine levels as soon as possible as well as an electrocardiogram. Obtain chest x-ray examination and cultures as needed. ‡Serum Na should be corrected for hyperglycemia (for each 100 mg/dl glucose > 100 mg/dl, add 1.6 mEq to sodium value for corrected serum value). IV, intravenous, NPO, nothing by mouth, SC, subcutaneous. *(From Hyperglycemic crises in patients with diabetes mellitus. Diabetes Care 26(suppl):5109-5117, 2003.)*

transition from insulin infusion to SC administration of insulin is made as described for DKA. If oral medications are appropriate, they may be started once the patient has been stable for 24 hours, and is tolerating oral feeding. Further adjustment in therapy may be made as an outpatient, and it is critical that these patients have appropriate follow-up arranged prior to discharge from the hospital.

The same considerations for potassium replacement that apply to patients with DKA

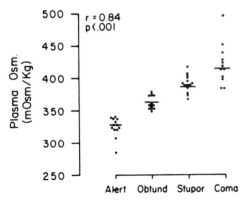

FIGURE 6-9. Relationship between state of consciousness and measured plasma osmolarity in 53 patients in hyperosmolar nonketotic coma. States of consciousness were defined as follows: (1) alert—the patient responds immediately and appropriately to normal stimuli; (2) obtundation—the patient is in a state of dull indifference in which increased stimulation is required to evoke a response; (3) stupor—the patient can be aroused only by vigorous and continuous stimulation; and (4) coma—the patient exhibits little or no response to stimulation. For calculation of the correlation coefficient (r), scores of 1 though 4 were given for each state of consciousness, respectively. For each group, plasma osmolarity was significantly different (P < 0.01) from that of the adjacent group(s). *(From Arieff AI, Carrol H: Cerebral edema and depression of sensorium in nonketotic hyperosmolar coma. Diabetes 23:525, 1974.)*

are pertinent to those in HHS, with two caveats. Because more patients in HHS may have underlying renal disease, urinary potassium losses may be lower. Bicarbonate therapy is obviously inappropriate for patients in HHS. These two factors lessen the possibility of hypokalemia. However, because patients with preexisting heart disease may be more susceptible to the effects of potassium, potassium replacement must still be monitored carefully.

Phosphate homeostasis follows a pattern similar to that in DKA. Because many of these patients also have underlying renal disease, close monitoring of phosphate concentrations is required before administering phosphate. The same general approach for phosphate replacement in HHS as in DKA should be used.

PROGNOSIS

The prognosis for patients in HHS is worse than that for those with DKA. Older mortality reports ranged from 15% to 60%, with most values between 30% and 50%. More recent reports have suggested a lower mortality, between 10% and 20%.[54,83,84] This improvement may be related to earlier recognition of HHS and more aggressive fluid administration.[76] Early mortality (<72 hours) is usually due to sepsis, progressive shock, or an underlying illness, whereas later mortality is usually caused by thromboembolic events or the effects of treatment.[77] An unfavorable outcome is more likely in older patients, with higher degrees of dehydration (as evidenced by the BUN level), higher sodium level, higher serum osmolality (which reflects the length of the prodromal period), and lower level of consciousness.[73] Although elevated levels of CPK reflecting rhabdomyolysis are common, especially in those patients with very high serum osmolalities, myoglobinuric acute tubular necrosis is rare, usually occurring in the presence of shock or preexisting renal disease.[77]

The causes of death are usually related to associated conditions rather than to the metabolic derangements per se. Gram-negative sepsis and pneumonia are particularly lethal to patients in HHS. In addition to infections, vascular events (e.g., thrombosis) are frequent causes of death. Renal failure is often present in these patients. As mentioned earlier, the presenting neurologic symptoms may take 3 to 5 days to resolve completely, even though the metabolic parameters may long since have returned to normal.

Finally, in contrast to patients with DKA, all of whom eventually require insulin therapy after recovery, many patients who recover from HHS can be treated with oral antidiabetic medications and/or dietary therapy alone. These approaches are particularly effective in patients whose initial manifestation of diabetes was HHS.

To help summarize the salient features of DKA and HHS and the basic differences between these conditions, refer to Table 6-10.

HYPOGLYCEMIA

Hypoglycemia is the clinical syndrome that results because of low plasma glucose levels. Although symptoms vary from person to person and range in severity, there are common complaints associated with hypoglycemia. Despite significant advances in medical therapies for diabetes, hypoglycemia is still a common problem among patients who are trying to achieve better control. In large-scale studies such as the Diabetes Control and Complications Trial (DCCT), low blood sugars occurred more commonly in patients treated with intensive management. Although their A1C levels were lower, affording them better outcomes in regard to complications such as eye disease, kidney disease, and nerve damage, they also endured more episodes of low blood sugars.[85] This is important to note, especially because as goals for successful treatment become tighter, the risk for hypoglycemia increases in everyday practice.

The brain depends on glucose almost exclusively for energy.[86] The major exception is prolonged fasting, a situation in which ketone bodies can provide some energy by default. Because the brain cannot synthesize glucose on its own, it depends on circulating glucose in the body. If plasma glucose falls below a certain level, or conversely, if the brain's demands increase, glucose transport from the blood to the brain becomes rate limiting, and thus an impairment in brain function may ensue.[87]

When circulating blood glucose levels fall, the brain senses this change and triggers a series of events, which includes changes in hormonal and sympathetic responses aimed at increasing circulating plasma glucose. Insulin levels decrease, and counter regulatory hormones such as glucagon, epinephrine, cortisol, and growth hormone increase levels[88] (Figure 6-10). These hormones are released in an attempt to prevent or correct the hypoglycemia. These regulatory systems are usually activated at glycemic levels of 68 mg/dl. This threshold provides a safety net, because it is above the levels for theoretical hypoglycemic symptoms (54 mg/dl) and cognitive dysfunction (49 mg/dl). Many other hormones also increase, such as prolactin, vasopressin, aldosterone, atrial natriuretic hormone, and gastrin, although the physiologic relevance of these increases is unclear.

Hypoglycemia in patients on insulin has been classified as follows[87]: asymptomatic or

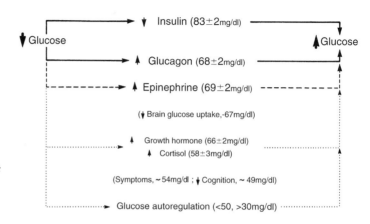

FIGURE 6-10. Normal glucose counterregulation. *(Adapted from Cryer PE: Glucose counterregulation: The prevention and correction of hypoglycemia in humans. Am J Physiol 264:E149, 1993.)*

biochemical hypoglycemia, mild to moderate symptomatic hypoglycemia, and severe hypoglycemia. This last category is defined by the inability of patients to treat themselves and the need for assistance. The classification provides a starting point for a discussion with patients, and is a good teaching tool; however, the practical importance is debatable, especially because the lack of symptoms may actually be a very dangerous event related to hypoglycemia unawareness.

Symptoms of hypoglycemia are varied in severity, character, and presentation. In type 1 and type 2 diabetes, the presentation of hypoglycemia seems to be idiosyncratic. The most common symptoms reported have been compiled in a review and include sweating (47% to 84%), trembling (32% to 78%), weakness (28% to 71%), visual changes (24% to 60%), hunger (39% to 49%), palpitations (8% to 62%), difficulty speaking (7% to 41%), perioral tingling (10% to 39%), dizziness (11% to 41%), headache (24% to 36%), anxiety (10% to 44%), and difficulty concentrating (31% to 75%).[89] Other symptoms reported include nausea, tiredness, drowsiness, and confusion. There is some debate about symptoms differing in patients on insulin versus oral agents, but this has yet to be clarified. Hypoglycemia does not occur in patients who are treated solely with lifestyle modifications. There is a caveat, however. In some patients with type 2 diabetes, who, by definition, have high circulating levels of insulin, a decrease in carbohydrate intake or problems with digesting foods may lead to unopposed high levels of insulin, and symptoms of hypoglycemia. Although this situation and its cause are debatable among endocrinologists, patients may have symptomatic complaints suggesting hypoglycemia. Hypoglycemia is also rare in patients treated with drugs such as acarbose (Precose), metformin, Avandia (rosiglitazone), and Actos (pioglitazone). However, when these drugs are used in combination with drugs such as glyburide, or other drugs in the sulfonylurea family and rapid-acting insulin secretagogues such as Prandin (repaglinide) or Starlix (nateglinide), hypoglycemia may occur. Hypoglycemia may also occur when sulfonylurea agents or rapid-acting insulin secretagogues are used on their own, with the risk being higher in sulfonylurea agents. Risk factors for iatrogenic hypoglycemia on oral agents include advancing age, poor nutritional status, drug interactions, liver disease, and kidney disease.[90] In addition, drugs with longer half-lives, such as first-generation sulfonylurea agents, are higher risk. In cases of oral agents causing hypoglycemia, the resulting recovery phase may be prolonged. Days of hospitalization with IV glucose infusions are not uncommon in these cases.

The symptoms of hypoglycemia are often divided into two categories (Table 6-11). The first category results from the brain getting a reduction in fuel source (the brain needs glucose as its fuel). These are known as neuroglycopenic symptoms. The second category results from the body's response to the physiologic stress of having low levels of circulating blood glucose. This is known as the *neurogenic response,* and occurs before the neuroglycopenic symptoms in most cases. The neurogenic symptoms include shakiness, palpitations, anxiety and nervousness, sweating, and hunger, whereas the neuroglycopenic symptoms include confusion, drowsiness, weakness, dysarthria, incoordination, odd behavior, and more severe symptoms such as coma and seizure.[91] The symptoms usually occur gradually and, if ignored, blood glucose levels continue to fall; severity increases; and seizure, coma, and death may ensue. Although most patients have never experienced such severe symptoms, those who have recurrent severe episodes may suffer from long-term consequences.

The diagnosis of hypoglycemia is classically made by employing Whipple's triad: symptoms consistent with hypoglycemia in the presence of a low plasma glucose

TABLE 6-11 SIGNS AND SYMPTOMS OF HYPOGLYCEMIA	
Autonomic[*]	**Neuroglucopenic**[†]
Weakness	Headache
Sweating	Hypothermia
Tachycardia	Visual disturbances
Palpitations	Mental dullness
Tremor	Confusion
Nervousness	Amnesia
Irritability	Seizures
Tingling of mouth and fingers	Coma
Hunger	
Nausea[‡]	
Vomiting[‡]	

[*]Caused by increased activity of the autonomic nervous system.
[†]Caused by decreased activity of the central nervous system.
[‡]Unusual.

concentration that resolve with the normalization of plasma glucose levels. Home blood glucose monitoring, although inaccurate at low levels of plasma glucose, still provides the best tool for diagnosing hypoglycemic episodes.[92] A relationship between meal patterns and medications can be derived from the data obtained using home glucose monitoring, especially in the presence of symptoms. If it is not practical to check a glucose level, it is reasonable to treat based on symptoms. Rigid definitions of asymptomatic hypoglycemia are not useful in individual cases. In some patients, a level of 70 may prompt treatment, particularly if a coexisting heart condition or other comorbidities are present. In others, a level of 60 mg/dl may be the limit, and 50 mg/dl should prompt treatment in all patients regardless of symptoms.

Risk factors for hypoglycemia include the following: excessive insulin or the wrong type of insulin administration, missing meals or snacks, excessive exercise, alcohol ingestion leading to a decrease in endogenous glucose production, an increased sensitivity to insulin, and renal insufficiency—where insulin's half life is prolonged because of decreased clearance. A defective ability to generate glucose counter regulation (such as with autonomic failure) may also play a role.

The frequency of asymptomatic hypoglycemia has been noted as being inversely related to the median plasma glucose concentration.[93] If the median blood glucose level was documented as 90 mg/dl, data predicts glucose levels of less than 54 mg/dl approximately 10% of the time. Asymptomatic hypoglycemia is more common an occurrence during the nighttime hours.[94] Of patients with type 1 diabetes, 56% were noted as having blood glucose levels of <36 mg/dl during overnight sampling, and only 36% of these patients reported symptoms. In general, these values of hypoglycemia are directly related to bedtime and morning glucose levels. With mild to moderate symptomatic hypoglycemia, data has shown that in a sample of 411 patients on insulin, the average symptomatic episodes of hypoglycemia was 1.8 per week.[95] It is important to note that as a group, these patients were not being treated aggressively. This data would amount to thousands of episodes over a lifetime, and it is reasonable to assume the incidence in intensively treated patients may be significantly higher. Severe episodes of hypoglycemia range from 4.5% to 44% of patients per year and from 5 to 140 episodes per 100 patients per year.[96] Such a wide range may be the result of differing definitions of "severe." In the DCCT,[97] 10% of 132 conventionally treated patients suffered at least one episode of hypoglycemia and 25% of 146 intensively managed patients suffered from severe hypoglycemia. In this latter group, 20% had hypoglycemia coma, versus 6%. As is evident, aggressive treatment of diabetes carries significant risk of hypoglycemia and its sequelae.

The concerns of hypoglycemia relate to its impact on physical morbidity and even mortality. As mentioned earlier, signs and symptoms arise based on the severity of glucose levels. A recent study showed that cognitive recovery from an acute severe hypoglycemic episode takes 1.5 days, whereas the cognitive decrements and altered mood states may be persistent and a consequence of previous exposure to hypoglycemia.[98] Rarely, there may be permanent focal or generalized neurologic sequelae.[99] The determination of this most likely depends on both the depth and length of hypoglycemia. Recurrent episodes of hypoglycemia have also been linked to cognitive impairment.[100] Earlier studies showed that

intelligence quotient scores in those with recurrent hypoglycemia tend to be lower. Other data[101] showed no difference in cognitive function between an intensively treated group and a conventionally treated group of subjects with diabetes, and the DCCT supported this finding.[102] The psychologic effect of hypoglycemia ranges from fear, anxiety, and depression to guilt about being fearful. The effect extends to others directly and indirectly as well. Hypoglycemia concerns families, friends, employers, and colleagues, as well as the Department of Motor Vehicles.

Management of these patients should be aimed at the acute episode, and also at preventing future episodes. Therapeutic goals should be individualized, and a team-based approach should be used. Strategies for treating hypoglycemia are shown in Table 6-12. The expertise of a nurse educator and nutritionist is very valuable in these cases.

TABLE 6-12 MANAGEMENT STRATEGIES FOR HYPOGLYCEMIA

Situation	Treatment
Adults	
Mild or documented asymptomatic hypoglycemia: *not* on alpha glucosidase inhibitors	• 10–20 g glucose in the form of juice, soda, liquid glucose, or glucose tablets. • Check SMBG and repeat q10–20 min as needed
Adults	
Mild or documented asymptomatic hypoglycemia: *on* alpha glucosidase inhibitors	• Liquid or tablet glucose (cannot break down carbohydrate)
Adults	
Severe hypoglycemia	• Glucagon intramuscular injection (1.0 mg) or IV glucose
Children	
Mild or documented asymptomatic hypoglycemia	• Glucose in the form of juice, soda, liquid glucose, or glucose tablets at a dose of 0.3 g/kg
Children	
Severe hypoglycemia	• 15 µg/kg/dose intramuscular glucagon or IV glucose

IV, intravenous; SMBG, self-monitoring of blood glucose.

TABLE 6-13 COMMONLY AVAILABLE SOURCES OF 10 g OF GLUCOSE	
Orange juice	1 cup*
Grape juice	½ cup
Table sugar	4 teaspoons†
Honey	3 teaspoons
Lifesavers	10
B-D glucose tablets	2
DextroEnergy glucose tablets	3
Dex 4 glucose tablets	2.5
Glucose tablets	2

*1 cup = 8 ounces (fluid).

†1 tablespoon = 3 teaspoons.

Most hypoglycemic episodes can be treated with juice, soda, or candy. Common sources for appropriate forms of glucose are listed in Table 6-13. A 20-g glucose dose is recommended for adults, whereas in children, 0.3 g/kg is advised.[103] In general, this amount of oral glucose has been shown to raise plasma glucose from 58 mg/dl to 122 mg/dl over 45 minutes, with peak response at 15 minutes, and a decline resulting by 60 minutes. Glucagon stimulates hepatic glucose production by both increasing glycogenolysis and gluconeogenesis. It is not as effective in patients with glycogen depleted stores and may not be beneficial in patients on metformin. The standard dose is 1.0 mg (or 15 μg/kg in children). The response lasts for about 90 minutes. In cases in which failure to stabilize the glycemic profile by these methods is seen, IV glucose administration is required. For long-term goals, self-management is really the key, and patients require a significant amount of individualized education to be proficient in their management of hypoglycemia. Patients should be taught how to recognize hypoglycemia, and how to treat it effectively. They should be advised to keep rapidly absorbable glucose-containing treatments with them, and be taught how much to give. Those who support the patient, both family and friends, should be educated about hypoglycemia and its treatment. In certain cases, the use of par-enteral glucagon should be taught to these individuals in cases in which patients are unable to help themselves. All attempts should be made to minimize risk factors, such as insulin administration errors, meal omissions, variable surges in activity, and excessive alcohol consumption.

REFERENCES

1. DeFronzo RA, Matsuda M, Barrett EJ: Diabetic ketoacidosis: A combined metabolic-nephrologic approach to therapy. Diabetes Rev 2:209, 1994.
2. Matz R: Hypothermia in diabetic acidosis. Hormones 3:36, 1972.
3. Munro JF, Campbell IW, McCuish AC, Duncan LJP: Euglycaemic diabetic ketoacidosis. BJM 2:578, 1973.
4. Brandt KR, Miles JM: Relationship between severity of hyperglycemia and metabolic acidosis in diabetic ketoacidosis. Mayo Clin Proc 63:1071, 1988.
5. American Diabetes Association: Hyperglycemic crisis in patients with diabetes mellitus. Position statement. Diabetes Care 25[suppl 1]:S100-S108, 2002.
6. Stephens JM, Sulway MJ, Watkins PJ: Relationship of blood acetoacetate and 3-hydroxybutyrate in diabetes. Diabetes 20:485, 1971.
7. Owen OE, Block BS, Patel M et al: Human splanchnic metabolism during diabetic ketoacidosis. Metabolism 26:381, 1977.
8. Reichard GA, Skutches CL, Hoeldtke RD et al: Acetone metabolism in humans during diabetic ketoacidosis. Diabetes 35:668, 1986.
9. Sanders G, Boyle G, Hunter S et al: Mixed acid-based abnormalities in diabetes. Diabetes Care 1:362, 1978.
10. Walsh CH, Baylis PH, Malins JM: Plasma arginine vasopressin in diabetic ketoacidosis. Diabetologia 16:93, 1978.

11. Katz MA: Hyperglycemia-induced hyponatremia calculation of expected serum sodium depression. N Engl J Med 289:843, 1973.

12. Slovis CM, Mork VGC, Kandall JS et al: Diabetic ketoacidosis and infection: Leukocyte count and differential as early predictors of serious infection. Am J Emerg Med 5:1, 1987.

13. Nsien EE, Steinberg WM, Borum M et al: Marked hyperlipasemia in diabetic ketoacidosis: A report of three cases. J Clin Gastroenterol 15:117, 1992.

14. Warsha A, Feller ER, Lee KHG: On the cause of raised serum-amylase in diabetic ketoacidosis. Lancet 1:929, 1977.

15. Vinicor F, Lehrner LM, Karn RC, Marritt AD: Hyperamylasemia in diabetic ketoacidosis: Sources and significance. Ann Intern Med 91:200, 1979.

16. Salen MM, Mujais SK: Gaps in the anion gap. Arch Intern Med 153:1625, 1992.

17. Wäldhausl W, Kleinberger G, Korn A et al: Severe hyperglycemia: Effects of rehydration on endocrine derangements and blood glucose concentration. Diabetes 28:577, 1979.

18. Clements RS Jr, Vourganti B: Fatal diabetic ketoacidosis: Major causes and approaches to their prevention. Diabetes Care 1:314, 1978.

19. Kitabchi AE, Ayyagari V, Guerra SMO, Medical House Staff: The efficacy of low-dose versus conventional therapy of insulin for treatment of diabetic ketoacidosis. Ann Intern Med 84:633, 1976.

20. Piters KM, Kumar D, Pei E, Bessman AN: Comparison of continuous and t-intermittent intravenous insulin therapies for diabetic ketoacidosis. Diabetologia 13:317, 1977.

21. Pfeifer MA, Samols E, Wolter CF, Winkler CF: Low-dose versus high-dose insulin therapy for diabetic ketoacidosis. South Med J 72:149, 1979.

22. Soler NG, Wright AD, FitzGerald MG, Malins JM: Comparative study of different insulin regimens in management of diabetic ketoacidosis. Lancet 2:1221, 1975.

23. Shappard MC, Wright AD: The effect on mortality of low-dose insulin therapy for diabetic ketoacidosis. Diabetes Care 5:111, 1982.

24. Peterson L, Caldwell J, Hoffman J: Insulin adsorbance to polyvinylchloride surfaces with implications for constant-infusion therapy. Diabetes 25:72, 1976.

25. Adrogue HJ, Lederer ED, Suki WN et al: Determinants of plasma potassium levels in diabetic ketoacidosis. Medicine 65:163, 1986.

26. Kanter Y, Gerson JR, Bessman AN: 1, 3-Diphosphoglycerate, nucleotide phosphate, and organic and inorganic phosphate levels during the early phases of diabetic ketoacidosis. Diabetes 26:429, 1977.

27. Gibby OM, Veale KEA, Hayes TM et al: Oxygen availability from the blood and the effect of phosphate replacement on erythrocyte 2,3-diphosphoglycerate and haemoglobin-oxygen affinity in diabetic ketoacidosis. Diabetologia 15:381, 1978.

28. Keller U, Berger W: Prevention of hypophosphatemia by phosphate infusion during treatment of diabetic ketoacidosis and hyperosmolar coma. Diabetes 29:87, 1980.

29. Fisher JN, Kitabchi AE: A randomized study of phosphate therapy in the treatment of diabetic ketoacidosis. J Clin Endocrinol Metab 57:177, 1983.

30. Wilson HK, Keuer SP, Lea AS et al: Phosphate therapy in diabetic ketoacidosis. Arch Intern Med 142:517, 1982.

31. Ditzel J, Standl E: The problems of tissue oxygenation in diabetes mellitus. Acta Med Scand 578(suppl):49, 1975.

32. Zipf WB, Bacon GE, Spencer ML et al: Hypocalcemia, hypomagnesemia, and transient hypoparathyroidism during therapy with potassium phosphate in diabetic ketoacidosis. Diabetes Care 2:265, 1979.

33. Lavis VR: Treatment of diabetic ketoacidosis. Diabetes Care 2:385, 1979.

34. Fisher JN, Kitabchi AE et al: A randomized study of phosphate therapy in the treatment of diabetic ketoacidosis. J Clin Endocrinol Metab 57:177, 1983.

35. Knochel JP: The pathophysiology and clinical characteristics of severe hypophosphatemia. Ann Intern Med 137:203, 1977.

36. Lentz RD, Brown DM, Kjellstrand CM: Treatment of severe hypophosphatemia. Ann Intern Med 89:941, 1978.

37. Barnes EV, Cohen RD, Kitabchi AE et al: When is bicarbonate therapy appropriate in treating metabolic acidosis including diabetic ketoacidosis? In Gitnick G, Barnes HV, Duffy TP et al (eds). Diabetes in Medicine. Chicago, Yearbook, 1990, p. 172.

38. Posner JB, Plum F: Spinal-fluid pH and neurologic symptoms in systemic acidosis. N Engl J Med 297:605, 1967.

39. Ohman JL Jr, Marliss EB, Aoki TT et al: The cerebrospinal fluid in diabetic ketoacidosis. N Engl J Med 284:283, 1971.

40. Matz R: Diabetic acidosis, rationale for not using bicarbonate. NY State J Med 76:1299, 1976.

41. Dorin RI, Crapo LM: Hypokalemic respiratory arrest in diabetic ketoacidosis, JAMA 257:1517, 1987.

42. Assal J-Ph, Aoki TT, Manzano FM, Kozak GP: Metabolic effects of sodium bicarbonate in management of diabetic ketoacidosis. Diabetes 23:405, 1974.

43. Bureau MA, Begin R, Berthiaume Y et al: Cerebral hypoxia from bicarbonate infusion in diabetic acidosis. J Pediatr 96:968, 1980.

44. Okuda Y, Adrogue HJ, Field JB et al: Counterproductive effects of sodium bicarbonate in diabetic ketoacidosis. J Clin Endocrinol Metab 81:314, 1996.

45. Lever E, Jaspan JB: Sodium bicarbonate therapy in severe diabetic ketoacidosis. Am J Med 75:263, 1983.

46. Morris LR, Murphy MB, Kitabchi AE: Bicarbonate therapy in severe diabetic ketoacidosis. Ann Inter Med 105:836, 1986.

47. Narins R: Acid-base disorders: Definitions and introductory concepts. In Narins R (ed): Clinical

Disorders of Fluid and Electrolyte Metabolism. McGraw-Hill, New York, 1994, pp. 755-767.

48. Sulway MJ, Malins JM: Acetone in diabetic ketoacidosis. Lancet 2:736, 1970.

49. Oh MS, Carroll HJ, Goldstein DA, Fein IA: Hyperchloremic acidosis during the recovery phase of diabetic ketosis. Ann Intern Med 89:925, 1978.

50. Oh MS, Banerji MA, Carroll HJ: The mechanism of hyperchloremic acidosis during the recovery phase of diabetic ketoacidosis. Diabetes 30:310, 1981.

51. Halperin ML, Bear RA, Hannaford MC, Goldstein MB: Selected aspects of the pathophysiology of metabolic acidosis in diabetes mellitus. Diabetes 30:781, 1981.

52. Androgué HJ, Wilson H, Boyd AE III et al: Plasma acid-base patterns in diabetic ketoacidosis. N Engl J Med 307:1603, 1982.

53. Gale EAM, Dornan TL, Tattersall RB: Severely uncontrolled diabetes in the over-fifties. Diabetologia 21:25, 1981.

54. Carroll P, Matz R: Uncontrolled diabetes mellitus in adults: Experience in treating diabetic ketoacidosis and hyperosmolar nonketotic coma with low-dose insulin and uniform treatment regimen. Diabetes Care 6:579, 1983.

55. Carroll P, Matz R: Adult respiratory distress syndrome complicating severely uncontrolled diabetes mellitus: Report of 9 cases and a review of the literature. Diabetes Care 5:574, 1982.

56. Beigelman PM: Severe diabetic ketoacidosis (diabetic "coma"): 482 episodes in 257 patients; experience of three years. Diabetes 20:490, 1971.

57. Singhal PC, Abramovici M, Venkatesan J: Rhabdomyolysis in the hyperosmolal state. Am J Med 88:9, 1990.

58. Wang L-M, Tsai S-T, Ho L-T et al: Rhabdomyolysis in diabetic emergencies. Diabetes Res Clin Pract 26:209, 1994.

59. Caramori MLA, Gross JL, Friedman R et al: Pneumomediastinum and subcutaneous emphysema in diabetic ketoacidosis. Diabetes Care 18:1311, 1995.

60. Hammond P, Wallis S: Cerebral oedema in diabetic ketoacidosis: still puzzling—and often fatal. BMJ 305:203, 1992.

61. Rosenbloom AL: Intracerebral crises during treatment of diabetic ketoacidosis. Diabetes 13:22, 1990.

62. Bello FA, Stone JF: Cerebral edema in diabetic ketoacidosis in children. Lancet 336:64, 1990.

63. Clements RS Jr, Blumenthal SA, Morrison AD, Winegrad AI: Increased cerebrospinal-fluid pressure during treatment of diabetic ketosis. Lancet 2:671, 1971.

64. Fein IA, Rackow EC, Sprung CL, Grodman R: Relation of colloid osmotic pressure to arterial hypoxemia and cerebral edema during crystalloid volume loading of patients with diabetic ketoacidosis. Ann Intern Med 96:570, 1982.

65. Krane EJ, Rockoff MA, Wallman JK et al: Subclinical brain swelling in children during

treatment of diabetic ketoacidosis. N Engl J Med 312:1147, 1985.

66. Hoffman WH, Steinhart CM, El Gammal T et al: Cranial computed tomography in children and adolescents with diabetic ketoacidosis. J Neuroradiol 9:733, 1988.

67. Durr JA, Hoffman WH, Sklar AH et al: Correlates of brain edema in uncontrolled IDDM. Diabetes 41:627, 1992.

68. Glasgow AM: Devastating cerebral edema in diabetic ketoacidosis before therapy. Diabetes Care 14:77, 1991.

69. Couch RM, Acott PD, Wong GWK: Early onset fatal cerebral edema in diabetic ketoacidosis. Diabetes Care 14:78, 1991.

70. Harris GD, Fiordalisi I, Harris WL et al: Minimizing the risk of brain herniation during treatment of diabetic ketoacidemia: A retrospective and prospective study. J Pediatr 117:22, 1990.

71. Harris GD, Fiordalisi I: Physiologic management of diabetic ketoacidemia: A 5-year prospective pediatric experience in 231 episodes. Arch Pediatr Adolesc Med 148:1046, 1994.

72. Duck SC, Wyatt DT: Factors associated with brain herniation in the treatment of diabetic ketoacidosis. J Pediatr 113:10, 1988.

73. Ennis ED, Stahl EJVB, Kreisberg RA: The hyperosmolar hyperglycemic syndrome. Diabetes Rev 2:115-126, 1994.

74. Wachtel TJ, Tetu-Mouradijian LM, Goldman DL et al: Hyperosmolarity and acidosis in diabetes mellitus: A three-year experience. J Gen Internal Med 6:495, 1991.

75. Turpin BP, Duckworth WC, Solomon SS: Stimulated hyperglycemic hyperosmolar syndrome. Impaired insulin and epinephrine effects upon lipolysis in the isolated rat fat cell. J Clin Invest 63:403, 1979.

76. Matz R: Hyperosmolar nonacidotic uncontrolled diabetes: Not a rare event. Clin Diabetes 6:25, 1988.

77. Lorber D: Non-ketotic hypertonicity in diabetes. Endocrinologist 3:29, 1993.

78. Maccario M: Neurological dysfunction associated with nonketotic hyperglycemia. Arch Neurol 16:525, 1968.

79. Guisado R, Arieff AI: Neurologic manifestations of diabetic comas: Correlation with biochemical alterations in the brain. Metabolism 24:665, 1975.

80. Morres CA, Dire DJ: Movement disorders as a manifestation of nonketotic hyperglycemia. J Emerg Med 7:359, 1989.

81. Gerich JE, Martin MM, Recant L: Clinical and metabolic characteristics of hyperosmolar nonketotic coma. Diabetes 20:228, 1971.

82. Arieff AI: Cerebral edema complicating nonketotic hyperosmolar coma. Miner Electrolyte Metab 12:383, 1986.

83. Khardori R, Soler NG: Hyperosmolar hyperglycemia nonketotic syndrome. Am J Med 77:899, 1984.

84. Wachtel TJ, Silliman RA, Lamberton P: Predisposing factors for the diabetic hyperosmolar state. Arch Intern Med 147:499, 1987.

85. Diabetes Control and Complications Trial Research Group: The effect of intensive treatment of diabetes on the development and progression of long-term complications in insulin-dependent mellitus. N Engl J Med 329:977, 1993.

86. McCall AL: Effects of glucose deprivation on glucose metabolism in the central nervous system. In Frier BM, Fisher BM (eds): Hypoglycemia and Diabetes. Edward Arnold, London, 1993, pp. 59-71.

87. Cryer PE: Glucose counterregulation: The prevention and correction of hypoglycemia in humans. Am J Physiol 264:E149, 1993.

88. Cryer PE, Fisher JN, Shamoon H et al: Hypoglycemia. Technical Review. Diabetes Care 17(7):734-755, 1994.

89. Hepburn DA: Symptoms of hypoglycaemia. In Frier BM, Fisher BM (eds): Hypoglycemia and diabetes. Edward Arnold, London, 1993, pp. 93-103.

90. Campbell IW: Hypoglycaemia and type 2 diabetes: Sulfonylureas. In Frier BM, Fisher BM (eds): Hypoglycemia and diabetes. Edward Arnold, London, 1993, pp. 387-392.

91. Towler DA, Haulin CE, Craft S et al: Mechanism of awareness of hypoglycemia. Perception of neurogenic (predominately cholinergic) rather than neuroglycopenic symptoms. Diabetes 42(12):1791-1798, 1993.

92. Tieszen KL, Patrick AW, Smith E et al: Accurate and precise blood glucose measurements in the hypoglycaemic range. Diabet Med 10(6)560-563, 1993.

93. Thorsteinsson B, Pramming S, Lauritzen T, Binder C: Frequency of daytime biochemical hypoglycemia in insulin treated diabetics:

Relationship to daily median blood glucose concentrations. Diabetic Med 3:147, 1986.

94. Gale EAM, Tattersall RB: Unrecognized nocturnal hypoglycaemia in insulin-treated diabetes. Lancet 1:1049-52, 1979.

95. Pramming S, Thorsteinsson B, Bendtson I, Binder C: Symptomatic hypoglycaemia in 411 type 1 diabetic patients. Diabetic Med 8:217, 1991.

96. Tattersall RB: Frequency and causes of hypoglycaemia. In Frier BM, Fisher BM (eds): Hypoglycaemia and Diabetes. Edward Arnold, London, 1993, pp.176-189.

97. Diabetes Control and Complications Trial Research Group: Epidemiology of severe hypoglycemia in the Diabetes Control and Complications Trial. Am J Med 90:450, 1991.

98. Strachan MWJ et al: Recovery of cognitive function and mood after severe hypoglycemia in adults with insulin treated diabetes. Diabetes Care 23:305, 2000.

99. Chalmers J, Risk MTA, Kean DM et al: Severe amnesia after hypoglycemia. Diabetes Care 14:922, 1991.

100. Deary IJ, Langan SJ, Graham KS et al: Recurrent severe hypoglycaemia, intelligence and speed of information processing. Intelligence 16:337, 1992.

101. Reichard P, Brita A, Rosenquist U: Intensified conventional insulin treatment and neuropsychological impairment. BMJ 303:1439, 1991.

102. Austin EJ, Deary IJ et al: Effects of repeated hypoglycemia on cognitive function. A psychometrically validated reanalysis of the Diabetes Control and Complications Trial date. Diabetes Care 22:1273, 1999.

103. Brodows RG, Williams C, Amatruda JM: Treatment of insulin reaction in diabetics. JAMA 252:3378, 1984.

CHAPTER 7

COMPLICATIONS OF DIABETES MELLITUS: PRIMARY CARE IMPLICATIONS

Although by definition diabetes is characterized by elevated glucose concentrations, the impact of diabetes, on both the health of individuals and on health care systems, resides almost entirely in the complications of diabetes. The effect of acute hyperglycemia and its associated ketoacidosis (primarily type 1 diabetes) or hyperosmolar hyperglycemic state (HHS) (type 2 diabetes) has a very small role in the total mortality, morbidity, and costs ascribed to diabetes mellitus. It has been estimated that diabetes and its associated vascular complications are the fourth leading cause of death in this country. Diabetes is the leading cause of blindness in individuals between 20 and 74 years of age in industrialized countries. Almost half of new patients undergoing dialysis have diabetic nephropathy. More than half of all nontraumatic lower extremity amputations take place in patients with diabetes. On a relative basis, people with diabetes are 25 times more likely to develop blindness, 17 times more likely to develop kidney disease, 20 times more likely to develop gangrene, 30 to 40 times more likely to undergo a major amputation, two (males) or four (females) times more likely to develop coronary artery disease, and twice as likely to suffer a stroke than are

individuals without diabetes. The total direct and indirect cost of diabetes in 2002 was estimated at \$132 billion dollars,[1] which accounts for one of every seven health care dollars spent in the United States!

Because over 90% of patients with diabetes are cared for by primary care physicians (PCPs), it is obvious that major inroads into improving the situation for patients with diabetes will have to be initiated by nonspecialists. In the past, it was not clear if anything could be done to ameliorate these complications. As discussed previously in this book, it has now been irrefutably demonstrated that strict diabetic control has an important beneficial effect on delaying (and possibly preventing) the appearance of the early changes in diabetic retinopathy, nephropathy, and neuropathy, as well as in slowing progression of existing complications. In addition to blood glucose lowering, a number of other approaches should be employed to help prevent, recognize, and/or treat diabetic complications.

The complications of diabetes are best considered in three separate categories: (1) microvascular (small vessel) disease, the clinical manifestations of which are diabetic retinopathy and diabetic nephropathy; (2) neuropathy (involvement of both the peripheral and autonomic nervous systems), the clinical manifestations of which can lead to various problems; and (3) macrovascular (large vessel or atherosclerotic) disease, the clinical manifestations of which are angina and myocardial infarctions, cerebrovascular accidents, and peripheral vascular disease. This chapter describes the microvascular, neuropathic, and macrovascular complications of diabetes. Chapter 8 also discusses the risk for macrovascular disease.

DIABETIC RETINOPATHY

Although the majority of concern with diabetic eye disease is centered on the retinal changes that occur with diabetes, it is important to realize that the outer (lens) and middle (vitreous) chambers of the eye can also be affected by diabetes. The lens may change shape with marked changes in blood glucose concentration, leading to temporary blurring of vision. Glucose concentrations equilibrate between the lens and the aqueous humor surrounding it, leading to shifts in water, which alters the shape of the lens. Hyperglycemia in the aqueous humor draws fluid out of the lens, resulting in an artificial myopia or nearsightedness. Return of glucose levels to a more normal concentration in the aqueous humor causes water to move into the lens. This results in a transient hyperopia, or farsightedness. Both can occur, the former when a patient's hyperglycemia is evolving and the latter as treatment lowers glucose levels. It can take up to 1 month before baseline vision is restored, although most patients note a significant improvement within a few weeks.

The lens is also more prone to cataract formation in diabetic patients. A rare occurrence is a "snowflake" or "Christmas tree" type of cataract (sometimes called the *diabetic cataract*) in which a pattern resembling these kinds of structures can be seen in the middle of the lens. Because this type of cataract is usually associated with episodes of

severe diabetic ketoacidosis, it is rarely seen today. Although more typical "senile" cataracts may not be more common in the diabetic population, they are approximately five times more likely to develop at a younger age than in the normal population. Diabetic control (as reflected in glucose levels) does not seem to have a role in the development of these cataracts.

With regard to retinal involvement, the first observable diabetic changes on the retina are a subtle dilatation of the major retinal veins. The retinal veins normally are 1.5 times the size of the retinal arteries (a 2:3 artery/vein ratio). In these early changes, the arteries remain normal but the veins become distended and may become two to three times the size of the arteries. This phase, termed *preretinopathy*, is generally present for less than 2 years before the retinal changes progress to the classic background stage.

The next phase is called *background, simple,* or *nonproliferative* diabetic retinopathy. These changes occurring within the retina are characterized by microaneurysms, hemorrhages, and hard exudates (Figure 7-1). Microaneurysms, usually the first sign of background retinopathy, appear as tiny round red dots, which, as the name implies, are small aneurysmal outpouchings or sacculations of the retinal capillaries. If hemorrhage from these weakened areas of the capillary occurs in the superficial retinal layers, they appear flame-shaped. Those occurring in the deeper retinal layers have the appearance of dots and blots. Although the smaller ones may be difficult to distinguish from microaneurysms, most are large enough to be differentiated. In addition, the capillaries become permeable to plasma, which leaks out and precipitates in the retinal layers. This leads to the formation of hard exudates, which are seen as sharply defined, glistening, yellowish deposits. Such leakage involves only plasma, not red blood cells. These changes (microaneurysms, hemorrhages, and exudates) wax and wane.

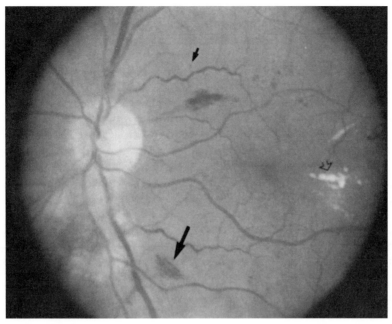

FIGURE 7-1. Background diabetic retinopathy. Note the microaneurysm (short dark arrow), hard exudate (open arrow), and hemorrhage (long dark arrow). *(Courtesy of Albert Sheffer, MD.)*

They do not impair vision unless the plasma leakage occurs near or in the macular area. There, the pattern is often of a ring of hard exudates surrounding the macula (Figure 7-2). Because this is the central vision area, exudates here with the associated swelling (termed *macular edema*) can diminish vision. Macular edema is much more common in older patients. Background retinopathy is not usually seen until approximately 10 years after the diagnosis of diabetes. (However, because the diagnosis is often delayed in persons with type 2 diabetes, background retinopathy is found in approximately 20% of patients when first diagnosed.) With our current results of controlling glucose levels, it eventually appears in up to 80% of diabetic patients (Figure 7-3).

The next stage is called *preproliferative diabetic retinopathy.* The veins now have an irregular caliber, often looking like a string of sausages. A particularly important sign is the appearance of cotton wool spots or soft exudates (Figure 7-4). They represent evidence of capillary closure with resultant hypoxia (lack of oxygen) to parts of the retina. Soft exudates are pale yellow patches with poorly defined margins that do not contrast well with the normal retina (i.e., they may be difficult to see with an ophthalmoscope). The other finding of particular significance is intraretinal microvascular abnormalities (IRMAs). IRMAs are tufts of new capillaries that are still located beneath the inner limiting membrane of the retina—that is, they have not yet broken through to lie on the surface of the retina.

Although it may be difficult (except by special tests) to distinguish between IRMAs and neovascularization (i.e., new vessels that either lie on the surface of the retina or are growing out into the vitreous), the differentiation is not clinically important because either one should trigger an immediate referral to a qualified ophthalmologist.

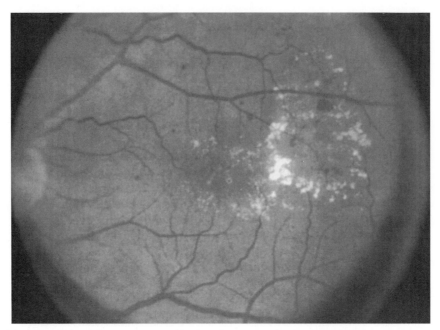

FIGURE 7-2. Macular edema. Circinate pattern of hard exudates in macular area. Note the other characteristics of background retinopathy (microaneurysms, hemorrhage). *(Courtesy of Albert Sheffer, MD.)*

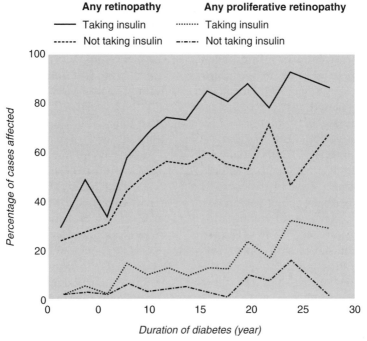

FIGURE 7-3. Frequency of retinopathy (any degree) and proliferative retinopathy by duration of diabetes in people with diabetes diagnosed at age 30 or under, according to insulin treatment. *(From Watkins PJ: Retinopathy. BMJ 326(7395):924–926, 2003.)*

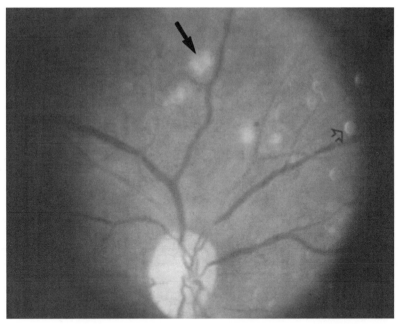

FIGURE 7-4. Preproliferative retinopathy. The soft or cotton wool exudate (dark arrow) has indistinct margins in contrast to the hard exudates in Figures 7-1 and 7-2, which have sharp margins and are brighter. The round structures with distinct margins (open arrow) are artifacts. *(Courtesy of Albert Sheffer, MD.)*

These preproliferative changes are the immediate forerunner to proliferative diabetic retinopathy (in which changes take place outside of the retina), which occurs in 5% to 10% of patients with diabetic retinopathy. New vessel growth occurring on the surface of the retina or growing from there into the vitreous is its distinguishing feature. These new vessels (Figure 7-5) are structurally weak and likely to hemorrhage, thereby obscuring vision. This often leads to formation of fibrous tissue as the blood is resorbed. This scar tissue obscures the retina and places traction on it, and a retinal detachment can result. If the process is allowed to continue untreated, the neovascularization can eventually involve the front part of the eye—namely, the iris and the anterior chamber angle. This angle is functionally very important because it contains a channel that drains to the outside the aqueous humor that is constantly secreted in the eye. If neovascularization occurs in the angle, this drainage channel becomes occluded, resulting in a drastic rise in the intraocular pressure (i.e., neovascular glaucoma), which usually leads to a blind and painful eye.

Vision-threatening retinal involvement almost never occurs within the first 5 years of diagnosis in a patient with type 1 diabetes, or before puberty. However, over the following 20 years, nearly all patients with type 1 diabetes develop some degree of retinopathy, although the more normal the blood glucose levels, the less the chance of developing clinically significant retinopathy. The situation is different in those with type 2 diabetes. In these cases, diabetes may have been present but undetected for years. As a result, approximately 1 in 4 patients with type 2 diabetes have retinopathy at the time of diagnosis. There are an estimated 700,000 people with proliferative diabetic retinopathy in the United States, and approximately 500,000 with macular edema.[2,3] Fortunately, the natural history of diabetic retinopathy does not have to occur in appropriately

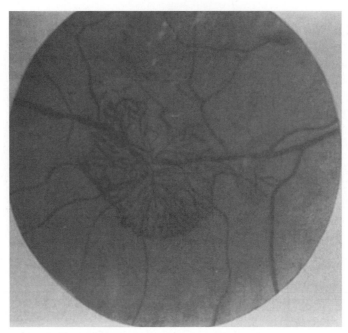

FIGURE 7-5. Proliferative retinopathy with a large area of neovascularization. Note the presence of background retinopathy (microaneurysms, hard exudates, hemorrhage) as well.

screened and treated patients. The Diabetes Control and Complications Trial (DCCT) illustrated a significant relationship between glycemic control and development of retinopathy. In the more intensively treated group (which achieved tighter glycemic control), there was a reduction or prevention in the development of retinopathy by 27% compared with conventional treatment. Intensive therapy also reduced the progression of already present retinopathy by 34% to 76%.[4] The difference in average hemoglobin A_{1c} (A1C) between the intensive group and conventional group was 7.2% and 9.0% respectively. In the United Kingdom Prospective Diabetes Study (UKPDS), patients with type 2 diabetes also had a reduction in the risk of developing retinopathy and other microvascular complications. The overall reduction in complications was 25% in those receiving intensive therapy versus conventional therapy. Furthermore, for every percent decrease in Hgb A_{1c} level, there was a

35% reduction in the risk of microvascular complications.

Thus maintaining near-normal glucose control can greatly delay the onset and progression of retinopathy. This may be a difficult goal, and in some people retinopathy may still progress. The sequelae of eye disease can be averted with appropriate therapy. Unfortunately, this is not always implemented. In one study, 55% of patients with high-risk proliferative retinopathy and/or clinically significant macular edema never had the needed laser photocoagulation, which is treatment of choice (as discussed later).[5] A full ophthalmic evaluation includes a comprehensive examination, including pupillary dilation, slit-lamp evaluation, and indirect ophthalmoscopy. Because of the complexities involved, it is recommended that all patients with diabetes should have a dilated ocular examination by an eye care provider familiar with diabetic eye disease. For reasons previously stated, the current recommendation for initial ophthalmologic examination is within 3 to 5 years after the diagnosis of type 1 diabetes once patients are 10 years of age or older. For those with type 2 diabetes, initial ophthalmic examination is recommended beginning at the time of diagnosis of type 2 diabetes.[3] This interaction between subspecialists and generalists in the management of diabetes is fundamental to the care of the patient, and to afford them the best opportunity for health.

In addition to a comprehensive eye evaluation, the primary care provider must remember that careful management of the metabolic and pathologic aspects of diabetes also impact positively on the patients visual prognosis. Ability to reduce microalbuminuria,[6] cholesterol concentrations,[7] and blood pressure (BP),[8] in addition to blood glucose levels, affects the onset and progression of eye disease in diabetes.

Diabetic retinopathy can take an aggressive turn during pregnancy[9] as a result of multiple hormonal influences and growth factors. When planing a pregnancy, women with preexisting diabetes should have a comprehensive eye examination and should be counseled on the risk of development and/or progression of eye disease. Close follow-up throughout pregnancy is necessary, with a comprehensive eye examination in the first trimester. Further examinations are based on the findings during this examination. Women who develop gestational diabetes are not at risk for developing diabetic retinopathy.

Photocoagulation has been shown to slow and often arrest the two processes that lead to severe visual loss. These are the proliferation of new vessels with subsequent bleeding (leading to vitreous opacities, the formation of scar tissue obscuring the retina, possibly causing a retinal detachment) and macular edema. In regard to the former mechanism, 1727 patients with proliferative retinopathy were randomized to receive either immediate photocoagulation or careful observation in the Diabetic Retinopathy Study.[10] Severe visual loss was defined as vision worse than 5/200 at two or more consecutively completed visits at 4-month intervals. The incidence of severe visual loss was decreased by 50% throughout a 6-year follow-up starting almost immediately. After 6 years, approximately 30% of the untreated eyes had suffered severe visual loss, compared with approximately 15% of the treated eyes.

The results of therapy for macular edema in the Early Diabetic Retinopathy Study[11] were similar. Focal photocoagulation of the macular area was carried out in 754 eyes with macular edema, and 1490 untreated eyes served as controls. The endpoint was a 50% deterioration of vision (e.g., 20/40 to 20/80) when evaluated by a visual acuity chart. At the end of 3 years, 12% of the treated eyes had deteriorated, compared with 24% of the untreated eyes. Further analysis revealed that only eyes with "clinically significant macular edema" needed to be treated because the rate of visual loss was very low in eyes with milder macular changes, and there was no evidence of benefit from treatment of this earlier process. Retinal thickening that occurs at or near the center of the macula is the hallmark of clinically significant macular edema. This can only be assessed by stereo contact lens biomicroscopy and stereo photography, procedures not available to nonophthalmologists. To complicate matters further, initial visual acuity does not help select patients for further investigation. Even patients with normal visual acuity and clinically significant macular edema were helped by focal macular photocoagulation. Thus appropriate treatment might be denied patients who were not referred to an ophthalmologist either until some visual loss occurred or until lesions could be appreciated by direct ophthalmoscopy.

What then is the role of PCPs in regard to diabetic eye disease? The primary goal is to reduce the risk of visual loss by implementing appropriate treatment. Strict diabetes and hypertension control forestalls the development of diabetic retinopathy, and it is the physician's responsibility to discuss this fact with patients and to give direct diabetic care to achieve the best control possible, given the limitations of patients' adherence and circumstances. In regard to the diagnosis of diabetic retinopathy, most PCPs do not dilate the pupils before examination with an ophthalmoscope, if they examine the retina at all. Even if direct ophthalmoscopy is performed through dilated pupils, diabetic retinopathy is diagnosed poorly by nonophthalmologists, including diabetologists. For instance, senior medical residents and board-certified internists missed proliferative retinopathy approximately 50% of the time, and diabetologists missed it 33% of the time.[12] These and similar observations lead to the conclusion that diabetic retinopathy should be diagnosed (at an early stage for appropriate follow-up and treatment) by an ophthalmologist, preferably one who is a retinal specialist.

The American Diabetes Association (ADA)[13] has promulgated the following guidelines: (1) care of the eyes in a diabetic patient reflects a partnership between the PCP and the ophthalmologist; (2) the former has a fundamental role in the medical management, appropriate referrals, and coordination of care, and the latter determines the diagnosis and treatment of diabetic retinopathy; and (3) it is the responsibility of the PCP to inform the patient of the potential for visual loss in diabetes and that early detection and treatment greatly reduce this risk, and to refer the patient appropriately to a qualified ophthalmologist. As mentioned previously, patients with type 1 diabetes should be referred within 3 to 5 years after diagnosis of diabetes once patient is ≥10 years of age and type 2 patients should see an ophthalmologist at the time of diagnosis. The latter procedure is recommended because many patients with type 2 diabetes have their disease for approximately 10 years before the diagnosis is made.[14] The PCP should also inform the patient about

the pros and cons of exercise in those with retinopathy. Although general activity has not been shown to accelerate diabetic retinopathy (and we know that physical exercise has a beneficial impact on reducing the risk of diabetic complications and helping to control blood glucose levels) strenuous activity in patients with active proliferative retinopathy can precipitate hemorrhaging.[15,16] There is no consensus on this topic at present; however, it is wise for PCPs to advise their patients with active proliferative retinopathy against strenuous activity, especially those that involve Valsalva maneuvers or jarring of the head.[17] In addition, because the ADA has guidelines for aspirin therapy, it is important to inform patients that aspirin therapy does not alter the course of diabetic retinopathy. In summary, although aspirin does not reduce the risk of visual loss, it also does not promote vitreous hemorrhage. Thus there are no ocular contraindications to the use of aspirin if indicated for other medical conditions.

PCPs may interact with the patient in one more circumstances regarding diabetic retinopathy. They are often called when a patient develops a vitreous hemorrhage. This typically involves a rather sudden, painless loss of vision, the amount depending on the size of the hemorrhage. If total vision is not obscured, the patient describes a dark area moving around in the field of vision. The hemorrhage tends to spread out inferiorly, especially if the patient remains upright. Activity should be restricted, and the head should be elevated during sleep. Patients who note the sudden onset of floaters (possible small vitreous hemorrhage) or the sudden onset of blurring of vision (possible large vitreous hemorrhage) should be referred immediately to an ophthalmologist, preferably a retinal specialist. Although many may have hemorrhages that are too large (thus obscuring the vitreous) for immediate treatment, some may have small hemorrhages that are easier to treat early while the clot is organized and has not yet had the opportunity to spread out diffusely throughout the vitreous space. Gradual onset of blurring of vision may be due to changes in the lens secondary to changing glucose concentrations or to macular edema.

DIABETIC RENAL DISEASE

The clinical course of diabetic nephropathy for type 1 patients is depicted in Figure 7-6. Screening tests for diabetic nephropathy are shown in Table 7-1. The risk of nephropathy and progression is similar in type 1 and type 2 diabetes.[18] According to recent data, there has been an increase among patients with diabetes who progress to end-stage renal disease (ESRD). From 1982 to 1992 the proportion of patients with both ESRD and diabetes rose from 27% to 36%[19] and in 2002 increased to 43%.[20] This trend is being seen in other developed countries as well, and may be a result of medical ability to prolong life by improving cardiovascular mortality so that more of this population has time to progress in other morbidities related to diabetes. It is also important to note that

up to 20% of patients with type 2 diabetes who have ESRD have a nondiabetic form of kidney disease.[21] Physicians must be aware that diseases coexist, and there may be a role to investigate a decline in renal function as something other than diabetes-related. There is a genetic basis for the development of nephropathy in those with diabetes. Familial clusterings are noted[22] and the risk of nephropathy has been linked to specific chromosomal sites,[23] although genes have not yet been identified. The angiotensin converting enzyme gene is not a predictor of development of renal failure, but may influence the progression of disease.[24]

CLASSIFICATION

Diabetic nephropathy can be divided into five stages.[25,26] Stage I occurs at the onset of the disease. It is characterized by a 30% to 40% increase in the glomerular filtration rate (GFR) above normal and has been documented primarily in patients with new-onset type 1 diabetes. The elevated GFR does not reverse acutely with institution of insulin therapy, but may return to normal within several weeks to a few months. This

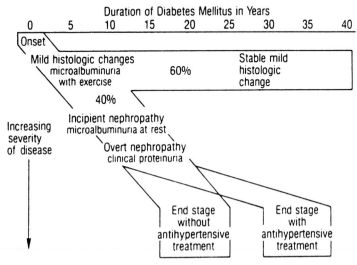

FIGURE 7-6. Clinical course of diabetic nephropathy. (See text for discussion.) *(From Omachi R: The pathogenesis and prevention of diabetic nephropathy. West J Med 145:222, 1986.)*

| TABLE 7-1 SCREENING OF DIABETIC NEPHROPATHY |||
Test	When	Desired Range
Blood pressure	Each office visit	<130/80 mmHg
		Children: <90th percentile
Urinalysis	At diagnosis*	Normal
Urine albumin	Yearly*	<30 mg/24 h
		<30 µg/mg creatinine
		<20 µg/min (timed)

*In children, start at puberty or after 5 years of diabetes.

hyperfiltration is associated with enlarged kidneys and increased intraglomerular pressure, which may cause a transient increase in albumin excretion. One current theory about the development of renal insufficiency involves intraglomerular hypertension causing subsequent nephron loss. This has several important prognostic and therapeutic implications (discussed later).

Stage II is characterized by normal excretion of albumin (<20 µg/min or 30 mg/24 h) regardless of the duration of the disease. Some patients maintain their hyperfiltration, which may be a poor prognostic indicator for subsequent development of diabetic nephropathy.[27] In general, these individuals are usually in poor diabetic control, whereas those whose GFRs return to normal have generally lower glycated hemoglobin levels.[26]

Stage III, or incipient diabetic nephropathy, is characterized by microalbuminuria at rest. This is defined as elevated excretion rates of albumin between 20 and 200 µg/min (30 and 300 mg/24 h). In general, patients with lower amounts of microalbuminuria (20 to 70 µg/min) have either elevated or normal GFRs that are higher than those with more microalbuminuria (70 to 200 µg/min). In a 2-year prospective study,[28] patients with either normal albumin excretion rates (<30 mg/24 h) or mild microalbuminuria (30 to 100 mg/24 h) had no change in their GFR, whereas those with more marked microalbuminuria (101 to 300

mg/24 h) showed a significant reduction. This suggests that the GFR begins to decline during the incipient stage of diabetic nephropathy. At this stage, BPs are often higher (although in the normal range) than in nondiabetic subjects and may increase to abnormally high levels during exercise. In general, BPs increase 3 to 4 mm Hg per year. In the past, approximately 80% of patients with microalbuminuria progressed within 7 to 14 years to clinical proteinuria or overt diabetic nephropathy (discussed later); only 5% without microalbuminuria did so.[26] Control of glucose levels and BP (especially with use of angiotensin-converting enzyme inhibitors [ACEIs] and/or angiotensin receptor blockers [ARBs]) reduces or eliminates microalbuminuria.[29,30] More recently, with strict diabetic control, less than 20% of patients with type 1 diabetes with microalbuminuria progressed to overt nephropathy in a 10-year period.[31] The majority reverted to normoalbuminuria. This is very encouraging because patients with normal albumin excretion rates maintain normal GFR and BP even after 20 years of follow-up.[29]

Stage IV, or overt diabetic nephropathy, is characterized by clinical proteinuria; that is, a level of urinary protein that is detectable (dipstick-positive) by simple tests. These semiquantitative methods are much less sensitive than the specially developed ones used to measure microalbuminuria. Thus overt diabetic nephropathy is defined by urinary protein excretion exceeding 0.5 g/24 h.

Because albumin is not the only protein excreted at this stage, clinical proteinuria corresponds to albumin excretion rates exceeding 200 µg/min or 300 mg (0.3 g)/24 h. Overt diabetic nephropathy develops in approximately 30% to 40% of patients with type 1 diabetes,[29,32] although more recently, when patients were kept in strict diabetic control, less than 10% did so.[33] Genetics also has a role at least in type 1 diabetes. Two independent predictors for type 1 diabetic patients to develop overt nephropathy are positive family histories of renal disease[34] or hypertension.[35] Smoking is also an independent risk factor in both type 1[36] and type 2[37] diabetes.

Early in the clinical course of overt diabetic nephropathy, the GFR may be in the normal range, but usually declines slowly but steadily. Although the rate of fall in GFR may vary markedly among patients, the decrease in GFR is fairly constant within each patient. This is shown in Figure 7-7, in which the GFR is approximated by the inverse of the serum creatinine concentration. There is a linear relationship between the two once the serum creatinine level reaches 2.3 mg/dl (200 µmol/L). The average GFR decline is approximately 1 ml/min/month. During this stage of diabetic nephropathy, BP increases approximately 7 mm Hg per year; thus hypertension eventually occurs in almost all patients. Aggressive treatment of elevated BP slows the rate of decline of the GFR[18] (Figure 7-8). Use of medications such as ACF-1 and/or ARBs (Figure 7-9) can also slow progression to nephropathy. At this point, aggressive treatment of elevated glucose concentrations has little effect. Once the process of nephron destruction is under way, it seems independent of the inciting cause (in many types of renal disease, not just diabetic nephropathy), although lowering the BP is definitely helpful.

Stage V, or ESRD, is similar to kidney failure resulting from any other cause. However, a disproportionate share have diabetic nephropathy. Although only 3% of the population is known to have diabetes, nearly 50% of patients starting dialysis have renal failure caused by diabetes. Signs and symptoms include progressive weakness, lethargy, fluid retention (possibly leading to congestive heart failure), anorexia, nausea, vomiting, diarrhea, hiccups, pruritus, difficulty in controlling hypertension, anemia, and electrolyte disturbances. The clinical impression, however, is that patients with ESRD resulting from diabetes are more symptomatic at higher levels of GFR than patients with nondiabetic causes of kidney failure—that is, the GFR does not have to be as low for diabetic patients to start experiencing difficulties. Therefore dialysis is usually

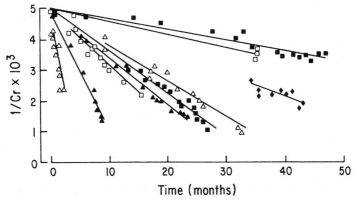

FIGURE 7-7. Progression of renal failure in nine diabetic patients. Inverse of serum creatinine (µmol/L) plotted against time. *(From Jones RH, McKay JD, Hayakawa H et al: Progression of diabetic nephropathy. Lancet 1:1105, 1979.)*

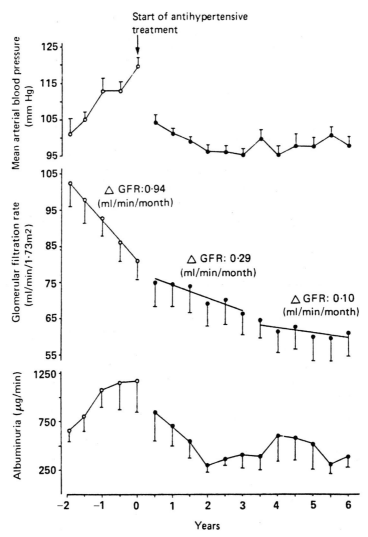

FIGURE 7-8. Changes in mean arterial pressure, glomerular filtration rate, and albuminuria before (open circles) and during (closed circles) long-term effective antihypertensive treatment of nine type I diabetic patients with diabetic nephropathy. *(From Parving HH, Andersen AR, Smidt UM et al: Effect of antihypertensive treatment on kidney function in diabetic nephropathy. BMJ 294:1443, 1987.)*

started earlier in patients with diabetes. Patients with diabetes who have renal insufficiency should be referred to a nephrologist when the serum creatinine level reaches 3 mg/dl or if the patient has refractory hypertension (BP >130/80 in spite of pharmacologic therapy). Diabetic patients undergoing dialysis have a worse prognosis than nondiabetic patients. For this reason, kidney transplantation is considered the preferred method of treatment, especially if a close relative can donate a kidney. Despite successful treatment for ESRD, many of these patients succumb to their associated macrovascular disease.

With this background for the development of diabetic nephropathy, what part can the PCP play? Medical management of dia-

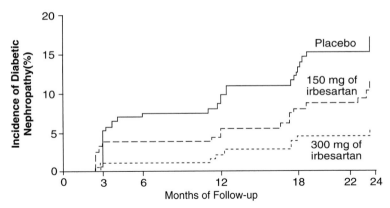

FIGURE 7-9. Incidence of progression to diabetic nephropathy during treatment with 150 mg of irbesartan daily, 300 mg of irbesartan daily, or placebo in hypertensive patients with type 2 diabetes and persistent microalbuminuria. The difference between the placebo group and the 150-mg group was not significant ($P = 0.08$ by the long-rank test), but the difference between the placebo group and the 300-mg group was significant ($P < 0.001$ by the long-rank test). *(From Parving HH, Lehnert H, Brochner-Mortensen J et al:The effect of irbesartan on the development of diabetic nephropathy in patients with type 2 diabetes. N Engl J Med 345:870–878, 2001.)*

betic patients is a critical factor not only in their propensity to develop diabetic retinopathy, but also in the subsequent course. As discussed in Chapter 2 and shown in Figure 2-10, tight diabetic control has a marked impact on delaying and possibly preventing clinical proteinuria. Once persistent proteinuria occurs, elevation of serum creatinine levels is much more likely in hypertensive patients than in normotensive ones.[38] The 10-year mortality rate in patients with diabetes who have overt diabetic nephropathy is three to four times lower if effective hypertensive treatment is given.[39] Thus the PCP has an overriding responsibility to ensure that the blood glucose and BP are meticulously controlled to the level that patients' compliance and disease allow. The limiting factor should be the patient, not the physician. The PCP can also play an important role in helping to modify other risk factors that contribute to the development of diabetic kidney disease, as discussed later. It should be noted that patients with hypertension and diabetes often require use of three or more agents for the treatment of their hypertension (UKPDS)[8] and that patients should be

encouraged to take all of their medication regularly.

MICROALBUMINURIA

The development of ESRD proceeds along a continuum from normoalbuminuria to microalbuminuria to clinical proteinuria to a progressive decline in renal function (Figure 7-10). Virtually all of the longitudinal studies have been carried out on patients with type 1 diabetes because the onset of diabetes usually can be accurately determined. The few studies enrolling patients with type 2 diabetes strongly suggest that, in general, the same progression occurs in these patients as well, although the high prevalence of hypertension has an additional important role.[40] Microalbuminuria is rare during the first 5 years of diabetes. It generally occurs 8 to 10 years after the onset of diabetes and precedes clinical proteinuria by 5 to 8 years. Thus, as discussed earlier, the microalbuminuria, if left untreated, predicts the subsequent development of clinical proteinuria in approximately 30% of patients after 5 years and in as many as 80% 10 to 14 years later. Fewer than 5% of diabetic

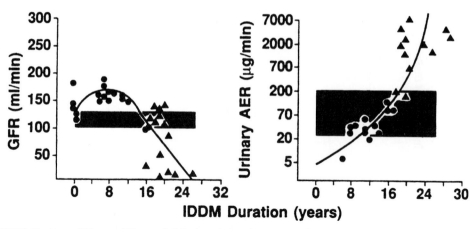

FIGURE 7-10. Natural history of 20 type 1 diabetic patients who progressed to overt diabetic nephropathy (see text for definition of overt nephropathy) in a 12-year period. (•), initial values; (▲), follow-up values; AER, albumin excretion rate; GFR, glomerular filtration rate; IDDM, insulin-dependent diabetes mellitus (type 1 diabetes); shaded areas show normal range. *(From DeFronzo RA: Diabetic nephropathy etiologic and therapeutic considerations. Diabetes Rev 3:510, 1995.)*

patients without microalbuminuria develop clinical proteinuria 7 to 14 years later.[26] In a study on patients with type 1 diabetes with microalbuminuria, regression was frequent with a six-year cumulative incidence of 58%. The use of angiotensin-converting-enzyme inhibitors was not associated with the regression of microalbuminuria. However, microalbuminuria of short duration, A1C levels less than 8%, low systolic blood pressure (less than 115 mg Hg), and low levels of both cholesterol and triglycerides were independently associated with the regression of microalbuminuria.[41]

Because of these considerations and the fact that microalbuminuria is treatable, it is very important for the PCP to accurately assess whether microalbuminuria is present. Other nondiabetic causes of microalbuminuria must be kept in mind, and before microalbuminuria is assumed to reflect incipient diabetic nephropathy, they must be ruled out. These causes are (1) poor diabetic control, (2) systemic or urinary tract infection, (3) fever (per se), (4) congestive heart failure, (5) elevated BP, and (6) exercise.

Five methods are available for assessing for the presence of microalbuminuria: (1) measuring albumin in urine collected during a 24-hour period, (2) measuring albumin in a specifically timed shorter urine collection period (e.g., over 4 hours), (3) measuring albumin in urine collected overnight (i.e., between going to sleep and waking up in the morning), (4) measuring the albumin-to-creatinine ratio in a random urine sample, and (5) measuring the albumin concentration. The latter can be performed either quantitatively or semiquantitatively with a strip (Micral, Boehringer Mannheim, Indianapolis, IN) specifically adapted to very low concentrations of albumin. A concentration ≥20 mg/L has been accepted as being positive for microalbuminuria. However, an albumin concentration exceeding this value must be confirmed by one of the other methods before a diagnosis of microalbuminuria can be made. Because urinary volume is so critical to the concentration of albumin measured, simply measuring the albumin concentration is not generally recommended as a screening test if one of the other approaches is available.[42]

A single abnormal value is not sufficient to make the diagnosis of microalbuminuria. Because of as much as a 40% to 50% day-to-day variation in albumin excretion, an abnormal result mandates a repeat test to confirm the abnormal value. This is especially important in patients whose results are in the lower microalbuminuric range. Timed urine collections and 24-hour urine collections are the least convenient for patients. An overnight urine collection is less inconvenient, but because of recumbency and little activity, the albumin excretion rate overnight is approximately 25% less than during the day (upright posture and exercise increase albumin excretion). This may not be a drawback because an abnormal value in an overnight collection is more certain to be a valid diagnosis (values in the lower microalbuminuric range are much more likely to be normal on retesting). The albumin/creatinine ratio is the simplest of the four valid tests to assess microalbuminuria. Albumin/creatinine ratios of 30 µg/mg (3.5 µg/µmol) or higher have a high degree (95% to 100%) of both sensitivity and specificity in predicting microalbuminuria when measured by 24-hour or timed urine collections.[43,44] A ratio measured in a sample collected on rising in the morning correlates much more closely with microalbuminuria measured by other means than does a sample collected randomly during the day.[45] The Council on Diabetes Mellitus of the National Kidney Foundation[46] has recommended the simpler albumin/creatinine ratio over other methods. A diagnosis of microalbuminuria requires two values between 30 and 300 µg/mg within a 3-month period. Values of 300 µg/mg or higher diagnose clinical proteinuria. However, a more cost-effective approach is to initially test a random urine sample with a standard dipstick for protein. If that result is positive (and confirmed), the patient has clinical proteinuria and further work-up for microalbuminuria is unnecessary. The distinction between the upper end of the microalbuminuric range

and the lower end of the clinical proteinuria range is not important because the clinical approach is the same. All patients with diabetes, with the exception of those with type 1 diabetes within the first 5 years of diagnosis, should be tested for the presence of albumin in the urine. If the test result for microalbuminuria is negative, evaluation should be repeated on a yearly basis.

Another aspect of microalbuminuria is noteworthy.[29,47] It predicts not only the development of clinical proteinuria, but also cardiovascular mortality in patients with type 2 diabetes, perhaps as a marker for endothelial damage. For instance, Figure 7-11 shows a progressive increase in mortality after 9.5 years as the level of microalbuminuria increased in patients with type 2 diabetes compared with age-matched controls. Although these patients have other risk factors for cardiovascular disease (CVD), the excess mortality is only partially explained by them. It has long been well documented that clinical proteinuria in type 1 diabetes is a powerful predictor of mortality resulting from coronary artery disease.

Microalbuminuria and clinical proteinuria also predict increased cardiovascular mortality in nondiabetic populations. One hypothesis to explain this association is that albuminuria simply reflects vascular damage that has occurred throughout the body.[28] The increased permeability of vessels would allow atherosclerotic lipoproteins to penetrate the walls of large vessels and would account for the leakage of retinal blood vessels in diabetic patients. This theory is supported by the markedly increased transcapillary escape of albumin[48] and fibrinogen in diabetic patients with microalbuminuria.

RISK FACTORS FOR DEVELOPMENT OF NEPHROPATHY IN DIABETES

Smoking

Smoking actually has adverse effects on many types of renal disease, including diabetic

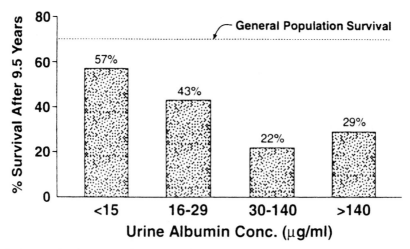

FIGURE 7-11. Survival after 9.5 years in 76 patients with type 2 diabetes with various degrees of microalbuminuria (based on urinary albumin concentration) compared with an age-matched population. *(From DeFronzo RA: Diabetic nephropathy: Etiology and therapeutic considerations. Diabetes Rev 3:510, 1995.)*

nephropathy. Patients with type 2 diabetes who smoke have a greater risk of microalbuminuria than those who do not smoke, and their rate of progression to ESRD is approximately twice as fast. In addition, there is data in type 1 diabetes that the cessation of smoking results in a slower rate of decline in renal function than in those who continue to smoke.[49] PCPs should explore options with patients to aide in smoking cessation, and revisit this issue frequently to encourage compliance.

Protein Intake

The evidence that a diet high in protein contributes to the decline in renal function in diabetes is suspect and debated widely, and unfortunately, good controlled studies are lacking. There is some evidence to indicate that patients with type 1 diabetes who consume less protein have a lower prevalence of microalbuminuria.[50] As a result, PCPs should advise against excessive protein consumption. However, protein restriction cannot be advocated in most cases, because the effect of dietary protein restriction is minimal.[51] In general, convention states that

0.8 to 1.0 g/kg of body weight is an appropriate recommendation. This amounts to about 60 to 70 g of protein per day in most cases. This does not apply to patients in overt renal failure or ESRD.

Glycemic Control

Although intuitively obvious, it has now been proven that the glycemic control in both type 1 and type 2 diabetes directly affects the rate of progression of and the risk of development of microalbuminuria. Both the DCCT[52] in patients with type 1 diabetes, and the UKPDS in patients with type 2 diabetes[53] have shown conclusively that glycemic control is important in preventing and retarding the progression of renal disease in diabetes. In the DCCT, intensive treatment reduced the development of microalbuminuria by 34% (P < 0.04) in the primary prevention cohort and by 43% (P < 0.001) in the secondary intervention cohort. The risk of dipstick proteinuria was reduced by 56% (P < 0.01) in the secondary intervention cohort. Another important note for the PCP to take from the UKPDS trial is that the actual agent used to achieve glycemic control was not important; only the end result of actual control played a role in prevention.

Hyperlipidemia

Hypercholesterolemia may be regarded as a factor in the progression of segmental glomerulosclerosis and dietary increased of cholesterol supplementation accelerate glomerular injury.[54] Diabetic dyslipidemia, which is associated with elevated triglycerides (TGs) and low high-density lipoprotein (HDL) levels, has been shown to be a predictor of a more rapid rate of progression of microalbuminuria in patients with controlled hypertension.[55] Tonolo et al.[56] studied the long-term effects of simvastatin on urinary albumin excretion rate in patients with type 2 diabetes who were normotensive with microalbuminuria. They found that the 3-hydroxy-3-methylglutaryl coenzyme A (HMG CoA) reductase inhibitor decreased low-density lipoprotein (LDL) and total cholesterol levels at 1 year, and decreased urinary albumin excretion by 25% from baseline. Although the use of a statin simply for the potential renal benefits is not advocated, the primary physician should pay close attention to the cholesterol profiles of their patients with diabetes, and realize that institution of therapy early is appropriate, and also has additional benefits.

Hypertension

Aggressive treatment of hypertension is critical for maintaining normal renal function in patients with diabetes. ACEIs and ARBS should be first-line agents in the treatment of hypertension in the patients with diabetes and is discussed later.

HYPORENINEMIC HYPOALDOSTERONISM

Another situation with which PCPs may have to deal is the syndrome of hyporeninemic hypoaldosteronism.[56a] Patients with this condition present with hyperkalemia that is asymptomatic approximately 75% of the time. Symptoms in the other 25% are muscle weakness and/or cardiac arrhythmias. Approximately half of patients have a hyperchloremic acidosis. This syndrome usually occurs in older patients. This fact may not be surprising because aging is associated with decreased secretion of both renin and aldosterone. Most patients have mild to moderate renal insufficiency and/or diabetes mellitus.

The pathogenesis of this enigmatic syndrome is not clear, and this is not the place to discuss the various hypotheses. The problem for PCPs is one of management. One must keep in mind that most of these patients are older and have associated medical conditions such as diabetes, renal failure, macroangiopathy, and/or hypertension. Therefore the side effects of any therapeutic interventions must be weighed against the possible benefits of lowering the serum potassium level. Obviously, drugs that may raise potassium levels (e.g., potassium-sparing diuretics, ACEIs) should be used with caution. An asymptomatic patient with a potassium level lower than 6 mEq/L does not generally require treatment as long as no changes of hyperkalemia are noted on the electrocardiogram (ECG). If therapy is deemed necessary, either mineralocorticoid (fludrocortisone acetate [Florinef]) administration or sodium-potassium exchange resins can be tried. Sodium retention leading possibly to congestive heart failure may occur with both therapies (high doses of fludrocortisone acetate [0.2 to 0.5 mg] are often required). Potassium-wasting diuretics may be helpful. The mild acidosis may be treated with oral sodium bicarbonate, which may also improve potassium excretion, but once again an increased sodium load may be a problem.

The final circumstance to be discussed involving diabetic nephropathy concerns radiocontrast-induced acute renal failure.

Because of their coronary artery and peripheral vascular diseases, patients with diabetes are likely to undergo dye studies. Unfortunately, patients with diabetes, congestive heart failure, and/or renal insufficiency are at an increased risk for radiocontrast-induced renal dysfunction. Patients with diabetes with renal insufficiency are particularly susceptible.[57] The higher the prestudy serum creatinine concentration, the more likely it is that acute renal failure will occur and that dialysis may be necessary for temporary treatment.[58,59] For example, in a cohort of patients with a mean serum creatinine level of 2.4 mg/dl, 40% manifested radiocontrast-induced renal failure despite previous hydration.[58] In two other studies,[57-60] the prevalence of acute renal failure was 2% to 5% in low-risk patients and 9% to 16% in high-risk patients, with *high risk* defined as the presence of diabetes mellitus, preexisting renal insufficiency, or congestive heart failure. None of these patients required dialysis. Unfortunately, using the newer, non-ionic, low-osmolality radiocontrast materials did not protect the patients from acute renal failure.[57,60,61]

What then is the role of PCPs under these circumstances? First, be certain that the dye study is really necessary and that equivalent information could not be obtained by other imaging techniques. Second, because plasma volume contraction and decreased renal plasma flow are extremely important risks, withhold diuretics, nonsteroidal anti-inflammatory agents, and metformin the day before the procedure. Third, ensure adequate hydration by infusing saline to induce a gentle diuresis ($\geq$75 ml/h).[58,62] Some physicians begin this several hours before the study; others begin the hydration after the study is completed. In either case, it should be continued for approximately 4 hours after the procedure. Although centers also use concomitant administration of furosemide or mannitol, a prospective controlled study demonstrated that these agents may actually increase nephrotoxicity.[62]

DIABETIC NEUROPATHY

Neuropathy is the most frequent symptomatic complications of diabetes. The high prevalence of neuropathy in patients with diabetes and its often serious sequelae make it an important issue of which primary care givers need to be aware. Diabetic neuropathy (Table 7-2) has an important role in the increased morbidity and mortality suffered by individuals with diabetes. Diabetic neuropathy is reported to affect greater than 50% of patients with a history of diabetes for 25 years or more.[63] A large series reported 7.5% of patients had neuropathy at the time of diagnosis.[63] Although the exact mechanism is not known, it is generally believed that long-term hyperglycemia is the cause (except as noted).

Although many classifications of neuropathy have been proposed over the years, one of the most popular was proposed by Thomas[64] and is based on whether the neuropathy is diffuse or local. If diffuse, the subclassifications include distal symmetric sensorimotor polyneuropathy, symmetric proximal lower limb motor neuropathy (amyotrophy), and autonomic neuropathy. This latter category is further divided into sudomotor, cardiovascular, gastrointestinal, genitourinary. Local disease is subclassified as cranial neuropathy, radiculopathy, entrapment neuropathy, and asymmetric lower limb motor neuropathy (amyotrophy).

Peripheral (Distal Symmetric) Neuropathy

Peripheral neuropathy or distal symmetric neuropathy is the earliest, most widely recognized, and probably the most common form of diabetic neuropathy. It is a common complication intimately related to the duration of diabetes (Figure 7-12). The overall prevalence in the diabetic population is 25% to 35%.[65,66]

Peripheral neuropathy is a generalized, sensorimotor polyneuropathy of gradual onset that is usually progressive.[67] The legs

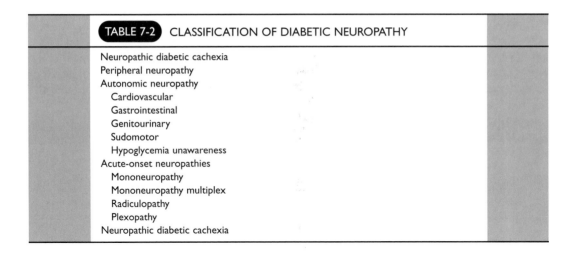

TABLE 7-2	CLASSIFICATION OF DIABETIC NEUROPATHY

Neuropathic diabetic cachexia
Peripheral neuropathy
Autonomic neuropathy
    Cardiovascular
    Gastrointestinal
    Genitourinary
    Sudomotor
    Hypoglycemia unawareness
Acute-onset neuropathies
    Mononeuropathy
    Mononeuropathy multiplex
    Radiculopathy
    Plexopathy
Neuropathic diabetic cachexia

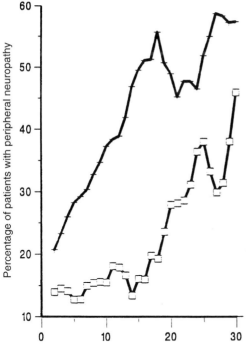

FIGURE 7-12. The prevalence of peripheral neuropathy in type 1 (Δ) and type 2 (+) diabetic patients by duration of disease. *(From Young MJ, Boulton AJM, Macleod AF et al: A multicentre study of the prevalence of diabetic peripheral neuropathy in the United Kingdom hospital clinic population. Diabetologia 36:150, 1993.)*

are almost always affected earlier than the hands. Many patients are asymptomatic or only mildly symptomatic, and the neuropathy is only detected by careful examination. Those that are symptomatic initially experience sensory manifestations (e.g., paresthesias, burning sensations, and hyperesthesia), which can be quite uncomfortable. Pain, especially in the legs, appears more severe at night.[68] The hyperesthesia may be profound and out of proportion to the clinical findings. On examination, early loss of tendon reflexes, decreased vibration sense, and sense of touch are noted. As the peripheral neuropathy progresses, the feet become numb and the patient is unable to appreciate trauma. Additionally, involvement of motor fibers can cause muscle weakness and atrophy. This can cause deformities of the feet, leading to areas that receive increased pressure and are manifested initially by callus formation. A further serious cause of foot deformities and areas receiving increased pressure is Charcot's arthropathy (joint destruction secondary to unappreciated trauma). This repeated unrecognized trauma to the foot may destroy the joint structures, with subsequent flattening of the foot arch (Figure 7-13). Because patients have decreased sensation in the foot, these areas can ulcerate. Once the integrity of the skin has been breached, the chances for a serious infection are increased, especially if a patient is very hyperglycemic. Any

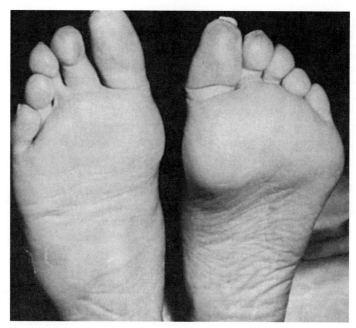

FIGURE 7-13. Charcot's joint resulting in flattening of the arch.

impairment of circulation to the foot because of peripheral vascular disease compounds the problem. The combination of loss of sensation leading to ulceration of the skin (regardless of whether foot deformities are involved) and diminished circulation is the root cause of the large number of lower extremity amputations in diabetic patients (50% to 75% of total nontraumatic amputations in the United States).

Both retrospective and prospective studies have shown a relationship between hyperglycemia and the development and severity of diabetic neuropathy. The DCCT has shown the benefit of tight glycemic control on the reduction of neuropathy.[69]

The *pain of peripheral neuropathy* is particularly vexing to the patients and is not easy to treat. The first thing to emphasize to patients is that near euglycemia often alleviates the pain of peripheral diabetic neuropathy,[70] especially in its early stages. This discomfort often motivates patients to work to achieve strict diabetic control. Although many patients do not respond to ordinary analgesics, these should be tried first (as a patient is attempting to improve diabetic control) because some will respond.[71] Nonsteroidal antiinflammatory drugs, however, should not be used on a long-term basis because of their potential to reduce renal function. Narcotics should be avoided because these drugs often do not satisfactorily control the pain and addiction is a potential problem. However, if other approaches fail, small doses of narcotics, best given intermittently, can take the edge off the pain.

Most patients with marked pain have difficulty sleeping through the night and are often depressed as well. Sleeping medication is usually not helpful. However, small amounts of the antidepressants imipramine (Tofranil), amitriptyline (Elavil), desipramine or venlafaxine (Effexor XR)[72] may improve the pain, disturbed sleeping patterns, and associated depression.[73-75] The beneficial effect of the antidepressants on the pain of diabetic peripheral neuropathy is independent of their antidepressant effects.[75] Because nighttime pain is usually more severe, the drugs are given before bed, starting with small doses and gradually increasing as necessary. Patients should be warned about the side effects (sedation and anticholinergic symptoms). Patients usually respond within 1 week (which is faster than the antidepressant effect of higher doses). Tricyclic antidepressants are contraindicated in patients with heart block, recent myocardial infarctions, congestive heart failure, urinary tract obstruction, orthostatic hypotension, or narrow-angle glaucoma. They should be stopped slowly to avoid withdrawal symptoms (e.g., rebound insomnia, headache, excessive salivation, diarrhea, malaise, anorexia, and fatigue), although these are less likely with the lower doses used to treat diabetic neuropathy.

Gabapentin has also been shown to be effective[76] with few side effects. A small dose (300 mg at bedtime) is initially used, with dosage titrated up as needed. The maximum dose is 2400 mg per day, often given three times daily. Patients should be warned that they will not have an immediate improvement, but rather a gradual lessening of their pain. Adverse events include dizziness, sleepiness, headache, and diarrhea. Sleepiness can often be dealt with by giving the drug initially only at night.

Other drugs can be tried if antidepressants and gabapentin were ineffective. Although phenytoin (Dilantin) was advocated many years ago[77] (and carried along in textbooks and reviews ever since), a small double-blind, placebo-controlled study refuted the value of the drug.[78] Anecdotal experience supports this lack of an effect. The second-line drug most often used is carbamazepine (Tegretol). Several double-blind studies have demonstrated its efficacy in painful diabetic neuropathy.[79,80] The usual effective dose of carbamazepine ranges between 400 and 800 mg/day in divided doses, although for some patients up to 1200 mg/day may be required. The initial dose is 100 mg twice a day; this should be gradually increased every day or two to yield therapeutic plasma levels of 4 to 10 µg/ml. Baseline blood and platelet counts, urinalysis, and hepatic and renal function tests are advisable before starting treatment. Carbamazepine may cause leukopenia and a complete blood cell count should be checked at baseline and then repeatedly over the next 3 months

Aldose reductase inhibitors (not available in the United States) work by inhibiting the influx of glucose through the polyol pathway. The result is a reduction of sorbitol. Sorbitol is an organic osmolyte that helps cells adapt to osmotic stress. Results are not clear as of yet; some studies have shown a reduction in pain,[81,82] whereas others have not.[83] Linoleic acid, an essential fatty acid, is metabolized to dihomogamma-linolenic acid (GLA), which in turn is an important membrane phospholipid and also a substrate for prostaglandin E (which may help to preserve nerve blood flow). In patients with diabetes the conversion to GLA is impaired. GLA administration to patients with diabetes has shown subjective and objective benefits.[84] Aminoguanidine inhibits the formation of advanced glycosylation end products, which are thought to play an important role in diabetic neuropathy. Although animal studies are promising, there is no data to support its use in humans at this time. N-acetyl-L-carnitine and alpha lipoic acid are also possible treatments, but at present are not fully studied. Myo-Inositol supplementation may improve subjective symptoms,[85] but benefits may take up to 6 months to be seen.

A locally applied cream, 0.075% capsaicin, may be helpful for the superficial (as opposed to the deep, gnawing, "toothache") type of pain of diabetic peripheral neuropathy.[86] Capsaicin (naturally found in red peppers and used as a folk remedy for centuries to treat pain) is thought to work by depleting substance P, a neurotransmitter of pain, from peripheral nerve endings. It should be applied to the painful areas three to four times a day. Patients should be cautioned not to use excessive amounts because of its tendency to aerosolize and induce coughing and sneezing. Great care must be taken to avoid exposing mucous membranes (e.g., eyes and mouth) to the drug by either wearing gloves when applying it or thoroughly washing one's hands afterward to prevent a burning sensation in those areas. Because the mechanism of action of capsaicin is to deplete the nerve endings of substance P, thereby alleviating pain, it is not surprising that many patients experience a local exacerbation of pain after the initial applications until the neurotransmitter has been depleted. This usually abates after the first week if the patient uses the cream consistently. Although statistically significant differences have been found between capsaicin and its vehicle in published studies, the high placebo response (approximately 50%) makes interpretation difficult. Its role in the treatment of painful diabetic neuropathy remains uncertain because it can take up to 4 weeks to be effective and many patients stop using it.

Diabetic patients often complain of *leg cramps*. These can occur at rest (and therefore are not related to intermittent claudication) and seem to be more frequent overnight. It is commonly stated that these may be a manifestation of diabetic neuropathy, although little direct evidence supports this. Patients should know that, although painful, these cramps do not represent a serious abnormality. Sometimes treatment for diabetes neuropathy can improve the frequency of leg cramps.

The treatment of *Charcot's arthropathy* previously was total immobilization (usually by casting) and surgery to correct the deformities resulting from bone destruction. Although immobilization can arrest the condition in its early stages, it most often recurs on weight bearing. These patients need to be closely followed by a podiatrist who is an expert in diabetic feet.

Most of the previously mentioned therapies can be administered by PCPs. If there is concern over complications, and hesitancy to prescribe these agents in this setting, the involvement of a neurologist may be appropriate. The adjunct care provided by a neurologist also allows for specialized testing, including peripheral nerve biopsy, quantitative sensory testing, and electrophysiologic testing for the diagnosis and continual assessment of diabetic peripheral neuropathy. The PCP in conjunction with the specialist may be the best option to provide optimal care to patients with neuropathy.

Autonomic Neuropathy

Autonomic neuropathy can be a very serious problem in diabetes, and in fact, more than one in four patients with type 1 diabetes have evidence of autonomic dysfunction at the time of diagnosis.[87] The presentations are extremely variable, and include abnormalities in sweating, sexual dysfunction, gastrointestinal symptoms, and orthostasis. Although various tests may reveal abnormalities in the functioning of the autonomic nervous system (both sympathetic and parasympathetic) early in the course of diabetes, clinical signs and symptoms appear much later and almost always after peripheral neuropathy is established. Cardiac autonomic dysfunction can be diagnosed at the bedside by relatively simple clinical maneuvers outlined in a landmark paper by Ewing et al.[88] These authors describe techniques to assess heart rate variability with Valsalva's maneuver, hand grip, and positioning, along with respiratory variations with inspiration and ECG changes in respiratory rate (RR) variability to detect early autonomic involvement. Normally, parasympathetic activity decreases the heart rate while sympathetic activity increases the heart rate and the force of cardiac contraction (leading to a rise in cardiac output) and redirects blood flow from the viscera to skeletal muscle by increasing splanchnic resistance more than peripheral resistance. The parasympathetic arm of the autonomic nervous system is often affected earlier and more profoundly than the sympathetic one. Therefore a *resting tachycardia* is usually the initial clinical cardiovascular effect of autonomic neuropathy. *Exercise intolerance* may occur when the sympathetic nervous system is affected, because the necessary increase in cardiac output and skeletal blood flow is blunted. When one arises from a lying to sitting to standing position, the sympathetic nervous system is responsible for the maintenance of the BP via stimuli from the baroreceptors. Therefore autonomic neuropathy may cause *postural (orthostatic) hypotension,* which has been defined in two ways: either a 30 mm Hg decrease in systolic BP or a 10 mm Hg fall in diastolic BP 2 minutes after standing. Clinically, patients complain of sudden dizziness (lightheadedness), weakness, nausea, and occasionally vomiting or syncope after standing up quickly.

Although many of the problems caused by *autonomic neuropathy* may be handled by the appropriate specialist (neurologist, urologist, gastroenterologist, cardiologist), PCPs should be aware of certain treatment options in which they may be involved. It is important to note that there is a possible role of persistently high cardiac output in these patients that may lead to an increased risk of cardiac events in an already high-risk population. Reduced vagal tone may be a contributing factor to sudden cardiac death and infarction. Most of the cardiovascular manifestations of the autonomic nervous system do not require treatment except for the *orthostatic hypotension.* A number of nonpharmacologic measures can be very helpful in this difficult situation.[89] Attempts to increase venous return by using compressive stockings may help. If drugs are necessary, the use of fludrocortisone acetate (0.05 to 0.1 mg daily) to increase the intravascular volume is usually tried first. If a small dose is ineffective, larger amounts may be tried, but excessive sodium retention with edema and

possibly congestive heart failure often limit this approach. Hypokalemia may also be a confounding side effect of therapy. Other drugs that may be helpful are midodrine[90,91] (an orphan drug), diltiazem,[92] erythropoietin,[93] and octreotide (somatostatin).[94]

Autonomic neuropathy can involve all parts of the gastrointestinal tract: esophagus, stomach, gallbladder, small intestine, and large intestine. Esophageal and gallbladder dysfunction do not usually cause any symptoms. In fact, hyperglycemia itself in the absence of diabetes is known to produce disruption in function of all levels of the digestive tract; however, the most common gastrointestinal diagnoses are gastroesophageal reflux disease, gastric dysfunction, and altered bowel habits (diarrhea or constipation.)

In patients with gastric involvement, this can range in severity. Studies of gastric physiology have shown that up to 85% of diabetics have measurable gastric dysfunction, although a minority of these patients have symptomatic disease.[95] The extreme form of diabetic gastropathy is diabetic gastroparesis *(gastroparesis diabeticorum).* This diagnosis is often overcalled. In this condition, the stomach is large, dilated, and hypotonic. Symptoms include anorexia, postprandial bloating, early satiety, nausea, vomiting, and gastric reflux. Abdominal pain is remarkably rare. Also, because the ingested food remains in the stomach and is delayed in entering the small intestine, the vomitus may include undigested food eaten many hours earlier. This problem is a particularly difficult one for patients who require insulin, who need a predictable response to meals to cover the action of the injected insulin.

More commonly, diabetic gastropathy is milder. These milder forms often involve the effect of hyperglycemia on gastric pacemaker activity.[88] Hyperglycemic clamp of normal subjects can produce symptomatic gastric dysrhythmia that is reversible and therefore does not represent a "paresis" as would be seen with the end-stage gastro-paretic. These patients often complain more of nausea and vomiting on an empty stomach in addition to postprandially.

Treatment of symptomatic *gastroparesis diabeticorum*[96] can be difficult and frustrating. The modalities of treatment are diet, glycemic control, drugs, and, in severe cases, nutritional support. Although hyperglycemia delays gastric emptying, near euglycemia improves it. Because the control of gastric emptying determines the rate of glucose delivery to the small intestine, glucose control becomes even more erratic when gastric emptying is abnormal. Hyperglycemia then further impairs gastric emptying and a vicious cycle ensues. Hyperglycemia actually results in a dysrhythmia of the stomach as seen on electrogastrographic studies.[88] With resolution of dysrhythmia, gastroparetic findings such as nausea and vomiting may subside dramatically. In true diabetic gastroparesis, frequent small meals (six to eight feedings per day) with a low-fat and low-fiber content and especially liquids and foods of soft consistency are best. Because absorption of carbohydrate is delayed, it may be helpful not only to inject regular insulin just before eating or even after the meal (instead of the recommended 30 minutes prior) but also to move the site of injection from the abdomen to the arms, thighs, or buttocks, where absorption of insulin is slower. Newer analogs such as lispro (Humalog) or aspart (Novolog) may allow for better control, as may pump therapy because these modalities allow for more patient flexibility. Drug treatments include metoclopramide (Reglan) and erythromycin. Metoclopramide is cholinergic and anti-dopaminergic. The former action increases gastric emptying and the latter accounts for its antiemetic properties by inhibiting the central vomiting center. Metoclopramide has little effect on gastric emptying of a liquid meal, and many patients develop tachyphylaxis to the effect of the drug on accelerating gastric emptying of more solid meals. Despite this, metoclopramide often produces sustained relief of symptoms, probably related to its central antiemetic properties. The usual dose is 5 to 20 mg given 15 to 60 minutes before each meal and at bedtime. It can also be administered as a suppository. If the symptoms are mild and intermittent, the drug should be given only during symptomatic intervals to avoid the long-term side effects. These occur in as many as 20% of patients, in whom reversible neurologic symptoms (sedation, restlessness, anxiety, fatigue) develop. Extrapyramidal signs (tremor and even tardive dyskinesia) can be a problem, as can the neuroendocrine side effects of hyperprolactinemia and occasionally galactorrhea. Another prokinetic, bethanecol, has demonstrated good efficacy in gastric delay of diabetes with little or no central nervous system side effects. It is, unfortunately, not available in the United States. Bethanecol is given at a dose of 10 to 20 mg before each meal.

Erythromycin stimulates gastrointestinal motor activity via its binding to the motilin receptor. Through that mechanism, it accelerates gastric emptying of both liquid and solid meals, and improves the symptoms related to gastroparesis diabeticorum.[97,98] Erythromycin has an added benefit of stimulating housekeeper waves during fasting, which are responsible for clearing the digestive system of undigested debris. The effective dose for these effects is 50 mg intravenously or orally three to four times a day. Tachyphylaxis may also be a problem with erythromycin if used too frequently. The side effects (nausea, bloating, abdominal cramps, diarrhea) seem to be dose related, allowing the possibility that a dose reduction might alleviate the side effects without eliminating the beneficial therapeutic effect.[96] Recently, smaller doses of erythromycin have been used in suspension form with good results. For hyperglycemic dysrhythmias, the treatment is glycemic control.

Autonomic neuropathy of the intestine (enteropathy) leads to constipation (most common), diarrhea, or alternating constipation and diarrhea. Diabetic diarrhea is often nocturnal and can be associated with fecal incontinence (caused by neurogenic impairment of rectal sensation). *Diabetic diarrhea* is a diagnosis of exclusion to be made only when other causes of diarrhea have been ruled out. Because the pathogenesis is unknown, treatment is necessarily empirical. The antidiarrheal agents loperamide and diphenoxylate can decrease the number of stools per day.

One form of diarrhea that may need to be ruled out in diabetes is small intestinal bacterial overgrowth. A lactulose hydrogen breath test may be a useful tool for diagnosis of this condition, and treatment involves broad-spectrum antibiotics (tetracycline, cephalosporins, quinolones, metronidazole) can be helpful. However, bacterial overgrowth can be a recurring phenomenon resulting in repeated courses of antibiotics leading to bacterial resistance. Some clinicians advocate rotating courses of antibiotics to prevent resistance, although there is little evidence that this works. Clonidine (started in a low dose, 0.1 mg twice daily and gradually increased up to 0.5 or 0.6 mg twice daily as necessary) has been shown to be effective for unexplained diarrhea.[99] Others have successfully used topical clonidine[100,101] to avoid the side effects of the oral formulation that would be particularly troublesome in these patients (orthostatic hypotension and delay of gastric emptying). Finally, 50 to 75 µg of octreotide, the long-acting somatostatin analogue, injected twice a day has been very beneficial in some patients[94,102,103] and may be given in the same syringe with insulin.[103] The major drawback to octreotide is reduced gallbladder contractility leading to cholelithiasis in the setting of already increased risk because of the underlying diabetes.[88]

Constipation is more common than diarrhea and can be very difficult for patients.

Management should include bulk or osmotic laxatives, but cathartics should be avoided. Stimulants of colonic motility, such cholinergic agonists (e.g., bethanechol) may be helpful in some patients. If all else fails and the constipation is severe, an enema program may be necessary.

Bladder dysfunction (cystopathy) and, in men, retrograde ejaculation and impotence are the result of autonomic neuropathy involving the genitourinary tract. As in the intestinal tract, the parasympathetic nervous system mediates the sensation of bladder fullness and contraction of bladder smooth muscle. The necessary involuntary relaxation of the bladder sphincters during urination is under control of the sympathetic nervous system. Patients with a neurogenic bladder may not be able to sense when their bladders are full. The initial symptom is decreased frequency of urination as the bladder capacity increases before contraction occurs. This progresses to overflow incontinence associated with urgency and dribbling, incomplete emptying of the bladder, and finally inability to void. The retained urine is a prime source for infection, which, if it travels in a retrograde direction up the ureter, can lead to serious kidney infections. PCPs should instruct patients on Credé's maneuver, which involves squeezing the bladder from all sides in a downward motion to start the flow of urination. Parasympathomimetic agents such as bethanechol are sometimes helpful, and doses are usually 5 to 10 mg initially and then hourly until a maximum of 50 mg is given, or a good response has occurred. This dose is then divided into a three times daily or four times daily maintenance dose. Self-catheterization may also be needed, and alpha 1 blockers such as doxazosin may also be required.

Unfortunately, impotence *(erectile dysfunction)* is a common problem in male patients with diabetes and can eventually occur in over 50%. The usual situation is a slowly progressive inability initially to maintain and eventually to achieve a satisfactory erection. This usually occurs (at least initially) in association with normal libido and ejaculation. However, as satisfactory intercourse becomes more difficult, the accompanying anxiety and depression may secondarily impair libido. Other causes of impotence must be ruled out, especially a primary psychogenic cause and, importantly in patients with diabetes, vascular insufficiency. As mentioned earlier, certain antihypertensive medications may be a contributing factor.

Normal functioning of the parasympathetic nervous system is necessary for an erection by dilating the penile blood vessels. The sympathetic nervous system is responsible for muscle contractions resulting in ejaculation. If the internal bladder sphincter (which is innervated by the sympathetic nervous system) does not close appropriately during orgasm, the ejaculate enters the bladder *(retrograde ejaculation)*. The sensory component of orgasm (as opposed to the ejaculatory aspect) is mediated by nervous pathways that are not part of the autonomic nervous system. Thus the pleasurable sensation of orgasm remains intact. Involvement of the parasympathetic nervous system occurs more readily than impairment of the sympathetic component. Therefore the inability to achieve a satisfactory erection to complete the act of sexual intercourse successfully is much more common than retrograde ejaculation. The latter is uncommon by itself. When it does occur, it is almost always in conjunction with erectile dysfunction.

Most genitourinary complications are managed by a urologist. However, the problem of *impotence* is almost always shared first with the PCP. Although the work-up of impotence[104] is beyond the scope of this chapter, the primary cause usually falls within the following categories: endocrine, psychogenic, autonomic neuropathy, vascular, or drug-related. In diabetic patients, two or all three of the latter three may be involved. The first step is to evaluate whether drugs[105] (usually antihypertensive agents) may be contribut-

ing. Assuming that this is not the case and that an appropriate evaluation rules out endocrine and primarily psychogenic causes, one needs to discuss treatment options. Although sophisticated evaluation by urologists for impotence is sometimes able to pinpoint a vascular cause for which surgical intervention may be helpful, a National Institutes of Health consensus conference on impotence recommended that this approach be limited to very select patients (e.g., those with congenital or traumatic vascular abnormalities) and restricted to clinical investigation settings in medical centers with experienced personnel.[106] Therefore the treatment for erectile dysfunction is necessarily nonspecific. Because the sensation of orgasm is retained, it is important for the physician to remind the patient that it is possible for both the patient and his sexual partner to achieve sexual gratification in ways not requiring vaginal penetration by the erect penis.

The use of phosphodiesterase (PDE) 5 inhibitors such as sildenafil (Viagra) have moved to the forefront of therapy in patients with erectile dysfunction. It is taken at a dose of 25 to 100 mg (most patients with diabetes require the 100 mg dose) 1 hour before intercourse. The major concern is its interaction with nitrates (it can cause severe hypotension); it should not be used in patients who take nitrates. Sildenafil is effective in approximately 50% of patients with diabetes. When used, it should not be given more than once in a 24-hour period. Patients need to be aware that in addition to the medication, sexual stimulation is still necessary for arousal. Patients may also need to try it on several different occasions until they start to notice a response. It is most fully absorbed on an empty stomach. Alternatively, newer agents such as tadalafil (Cialis) and vardenafil (Levetra), which have different parmacokinetic profiles, may be tried.[107]

Intracavernosal injection of vasodilators can be effective, but is a technique many men would prefer to avoid. Injection of vasodilatory substances, papaverine, phentolamine, and alprostadil[108] (a synthetic prostaglandin E$_1$) alone or in various combinations is successful in 65%[109] to 85%[108] of patients with various causes of erectile dysfunction. However, in a small study of diabetic men, age was an important predictor of success, which was less than in the general population of impotent men.[110] Only 1 of 14 patients older than 60 years had a satisfactory response to phentolamine-papaverine intracavernosal injections, whereas 11 of 19 younger than 60 years had a favorable response. Solutions containing prostaglandin E$_1$ are replacing those with papaverine because of a lower incidence of priapism and penile scarring. Priapism and penile fibrosis occur in less than 5% of patients, but dose-related pain occurs at the injection site 10% of the time after injection of the prostaglandin E$_1$ analogue. The first injection of these agents should take place under a physician's supervision in a private examination room while instructing the patient on how to administer the injections at home. This initial demonstration often helps to alleviate some of the patient's anxiety about self-administering intracavernosal injections and helps to determine the appropriate dose to achieve an erection. Intraurethral instillation of alprostadil (medicated urethral system for erection [MUSE]) has been used successfully in some individuals.

Implantation of a penile prosthesis is considered second-line therapy for erectile dysfunction.[106] Use of testosterone is indicated only in patients in whom a hypogonadal state has been documented; it is ineffective otherwise. Similarly, oral yohimbine, an α$_2$-blocker, although widely used, was shown to be ineffective in the single double-blind study.[104]

Patients with autonomic dysfunction may also have *sudomotor dysfunction*. Areas of anhidrosis and hyperhidrosis are usually distributed over the body, with the former more common in the lower extremities and the latter usually occurring over the trunk and face. The probable explanation is that lack of perspiration over one area leads to a compensatory increase over other areas to accomplish overall heat regulation. Regrowth of damaged autonomic nerve fibers has also been suggested. Excessive sweating often occurs at mealtime, at night, or under stress. Although sudomotor dysfunction is usually not bothersome, an uncommon but troublesome symptom is profuse facial perspiration when the patient starts to eat *(gustatory sweating)*.

The final manifestation of autonomic dysfunction may be *hypoglycemic unawareness*, which can lead to hypoclycemia-associated autonomic failure (Figure 7-14).[111] Hypoglycemic unawareness secondary to autonomic neuropathy is mainly restricted to type 1 diabetic patients for the following reason. The normal hormonal counterregulatory responses to hypoglycemia are secretion of glucagon from the α-cells in the pancreatic islets of Langerhans, epinephrine from the adrenal medulla, cortisol from the adrenal cortex, and growth hormone from the pituitary gland. The first two are secreted rapidly and have immediate but short-lived effects to restore glucose levels toward normal. Not only is there an approximately 30-minute delay before the latter two are secreted, but their effects are also delayed and prolonged. As long as the glucagon response is intact, glucose concentrations will be restored. If glucagon is not secreted, epinephrine will raise glucose levels. If both of these normal responses are absent, hypoglycemic levels will be maintained (or continue to drop) because the effects of growth hormone and cortisol are too delayed to reverse the situation.

For unknown reasons, the glucagon response to hypoglycemia starts to wane shortly after the onset of type 1 (but not type 2) diabetes and is mostly gone 5 years later. Epinephrine secretion remains as the patient's only effective rapid counterregulatory response to combat hypoglycemia. Secretion of epinephrine also causes the autonomic signs and symptoms of

Hypoglycemia-Associated Autonomic Failure

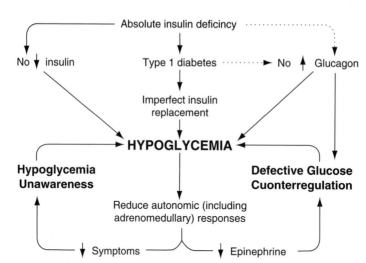

FIGURE 7-14. Schematic diagram of proposed mechanics for hypoglycemia-associated autonomic failure in patients with diabetes. *(From Cryer PE, Davis SN, Shamoon H: Hypoglycemia in diabetes. Diabetes Care 26:1902–1912, 2003.)*

hypoglycemia (weakness, sweating, tachycardia, palpitations, hunger, tremor, nervousness, tingling of mouth and fingers). Because epinephrine secretion by the adrenal medulla is mediated by autonomic innervations, autonomic neuropathy blunts and eventually abolishes this counterregulatory response. Not only does this leave patients without any warning of hypoglycemia so that they may eat to counteract it, but epinephrine is not present to reverse the hypoglycemia. Therefore the neuroglucopenic signs and symptoms (visual disturbances, bizarre behavior, mental dullness, confusion, amnesia, seizures, coma) often occur without warning in these patients. Even though autonomic neuropathy would also impair the catecholamine response to hypoglycemia in patients with type 2 diabetes, preservation of the glucagon response usually prevents severe hypoglycemia requiring the assistance of another person by increasing hepatic glucose production before glucose concentrations fall to extremely low levels. Severe hypoglycemia does occasionally occur in sulfonylurea agent-induced hypoglycemia

because the effect of the drug persists and overwhelms the ability of the liver to produce enough glucose.

DIABETIC AMYOTROPHY

The descriptive term *amyotrophy* is sometimes used to describe a syndrome of asymmetric pain and weakness usually involving the pelvic girdle and thigh muscles. It is commonly encountered in older individuals and could be the result of lesions classified as a mononeuropathy, mononeuropathy multiplex, or plexopathy. The acute-onset neuropathies are likely caused by acute thrombosis or ischemia of the vessels nourishing the particular nervous system structures involved rather than by chronic hyperglycemia.

FOCAL NEUROPATHIES

Certain neuropathies seem to develop rapidly. In addition to their rather acute onset, they are usually associated with pain and a self-limited course of 1 to 3 months' duration for cranial nerve palsies, but up to 1 year or more for the others, with eventual spontaneous resolution of both cranial and peripheral nerve dysfunction. They may occur in patients without peripheral or autonomic neuropathy. Indeed, the most common one, a third cranial nerve palsy (Figure 7-15) (fourth, sixth, and rarely seventh nerve palsies may also occur), may herald the onset of diabetes. Also classified under acute-onset neuropathies are lesions of several nerves (mononeuropathy multiplex) and focal lesions of the lumbosacral (or rarely brachial) plexus (plexopathy) or of the nerve roots (radiculopathy). In addition to the pain in the distribution of the affected nerve structures, motor weakness in the muscles innervated by involved nerve(s) also commonly occurs. For the *acute-onset neuropathies* and *neuropathic diabetic cachexia*, the PCP can only provide reassurance about the eventual outcome and palliative measures (as discussed earlier) for the associated pain and depression.

NEUROPATHIC DIABETIC CACHEXIA

A very unusual syndrome, occurring mostly in older men with relatively mild type 2 diabetes, consists of anorexia, painful neuropathy, depression, and profound weight loss (neuropathic diabetic cachexia). The weight loss is so dramatic that an occult malignancy is usually suspected. Spontaneous recovery occurs gradually within 12 to 18 months.

PREVENTION OF NEUROPATHY

Given this litany of the deleterious effects of diabetic neuropathy, what can PCPs do to help their patients with this complication of diabetes? The primary role is one of prevention, for once manifestations of diabetic neuropathy occur, our interventions are palliative at best. As discussed in Chapter 2 and shown in Figure 2-11, tight diabetic control not only forestalls (and possibly prevents) the development of diabetic neuropathy, but also reverses the early painful symptoms. Once the peripheral neuropathy progresses

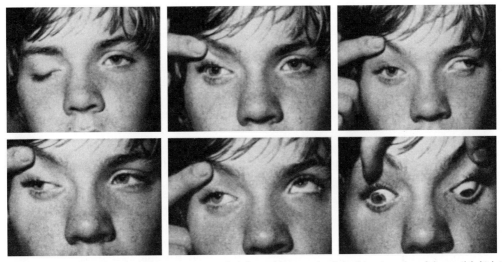

FIGURE 7-15. Right third nerve palsy in a patient with diabetes. Note ptosis of the lid and sparing of the pupil (which is a distinguishing characteristic of diabetic origin compared with more serious causes, which usually affect the pupil). The patient is unable to turn the eye inward. Although the eye can turn outward, it cannot be raised or lowered normally in the lateral position. *(From Miller NR: Walsh and Hoyt's Clinical Neuro-Ophthalmology, 3rd ed. Williams & Wilkins, Baltimore, 1969, p. 668.)*

to numbness of the feet, patients are at an increased risk of developing diabetic foot ulcers over areas receiving increased pressure (Figure 7-16). These are entirely preventable by appropriate education and by examination of the feet. Unfortunately, physicians examine the feet of their diabetic patients only approximately 15% of the time.[112,113] Even when a nurse or aide removes the patient's shoes and socks, examinations were performed only two thirds of the time.[112] Callus formation should alert the physician to increased pressure. Appropriate advice about properly fitting shoes and general foot care[114] should be given. Patients with high-risk feet (loss of sensation and/or bony deformities and/or poor circulation and/or history of prior ulcer formation) may be eligible to receive special orthotic shoes and inserts designed to help protect vulnerable feet. Therefore

referral to a podiatrist should be considered for high-risk patients.

MACROVASCULAR COMPLICATIONS

Patients with diabetes have a markedly increased risk for macrovascular disease. A patient with diabetes, with no known CVD, has the same risk as a person with diabetes who has already had a CVD event.[115] It is because of this high risk that in the National Cholesterol Education Program (NCEP) Adult Treatment Panel (ATP) III guidelines diabetes is considered a CVD equivalent—that is, the same risk and need for treatment as someone who traditionally would have been considered in a "secondary prevention" category.[116] Hypertension is also common and eventually occurs in approximately 50% of diabetic patients. Although appropriate treatment of hypertension eliminates it as a risk factor, it is estimated that at least 25% of all hypertensive patients do not take their medications. Like diabetes, hypertension is a silent killer without symptoms, which must be treated aggressively by the patient's team of health care providers.

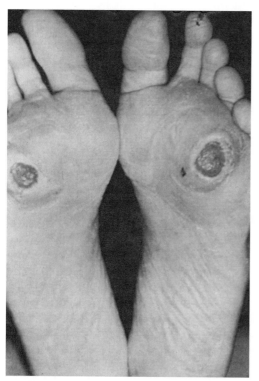

FIGURE 7-16. Diabetic foot ulcers. Note the callus formation surrounding the ulcerations.

LIPIDS

The classic diabetic dyslipidemia is characterized by a high TG level and low HDL cholesterol level (which is usually associated with an increase in small, dense LDL particles, which are more atherogenic than larger LDL particles).[117] In addition, patients may have slightly elevated LDL cholesterol levels (and in patients with diabetes, an LDL cholesterol level higher than 100 mg/dl is considered elevated). Overall, the evidence regarding elevated cholesterol levels as a risk factor is very strong. This evidence has been summarized in the First NCEP) ATP I(1988), and updated in 1993 (ATP II). Both reports concurred with the conclusions of observational studies that an elevated level of LDL cholesterol increases risk of coronary heart disease (CHD), and that lowering LDL cholesterol reduces this risk. Since then, findings from large-scale clinical trials[118-122] have significantly demonstrated the benefit of LDL-lowering therapy in the prevention and treatment of CHD, and are incorporated into the newest report, the ATP III. Similar data went into the development of the guidelines for lipid management by the ADA.[123]

All patients with diabetes should have a yearly fasting lipid panel measured, consisting of a total and HDL cholesterol level and TG level. Although a method of measuring LDL cholesterol concentrations directly has become available in most laboratories, the LDL cholesterol level is often calculated from the results of a lipoprotein analysis in which total and HDL cholesterol as well as TG concentrations are measured. LDL cholesterol concentrations are estimated from the following relationship:

$$LDL\ cholesterol = total\ cholesterol - HDL\ cholesterol - TG\ level/5$$

TG levels should be measured after an overnight fast (12 hours or more is preferable). If TG concentrations are ≥400 mg/dl, the relationship depicted earlier becomes less and less accurate, and the formula should not be used.

Non-HDL cholesterol is defined as the sum of LDL cholesterol and very-low-density lipoprotein cholesterol, and is calculated as total cholesterol minus HDL cholesterol (*non-HDL cholesterol = total cholesterol − HDL cholesterol*). Treating non-HDL cholesterol is recommended when elevated TG levels (≥200 mg/dl) cannot be lowered to <150 mg/dl. High TG levels are indicative of increased levels of TG-rich remnant lipoproteins, which appear to have an atherogenic potential similar to LDL cholesterol. The therapeutic goal for non-HDL cholesterol is approximately 30 mg/dl greater than that for LDL cholesterol in each risk category (so that in patients with diabetes, non-HDL cholesterol levels should be less than 130 mg/dl). See Tables 7-3, 7-4, and 7-5 for the definitions of normal and elevated lipid levels.

Diabetes imposes an increased risk for CVD mortality over and beyond what would be expected in the presence of one to three of the more important classic risk factors. Although it is not known for certain what causes this enhanced tendency for macrovascular disease in diabetic patients, a clue may be found in the association of coronary artery disease with a number of other factors. Because insulin resistance seems to be the underlying feature, this clustering of risk factors (in addition to the classic ones mentioned earlier) has been termed the

TABLE 7-3 ATP III CLASSIFICATION OF LDL CHOLESTEROL

LDL Cholesterol Level (mg/dl)	Category
<100	Optimal
100–129	Near or above optimal
130–159	Borderline high
160–189	High
≥190	Very high

ATP, Adult Treatment Panel; LDL, low-density lipoprotein.

Adapted from Expert Panel on Detection, Evaluation, and Treatment of High Blood Cholesterol in Adults: Executive summary of the third report of the National Cholesterol Education Program (NCEP) Expert Panel on Detection, Evaluation, and Treatment of High Blood Cholesterol in Adults (Adult Treatment Panel III). JAMA 285:2486, 2001.

TABLE 7-4 ATP III CLASSIFICATION OF TRIGLYCERIDES	
Triglyceride Level (mg/dl)	**Category**
<150	Normal
150–199	Borderline high
200–499	High
≥500	Very high

ATP, Adult Treatment Panel.

Adapted from Expert Panel on Detection, Evaluation, and Treatment of High Blood Cholesterol in Adults: Executive summary of the third report of the National Cholesterol Education Program (NCEP) Expert Panel on Detection, Evaluation, and Treatment of High Blood Cholesterol in Adults (Adult Treatment Panel III). JAMA 285:2486, 2001.

TABLE 7-5 ADA CLASSIFICATION OF HDL CHOLESTEROL LEVELS	
HDL Cholesterol Level (mg/dl)	**Risk**
>45	Normal
35–45	Borderline high
<35	High

ATP, Adult Treatment Panel; HDL, high-density lipoprotein.

From American Diabetes Association: Management of dislipidemia in adults with diabetes. Diabetes Care 26:580–583, 2003.

insulin resistance syndrome and is described in Chapter 8.

Because of the increase in coronary artery disease imposed by diabetes (approximately three quarters of deaths in patients with type 2 diabetes are due to macrovascular disease), it behooves all of us (physicians, other health care providers, and, most importantly, patients) to reduce the reversible risk factors as much as possible. In regard to lipids, aggressive treatment is needed. Multiple studies provide evidence for benefits of lipid lowering in patients with diabetes. The Heart Protection Study[124] deserves special mention. In this study patients with diabetes had a reduction in the risk of cardiovascular risk *regardless* of the their initial LDL cholesterol level when treated with statin therapy. Therefore, much as with the benefit of ACEIs in the Heart Outcomes Prevention Evaluation (HOPE) trial (see following text) it appears that most patients with diabetes, particularly type 2 diabetes, benefit from statin therapy. Figure 7-17 provides the suggested pathway for the treatment of dyslipidemia in the high risk individual.

THERAPEUTIC LIFESTYLE CHANGES

Lifestyle changes are first-line therapy in the management of high cholesterol. The NCEP-recommended Therapeutic Lifestyle Changes (TLC) program is a multifaceted lifestyle approach to reduce CHD risk. Its essential features are the following:

- Reduced intake of saturated fats (<7% of total calories) and cholesterol (<200 mg/day)
- Therapeutic options for enhancing LDL lowering, such as plant stanols/sterols (2 g/day) and increased soluble fiber (10 to 25 g/day)
- Weight reduction
- Increased physical activity.

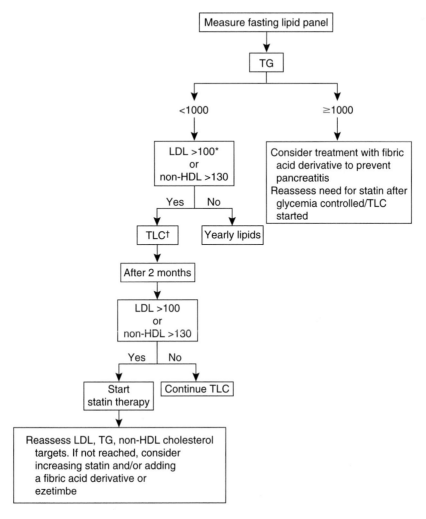

FIGURE 7-17. A general approach for the treatment of lipid disorders in the patient with diabetes. HDL, high-density lipoprotein; LDL, low-density lipoprotein; TG, triglyceride; TLC; Therapeutic Lifestyle Changes.

The TLC diet is the focus of the program. Total fat intake is encouraged to range from 25% to 35% of total intake (as long as saturated and trans fats are kept low), because a higher intake of unsaturated fat may help lower TGs and raise HDL cholesterol in patients with the metabolic syndrome.[116] At all stages of dietary therapy, clinicians are encouraged to refer patients to registered dietitians or nutritionists for nutritional intervention and guidance.

ATP III recommends that a 3-month trial of TLC should precede the use of drug therapy. However, for patients with CHD or

CHD risk equivalents (in particular, diabetes) and an LDL cholesterol level of 130 mg/dl or higher, an LDL-lowering drug may be started simultaneously with TLC to achieve the LDL goal of less than 100 mg/dl. The NCEP-recommended cutpoints for initiating TLC and drug therapy and their respective LDL cholesterol goals are shown in Table 7-6.

PHARMACOLOGIC TREATMENT

Description of Drugs

Five classes of drugs are used in the treatment of hyperlipidemia (Table 7-7 and Table 7-8). These are (1) HMG-CoA reductase inhibitors, (2) bile acid resins, (3) nicotinic acid, and (4) fibric acid derivatives, and (5) inhibitors of cholesterol absorption. Not all are recommended for patients with diabetes. Estrogen was once considered a drug to be used in postmenopausal patients. It reduces LDL cholesterol levels by approximately 15% in nondiabetic women and can increase HDL cholesterol levels as much as 15% as well. However, the cardiovascular benefits of hormone replacement therapy (HRT) is in question (see the following text), and these agents should no longer be used solely to lower cardiovascular risk.

The *HMG-CoA reductase inhibitors (statins)* inhibit the rate-limiting enzyme of cholesterol synthesis. This decrease of cellular cholesterol, especially in the liver, up-regulates LDL receptors and thus increases the clearance of LDL cholesterol. As a single-drug therapy, the statins are the most effective LDL cholesterol–lowering agents and are the recommended first-line therapy for the treatment of the diabetic dyslipidemia in the majority of cases. TG levels may decrease slightly and HDL concentrations increase somewhat, but these effects are not consistent. Because hepatic cholesterol synthesis is more active overnight, these drugs are more effective if taken at bedtime. Side effects are uncommon and include abnormal results of liver function tests, headaches, sleep disturbances, and rarely creatine phosphokinase

elevations and myositis (especially with gemfibrozil, nicotinic acid, cyclosporine, erythromycin, or renal failure). There is no effect on glycemia.

The *fibric acid derivatives* available in this country are gemfibrozil and fenofibrate. These drugs lower TG concentrations by increasing their clearance, although the mechanism is not clear. HDL cholesterol levels rise slightly. In general, LDL cholesterol concentrations increase in hypertriglyceridemic patients, but decrease in normotriglyceridemic patients. The increase in LDL cholesterol levels, however, is associated with a potentially favorable change in the composition of the LDL particle, which increases in size and decreases in density (i.e., a shift from pattern B to pattern A—see the earlier discussion of dyslipidemia in insulin resistance syndrome for significance). Side effects include rash, nausea, abdominal pain, and cholelithiasis. Myositis occurs rarely in patients in renal failure or also taking a statin.

Bile acid resins are not absorbed. They act in the gastrointestinal tract by binding bile acids. This interferes with the enterohepatic circulation of cholesterol and forces the liver to utilize stored cholesterol. The result is an up-regulation of LDL receptors that increases LDL clearance. Side effects include constipation, bloating, flatulence, nausea, abdominal pain, hemorrhoids, and drug interactions. Therefore these drugs should not be used by patients with autonomic neuropathy and constipation. Because the bile acid resins interfere with the absorption of other drugs (e.g., digoxin, warfarin, diuretics, β-blockers, iron, thyroid hormone, tetracycline, vancomycin, barbiturates), it is recommended that other drugs be taken at least 1 hour before or 4 hours after these cholesterol-lowering agents. Bile acid resins raise TG concentrations and are (relatively) contraindicated in patients with TG levels exceeding 400 mg/dl.

Nicotinic acid lowers both LDL cholesterol and TG concentrations and raises HDL cholesterol levels. Its mechanism of action is not clear. The drug has significant side effects

TABLE 7-6	WHEN TO START TLCS AND DRUG THERAPY, AND LDL CHOLESTEROL GOALS		
Risk Category	**LDL Level to Initiate TLC (mg/dl)**	**LDL Level to Start Drug Therapy (mg/dl)**	**LDL Goal (mg/dl)**
CHD or CHD risk equivalents (e.g., diabetes)	≥100	≥130 (100–129: drug optional)*	<100

CHD, coronary heart disease; LDL, low-density lipoprotein; TLC, therapeutic lifestyle changes.

*Many authorities recommend use of LDL-lowering drugs in this category if an LDL cholesterol level of <100 mg/dl cannot be achieved by TLC.

Adapted from Expert Panel on Detection, Evaluation, and Treatment of High Blood Cholesterol in Adults: Executive summary of the third report of the National Cholesterol Education Program (NCEP) Expert Panel on Detection, Evaluation, and Treatment of High Blood Cholesterol in Adults (Adult Treatment Panel III). JAMA 285:2486, 2001.

including flushing, pruritus, gastritis, peptic ulcer, hepatitis, cholestatic jaundice, hyperuricemia, and, in higher doses, worsening of glycemia. For the last reason, it is recommended for use by patients with diabetes or insulin resistance only with close follow-up of glucose levels.

Ezetimibe is a selective *inhibitor of cholesterol absorption* that reduces the overall delivery of cholesterol to the liver, thereby promoting the synthesis of LDL receptors, with a subsequent reduction of serum LDL-C. Its mechanism of action is different from that of other intestinal-acting lipid-altering agents such as phytosterols/phytostanols, resins, and polymers.[125] Ten milligrams of ezetimibe given once daily produces an approximately 20% reduction in LDL-cholesterol levels. It has been shown to act synergistically with statins and can be combined with them for additional cholesterol lowering. It has few side effects and is generally well tolerated. Figure 7.18 shows the lipid benefits of ezetimibe when it is added to atorvastatin therapy.[126]

PHARMACOLOGIC TREATMENT

General Approach

If nonpharmacologic methods have failed to lower TG and/or LDL concentrations to below target levels in 2 months, drug treatment should be initiated (if not started initially). The approach to the drug treatment of the dyslipidemia in diabetes is complex and is depicted in Figure 7-18. In the patient with TG concentrations lower than 1000 mg/dl, treatment of the LDL or total non-HDL cholesterol tends to dictate treatment and usually requires use of a statin. If the TG levels are higher than 1000 mg/dl patients may need initial therapy with a fibric acid derivative to bring this level down. However, if a patient is in poor glycemic control, rapid normalization of glucose levels (with or without the use of pioglitazone, which can lower both glucose and TG levels) often brings the TG levels into a normal range. When approaching drug therapy of dyslipidemia in a patient with diabetes, it is always important to remember that statin therapy provides the greatest cardiovascular risk reduction as a result of their lipid lowering as well as nonlipid lowering effects.[127]

TG levels exceeding 1000 mg/dl are occasionally found in patients with uncontrolled diabetes. These patients are at increased risk for pancreatitis. Therefore drug therapy with a fibric acid derivative should be started immediately without waiting for a lower-fat diet and treatment of the hyperglycemia to have an effect on the TG levels. Patients with elevated TG levels should be counseled to avoid consumption of alcohol.

TABLE 7-7   LIPID-LOWERING AGENTS

Drug Class	Average Lipid/Lipoprotein Effects	Side Effects	Contraindications	Clinical Trial Results
HMG-CoA reductase inhibitors (statins)[a]	LDL-C ↓18%–60% HDL-C ↑5%–15% TG ↓7%–37%	Myopathy Increased liver enzymes	Relative: Active or chronic liver disease Concomitant use with certain drugs[b]	Reduced major coronary events, CHD deaths, need for coronary procedures, stroke, and total mortality
Bile acid sequestrants[c]	LDL-C ↓15%–30% HDL-C ↑3%–5% TG No change, or an increase	GI distress Constipation Decreased absorption of other drugs	Absolute: Dysbetalipoproteinemia TG > 400 mg/dl Relative: TG > 200 mg/dl	Reduced major coronary events and CHD deaths CHD deaths
Nicotinic acid[d]	LDL-C ↓5%–25% HDL-C ↓20%–50% TG ↑15%–35%	Flushing Hyperglycemia Hyperuricemia (or gout) Upper GI distress Hepatotoxicity	Absolute: Chronic liver disease Severe gout Relative: Diabetes Hyperuricemia Peptic ulcer disease	Reduced major coronary events, and possibly total mortality
Fibric acid derivatives[e]	LDL-C ↓5%–20% (May be increased in patients with high TG) HDL-C ↑10%–20% TG ↓20%–50%	Dyspepsia Gallstones Myopathy Unexplained non-CHD deaths in WHO study with clofibrate	Absolute: Severe renal disease Severe hepatic disease	Reduced major coronary events
Inhibitors of cholesterol absorption[f]	LDL-C ↓18%–20% HDL-C ↑3% TG ↓5%	No major side effect	Contradictions: Active or chronic liver disease	Pending

CHD, coronary heart disease; GI, gastrointestinal; HDL, high-density lipoprotein; HMG-CoA, hydroxymethylglutaryl coenzyme A; LDL, low-density lipoprotein; TG, triglyceride; WHO, World Health Organization.

[a]Atorvastatin (10–80 mg), fluvastatin (20–80 mg), lovastatin (20–80 mg), pravastatin (20–40 mg), simvastatin (20–80 mg), rosuvastatin (pending).

[b]Cyclosporine, macrolide antibiotics, antifungal agents, and cytochrome P-450 inhibitors (fibrates and niacin should be used with appropriate caution).

[c]Cholestyramine (4–16 g), colestipol (5–20 g), colesevelam (2.6–3.8 g).

[d]Immediate-release (crystalline) nicotinic acid (1.5–3 g), extended-release nicotinic acid (1–2 g), and sustained-release nicotinic acid (1–2 g).

[e]Gemfibrozil (600 mg bid), fenofibrate (200 mg), clofibrate (1000 mg bid).

[f]Ezetimibe (10 mg)

Adapted from Expert Panel on Detection, Evaluation, and Treatment of High Blood Cholesterol in Adults: Executive summary of the third report of the National Cholesterol Education Program (NCEP) Expert Panel on Detection, Evaluation, and Treatment of High Blood Cholesterol in Adults (Adult Treatment Panel III). JAMA 285:2486, 2001, and prescribing information for statins.

TABLE 7-8 RECOMMENDED LIPID-LOWERING DRUGS FOR DIABETIC PATIENTS

Generic Name	Brand Name	Tablet Size (mg)	Initial Dose (mg)	Maximum Dose (mg)
		Statins[a]		
Lovastatin	Mevacor	10, 20, 40	10	80[b]
Pravastatin	Pravachol	10, 20, 40	10	40
Simvastatin	Zocor	5, 10, 20, 40	5	40
Fluvastatin[c]	Lescol	20, 40	20	40
Atorvastatin[d]	Lipitor	10, 20, 40	10	80
Rosuvastatin[d]	Crestor	10, 20, 40	10	80
		Fibric Acid Derivative		
Gemfibrozil	Lopid	300, 600	1200[c]	1200
Fenofibrate	Tricor	54, 160	54–160	160
		Bile Acid Resin		
Cholestyramine	Questran	4 g per packet	8 g	24 g
Colestipol	Colestid	5 g per packet	10 g	30 g
		Inhibitor of Cholesterol Absorbtion		
Ezetimide	Zetia	10	10	10

[a]Hydroxymethylglutaryl coenzyme A reductase inhibitors.

[b]Up to 40 mg is given at bedtime, and the rest taken in the morning; the other statins are usually taken only at bedtime.

[c]Fluvastatin is slightly less effective than the other statins; it is the only one to bind to the bile acid resins and therefore should be taken 4 hours after the evening dose of the resin when that combination is used.

[d]More effective than other statins; also lowers triglyceride levels.

[e]The usual dose is 600 mg bid except when combined with a statin. When a combination of statin and gemfibrozil is used, statin should be started at the lowest dose and gemfibrozil given at 300 mg bid to minimize the risk of rhabdomyolysis. The dosage for both drugs should be increased cautiously if low-density lipoprotein cholesterol or triglyceride levels remain elevated.

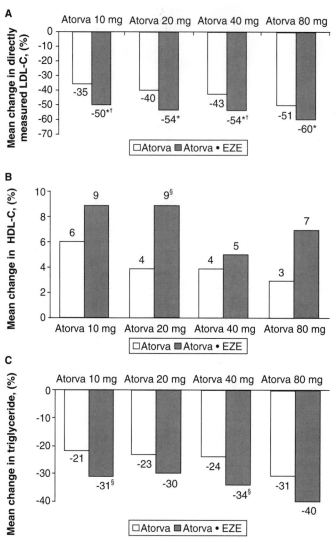

FIGURE 7-18. Change in direct LDL-C *(A)*, HDL-C *(B)*, and triglyceride *(C)* concentrations. Atorva, atorvastatin; EZE, ezetimibe. *P* < 0.01 for combination therapy vs *corresponding dose of atorvastatin alone, †atorvastatin (20 mg or 40 mg) alone, and ‡atorvastatin (40 mg) alone. §, *P* < 0.05 for combination therapy vs corresponding dose of atorvastatin alone. *(From Ballantyne CM, Houri J, Notarbartolo A, et al, Ezetimibe Study Group: Effect of ezetimibe coadministered with atorvastatin in 628 patients with primary hypercholesterolemia: A prospective, randomized, double-blind trial. Circulation 107(19):2409–2415, 2003, Figure 2.)*

In addition to abdominal pain (with or without documented pancreatitis), patients may also have eruptive xanthomata, lipemia retinalis, mental confusion, myalgias, and arthralgias (often in the hands). This is termed the *chylomicronemia syndrome* and is potentially very serious. In this situation,

fat intake may need to be decreased to <20% of total calories until the TG levels fall to three-digit numbers. Treatment of the uncontrolled diabetes (usually with insulin) is also important. TG levels of this magnitude are invariably superimposed on either a familial or another cause of hypertriglyceridemia.

Hormone Replacement Therapy

A consideration of hormonal status must be considered in women. This literature has become increasingly complicated, because not all studies show the same benefits of hormone replacement. Observational studies have long suggested a benefit of estrogen and/or HRT in women. The potential benefits of estrogen on the cardiovascular system are myriad. These include changes in lipid metabolism, carbohydrate metabolism, coagulation factors, and endothelial function.[128,129] In the Postmenopausal Estrogen/Progestin Intervention Trial, the effects of unopposed estrogen compared with a variety of combinations of estrogen and progesterone were studied in healthy postmenopausal women.[130] This trial showed that unopposed estrogen was the optimal regimen for elevation of HDL cholesterol. However, there was a 10% per year rate of adenomatous or atypical endometrial hyperplasia in women with an intact uterus on unopposed estrogen.

Observational studies have suggested a 35% to 50% reduction in coronary events among current hormone users. In the Nurses' Health Study the improvement in risk was particularly evident in women at high risk for CHD.[131] A decrease in carotid intimal medial thickening—a marker for atherosclerotic risk—was seen in women with diabetes who were past or current users of HRT.[132] However, observational studies may be biased by the factor that more compliant patients tend to take HRT and this positive health-related behavior is likely to be associated with other healthy lifestyle modifications. There may also be a selection bias, because healthier women tend to be more likely to be prescribed estrogen replacement.

The Heart and Estrogen/Progestin Replacement Study[133] was designed to prospectively evaluate the effects of HRT in postmenopausal women who had known coronary artery disease. It was a multicenter, placebo-controlled study involving 2763 women. The HRT regimen used was continuous conjugated equine estrogen at a dose of 0.625 mg/day and medroxyprogesterone acetate at a dose of 2.5 mg/day. These patients were followed for 4 years and, unexpectedly, those on HRT had the same rates of CVD events as did the women on placebo. This may have occurred as a result of the prothrombotic effects of estrogen, and the group on HRT had higher rates of thrombolic embolic disease. Subsequent 6-year follow-up data from this trial did not show any positive benefit from HRT.[134] Because patients with diabetes are considered to have a high risk for CVD, these data may be applicable to this population, as well.

Finally, the Women's Health Initiative,[135] a large, prospective randomized trial, showed that estrogen and progesterone therapy increased the risk of breast cancer, stroke, and cardiovascular events in postmenopausal women with an intact uterus. The risks increased over time on the treatment. The risks for fracture and colon cancer decreased (Table 7-9). This study provides the most thorough data to date on the risks and benefits of HRT, at least when used as an estrogen/progesterone combination.

From a practical perspective, it is important to individualize postmenopausal hormonal therapy. Women should *not* start it with the desire to lower their cardiovascular risk. In fact, women with diabetes should be sure to have their medication regimen maximized prior to starting HRT. This may involve use of aspirin, statin therapy, and ACEI therapy, among others, depending on the patient's circumstances. Women who wish to start on HRT may chose to do so to ameliorate the acute symptoms of menopause and perhaps to prevent bone loss and osteoporosis (although other therapies such as raloxifene or bisphosphonates can treat osteoporosis). Women should probably not take HRT for more than a few years, although much more data is needed to evaluate different forms and doses of estrogen. Additionally, women without a

TABLE 7-9	RESULTS OF THE WOMEN'S HEALTH INITIATIVE— TREATMENT OF 16,000 POSTMENOPAUSAL WOMEN WITH ESTROGEN/PROGESTIN VERSUS PLACEBO

Estrogen/progestin therapy resulted in:
- 26% increase in breast cancer
- 41% increase in strokes
- 29% increase in heart attacks
- Doubled rates of blood clots in legs and lungs
- 37% less colorectal cancer
- 34% fewer hip fractures and 24% fewer total fractures

uterus on estrogen alone may not have an increase in risk for adverse outcomes on hormonal therapy.

HYPERTENSION

Diabetes and hypertension are linked in many ways. Hypertension, glucose intolerance, obesity and dyslipidemia occur together in the metabolic syndrome. Underlying diabetic nephropathy can result in hypertension, and conversely, both systolic and diastolic hypertension markedly accelerate the progression of diabetic nephropathy. An aggressive attempt to reduce hypertension can decrease the rate of GFR decline. This is based on the theory that hemodynamic factors seen in hypertension cause changes in the microcirculation resulting in hyperfiltration of the glomeruli, increasing glomerular pressure, and an increased sensitivity to angiotensin II. Ideally, an appropriate antihypertensive agent should not increase insulin resistance, promote hypoglycemia, mask the symptoms of hypoglycemia, potentiate impotence, enhance orthostatic hypotension, aggravate macrovascular disease, or increase dyslipidemia, and it should offer specific preservation of renal function.

The ADA recommendations on the treatment of hypertension in adults with diabetes state that the primary goal of therapy in adults is to maintain a systolic pressure lower than 130 mm Hg and a diastolic pressure less than 80 mm Hg.[136] Joint National

Committee (JNC) VI[137] suggests that to detect evidence of autonomic dysfunction and orthostatic hypotension, BP should be measured in the supine, sitting, and standing positions in all patients with diabetes mellitus. It also notes that automated ambulatory BP monitoring may be especially helpful. In patients with isolated systolic hypertension, the systolic pressure is lowered in stages as tolerated. The importance of focused lowering of systolic blood pressure is discussed in JNC VII.[138] The physician should discuss lifestyle changed with the patient; specifically, weight loss, dietary salt reduction, and exercise should be emphasized.

The first line of therapy for treatment of hypertension in patients with diabetes are ACEIs (see Figure 8-5).[136] When given as monotherapy, the ACEIs are equally as effective as diuretics, β-blockers, and calcium antagonists in lowering BP. They enhance insulin sensitivity (i.e., decrease insulin resistance) and have no adverse effects on lipids. Although lowering insulin or sulfonylurea agent doses in an occasional patient is necessary to avoid hypoglycemia, for the most part this is unnecessary. Indeed, in large studies of use of ACEIs in patients with diabetes, few have shown improvements in long-term glycemic control, although in the HOPE trial patients on ACEIs developed diabetes at a lower rate than individuals without diabetes.[139] ACEIs reduce urinary protein excretion[140] in patients with both type 1 and type 2 diabetes and retard the deterioration of renal function.[141-144]

Angiotensin receptor blockers (ARBs) are also renoprotective in patients with type 2 diabetes.[145-148]

ACEIs may confer additional organ protection. The HOPE study provides evidence for ACEIs as conferring protection against vascular disease[149] and the Fosinopril Versus Amlodipine Cardiovascular Events Trial (FACET) study showed that fosinopril was associated with fewer vascular events than amlodipine.[150] In addition the Italian Study Group for the Prevention of Myocardial Infarction-3 (GISSI-3) study showed lisinopril treatment was associated with a reduction in mortality 1 month after a heart attack.[151] Clearly the benefits of ACEIs extend beyond their renal protection. This brings to mind a simple question. Should all patients with diabetes who have microalbuminuria (regardless of hypertension) be on ACEI therapy? A meta-analysis attempted to answer this question.[152] They reviewed raw data on 698 patients from 12 identified trials and analyzed effect of treatment at 2 years. They concluded that in normotensive patients with type 1 diabetes and microalbuminuria, ACEIs significantly reduced progression to macroalbuminuria and increased chances of regression. The benefits were lower at lower levels of microalbuminuria but were not related to other risk factors. This points to a further benefit of ACEIs beyond their BP lowering effects. To take one more step, a cost analysis was performed to see if treating all patients with type 2 diabetes with an ACEI was reasonable.[153] This study found that using ACEIs in all patients with type 2 diabetes would slow the progression of ESRD at a relatively low cost, and was cheaper than screening all patients for gross proteinuria or microalbuminuria. At present, we believe that patients with diabetes who have microalbuminuria, regardless of BP, should be treated with ACEIs (or ARBs, if ACEIs are not tolerated) and those with hypertension with or without microalbuminuria should also be treated with one of these agents.

If BP control is not achieved with a single agent, the stepwise addition of additional pharmacologic therapies is indicated. In Chapter 8, Figure 8-5 provides an approach to the treatment of hypertension in the patient with diabetes. If an ACEI is not tolerated, an ARB should be substituted. From there, sequential addition of antihypertensive agents should occur. Usually a diuretic is added next, then a calcium channel blocker (CCB) and/or a β-blocker (the latter is contraindicated in patients with hypoglycemia unawareness.) Agents are added sequentially and increased to the maximal tolerated dose until the BP is consistently below 130/80.

SPECIFIC ANTIHYPERTENSIVE THERAPIES

ACEIs are usually well tolerated. Hyperkalemia may occur, particularly in patients with diabetes who have an underlying type IV renal tubular acidosis. Because of this, monitoring serum potassium levels is recommended. Most nephrologists, however, are so convinced of the benefits of ACEIs in the treatment of hypertension and nephropathy in patients with diabetes that hyperkalemia is not considered limiting—if necessary, it is treated rather than stopping the ACEI. These drugs also may cause a cough, the incidence of which varies depending on the study. It is helpful to warn patients that a cough may develop, and patients should be asked whether or not they develop this symptom while on the drug. Rarely angioedema can occur, and patients who develop this side effect should not be treated with ACEIs.

Acute renal failure may occur in patients who have renal artery stenosis and are given these drugs. It is reversible if they are discontinued in time. Acute renal failure may also occur in a rare patient without renal stenosis. For these reasons, serum creatinine and potassium concentrations should be measured several weeks after starting an

ACEI. They are contraindicated in pregnancy because they may cause anomalies of the genitourinary tract in the fetus.

ARBs can be used if ACEIs are not tolerated or as a first-line agent in a patient with type 2 diabetes and microalbuminuria or clinical nephropathy. They have a similar antihypertensive and renoprotective effect. It has not yet been proven whether they provide the same cardiovascular protection as do the ACEIs. ARBs do not tend to cause a cough, although occasionally a cough can occur. They do cause hyperkalemia and therefore potassium levels should be monitored.

Some[154] have advocated the combination of ACEIs and ARBs. These are small studies, however, and maximal doses of drugs are not used. It may be just as effective to increase the ACEI to the maximum dose rather than to add in an ARB. Larger studies are underway to assess the benefit of this combination. The effects on potassium may also be additive, so monitoring for the development of hyperkalemia must occur.

A frequent second drug in the treatment of hypertension is the addition of a diuretic. Many of the ACEIs and ARBs are marketed as combination drugs with hydrochlorothiazide, lessening the burden of pills a patient has to take (it often takes three or more different agents to adequately treat hypertension in the patient with diabetes).[155] Diuretics have been shown to significantly reduce myocardial infarctions, strokes, and other cardiovascular events. Furthermore, they are inexpensive, are very effective, have few symptomatic side effects (especially when used in low doses), and have an additive effect when used with other antihypertensive agents.[156] They are a good choice for patients with diabetes because the hypertension associated with diabetes is linked to increased total body sodium, and therefore, not surprisingly, diuretics are as effective in diabetic patients as any other drug. Although somewhat less response is observed in young Caucasian males, diuretics work well in older individuals, African

Americans, and obese patients, as well as those with diabetes. In patients with renal impairment (GFR < 50 ml/min), however, thiazide diuretics are ineffective and loop diuretics must be used to control volume and BP.

A number of side effects have been associated with the use of diuretics. These include glucose intolerance in nondiabetic individuals, worsening glycemia in diabetic patients, transient increases in cholesterol and TG concentrations, sexual dysfunction, cardiac dysrhythmias, and even increased mortality in diabetic patients. It is now generally accepted, however, that these side effects are associated with high doses of thiazide diuretics and are minimal at doses equivalent to 25 mg hydrochlorothiazide.

β-Blockers

These agents competitively inhibit β-adrenergic receptors. Some agents are nonselective and inhibit both the β-1 and the β-2 receptors, whereas newer selective agents inhibit β-1 receptors. There is ample data that documents the benefit of β-blockers in patients with diabetes.[157-159] In the UKPDS, in which patients had new-onset type 2 diabetes, atenolol and captopril produced similar microvascular and macrovascular outcomes, although atenolol was less well tolerated than was captopril.[160] There is also a known benefit of β-blockers in patients who have had a myocardial infarction, with a 25% reduction in mortality when these agents are used.[161] Because patients with diabetes have higher mortality and morbidity rates after myocardial infarction then those without diabetes, the absolute benefit in patients with diabetes may actually be higher.

Older textbooks echoed a view that β-blockers should be used with caution (if at all) in patients with diabetes because the perception and recovery from hypoglycemia may be impaired as a result of the drug's effects on sympathetic function. In addition, in some studies β-blockers have been shown to have adverse effects on glucose and lipid levels, and may decrease peripheral blood flow.

Practically speaking, most patients with type 2 diabetes do not have hypoglycemic unawareness. In addition, in recent years, the advent of selective β-blockers even further minimizes this risk. The UKPDS did not show an increased incidence of hypoglycemia in the group treated with β-blockers. However, these agents should be used only with extreme caution patients on insulin who have known recurrent hypoglycemic events. However, in other groups of patients with diabetes, their usefulness supersedes potential risks. Moreover, there are additional reasons in addition to the treatment of hypertension for using β-blockers. These include angina, some cardiac dysrhythmias, migraine headache prophylaxis, tremors, and prevention of recurrent myocardial infarctions.

The efficacy of β-blockers as antihypertensive agents in diabetic patients is good, especially in young Caucasian individuals. However, glycemia can worsen in patients with type 2 diabetes taking β-blockers, especially the nonselective ones. This is, in part, because insulin secretion is mediated by the β_1-adrenoceptor. Additionally, although no studies of the effects on diabetic patients have been reported, β-blockers decrease insulin sensitivity in nondiabetic subjects. β-Blockers also increase TG concentrations and reduce HDL cholesterol levels. This is especially likely with the nonselective ones. Their effect on LDL cholesterol levels is less consistent. The agents with intrinsic sympathomimetic activity have little effect on lipid levels.

As mentioned previously, β-blockers can impair the recognition of the adrenergic symptoms of hypoglycemia and prolong the restoration of normal glucose concentrations. These adverse effects are more troublesome in patients with diabetes seeking near euglycemia; in these patients, hypo-

glycemia is more common. Again, nonselective agents are more likely to have this effect because both hepatic glycogenolysis and gluconeogenesis are mediated by the β_2-adrenoceptor. High doses of the selective ones, however, can also affect the recognition of and recovery from hypoglycemia.

Other adverse effects of β-blockers must also be considered; some may be more of a problem in patients with diabetes. These include decreased exercise tolerance (again, the nonselective agents are more likely to have this effect than the selective ones), less weight loss, bronchospasm, worsening of congestive heart failure, fatigue, lethargy, depression, altered sleep patterns, and hyperkalemia. (The latter is related to the fact that β-blockers decrease renin production by the juxtaglomerular apparatus in the kidneys and that β_2-adrenoceptors help mediate the shift of potassium from the extracellular to the intracellular space.) Therefore potassium levels should be monitored in patients receiving β-blockers, especially those also taking nonsteroidal antiinflammatory agents, those with renal impairment, and older adults.

Calcium Channel Blockers

CCBs inhibit calcium influx through voltage-dependent calcium channels, which results in a decrease in intracellular calcium and subsequent vasodilation.[162] CCBs can be divided into three subgroups that have different characteristics. Dihydropyridine CCBs (DCCBs) are mostly vasodilators and have minimal inotropic effects. They also exert little effect on the cardiac conduction system. Drugs in this group include amlodipine, felodipine, and nifedipine. The benzothiazepine subgroup have moderate vasodilatory effects, and moderate negative inotropic and chronotropic effects. The drug diltiazem falls into this group. The final subgroup is the phenylalkylamines, and this group has similar effects as the benzothiazepine group. The currently available drug in this group is verapamil. The benzothiazepine and phenylalkylamine groups are referred to collectively as the nondihydropyridine CCBs (NDCCBs).

DCCBs are good BP agents, and, although controversial, their benefit in cardiovascular protection has been shown in the Syst-Eur[163] and Hypertension Optimal Treatment (HOT)[164] trials. Controversy exists because in these trials, patients were also on either an ACEI or a β-blocker. The Appropriate Blood Pressure Control in Diabetes and FACET trials[88] show greater benefit for ACEIs than DCCBs in cardiovascular protection, and actually, nifedipine in short-acting preparations was shown to increase cardiovascular mortality.[165]

Diabetic nephropathy has been shown to worsen in the present of nifedipine use.[166] Specifically, the amount of proteinuria has been shown to increase under the influence of this agent in some studies, whereas other studies have not shown an adverse effect.[167] Amlodipine has also been found to be no different than placebo and less effective than the ARB, irbesartan.[168] Studies on the NDCCBs have been associated with an improvement in proteinuria,[169,170] but studies showing an improvement in GFR have not been performed as of yet.

CCBs are generally well tolerated, especially at low doses. The dihydropyridine derivatives may cause pedal edema, facial flushing, and tachycardia. Diltiazem and verapamil have negative inotropic and chronotropic effects on the heart. Both may precipitate or exacerbate congestive heart failure, especially in patients with decreased ejection fractions. In low doses, diltiazem is considered the best tolerated of the CCBs. The most common side effect at high doses is an atrioventricular conduction defect. Constipation is the most common side effect of verapamil at high doses. Both dihydropyridine and nondihydropyridine CCBs occasionally cause sexual dysfunction, orthostatic hypotension, and gingival hyperplasia.

Adrenergic Blockers

Centrally Acting (e.g., Alpha-Methyl-Dopa)

Centrally acting adrenergic blockers are not usually used as first-line therapy in diabetes with hypertension. They are, however, effective in lowering BP, and do so by decreasing central sympathetic outflow. As a side effect, orthostatic hypotension is seen, and thus they should be used with caution in patients who have diabetes-related autonomic dysfunction or dysregulation. Other side effects include drowsiness, impotence, and dry mouth. Rarely, a Coombs positive anemia has been noted with these agents. This class of antihypertensive agents has not been studied in detail with regard to effects on glycemic profile or microvascular and macrovascular disease in diabetes.

α-Adrenergic Blockers

α-Adrenergic blockers inhibit the alpha post-sympathetic adrenergic receptors.[171] There are no significant clinical trials at this time that look specifically at cardiovascular or renal outcomes on these agents. There is some evidence that α-blockers improve insulin sensitivity in[172] and modestly decrease[173] LDL. These agents may cause significant orthostatic hypotension, especially when used initially. There are recent reports that α-blockers may be linked to an increase in cardiovascular events when compared with diuretics, CCBs, β-blockers, and ACEIs.[173,174] However, to date, a subgroup analysis of patients with diabetes has not been performed. This class of agents has the added advantage of slightly improving insulin sensitivity, glycemic levels, the lipid profile, and urinary flow in older men, and it has the lowest prevalence of sexual dysfunction. To minimize the postural hypotension, it is recommended that the first dose of one of these drugs be given just before going to bed. Extra caution should be exercised in patients with nocturia. These agents may not be tolerated by patients with autonomic neuropathy and a tendency toward orthostatic hypotension.

REFERENCES

1. American Diabetes Association: Economic costs of diabetes in the United States in 2002. Diabetes Care 26:917–932, 2003.
2. Aiello LP, Garner TW, King GL et al: Diabetic retinopathy (Technical Review). Diabetes Care 21:143, 1998.
3. Fong D, Aiello L, Gardner TW et al: Diabetic Retinopathy. Diabetes Care 26:226–229, 2003.
4. Diabetes Control and Complications Trial Research Group: The relationship of glycemic exposure and progression of retinopathy in the Diabetes Control and Complications Trial. Diabetes 44:968, 1995.
5. Klein R, Klein BF, Moss SE, et al: The Wisconsin Epidemiologic Study of Diabetic Retinopathy. VI. Retinal photocoagulation. Ophthalmology 94:747–753, 1987
6. Gilbert RE, Cooper ME, McNally PG et al: Microalbuminuria: Prognostic and therapeutic implications in diabetes mellitus. Diabet Med 11:636, 1994.
7. Chew EY, Klein ML, Ferris FL III et al. Association of elevated serum lipid levels with retinal hard exudate in diabetic retinopathy. ETDRS report number 22. Arch Ophthalmol 114:1079, 1996.
8. United Kingdom Prospective Diabetes Study Group: Tight blood pressure control and risk of macrovascular and microvascular complications in type 2 diabetes: UKPDS 38. BMJ 317:708–713, 1998.
9. Klein BEK, Moss SE, Klein R et al: Effect of pregnancy on progression of diabetic retinopathy. Diabetes Care 13:34–40, 1990.
10. The Diabetic Retinopathy Study Group: Photocoagulation treatment of proliferative diabetic retinopathy: Clinical application of diabetic retinopathy study (DRS) findings. DRS report number 8. Ophthalmology 88:583, 1981.
11. Early Treatment Diabetic Retinopathy Study Research Group: Photocoagulation for diabetic macular edema: Early treatment diabetic retinopathy study report number 1. Arch Ophthalmol 103:1796, 1985.
12. Sussman EJ, William GT, Soper KA: Diagnosis of diabetic eye disease. JAMA 247:3231, 1982.
13. American Diabetes Association: Screening for diabetic retinopathy. Diabetes Care 20(suppl 1): S28, 1997.
14. Harris MI, Klein R, Welborn TA et al: Onset of NIDDM occurs at least 4–7 yr before clinical diagnosis. Diabetes Care 15:815, 1992.
15. Bernbaum M, Albert SG, Cohen JD et al: Cardiovascular conditioning in individuals with diabetic retinopathy. Diabetes Care 12:740, 1989.
16. Graham C, Lasko-McCarthy P. Exercise options for people with diabetic complications. Diabetes Educ 16:212, 1990.
17. Aiello LP, Cahill MT, Wong JS: Systemic considerations in the management of diabetic retinopathy. Am J Ophthomol 132:760–776, 2001.
18. Renal Data System. USRDS 1998 annual data report. Bethesda MD: National Institute of Diabetes and Digestive and Kidney Diseases, April 1998 (NIH publication no. 98-3176).
19. Ritz E, Orth SR: Nephropathy in patients with type 2 diabetes mellitus (review). N Engl J Med 341:1127, 1999.
20. American Diabetes Association: Facts and figures: Nephropathy. www.diabetes.org/main. Accessed July 10, 2003.
21. Ritz E, Stefanski A: Diabetic nephropathy in type II diabetes. Am J Kidney Dis 27:167, 1996.
22. Pettitt DJ, Saad MF, Bennett PH et al: Familial predisposition to renal disease in two generations of Pima Indians with type 2 (non-insulin-dependent) diabetes mellitus. Diabetologia 33:438, 1990.
23. Bowden DW, Sale M, Howard TD et al: Linkage of genetic markers on human chromosomes 20 and 12 to NIDDM in Caucasian sib pairs with a history of diabetic nephropathy. Diabetes 46:882–886, 1997.
24. Jeffers BW, Estacio RO, Raynolds MV et al: Angiotensin-converting enzyme gene polymorphism in non-insulin dependent diabetes mellitus and its relationship with diabetic nephropathy. Kidney Int 52:473, 1997.
25. Selby JV, FitzSimmons SC, Newman JM et al: The natural history and epidemiology of diabetic nephropathy. JAMA 263:1954, 1990.
26. Mogensen CE, Schmitz O: The diabetic kidney: From hyperfiltration and microalbuminuria to end-stage renal failure. Med Clin North Am 72:1465, 1988.
27. Rudberg S, Persson B, Dahlquist G: Increased glomerular filtration rate as a predictor of diabetic nephropathy: Results from an 8-year prospective study. Kidney Int 41:822, 1992.
28. Deckert T, Feldt-Rasmussen B, Borch-Johnsen K et al: Albuminuria reflects widespread vascular damage: The Steno hypothesis. Diabetologia 32:219, 1989.
29. DeFronzo RA: Diabetic nephropathy: Etiologic and therapeutic considerations. Diabetes Rev 3:510, 1995.
30. Vijan S, Hayward RA: Treatment of hypertension in type 2 diabetes mellitus: Blood pressure goals, choice of agents, and setting priorities in diabetes care. Ann Intern Med 138:593–602, 2003.
31. Bojestig M, Arnqvist HJ, Karlber BE et al: Glycemic control and prognosis in type 1 diabetes patients with microalbuminuria. Diabetes Care 19:313, 1996.
32. Rossing P, Rossing K, Jacobsen P et al: Unchanged incidence of diabetic nephropathy in IDDM patients. Diabetes 44:739, 1995.
33. Bojestig M, Arnqvist HJ, Hermansson G et al: Declining incidence of nephropathy in insulin-dependent diabetes mellitus. N Engl J Med 330:15, 1994.
34. Seaquist ER, Goetz FC, Rich S et al: Familial clustering of diabetic kidney disease: Evidence for genetic susceptibility to diabetic nephropathy. N Engl J Med 320:1161, 1989.
35. Krolewski AS, Canessa M, Warram JH et al: Predisposition to hypertension and susceptibility

to renal disease in insulin-dependent diabetes mellitus. N Engl J Med 318:140, 1988.

36. Sawicki PT, Didjurgeit U, Muhlhauser I et al: Smoking is associated with progression of diabetic nephropathy. Diabetes Care 17:126, 1994.

37. Klein R, Klein BEK, Moss SE: Incidence of gross proteinuria in older-onset diabetes. Diabetes 42:381, 1993.

38. Hassalacher Ch, Stech W, Wahl P et al: Blood pressure and metabolic control as risk factors for nephropathy in type I (insulin-dependent) diabetes. Diabetologia 28:6, 1985.

39. Parving HH, Hommel E: Prognosis in diabetic nephropathy. BMJ 299:230, 1989.

40. Ravid M, Savin H, Lang R et al: Proteinuria, renal impairment, metabolic control, and blood pressure in type 2 diabetes mellitus. Arch Intern Med 152:1225, 1992.

41. Perkins BA, Ficociello LH, Silva KH et al: Regression of microalbuminuria in type 1 diabetes. N Engl J Med 348:2285–2293, 2003.

42. Kouri TT, Viikari JSA, Mattila KS et al: Microalbuminuria: Invalidity of simple concentration-based screening tests for early nephropathy due to urinary volumes of diabetic patients. Diabetes Care 14:591, 1991.

43. Gatling W, Knight C, Hill RD: Screening for early diabetic nephropathy: Which sample to detect microalbuminuria? Diabet Med 2:451, 1985.

44. Nathan DM, Rosenbaum C, Protasowicki VD: Single-void urine samples can be used to estimate quantitative microalbuminuria Diabetes Care 10:414, 1987.

45. Gatling W, Knight C, Mullee MA et al: Microalbuminuria in diabetes: A population study of the prevalence and an assessment of three screening tests. Diabet Med 5:343, 1987.

46. Bennett PH, Haffner S, Kasiske BL et al: Screening and management of microalbuminuria in patients with diabetes mellitus: Recommendations to the scientific advisory board of the National Kidney Foundation from an ad hoc committee of council on diabetes mellitus of the National Kidney Foundation. Am J Kidney Dis 25:107, 1995.

47. Alzaid AA: Microalbuminuria in patients with NIDDM: An overview. Diabetes Care 19:79, 1996.

48. Nannipieri M, Rizzo L, Rapuano A et al: Increased transcapillary escape rate of albumin in microalbuminuric type II diabetic patients. Diabetes Care 18:1, 1995.

49. Sawicki PT, Didjurgeit U, Muhlhauser I et al. Smoking is associated with progression of diabetic nephropathy. Diabetes Care 17:126, 1994.

50. Toeller M, Buyken A, Heitkamp G et al: Protein intake and urinary albumin excretion rates in the EURODIAB IDDM complications Study. Diabetologia 40:1219, 1997.

51. Zeller K, Whittaker E, Sullivan L et al. Effect of restricting dietary protein on the progression of renal failure in patients with insulin dependent diabetes mellitus. N Engl J Med. 324:78, 1991.

52. The Diabetes Control and Complications Trial Research Group: The effect of intensive treatment of diabetes on the development and progression of long-term complications in insulin-dependent diabetes mellitus. N Engl J Med 329:977, 1993.

53. UK Prospective Diabetes Study (UKPDS) Group. Intensive blood glucose control with sulphonylureas or insulin compared with conventional treatment and risk of complications in patients with type 2 diabetes (UKPDS 33). Lancet 352:837, 1998.

54. Diamond JR., Karnovsky MJ: Focal and segmental glomerulosclerosis: Analogies to atherosclerosis. Kidney Int 33:917, 1988.

55. Smulders YM, Rakic M, Stenhouwer CDA et al: Determinants of progression of microalbuminuria in patients with NIDDM. Diabetes Care 20:999, 1997.

56. Tonolo G, Ciccarese M, Brizzi P et al: Reduction of albumin excretion rate in normotensive microalbuminuric type 2 diabetic patients during long-term simvastatin treatment. Diabetes Care 12:1891, 1997.

56a. DeFronzo RA: Hyperkalemia and hyporeninemic hypoaldosteronism. Kidney Int 17:118, 1980.

57. Parfrey PS, Griffiths SM, Barrett BJ et al: Contrast material-induced renal failure in patients with diabetes mellitus, renal insufficiency, or both: A prospective controlled study. N Engl J Med 320:143, 1989.

58. Brezis M, Epstein FH: A closer look at radiocontrast-induced nephropathy. N Engl J Med 320:179, 1989.

59. Manske CL, Sprafka M, Suon JT et al: Contrast nephropathy in azotemic diabetic patients undergoing coronary angiography. Am J Med 89:615, 1990.

60. Schwab SJ, Hlatky MA, Pieper KS et al: Contrast nephrotoxicity: A randomized controlled trial of a nonionic and an ionic radiographic contrast agent. N Engl J Med 320:149, 1989.

61. Moore RD, Steinberg EP, Powe NR et al: Nephrotoxicity of high-osmolality versus low-osmolality contrast media: Randomized clinical trial. Radiology 182:649, 1992.

62. Solomon R, Werner C, Mann D et al: Effects of saline, mannitol, and furosemide on acute decreases in renal function induced by radiocontrast agents. N Engl J Med 331:1416, 1994.

63. Pirart J: Diabetes mellitus and its degenerative complications: A prospective study of 4,400 patients observed between 1947 and 1973. Diabetes Care 1:168, 1978.

64. Thomas PK: Classification, differential diagnosis and staging of diabetic peripheral neuropathy. Diabetes 46(suppl 2):554–557, 1997.

65. Young MJ, Boulton AJM, Macleod AF et al: A multicentre study of the prevalence of diabetic peripheral neuropathy in the United Kingdom hospital clinic population. Diabetologia 36:150, 1993.

66. Harris M, Eastman R, Cowie C: Symptoms of sensory neuropathy in adults with NIDDM in the U.S. population. Diabetes Care 16:1446, 1993.

67. Simmons Z, Feldman EL: Update on diabetic neuropathy. Curr Opin Neurol 15:595–603, 2002.

68. Archer AG, Watkins PJ, Thomas PK et al: The natural history of acute painful neuropathy in diabetes mellitus. J Neurol Neurosurg Psychiatry 46:491, 1983.

69. The Diabetes Control and Complications Trial Research Group. The effect of intensive treatment of diabetes on the development an progression of long-term complications in insulin-dependent diabetes mellitus. N Engl J Med 329:977, 1993.

70. Boulton AJM, Drury J, Clarke B et al: Continuous subcutaneous insulin infusion in the management of painful diabetic neuropathy. Diabetes Care 5:386, 1982.

71. Cohen KL, Harris S: Efficacy and safety of nonsteroidal anti-inflammatory drugs in the therapy of diabetic neuropathy. Arch Intern Med 147:1442, 1987.

72. Davis JL, Smith RL: Painful peripheral diabetic neuropathy treated with venlafaxine HCl extended release capsules. Diabetes Care 22:1909, 1999.

73. Kvinesdal B, Molin J, Froland A et al: Imipramine treatment of painful diabetic neuropathy. JAMA 251:1727, 1984.

74. Young RH, Clarke BF: Pain relief in diabetic neuropathy: The effectiveness of imipramine and related drugs. Diabetic Med 2:363, 1985.

75. Max MB, Culnane M, Schafer SC et al: Amitriptyline relieves diabetic neuropathy pain in patients with normal or depressed mood. Neurology 37:589–596, 1987.

76. Backonja M, Beydoun A, Edwards KR et al: Gabapentin for the symptomatic treatment of painful neuropathy in patients with diabetes mellitus: A randomized controlled trial. JAMA 280:1831, 1998.

77. Ellenberg M: Treatment of diabetic neuropathy with diphenylhydantoin. N Y State J Med 68:2653, 1968.

78. Saudek CD, Werns S, Reidenberg MM: Phenytoin in the treatment of diabetic symmetrical polyneuropathy. Clin Parmacol Ther 22:196, 1977.

79. Rull RA, Quibrera R, Gonzalez-Millan H et al: Symptomatic treatment of peripheral diabetic neuropathy with carbamazepine (Tegretol): Double blind crossover trial. Diabetologia 5:215, 1969.

80. Wilton TD: Tegretol in the treatment of diabetic neuropathy. S Afr Med J 48:869, 1974.

81. Judzewitsch R, Jaspan J, Polonsky J: Aldose reductase inhibition improves nerve conduction velocity in diabetic patients. N Engl J Med 308:119, 1983.

82. Hotta N, Toyota T, Matsuoka K et al: SNK-860 Diabetic Neuropathy Study Group. Clinical efficacy of fidarestat, a novel aldose redctase inhibitor, for diabetic peripheral neuropathy: A 52-week multicenter placebo-controlled double-blind parallel group study. Diabetes Care 24:1776–1782, 2001.

83. Young R, Ewing D, Clarke B: A controlled trial of sorbinil, an aldose reductase inhibitor, in chronic painful diabetic neuropathy. Diabetes 32:938, 1983.

84. Keen H, Payan J, Allawi J et al: Treatment of diabetic neuropathy with gamma linolenic acid. Diabetes Care 16:8, 1992.

85. Gregersen G, Bertelsen B, Harbo H et al: Oral supplementation of myoinositol: Effects on peripheral nerve function in human diabetics and on the concentration in plasma, erythrocytes, urine and muscle tissue in human diabetics and normals. Acta Neurol Scand 67:164, 1983.

86. The Capsaicin Study Group: Treatment of painful diabetic neuropathy with topical capsaicin: A multicenter, double-blind, vehicle-controlled study. Arch Intern Med 151:2225, 1991.

87. Dyrberg T, Benn J, Christiansen JS et al: Prevalence of diabetic autonomic neuropathy measured by simple bedside tests. Diabetologia 20:190, 1981.

88. Ewing DJ, Martyn CN, Young RJ et al: The value of cardiovascular autonomic function tests: 10 years experience in diabetes. Diabetes Care 8:491–498, 1985.

89. Onrot J, Goldberg MR, Hollister AS et al: Management of chronic orthostatic hypertension. Am J Med 80:454, 1986.

90. Jankovic J, Gilden JL, Hiner BC et al: Neurogenic orthostatic hypotension: A double-blind placebo-controlled study with Midodrine. Am J Med 95:38, 1993.

91. Low PA, Gilden JL, Freeman R et al for the Midodrine Study Group: Efficacy of midodrine vs placebo in neurogenic orthostatic hypotension: A randomized, double-blind multicenter study. JAMA 277:1046, 1997.

92. Meyerhoff C, Sternberg F, Bischof F et al: Diltiazem for tachycardiac orthostatic hypotension in NIDDM. Diabetes Care 16:1628, 1993.

93. Hoeldtke RD, Streeten DHP: Treatment of orthostatic hypotension with erythropoietin. N Engl J Med 329:611, 1993.

94. Dudl RJ, Anderson DS, Forsyth AB et al: Treatment of diabetic diarrhea and orthostatic hypotension with somatostatin analogue SMS 201-995. Am J Med 83:584, 1987.

95. Mathur R, Pimentel M, Sam CL et al: Post prandial improvement of gastric dysrhythmia in patients with type 2 diabetes. Dig Dis Sci 46:705, 2001.

96. Nilsson P-H: Diabetic gastroparesis: A review. J Diabetes Complications 10:113, 1996.

97. Richards RD, Davenport K, McCallum RW: The treatment of idiopathic and diabetic gastroparesis with acute intravenous and chronic oral erythromycin. Am J Gastroenterol 88:203, 1993.

98. Erbas T, Varoglu E, Erbas B et al: Comparison of metoclopramide and erythromycin in the treatment of diabetic gastroparesis. Diabetes Care 16:1511, 1993.

99. Fedorak RN, Field M, Chang EB: Treatment of diabetic diarrhea with clonidine. Ann Intern Med 102:197, 1985.

100. Sacerdote A: Topical clonidine for diabetic diarrhea. Ann Intern Med 105:139, 1986.

101. Roof LW: Treatment of diabetic diarrhea with clonidine. Am J Med 83:603, 1987.

102. Nakabayashi H, Fujji S, Miwa U et al: Marked improvement of diabetic diarrhea with the somatostatin analogue octreotide. Arch Intern Med 154:1863, 1994.

103. Tsai S-T, Vinik Al, Brunner JF: Diabetic diarrhea and somatostatin. Ann Intern Med 104:894, 1986.

104. Korenman SG: Advances in the understanding and management of erectile dysfunction. J Clin Endocrinol Metab 80:1985, 1995.

105. Drugs that cause sexual dysfunction: An update. Med Lett Drugs Ther 34:73, 1992.

106. NIH Consensus Conference: Impotence. JAMA 270:83, 1993.

107. Gresser U, Gleiter CH: Erectile dysfunction: Comparison of efficacy and side effects of the PDE-5 inhibitors sildenafil, vardenafil and tadalafil—review of the literature. Eur J Med Res 7:435–446, 2002.

108. Linet OI, Ogring FG, for the Alprostadil Study Group: Efficacy and safety of intracavernosal alprostadil in men with erectile dysfunction. N Engl J Med 334:873, 1996.

109. Virag R, Shoukry K, Floresco J et al: Intracavernous self-injection of vasoactive drugs in the treatment of impotence: 8-year experience with 615 cases. J Urol 145:287, 1991.

110. Bell DSH, Cutter GR, Hayne VB et al: Factors predicting efficacy of phentolamine-papaverine intracorporeal injection for treatment of erectile dysfunction in diabetic males. Urology 40:36, 1992.

111. Cryer PE, Davis SN, Shamoon H: Hypoglycemia in diabetes. Diabetes Care 26:1902–1912, 2003.

112. Cohen SJ: Potential barriers to diabetes care. Diabetes Care 6:499, 1983.

113. Bailey TS, Yu HM, Rayfield EJ: Patterns of foot examination in a diabetes clinic. Am J Med 78:371, 1985.

114. Mooney V, Gottschalk F, Powell H: The diabetic foot ulcer: Treating one, preventing the next. Clin Diabetes 3:36, 1985.

115. Haffner SM, Lehto S, Ronnemaa T et al: Mortality from coronary heart disease in subjects with type 2 diabetes and in nondiabetic subjects with and without prior myocardial infarction. N Engl J Med 339:229, 1998.

116. Expert Panel on Detection, Evaluation, and Treatment of High Blood Cholesterol in Adults (Adult Treatment Panel III): Executive summary of the third report of the National Cholesterol Education Program (NCEP) Expert Panel on Detection, Evaluation, and Treatment of High Blood Cholesterol in Adults (Adult Treatment Panel III). JAMA 285:2486, 2001.

117. Garg A, Grundy SM: Lipid abnormalities in men and women. Diabetes Care 13:153, 1990.

118. Scandinavian Simvastatin Survival Study Group: Randomised trial of cholesterol lowering in 4444 patients with coronary heart disease: The Scandinavian Simvastatin Survival Study (4S). Lancet 344:1383, 1994.

119. Shepherd J, Cobbe SM, Ford I et al, for the West of Scotland Coronary Prevention Study Group: Prevention of coronary heart disease with pravastatin in men with hypercholesterolemia. N Engl J Med 333:1301, 1995.

120. Sacks FM, Pfeffer MA, Moye LA et al, for the Cholesterol and Recurrent Events Trial Investigators: The effect of pravastatin on coronary events after myocardial infarction in patients with average cholesterol levels. N Engl J Med 335:1001, 1996.

121. Downs JR, Clearfield M, Weis S, et al, for the AFCAPS/TexCAPS Research Group. Primary prevention of acute coronary events with lovastatin in men and women with average cholesterol levels: Results of AFCAPS/TexCAPS. JAMA 279:1615, 1998.

122. Long-Term Intervention with Pravastatin in Ischaemic Disease (LIPID) Study Group: Prevention of cardiovascular events and death with pravastatin in patients with coronary heart disease and a broad range of initial cholesterol levels. N Engl J Med 339:1349, 1998.

123. American Diabetes Association: Management of dyslipidemia in adults with diabetes. Diabetes Care 26:580–583, 2003.

124. Collins R, Peto R, Armitage J: The MRC/BHF Heart Protection Study: Preliminary results. Int J Clin Pract 56:53, 2002.

125. Bruckert E, Giral P, Tellier P: Perspectives in cholesterol-lowering therapy: The role of ezetimibe, a new selective inhibitor of intestinal cholesterol absorption. Circulation 107:3124–3128, 2003.

126. Ballantyne CM, Houri J, Notarbartolo A, et al, Ezetimibe Study Group: Effect of ezetimibe coadministered with atorvastatin in 628 patients with primary hypercholesterolemia: A prospective, randomized, double-blind trial. Circulation 1007:2409–2415, 2003.

127. McFarlane SI, Muniyappa R, Francisco R et al: Pleiotropic effects of statins: Lipid reduction and beyond. J Clin Endo Metab 87:1451, 2002.

128. Grady D, Rubin SM, Petitti DB et al: Hormone therapy to prevent disease and prolong life in postmenopausal women. Ann Intern Med 117:1016, 1992.

129. Humphrey LL, Chan BKS, Sox HC: Postmenopausal hormone replacement therapy and the primary prevention of cardiovascular disease. Ann Intern Med 137:E273–E289, 2002.

130. The Writing Group for the Postmenopausal Estrogen/Progestin Interventions (PEPI) Trial: Effects of estrogen or estrogen/progestin regimens on heart disease risk factors in postmenopausal women: The Postmenopausal Estrogen/Progestin Interventions (PEPI) Trial. JAMA 273:199, 1995.

131. Stampfer MJ, Colditz GA, Willet WC et al: Postmenopausal estrogen therapy and cardiovascular disease: Ten-year follow-up from the Nurses' Health Study. N Engl J Med 325:756, 1991.

132. Dubuisson JT, Wagenknecht LE, D'Agostino RB Jr et al: Association of hormone replacement therapy and carotid wall thickness in women with and without diabetes. Diabetes Care 21:1790, 1998.

133. Hully S, Grady D, Bush T et al, for the Heart and Estrogen/Progestin Replacement Study (HERS) Research Group: Randomized trial of estrogen plus progestin for secondary prevention of coronary heart disease in postmenopausal women. JAMA 280:605, 1998.

134. Grady D, Herrington D, Bittner V et al: Cardiovascular disease outcomes during 6.8 years of hormone therapy. Heart and estrogen/progestin replacement study follow-up (HERS II). JAMA 288:49, 2002.

135. Writing Group for the Women's Health Initiative Investigators: Risks and benefits of estrogen plus progestin in healthy postmenopausal women: Principal results from the Women's Health Initiative Randomized Controlled Trial. JAMA 288:321, 2002.

136. Arauz-Pacheco C, Parrott MA, Raskin P: The treatment of hypertension in adult patients with diabetes (technical review). Diabetes Care 25:134, 2002.

137. The sixth report of the Joint National Committee on prevention, detection, evaluation, and treatment of high blood pressure. Arch Int Med 159:2413, 1997.

138. Chobanian AV, Bakris GL, Black HR et al: National Heart, Lung, and Blood Institute Joint National Committee on Prevention, Detection, Evaluation, and Treatment of High Blood Pressure; National High Blood Pressure Education Program Coordinating Committee. The Seventh Report of the Joint National Committee on Prevention, Detection, Evaluation, and Treatment of High Blood Pressure: The JNC 7 report. JAMA 289:2560–2570, 2003.

139. Heart Outcomes Prevention Evaluation Study Investigators: Effects of ramipril on cardiovascular and microvascular outcomes in people with diabetes mellitus: Results of the HOPE Study and MICRO-HOPE substudy. Lancet 355:253, 2000.

140. Arauz-Pacheco C, Parrott MA, Raskin P: The treatment of hypertension in adult patients with diabetes. Diabetes Care 25(1):134–147, 2002.

141. Marre M, Chatellier G, LeBlanc II et al: Prevention of diabetic nephropathy with enalapril in normotensive diabetics with microalbuminuria. Br Med J 297:1092–1095, 1998.

142. Mathiesen ER, Hommel E, Giese J et al: Efficacy of captopril in postponing nephropathy in nmrotensive insulin-dependent diabetic patients with microalbuminuria. BMJ 303:81–87, 1991.

143. The ACE Inhibitors in Diabetic Nephropathy Trialist Group: Should all patients with type 1 diabetes mellitus and microalbuminuria receive angiotensin-converting enzyme inhlibitors? A meta-analysis of individual pateint data. Ann Intern Med 134:370–379, 2001.

144. Lewis EJ, Hunsicker Lg, Bain RP et al: The effect of angiotensin-converting enzyme inhibition on diabetic nephropathy. N Engl J Med 329:1456–1462, 1993.

145. Sasso FC, Carbonara O, Persico M et al: Irbesartan reduces the albumin excretion rate in microalbuminuric type 2 diabetic patients independently of hypertension: A randomized double-blind placebo-controlled crossover study. Diabetes Care 25:1909–1913, 2002.

146. Lewis EJ, Hunsicker LG, Clarke WR et al: Renoprotective effect of the angiotensin-receptor antagonist irbesartan in patients with nephropathy due to type 2 diabetes. N Engl J Med 345:851, 2001.

147. Brenner BM, Cooper ME, de Zeeuw D et al: Effects of losartan on renal cardiovascular outcomes in patients with type 2 diabetes and nephropathy. N Engl J Med 345:861–869, 2001.

148. Parving HH, Lehnert H, Brochner-Mortensen J et al: The effect of irbesartan on the development of diabetic nephropathy in patients with type 2 diabetes. N Engl J Med 345:870, 2001.

149. The Heart Outcome Prevention Evaluation Study Investigators: Effects of an angiotensin converting enzyme inhibitor, Ramipril, on cardiovascular events in high risk patients. N Engl J Med 342:145, 2000.

150. Tatti P, Pahor M, Byington RP et al: Outcome results of the Fosinopril versus Amlodipine Cardiovascular Events Randomized Trial (FACET) in patients with hypertension and NIDDM. Diabetes Care 21:597, 1998.

151. Zuanetti G, Latini R, Maggioni AP et al: Effect of the ACE inhibitor lisinopril on mortality in diabetic patients with acute myocardial infarction: Data from the GISSI-3 study. Circulation 96:4239, 1997.

152. Golan L, Birkmeyer JD, Welch HG: The cost-effectiveness of treating all patients with type 2 diabetes with angiotensin converting enzyme inhibitor. Ann Inter Med 131:660, 1999.

153. The ACE Inhibitors in Diabetic Nephropathy Trialist Group: Should all patients with type 1 diabetes mellitus and microalbuminuria receive angiotensin converting enzyme inhibitors? Ann Intern Med 134:370, 2001.

154. Jacobsen P, Andersen S, Rossing K et al: Dual blockade of the renin-angiotensin system in type 1 patients with diabetic nephropathy. Nephrology Dialysis Transplantation 17(6):1019–1024, 2002.

155. United Kingdom Prospective Diabetes Study Group: Tight blood pressure control and risk of macrovascular and microvascular complications in type 2 diabetes. UKPDS 38. BMJ 317:703, 1998.

156. The ALLHAT Officers and Coordinators for the ALLHAT Collaborative Research Group. Major outcomes in high-risk hypertensive patients randomized to angiotensin-converting enzyme inhibitor or calcium channel blocker vs diuretic: The Antihypertensive and Lipid-Lowering

Treatment to Prevent Heart Attack Trial (ALLHAT). JAMA 288:2981–2997, 2002.

157. Hansson L, Hedner T, Lund-Johansen P et al: Randomized trial of effects of calcium antagonists compared with diuretics and beta blockers on cardiovascular mortality in hypertension: The Nordic Diltiazem Study. Lancet 356:359, 2000.

158. Hansson L, Lindhol LH, Niskanen L et al: Effect of angiotensin converting enzyme inhibition compared with conventional therapy on cardiovascular morbidity and mortality in hypertension. The Captopril Prevention Project (CAPP) randomized trial. Lancet 353:611, 1999.

159. Nielsen FS, Rossing P, Gall MA et al: Long-term effect of lisinopril and atenolol on kidney function in hypertensive NIDDM subjects with diabetic nephropathy. Diabetes 46:1182, 1997.

160. United Kingdom Prospective Diabetes Study Group: Efficacy of atenolol and captopril in reducing the risk of macrovascular and microvascular complications in type 2 diabetes: UKPDS 39. BMJ 317:713, 1998.

161. Goldstein S: Beta blockers in hypertensive and coronary heart disease. Arch Intern Med 156:1267, 1996.

162. Kizer JR, Kimmel SE: Epidemiologic review of the calcium channel blocker drugs: An up-to-date perspective on the proposed hazards. Arch Int Med 161:1145–1158, 2001.

163. Tuomilehto J, Rastenyte D, Birkenhager WH et al: Effects of calcium channel blockade in older patients with diabetes and systolic hypertension. N Engl J Med 340:677, 1999.

164. Hansson L, Zanchetti A, Carruthers SG et al: Effects of intensive blood pressure lowering and low dose aspirin on patients with hypertension: Principal results of the Hypertension Optimal Treatment (HOT) randomized trial. Lancet 351:1755, 1998.

165. Furberg CD, Psaty BM, Meyer JV: Nifedipine: Dose-related increase in mortality in patients with coronary heart disease. Circulation 92:1326, 1995.

166. Melbourne Diabetic Nephropathy Study Group: Comparison between perindopril and nifedipine in hypertensive and normotensive diabetic patients with microalbuminuria. BMJ 302:210, 1991.

167. Pinol C, Cobos A, Cases A et al: Nitrendipine and enalapril in the treatment of diabetic hypertensive patients with microalbuminuria. Kid Int Suppl 55:S85, 1996.

168. Lewis EJ, Hunsicker LG, Clarke WR et al: Renoprotective effect of the angiotensin receptor antagonist irbesartan in patients with nephropathy due to type 2 diabetes. N Engl J Med 435:851, 2001.

169. Bakris GL: Effects of diltiazem or lisinopril on massive proteinuria associated with diabetes mellitus. Ann Intern Med 112:707, 1990.

170. Bakris GL, Mangrum A, Copley JB et al: Effect of calcium channel or beta blockade on the progression of diabetic nephropathy in African Americans. Hypertension 29:744, 1997.

171. Van Zwieten PA, Timmermans PB, Van Brummelen P: Role of alpha adrenoreceptors in hypertension and in antihypertensive drug treatments. Am J Med 77:17, 1984.

172. Pollare T, Sithell H, Selnius J et al: Application of prazosin is associated with an increase of insulin sensitivity in obese patients with hypertension. Diabetologia 31:41, 1988.

173. Kwan CM, Shepherd AM, Johnson J et al: Forearm and finger hemodynamics, blood pressure control and lipid changes in diabetic hypertensive patients treated with atenolol and prazosin: A brief report. Am J Med 86:55, 1989.

174. Messerli FH: Implications of discontinuation of doxazosin arm of ALLHAT: the Antihypertensive and Lipid Lowering Treatment to Prevent Heart Attack Trial. Lancet 355:863, 2000.

CHAPTER 8

REDUCING CARDIOVASCULAR RISK IN TYPE 2 DIABETES AND THE METABOLIC SYNDROME: THE EMERGING ROLE OF INSULIN RESISTANCE

DAVID M. KENDALL

Both type 2 diabetes and the metabolic syndrome are associated with a significant increase in the risk of cardiovascular disease (CVD)—including coronary heart disease (CHD), peripheral vascular disease, and stroke.[1-7] CVDs are arguably the most common and clinically important complications of diabetes in adults.[1-3,8,9] Clinical and epidemiologic data also support the strong association between the metabolic syndrome and increased CVD risk,[4-7] with CVD increased as much as threefold in those with this disorder.

Reducing the risk of CVD is of paramount importance and represents a key component of care for patients with diabetes or the metabolic syndrome. These two disorders share more in common than the increase in CVD risk. They also share a number of distinct and important CVD risk factors—many closely linked to the disorder of insulin resistance. The list of risk factors common in diabetes[10] and the metabolic syndrome[5-7,11] include the following:

1. Hypertension
2. Atherogenic dyslipidemia
3. Insulin resistance
4. Glucose intolerance
5. Vascular and hemodynamic abnormalities resulting from endothelial cell dysfunction
6. Hemostatic abnormalities that result in an increased risk for vascular thrombosis and acute coronary events

A better understanding of how these risk factors develop, combined with a systematic approach to management, is essential if we hope to limit cardiovascular risk in these patients. Priority should be given to therapies of demonstrated benefit, including use of statins for elevated low-density lipoprotein (LDL) cholesterol, use of fibrates for patients with low high-density lipoprotein (HDL) cholesterol and established CVD, use of aspirin, and aggressive glucose lowering. In addition, targeted treatment of insulin resistance may prove to be a central component of care in years to come.

In this chapter we review the current risk of CVD in diabetes and outline the relationship between diabetes and the metabolic (or insulin resistance) syndromes. A summary of the multiple risk factors present in these patients is included. A systematic approach to CVD risk management in these complex patients is then provided with a brief review of clinical trials supporting these interventions.

DEFINING THE PROBLEM— CVD RISK IN DIABETES AND THE METABOLIC SYNDROME

CVD risk in patients with type 2 diabetes is increased up to fivefold when compared with that in the general population.[9] Individuals with diabetes have a risk for CVD that is equivalent to that in patients with known coronary disease[8] and, as such, diabetes is now considered a CVD risk "equivalent" with a 10-year CVD risk equal to that in patients with established heart disease.[11] Cardiovascular complications develop in up to 80% of patients with diabetes and currently account for 75% of the mortality in diabetes.[1,3]. CVD events are responsible for three of four hospital admissions for patients with diabetes and account for more than 50% of health care spending on diabetes care.[12-15]

CVD is also common in patients with the so-called metabolic syndrome. The metabolic syndrome is defined as a constellation of risk factors—most of metabolic origin—that are now considered a critical CVD risk factor. The current diagnostic criteria defining the metabolic syndrome are summarized in Table 8-1. Although the various guidelines differ somewhat, all emphasize the constellation of CVD risk factors present in patients with this disorder.

The risk of CVD is increased two- to threefold in patients with the metabolic syndrome.[4-7] The metabolic syndrome also represents an increasingly important public health concern with recent studies suggesting that this disorder is present in approximately 25% of the adult population in the United States.[16] Metabolic syndrome patients account for up to 50% of patients admitted with acute coronary events.[4,6]

Type 2 diabetes and the metabolic syndrome are both closely linked to the generalized metabolic disorder of insulin resistance. Insulin resistance is a disorder of insulin action that results in numerous physiologic and vascular changes, and these changes appear to be responsible for the development of many of the CVD risk factors present in these patients. Insulin resistance is present in more than 90% of patients with type 2 diabetes[17] and the metabolic syndrome is commonly defined by markers of insulin resistancee.[11,18,19] Recent guidelines from the National Cholesterol Education Program (NCEP) describe the metabolic syndrome "as a constellation of lipid and non-lipid risk factors of metabolic origin . . . [all] closely linked to . . . insulin resistance."[11]

Type 2 diabetes and the metabolic syndrome are both thought to develop within this common background of insulin resistance (shown figuratively in Figure 8-1). Insulin resistance is linked not only to an increase in CVD risk but also to the development of the associated CVD risk factors listed.[20-24] The central role of insulin resistance in the development of hypertension, dyslipidemia, and glucose intolerance is well established.[24] In addition, many nonclassical CVD risk factors have been linked to insulin resistance as well.[25-30] These nonclassical risk determinants include abdominal (or central) adiposity, vascular inflammation, abnormal endothelial function, and a prothrombotic vascular milieu. The representation of type 2 diabetes and the metabolic syndrome shown in Figure 8-1 emphasizes the complex relationship of insulin resistance to these other disorders and suggests that insulin resistance represents a central defect responsible for both the constellation of CVD risk factors present and the development of CVD. It is

TABLE 8-1	CURRENT CRITERIA FOR THE DIAGNOSIS OF THE METABOLIC SYNDROME		
	WHO	**NCEP ATP III**	**AACE**
Hypertension	Current antihypertensive therapy and/or BP >160/90	BP >130/85	Hypertension
Dyslipidemia	Plasma triglycerides >1.7 mmol/L and/or HDL cholesterol <0.9mmol/L in men and <1.0 mmol/L in women	Plasma triglycerides> 150 mg/dl, HDL cholesterol <40mg/dl in men and <50 mg/dl in women	Dyslipidemia (HDL cholesterol <45 mg/dl in women, <35 mg/dl in men, or triglycerides >150 mg/dl)
Obesity	BMI >30 and/or waist/hip ratio >0.90 in males, >0.85 in females	Waist circumference >40 cm in males and >50 cm in females	Waist circumference >102 cm for men and >88 cm for women
Glucose	Type 2 diabetes or IGT	Fasting blood glucose >110 mg/dl	Impaired fasting glucose or type 2 diabetes
Other	Microalbuminuria = overnight urinary albumin excretion rate >20 μg/min		Insulin resistance (denoted by hyperinsulinemia relative to glucose levels) or acanthosis nigricans
Requirements for Diagnosis	Requires diagnosis of type 2 diabetes or IGT and any two of the previous criteria; if normal glucose tolerance, must demonstrate three other disorders	Requires any *three* of the previous disorders	Minor criteria including hypercoagulability, PCOS, vascular or endothelial dysfunction, microalbuminuria, and coronary heart disease

AACE, American Association of Clinical Endocrinology; BMI, body mass index; BP, blood pressure; HDL, high-density lipoprotein, IGT, impaired glucose tolerance; NCEP ATP III, National Cholesterol Education Program—Adult Treatment Panel III; PCOS, polycystic ovary syndrome; WHO, World Health Organization.

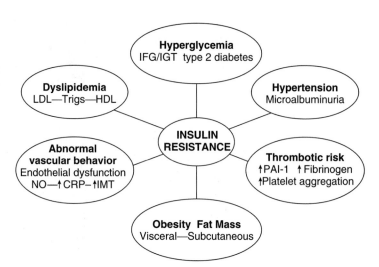

FIGURE 8-1. Clinical components in type 2 diabetes and the metabolic syndrome. Cellular insulin resistance is proposed to play a central role in the development of many of the associated features. CRP, C-reactive protein; HDL, high-density lipoproteins; IFG, impaired fasting glucose; IGT, impaired glucose tolerance; IMT, intima-media thickness; LDL, low-density lipoprotein; NO, nitrous oxide; PAI-1, plasminogen activator inhibitor type 1; Trigs, triglycerides. © *International Diabetes Center 2002. All rights reserved. Reprinted with permission.*

important to understand that although insulin resistance itself is not a disease, the physiologic changes that accompany IR significantly increase the risk of developing one or more of these associated abnormalities.

Figure 8-2 describes a theoretical "timeline" outlining the probable role of insulin resistance and other classic risk factors in the development of complications in dia-

betes. This figure suggests that type 2 diabetes and the metabolic syndrome are in fact disorders that exist on a continuum of disease.[31] Although the classic microvascular complications of diabetes are known to develop only *after* hyperglycemia occurs, individuals that develop type 2 diabetes are, even at the time of diagnosis, at significantly higher risk for CVD.[4-7] This observation sug-

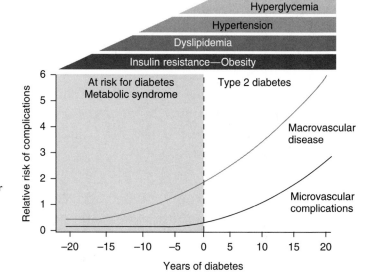

FIGURE 8-2. Theoretical timeline for the development of the insulin resistance syndrome, type 2 diabetes, and microvascular and macrovascular complications. © *International Diabetes Center 2001. All rights reserved. Reprinted with permission.*

gests that the metabolic syndrome is a prodrome of type 2 diabetes.[24] The period of "prediabetes" is classically characterized by the presence of insulin resistance, dyslipidemia, and hypertension, as well as by many of the other vascular disease risk factors listed in Figure 8-1. These metabolic abnormalities are present even in the absence of frank glucose intolerance. If such a timeline is in fact true, it follows that significant opportunity exists for targeting CVD risk both before *and* after the development of type 2 diabetes.

TARGETING CVD RISK— ESTABLISHING PRIORITIES

Cardiovascular risk reduction in patients with diabetes and the metabolic syndrome undoubtedly requires a comprehensive and aggressive approach to management. In the past decade, clinical trials have confirmed that specific interventions are of significant benefit to these patients, including treatment of elevated LDL cholesterol, aggressive management of blood pressure (BP), and the use of aspirin therapy. Other high-risk patient populations, such as those with the metabolic syndrome, are also likely to benefit from such therapies. More recently, clinical trials have suggested benefit from therapies for other risk factors present in patients with diabetes and the metabolic syndrome, including therapies designed to increase HDL cholesterol levels and lower triglycerides. The use of angiotensin-converting enzyme inhibitors (ACEIs) is also of established benefit in patients with markers of insulin resistance and the metabolic syndrome, even in the absence of BP elevations. In addition, accumulating evidence supports aggressive treatment of glucose intolerance and targeted IR in these CVD risk reduction efforts.

To ensure that patients receive high-quality comprehensive care, a clinically relevant approach to care is required. Such an approach is essential to provide clinicians with consistent diagnostic criteria, rational treatment targets, and clinically effective treatment recommendations.[31] Figure 8-3 and Table 8-2 outline management recommendations for patients with diabetes and the metabolic syndrome. Figure 8-3 describes each of the components of care, emphasizing the importance of baseline risk assessment. The figure establishes medical nutrition and lifestyle changes as central to our management, and it further details the specific areas for intervention, emphasizing treatments of established benefit. Although the figure itself is by no means all-inclusive, it provides practitioners with a simple depiction of a focused approach to care in these complex patients. To ensure that appropriate therapeutic interventions are applied, priorities of care must also be clearly identified. Table 8-2 describes specific interventions of particular importance in these patients. Details of each intervention are included in the following sections.

DIAGNOSIS AND SCREENING— DIABETES, THE METABOLIC SYNDROME AND CVD RISK

Early diagnosis of type 2 diabetes and the metabolic syndrome is critical if we are to initiate aggressive CVD risk reduction efforts as early as possible in this population. The importance of early diagnosis is supported by data suggesting that nearly one third of CVD events occur in patients with diabetes and that unrecognized glucose intolerance may be present in many CVD patients. Recent data from our institution suggest that up to 20% of patients admitted for coronary events or bypass surgery have undiagnosed diabetes or glucose intolerance.[32] Up to 50% of patients who suffer CVD events have clinical evidence of either IR or the metabolic syndrome, although this clinical diagnosis is rarely considered. The diagnostic criteria for diabetes are discussed elsewhere in this text and criteria for diagnosis of the metabolic syndrome are included in Table 8-1. Routine

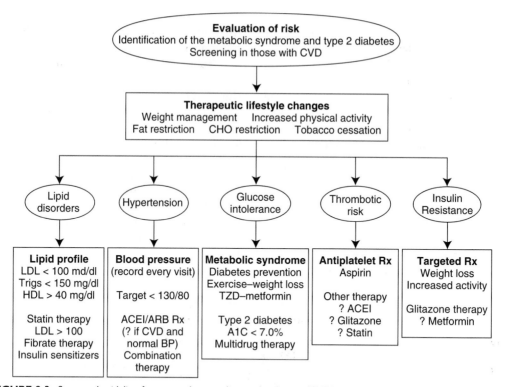

FIGURE 8-3. Suggested guideline for approach to cardiovascular disease (CVD) risk reduction in patients with type 2 diabetes and the metabolic syndrome. ACEI, angiotensin-converting enzyme inhibitor; BP, blood pressure; CHO, carbohydrate; HDL, high-density lipoprotein; LDL, low-density lipoprotein; Rx, prescription; Trigs, triglycerides; TZD, thiazolidinedione. © *International Diabetes Center 2002. All rights reserved. Reprinted with permission.*

TABLE 8-2 PRIORITIES OF CARE–REDUCING CVD RISK IN DIABETES AND THE METABOLIC SYNDROME

- Early identification of patients with diabetes, the metabolic syndrome or insulin resistance—screening of patients with established CVD is recommended
- Medical nutrition (therapeutic lifestyle changes) encouraged for all patients—emphasizing moderate weight loss (5%–10%), increased physical activity (<100 min/wk of aerobic activity), modest carbohydrate restriction, total and saturated fat restriction
- Patient education—instruction on risk factor management and modification and advice on screening for diabetes and additional CVD risk factors
- Statin therapy for patients with elevated LDL cholesterol (target LDL <100)
- Fibrate therapy for patient with low HDL cholesterol and established CVD (target HDL >40)
- Fibrate therapy and/or lifestyle changes for patients with triglyceride levels >150
- Aspirin therapy for all high risk patients >35 years
- Aggressive BP lowering—target BP <130/80; use of ACEI therapy preferred
- Lifestyle changes for any patient with clinical evidence of insulin resistance—consider glitazone therapy if very low HDL, early glucose intolerance or higher risk of CVD

ACEI, angiotensin-converting enzyme inhibitor; BP, blood pressure; CVD, cardiovascular disease; HDL, high-density lipoprotein; LDL, low-density lipoprotein.

screening of patients presumed to be at high risk or those admitted with evidence of CVD is advisable. Of note, the recent approval of a specific International Classification of Diseases 9 diagnostic code for the metabolic syndrome allows practitioners to diagnose and treat this condition more readily[19] and may permit earlier treatment of the many risk factors present.

THERAPEUTIC LIFESTYLE INTERVENTIONS

Therapeutic lifestyle changes are essential for all patients with type 2 diabetes and the metabolic syndrome. Careful instruction on the benefits of modest weight loss, carbohydrate and total fat restriction, and an increase in physical activity are of established benefit (see Figure 8-3). Obesity and physical inactivity are important risk factors for the development of these disorders and the associated cardiovascular risk factors. Central obesity is common in those with type 2 diabetes and is one of the key criteria used to identify the metabolic syndrome. Central obesity is often associated with insulin resistance as well.

Recent recommendations for management of diabetes[33] and the metabolic syndrome[11] clearly support the role of therapeutic lifestyle changes. Furthermore, such interventions play an important role in managing the associated dyslipidemia, hypertension, and hyperglycemia. Modest weight loss achieved through a reduction in total calorie and fat intake, when combined with an increase in physical activity, has also been shown to prevent type 2 diabetes.[34,35] Recent clinical trials demonstrated that therapeutic lifestyle changes reduce the risk of type 2 diabetes by more than 50%. Such prevention efforts are expected to significantly reduce the risk of both microvascular and macrovascular complications of diabetes. Many of the benefits of weight loss and activity in the metabolic syndrome and diabetes are likely related to their favorable effect on insulin sensitivity. Weight

reduction and changes in diet composition[36,37] improve insulin sensitivity. Dietary carbohydrate restriction lowers blood glucose and plasma triglyceride levels—often resulting in further improvements in insulin sensitivity. Physical activity increases insulin sensitivity by up to 25%. In addition, increased physical activity serves to lower BP and increase levels of HDL cholesterol.[38,39]

At present, the greatest difficulty we face with regard to lifestyle interventions is providing our patients with the both the incentive for change and specific methods by which they can achieve and sustain these changes. Unquestionably, education of patients is essential. Lifestyle interventions and education are of demonstrated benefit in patients with diabetes. The results of the recent diabetes prevention trial further underscore the need for supervised lifestyle interventions. At present, most health care insurance systems do not routinely provide financial coverage for lifestyle counseling or education outside the setting of diabetes. Yet many patients with the metabolic and insulin resistance will likely benefit significantly from education programs. Specific efforts to integrate educational and lifestyle interventions into the regular care of our patients is challenging but essential. We must challenge our patients to make every effort to establish these lifestyle changes. Doing so will not only limit the need for pharmacologic therapy, but will also provide added value to any drug therapy employed.

Tobacco use is also a critical cardiac risk factor in those with diabetes and the metabolic syndrome.[40,41] Tobacco cessation counseling should be included for all who use tobacco on a regular basis. A recent report confirmed that tobacco cessation efforts are a useful component of regular diabetes care and should be added to educational programs where appropriate.[41] Every effort should be made to counsel patients on tobacco cessation efforts. Pharmacologic therapy using nicotine replacement and/or bupropion (Zyban) should be considered in any patient refractory to nonpharmacologic options.

DYSLIPIDEMIA

Lipid disorders are common in adults with diabetes, with some abnormality of LDL cholesterol, HDL cholesterol, or triglycerides present in a majority of patients.[42] Similarly, lipid disorders are common in patients with the metabolic syndrome. Targeted treatment of elevated LDL cholesterol is recommended for any patient at high risk for CVD. However, the most common lipid disorder observed in these patients is the presence of high plasma triglycerides and low levels of HDL cholesterol. In fact, LDL cholesterol concentrations in insulin-resistant, type 2 diabetes patients are, in general, no different from those seen in healthy subjects. However, there are important qualitative changes in LDL cholesterol particles, with an increase in the number of small, dense LDL particles. Such changes render LDL particles more susceptible to both oxidation and uptake into the subendothelial space.

A suggested approach to the treatment of lipid disorders is outlined in Table 8-3. Annual lipid analysis is essential in any patient at high risk for CVD and is a standard of care for patients with diabetes and the metabolic syndrome (see Figure 8-3). This approach emphasizes the early and aggressive use of statin and fibrate therapy. It also suggests that alternative therapies will likely be needed and of considerable benefit in many patients. The LDL treatment target in any high-risk patient is <100 mg/dl. In its recent guidelines, the NCEP[11] also emphasized management of HDL cholesterol and triglycerides in patients with diabetes and the metabolic syndrome. Adjunctive treatment should be considered for any patient with HDL cholesterol levels <40 mg/dl. This recommendation is supported by both epidemiologic data[43] and recent clinical trials.[44,45] In addition, therapy should be considered if triglycerides levels are >150 mg/dl.

LDL Cholesterol

Lowering of LDL cholesterol is an essential component of care for all patients with dia-

TABLE 8-3	A SIMPLIFIED CLINICAL APPROACH TO THE TREATMENT OF DYSLIPIDEMIA IN DIABETES AND THE METABOLIC SYNDROME*		
	Normal HDL and/or TG <150	**HDL <40 and/or TG >150**	**HDL <40 and/or TG >400[†]**
LDL-C <100 (Optimal)	Emphasize glycemic control and treatment of other CVD risk factors	Fibrate therapy Pioglitazone	Fibrate therapy Glitazone
LDL-C >100	Statin	Statin Fenofibrate Statin + fibrate[b] Statin + pioglitazone Niacin	Statin + fibrate[b] Fenofibrate Statin + glitazone Statin + niacin

CVD, cardiovascular disease; HDL, high-density lipoprotein; TG, triglyceride.

*Medical nutrition therapy, including restriction of total and saturated fat, increased physical activity, and weight loss, is advised for all patients.

[†]Must counsel patients on the potential risk of myopathy with combination statin-fibrate therapy.

betes and those with CVD and the metabolic syndrome. Increased levels of LDL cholesterol have a greater negative effect for individuals with diabetes when compared with the nondiabetic population,[46,47] and a similar increase in risk is assumed for insulin-resistant patients with the metabolic syndrome. Based on the results of a number of landmark clinical trials, hydroxymethyl-glutaryl coenzyme A reductase inhibitor (statin) therapy to achieve LDL cholesterol levels below 100 mg/dl should be considered essential in any patient with established CVD, diabetes, or the metabolic syndrome. In both secondary and primary prevention trials, statin treatment in patients with type 2 diabetes significantly reduced the risk of CVD.[48-50] Indeed, the benefit for patients with diabetes was often greater than in those without diabetes. More recently, statin therapy administered even in those with normal LDL cholesterol levels has been shown to further reduce CVD risk.[51] Whether statin therapy should be provided to all patients with diabetes and the metabolic syndrome remains to be determined.

HDL and Triglycerides

Although lowering of LDL cholesterol is of established benefit for patients with diabetes and the metabolic syndrome, targeting LDL cholesterol alone does not address the most common lipid disorder found in these patients. Recent clinical trials suggest that targeted treatment of low HDL cholesterol is also of benefit for patients with known CVD, type 2 diabetes, and evidence of IR.[44,45,52] The Veterans Affairs HDL Intervention Trial[44] and the Diabetes Atherosclerosis Intervention Study[45] confirmed that use of the fibric acid derivatives (fibrates) is associated with a significant decrease in CVD risk. Importantly, the relative reduction in risk for patients receiving fibrate therapy was comparable with the risk reduction achieved with use of statin therapy in patients with elevated LDL levels. At present, it is not clear which

patients will benefit most from treatment of HDL over and above treatment for disorders of LDL cholesterol. From these studies, it is anticipated that a growing number of patients will likely benefit from combined treatment for LDL and HDL disorders.

A suggested approach to dyslipidemia management is provided in Table 8-3. These guidelines highlight the use of statin therapy for any patients with increased levels of LDL cholesterol who do not respond adequately to therapeutic lifestyle changes. Statins should be considered for any patient with established CVD and LDL >100.[11] Fibrate treatment should be considered for any patient with low HDL cholesterol or elevated triglycerides. Important treatment alternatives for patients with low HDL cholesterol and high triglycerides include high-dose statin therapy, niacin, and the insulin sensitizing medications. Niacin and the thiazolidinediones (TZDs or glitazones) may increase HDL levels by 20% or more, although niacin is associated with a modest increase in insulin resistance.

Given the high incidence of mixed lipid disorders, multidrug therapy may be needed for many patients. Combination therapy with statin-fibrate may be considered. However, despite the benefit of each therapy in separate clinical trials, the benefit of this combination has not been specifically tested. In considering use of this combination, the potential risk of drug-associated myopathy must be weighed against the potential benefit of combination treatment. In selected patients (particularly those with the lowest levels of HDL) addition of glitazone therapy (see later discussion) or niacin is also effective and avoids the potential risk of myopathy from combined fibrate-statin use.

Insulin Resistance and Dyslipidemia

IR is known to play an important role in the development of the dyslipidemia of diabetes and the metabolic syndrome.[53] The specific role of insulin resistance in lipid metabolism is depicted in Figure 8-4. Briefly, insulin resistance in adipose tissue results in increased breakdown of stored triglycerides. The increased levels of free fatty acids (FFAs) present in the circulation are transported to the liver, where they stimulate synthesis of triglyceride-rich very-low-density lipoprotein (VLDL) particles. Plasma VLDL then exchanges both cholesterol ester and triglyceride (via cholesterol ester transfer protein) with circulating HDL and LDL particles. This exchange results in lower plasma HDL and LDL cholesterol concentrations. However, in insulin resistant individuals, these triglyceride-rich LDL particles are subject to increased rates of lipolysis and small, dense LDL particles are created.

In addition to lowering glucose, therapies for insulin resistance can also improve the lipid profile in insulin-resistant individuals. As suggested by the recommendations in Table 8-3, glitazones can be used as adjunctive therapy to lower triglyceride levels, increase HDL concentrations, or both. The specific mechanism by which these agents exert these unique effects is not currently known, but likely relates to the effect of these therapies on insulin resistance and on FFA metabolism.[53,54] Both pioglitazone and rosiglitazone increase levels of HDL cholesterol, whether used alone or in combination with other drugs. However, clinical studies suggest that these agents differ with regard to their effect on plasma triglyceride levels.[53-56, 56a] Pioglitazone therapy is associated with a consistent reduction in triglyceride level, whereas rosiglitazone is reported to have a neutral or variable effect, with some studies demonstrating a reduction and others studies showing an increase in triglyceride levels. Rosiglitazone can significantly increase LDL concentrations, whereas studies with pioglitazone indicate that it does not alter LDL levels. Importantly, both agents reduce the frequency of small, dense LDL particles. Although glitazone therapy is not indicated for the primary treatment of lipid disorders, these agents represent a clinically useful alternative in the management of patients with low HDL and high triglyceride levels. One suggested clinical approach for statin-treated patients is to consider the addition a glitazone agent in lieu of com-

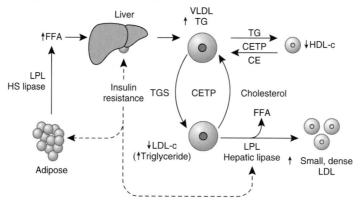

FIGURE 8-4. The role of insulin resistance in dyslipidemia. Insulin resistance results in increased plasma free fatty acid levels. In turn, hepatic insulin resistance increases production of triglyceride rich very-low-density lipoprotein (VLDL) particles. As a consequence, plasma proteins permit exchange of triglyceride and cholesterol between particles, resulting in lower concentrations of both high-density lipoproteins (HDL) and low-density lipoproteins (LDL). LDL particles are subject to further lipolysis, resulting in small, dense particle formation. CE, cholesterol ester; CETP, cholesterol ester transport protein; FFA, free fatty acid; HS, hormone sensitive; LPL, lipoprotein lipase; TG, triglyceride.

bined statin-fibrate treatment for adjunctive management of low HDL/high triglyceride disorders. Such an approach not only targets the dyslipidemia of insulin resistance, it also targets insulin resistance and may further lower blood glucose.

In summary, a significant number of patients with diabetes and the metabolic syndrome require pharmacologic treatment for a lipid disorder. Statin therapy is recommended for any patient with significant LDL cholesterol elevations and may be considered in *any* patient with established CVD, regardless of LDL level. Fibrate therapy should be considered for any patient with low HDL cholesterol and established CVD. Fibrates are also the therapy of choice for marked elevation in triglycerides. Alternatively, glitazone niacin therapy can be considered in any patient with low levels of HDL cholesterol—particularly in patients with clinical markers of insulin resistance, very low HDL levels, or contraindications to fibrate therapy.

HYPERTENSION

Elevated BP significantly increases the risk of both microvascular and macrovascular complications in diabetes. Even modest elevations in BP are associated with a marked increase in complications risk.[57] Hypertension is present in up to 70% of adult patients with diabetes. Elevated BP is also a defining characteristic of the metabolic syndrome. Although data are currently limited, it is estimated that hypertension is present in up to one third of those with the metabolic syndrome and is present in more than 20% with evidence of insulin resistance.

Regular BP measurement is essential in the routine care of patients with diabetes or the metabolic syndrome (see Figure 8-3). Any patient with BP values consistently above 130/80 should receive either non-pharmacologic or pharmacologic therapy to lower BP readings. The sixth report of the Joint National Committee on Prevention,

Detection, Evaluation, and Treatment of High Blood Pressure[58] recommends a BP goal of below 130/85 mm Hg, and recent data have led to the recommendation that the diastolic target be lowered to 80 mm Hg in patients with diabetes.[58a] Given the similar risk of CVD for individuals with insulin resistance and the metabolic syndrome, comparable diagnostic and treatment targets should be sought.[11]

Intensive treatment of BP using a wide variety of antihypertensive agents can reduce the risk of CVD—both in those with diabetes and those with hypertension in the absence of glucose intolerance. Treatment trials in patients with diabetes have demonstrated a significant reduction in rates of both microvascular *and* macrovascular complications with intensive BP management.[59-67] Given the lower treatment targets established, management of hypertension often requires the use of both pharmacologic and nonpharmacologic therapy. Figure 8-5 outlines a simplified treatment approach to hypertension management. Again, the use of nonpharmacologic interventions is emphasized and must include recommendations to increase physical activity, attempt prudent sodium restriction, and achieve modest weight loss.

ACEIs are recommended as initial therapy for virtually all patients with established CVD, and should also be used in any patient with microalbuminuria.[62-65] In this high-risk population, ACEI therapy has been shown to reduce CVD risk to a greater degree that most other antihypertensive therapies. The Heart Outcomes Prevention Evaluation Trial demonstrated that even individuals with normal BP (but at high risk for CVD such as those with diabetes and the metabolic syndrome) had fewer CVD events with expectant use of ACEI therapy.[62-63] Whether these data suggest that clinicians should recommend ACEI therapy for *all* high-risk patients remains unclear. From a practical perspective, ACEI therapy can and should be considered in any patient with diabetes and/or the metabolic syndrome with any of the following clinical characteristics:

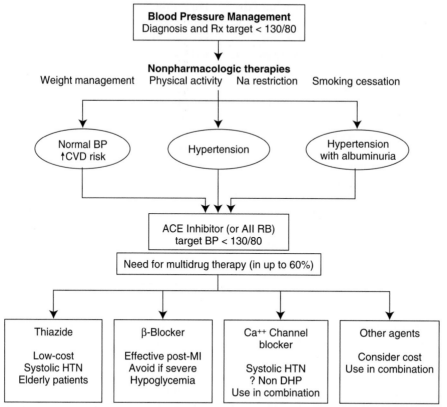

FIGURE 8-5. Suggested treatment approach to hypertension in patients with diabetes and the metabolic syndrome. Blood pressure (BP) thresholds for diagnosis and treatment are set at 130/80, given the higher baseline risk of BP elevations in these populations. Angiotensin-converting enzyme inhibitor (ACEI) therapy is preferred for all patients given the established benefit of such therapy. The figure describes common clinical scenarios and outlines guidelines for the use of antihypertensive therapies. AII RB, angiotensin II receptor blocker; CA++, ion calcium; CVD, cardiovascular disease; DHP, dihydropyridine; HTN, hypertension; MI, myocardial infarction; Na, sodium; Rx, prescription. © *International Diabetes Center 2001. All rights reserved. Reprinted with permission.*

- Hypertension
- Renal disease or microalbuminuria
- Congestive heart failure
- Recent CVD event
- Significant atherosclerosis or established CVD
- Diabetes and progressive or significant microvascular complications (retinopathy, nephropathy, neuropathy)

Angiotensin-2 receptor blockers (ARBs) have been reported to have similar benefits when compared to ACEIs and can now be considered acceptable alternatives for initial treatment of hypertension in these high-risk patients.[68,69] Recent data also suggest a potential role for combined ACEI-ARB treatment.

Effective treatment of hypertension in those with diabetes and the metabolic syndrome often requires the use of multidrug antihypertensive therapy. The need for multidrug therapy can be reduced by intensive attention to lifestyle modifications, including weight reduction; physical activity; and moderation of sodium, protein, and alcohol intake. However, these nondrug interventions have not been shown, by themselves, to reduce morbidity or mortality in those with diabetes, and as such, multidrug therapy should be used when needed.[70]

As shown in Figure 8-5, β-blockers can also be useful agents for patients with diabetes and the metabolic syndrome. In one recent study, β-blocker therapy was similarly beneficial when compared to ACEI therapy.[60] β-Blockers may be of particular benefit in those with symptomatic angina, established CVD, or congestive heart failure.[59,60,70] β-Blockers should be avoided in patients with diabetes who also have a history of recurrent and severe hypoglycemia because they may reduce hypoglycemia symptom awareness. Thiazide diuretics are also effective in patients with diabetes. Particular benefit has been demonstrated in older adults and in patients with systolic hypertension.[61] Calcium channel blockers (CCBs) are effective and, as with diuretics, are most effective in treating systolic hypertension. Despite evidence that CCBs have been associated with higher rates of CVD when compared with ACEIs,[64,65] CCBs do reduce the risk of CVD in high-risk populations with hypertension. CCB therapy may be particularly effective when used in combination with ACEIs. Some studies suggest that the nondihydropyridine agents may be preferred if a CCB is used. However, the recent Systolic Hypertension in Europe Trial[66] confirmed that aggressive BP treatment with a dihydropyridine is effective in reducing CVD risk. Regardless of the therapy employed, current treatment recommendations affirm that treatment of BP in these patients should be individualized according to clinical characteristics of the patient, tolerability of specific agents, clinical experience and preferences, and cost of therapy.[71]

The potential pathogenetic role of insulin resistance in hypertension has stimulated significant interest in recent years. Insulin resistance is associated with a number of changes in vascular endothelial and smooth muscle function—many of which are felt to

contribute to the development of hypertension. The potential mechanisms by which insulin resistance may cause hypertension include resistance to insulin-mediated vasodilatation, abnormal endothelial signaling (via nitric oxide–dependent pathways), sympathetic nervous system overactivity, sodium retention, and enhanced growth factor activity leading to proliferation of smooth muscle cells in the vessel wall. In addition to the known benefit of weight loss and activity, recent studies have suggested that treatment with glitazones can also lower BP.[72-77] The benefits of glitazone treatment on BP were greatest in those with baseline BP elevations. Although the BP reductions observed with glitazone therapy are often modest, these findings further support a central role for insulin resistance in the vascular disorders of diabetes and the metabolic syndrome. When taken with the beneficial impact of glitazone therapy on glucose tolerance and dyslipidemia, these findings suggest that glitazone therapy will likely play a much wider role in the clinical management of these patients in the years ahead.

GLUCOSE, GLYCEMIC CONTROL AND CARDIOVASCULAR RISK

Intensive glycemic control significantly reduces the risk of microvascular complications of diabetes.[78,79] However, the impact of intensive glucose lowering on CVD risk is, at present, unclear. Epidemiologic data support the assumption that lower blood glucose values are associated with the lowest rates of CVD events and mortality[79] and that maximal benefit is achieved as glucose levels approach normal. Which combination of glucose-lowering therapies will be of greatest benefit has not been determined, although some data support the use of metformin[78] and the insulin sensitizing medications.[74] Long-term studies of glucose lowering and its impact on CVD risk are essential if we are to fully understand the role of intensive glycemic control in managing CVD.

The benefit of intensive glycemic control has been demonstrated for patients hospitalized for treatment of an acute CVD event.[80] The Diabetes Insulin Glucose Infusion in Acute Myocardial Infarction trial assessed the impact of early and aggressive glucose lowering—by means of an insulin infusion—on CVD risk and mortality. In this trial, intensive therapy using insulin infusion was associated with reductions in total mortality. More recently, treatment of acutely ill patients without diabetes using insulin infusion was shown to lower in-hospital mortality.[81] Both studies suggest that intensive glucose lowering may indeed be necessary if we are to limit CVD risk in the acute care setting.

In contrast to those with diagnosed diabetes, patients with the metabolic syndrome often have only modest elevation in plasma glucose. Data from several clinical studies[82] confirm that even relatively modest changes in glucose tolerance may be associated with an increased risk of CVD. A such, the goal of treatment for patients with the metabolic syndrome should be to maintain levels of blood glucose as near normal as possible, particularly in the acute care setting. Whether this will indeed reduce the risk of CVD will require data from additional long-term studies. However, the potential benefit of sustained normoglycemia on microvascular disease risk is clear, and the emerging importance of blood glucose control in those with heart disease is compelling.

THROMBOTIC RISK

Many of the risk factors present in patients with diabetes, including insulin resistance, increasing the risk of atherosclerosis. However, CVD events are not only the result of the atherosclerotic process. Rather, most CVD events occur in individuals with small, nonflow–limiting vascular lesions. Acute thrombosis of a damaged vessel is now known to play a key role in triggering acute CVD events.

Diabetes and the metabolic syndrome are both disorders characterized by abnormalities of the vessel wall and plasma that significantly increase thrombotic risk. Factors contributing to a prothrombotic state include changes in the equilibrium between activators of plasminogen (primarily tissue type plasminogen activator) and inhibitors of such events such as plasminogen activator inhibitor type 1 (PAI-1).[25,26] Excessive inhibition of fibrinolysis increases the risk of abnormal coagulation and thrombosis. Plasma levels of PAI-1 are increased in insulin-resistant individuals, including obese subjects with and without diabetes.[25] A number of studies suggest a mechanistic link between insulin resistance and these abnormal fibrinolytic features.[26] In addition, diabetes and IR are associated with increased platelet aggregation. These observations suggest that antiplatelet therapy will play a critical role for patients with diabetes and insulin resistance.[83,84] Aspirin therapy is of recognized benefit. A recent report suggested that as many as 98% of adults with diabetes are candidates for aspirin therapy.[85] A dose of 81 to 325 mg per day is currently recommended for all high-risk patients with diabetes who are older than 35 years of age. Given that similar abnormalities of platelet function and fibrinolysis are present in those with insulin resistance and the metabolic syndrome, similar recommendations are appropriate for these patients as well.

INSULIN RESISTANCE

Throughout this review, we have emphasized the role of insulin resistance in the development of diabetes, the metabolic syndrome, and CVD risk. As described, insulin resistance is closely tied to most, if not all, of the important vascular changes that contribute to the risk of CVD in these patients. These vascular abnormalities include impaired vascular reactivity, procoagulant abnormalities (characterized by elevations in PAI-1, fibrinogen, and increased platelet aggregation), and abnormalities in endothelial function.

Drug treatment of insulin resistance has been shown to have a beneficial effect on many of these surrogate markers of CVD risk.[74] Glitazones not only improve glycemic control, they also correct dyslipidemia and have favorable effects on several of the vascular and procoagulant abnormalities of insulin resistance. Glitazones decrease the release of specific cytokines such as tumor necrosis factor (TNF)-α and reduce markers of vascular inflammation. Glitazones improve endothelial function and have an inhibitory effect on carotid artery intima-media thickness in patients with type 2 diabetes.[86] As such, these agents are likely to provide further protection against CVD. Although reductions in cardiovascular events have not yet been demonstrated, practitioners should consider early use of these agents. Glitazones may ultimately serve as therapy for glucose intolerance and treatment of insulin resistance itself. Such therapy will be useful both for the prevention of diabetes and as targeted therapy for the numerous vascular abnormalities of insulin resistance.

At present, use of these agents should be considered in any patient with clinical evidence of insulin resistance[87] and may be of particular benefit in patients with lipid disorders (particularly low HDL levels), established CVD, or evidence of vascular inflammation suggesting the presence of unstable atherosclerotic plaque.[88] At this time, a number of clinical trials are underway to assess the specific impact of glitazone therapy on dyslipidemia and the risk of CVD. Such trials will be invaluable in guiding the clinician's choice of initial therapeutic options.

PUTTING IT ALL TOGETHER—COMPREHENSIVE RISK FACTOR MANAGEMENT

Despite the enormous risk for CVD in patients with diabetes and the metabolic syndrome, putting these efforts in clinical practice presents an ongoing challenge. Most clinicians have a strong appreciation for the benefit of aggressive multirisk factor intervention. Yet, establishing which therapy to initiate and when remains difficult. In addition, the presence of multiple risk factors makes multidrug therapy necessary for most patients. A recent meta-analysis of studies assessing risk factor management supports the notion that such therapy will significantly decrease rates of death from CHD by lowering both BP and cholesterol[89] Indeed, although clinicians now recognize the need for multirisk–factor intervention in most patients, recent studies suggest that fewer than 10% of patients may achieve control of even two risk factors.[90] When all risk factors were considered, only 3.2% of patients met the combined American Diabetes Association treatment goals for BP, LDL cholesterol, and glycemic control.[90]

Despite the challenges, we as clinicians can and should make every effort to provide therapies of known benefit to our patients with diabetes and the metabolic syndrome. By employing a systematic approach to care, we can, over time, successfully address most, if not all of these risk factors. To do so will likely serve to achieve the aggressive treatment targets established. In the future, targeted treatment of insulin resistance and the metabolic syndrome, combined with changes in the delivery of education for our patients, will most certainly serve to reduce the immense risk of CVD in this population.

REFERENCES

1. Wingard DL, Barrett-Connor E: Heart disease and diabetes. In National Diabetes Data Group. Diabetes in America, 2nd ed. Washington, D.C.: Government Printing Office, 1995, pp. 429-448 (NIH publication no. 95-1468).
2. Stamler J, Vaccaro O, Neaton JD, Wentworth D: Diabetes, other risk factors, and 12-year cardiovascular mortality for men screened in the Multiple Risk Factor Intervention Trial. Diabetes Care 16:434, 1993.
3. Koskinen P, Manttari M, Manninen V et al: Coronary heart disease incidence in NIDDM patients in the Helsinki Heart Study. Diabetes Care 15:820, 1992.
4. Haffner SM, Valdez RA, Hazuda HP et al: Prospective analysis of the insulin resistance syndrome (syndrome X). Diabetes 41:715, 1992.
5. Isomaa B, Almgren P, Tuomi T et al: Cardiovascular morbidity and mortality associated with the metabolic syndrome. Diabetes Care 24:683, 2001.
6. Yip P, Facchini FS, Reaven GM: Resistance to insulin mediated glucose disposal as a predictor of cardiovascular disease. J Clin Endocrinol Metab 83:2773, 1998.
7. McFarlane SI, Banerji M, Sowers JR: Insulin resistance and cardiovascular disease. J Clin Endocrinol Metab 86:713, 2001.
8. Haffner SM, Lehto S, Ronnemaa T et al: Mortality from coronary heart disease in subjects with type 2 diabetes and in nondiabetic subjects with and without prior myocardial infarction. N Engl J Med 339:229, 1998.
9. Sowers JR: Diabetes mellitus and cardiovascular disease in women. Arch Intern Med 158: 617-621, 1998.
10. Turner RC, Millns H, Neil HA et al: Risk factors for coronary artery disease in non-insulin dependent diabetes mellitus: United Kingdom Prospective Diabetes Study (UKPDS: 23). Br Med J 316:823, 1998.
11. Executive Summary of The Third Report of The National Cholesterol Education Program (NCEP) Expert Panel on Detection, Evaluation, and Treatment of High Blood Cholesterol In Adults (Adult Treatment Panel III). JAMA 285:2486, 2001.
12. American Diabetes Association: Economic consequences of diabetes mellitus in 1997. Diabetes Care 21:296, 1998.
13. Brown JB, Pedula KL, Bakst AW: The progressive cost of complications in type 2 diabetes mellitus. Arch Intern Med 159:1873, 1999.
14. Rubin RJ, Altman WM, Mendelson DN: Health care expenditures for people with diabetes mellitus, 1992. J Clin Endocrinol Metab 78:809A, 1994.
15. Gilmer T, O'Conner P, Manning W et al: The cost to health plans of poor glycemic control. Diabetes Care 20:1847, 1997.
16. Ford ES, Giles WH, Dietz WH: Prevalence of the metabolic syndrome among US adults: Findings from the third National Health and Nutrition Examination Survey. JAMA 287:356, 2002.
17. Haffner SM Mykkanen L, Festa A, Burke JP, Stern MP: Insulin resistant prediabetic subjects have more atherogenic risk factors than insulin-sensitive prediabetc subjects. Circulation 101:975, 2000.
18. Alberti KGMM Zimmet PZ, for the World Health Organization Consultation: Definition, diagnosis and classification of diabetes mellitus and its complications Part 1: Diagnosis and classification of diabetes mellitus. Provisional report of a WHO consultation. Diabet Med 15:539, 1998.
19. American Association for Clinical Endocrinology: Information derived from organization web site. Available at http://www.aace.com/members/socio/syndromex.php.{Au: Please provide date accessed}
20. Pyorala M, Miettinen H, Laakso M, Pyorala K: Plasma insulin and all-cause, cardiovascular, and noncardiovascular mortality: The 22-year follow-up results of the Helsinki Policemen Study. Diabetes Care 23:1097, 2000.
21. Ruige JB, Assendelft WJ, Dekker JM et al: Insulin and risk of cardiovascular disease: A meta-analysis. Circulation 97:996, 1998.
22. Folsom AR, Szklo M, Stevens J, et al: A prospective study of coronary heart disease in relation to fasting insulin, glucose, and diabetes. The Atherosclerosis Risk in Communities (ARIC) Study. Diabetes Care 20:935, 1997.
23. Haffner SM, Stern MP, Hazuda HP et al: Cardiovascular risk factors in confirmed prediabetic individuals. Does the clock for coronary heart disease start ticking before the onset of clinical diabetes? JAMA 263:2893, 1990.
24. Stern MP: Diabetes and cardiovascular disease. The "common soil" hypothesis. Diabetes 44:369, 1995.
25. Sobel BE: Insulin resistance and thrombosis: A cardiologist's view. Am J Cardiol 84:37J, 1999.
26. Calles-Escandon J, Mirza SA, Sobel BE, Schneider DJ: Induction of hyperinsulinemia combined with hyperglycemia and hypertriglyceridemia increases plasminogen activator inhibitor 1 in blood in normal human subjects. Diabetes 47:290, 1998.
27. Hsueh WA, Law RE: Insulin signaling in the arterial wall. Am J Cardiol 84:21J, 1999.
28. Festa A, D'Agostino RJ, Howard G et al: Chronic subclinical inflammation as part of the insulin resistance syndrome: The Insulin Resistance Atherosclerosis Study (IRAS). Circulation 102:42, 2000.
29. Kahn BB, Flier JS: Obesity and insulin resistance. J Clin Invest 106:473, 2000.
30. Ruderman N, Chisholm D, Pi-Sunyer X, Schneider S: The metabolically obese, normal-weight individual revisited. Diabetes 47:699, 1998.
31. Kendall DM, Bergenstal RM: Comprehensive management of type 2 diabetes: Establishing priorities of care. Am J Manag Care 7 (Suppl): S327, 2001.

32. Fish LH, Weaver TW, Moore A et al: Post-Operative Blood Glucose Predicts Complications and Length of Stay in Patients after Coronary Artery Bypass Surgery. American Diabetes Association (late-breaking abstract) 2000.

33. American Diabetes Association: 2002 Clinical Practice Recommendations. Diabetes Care 25:Suppl 1, 2002.

34. Tuomilehto J, Lindstrom J, Eriksson JG et al: Prevention of Type 2 Diabetes Mellitus by Changes in Lifestyle among Subjects with Impaired Glucose Tolerance. N Engl J Med 344:1343, 2001.

35 Knowler WC, Barrett-Connor E, Fowler SE et al: Diabetes Prevention Program Research Group. Reduction in the incidence of type 2 diabetes with lifestyle intervention or metformin. N Engl J Med 346:393, 2002.

36. Riccardi G, Rivellese AA: Dietary treatment of the metabolic syndrome–the optimal diet. Br J Nutr 83 (Suppl 1):S143,2000.

37. Reaven GM: Diet and Syndrome X. Curr Atheroscler Rep 2:503, 2000.

38. Ross R, Dagnone D, Jones PJ et al: Reduction in obesity and related comorbid conditions after diet-induced weight loss or exercise-induced weight loss in men. A randomized, controlled trial. Ann Intern Med 18:92, 2000.

39. Perseghin G, Price TB, Petersen KF: Increased glucose transport-phosphorylation and muscle glycogen synthesis after exercise training in insulin-resistant subjects. N Engl J Med 335:1357, 1996.

40. Haire-Joshu D, Glasgow RE, Tibbs TL: Smoking and diabetes (Technical Review). Diabetes Care 22:1887, 1999.

41. Canga N, De Irala J, Vara E et al: Intervention study for smoking cessation in diabetic patients: A randomized controlled trial in both clinical and primary care settings. Diabetes Care. 10:1455, 2000.

42. Steiner G: Treating lipid abnormalities in patients with type 2 diabetes mellitus. Am J Cardiol. 88:37N, 2001.

43. Gordon T, Castelli WP, Hjortland MC et al: Highdensity lipoprotein as a protective factor against coronary heart disease. The Framingham Study. Am J Med 62:707, 1977.

44. Rubins HB, Robins SJ, Collins D et al: Gemfibrozil for the secondary prevention of coronary heart disease in men with low levels of high-density lipoprotein cholesterol. Veterans Affairs High-Density Lipoprotein Cholesterol Intervention Trial Study Group. N Engl J Med 341:410, 1999.

45. Diabetes Atherosclerosis Intervention Study Investigators:. Effect of fenofibrate on progression of coronary-artery disease in type 2 diabetes: the Diabetes Atherosclerosis Intervention Study, a randomised study. Lancet 357:905, 2001.

46. Rosengren A, Welin L, Tsipogianni A, Wilhelmsen L: Impact of cardiovascular risk factors on coronary heart disease and mortality among middle aged diabetic men: A general population study. BMJ 299:1127, 1989.

47. Markovic TP, Campbell LV, Balasubramanian S et al: Beneficial effect on average lipid levels from energy restriction and fat loss in obese individuals with or without type 2 diabetes. Diabetes Care 21:695, 1998.

48. Pyorala K, Savolainen E, Kaukola S et al: Cholesterol lowering with simvastatin improves prognosis of diabetic patients with coronary heart disease: Subgroup analysis of the Scandinavin Simvastatin Survival Study. Diabetes Care 20:614, 1997.

49. The Care Investigators: Cardiovascular events and their reduction with pravastatin in diabetic and glucose-intolerant myocardial infarction survivors with average cholesterol levels: Subgroup analyses in the cholesterol and recurrent events (CARE) trial. Circulation 98:2513, 1998.

50. Downs JR, Clearfield M, Weis S et al: Primary prevention of acute coronary events with lovastatin in men and women with average cholesterol levels: Results of AFCAPS/ TexCAPS. Air Force/Texas Coronary Atherosclerosis Prevention Study. JAMA 279:1615, 1998.

51. Collins R, Peto R, Armitage J: The MRC/BHF Heart Protection Study: Preliminary results. Int J Clin Pract 56:53, 2002.

52. Tenkanen L Manttari M, Manninen V: Some coronary risk factors related to the insulin resistance syndrome and treatment with gemfibrozil. Experience from the Helsinki Heart Study. Circulation 92:1779, 1995.

53. Ginsberg HN: Insulin resistance and cardiovascular disease. J Clin Invest 106:453, 2000.

54. Nass CM and Blumenthal RS: The effect of glitazones on lipid profiles. Am J Manag Care 6:S1247, 2000.

55. Gegick CG, Altheimer MD: Comparison of effects of thiazolidinediones on cardiovascular risk factors: Observations from a clinical practice. Endocr Pract 7:162, 2001.

56. Khan MA, St. Peter JV, Xue JL: A prospective, randomized comparison of the metabolic effects of pioglitazone or rosiglitazone in patients with type 2 diabetes who were previously treated with troglitazone. Diabetes Care 25:708, 2002.

56a.Boyle PJ, King AB, Olarsky L et al: Effects of pioglitazone and rosiglitazone on blood lipid levels and glycemic control in patients with type 2 diabetes mellitus: A retrospective review of randomly selected medical records. Clin Theraputics 24:378, 2002.

57. Geiss LS, Rolka DB, Engelgau MM: Hypertension in the US adult population: Where are we now? Diabetes 49(Suppl 1):A46 (Abstract 188), 2000.

58. Joint National Committee on Prevention, Detection, Evaluation and Treatment of High Blood Pressure: Sixth report. Arch Intern Med 157:2413, 1997.

58a.Chobanian AV, Bakris GL, Black HR et al: National Heart, Lung, and Blood Joint Institute National Committee on Prevention, Detection, Evaluation, and Treatment of High Blood

Pressure. National High Blood Pressure Education Coordinating Committee. The Seventh Report of the Joint National Committee on Prevention, Detection, Evaluation, and Treatment of High Blood Pressure: The JNC 7 Report. JAMA 289:2560, 2003.

59. United Kingdom Prospective Diabetes Study Group: Tight blood pressure control and risk of macrovascular and microvascular complications in type 2 diabetes: UKPDS 38. Br Med J 317:703, 1998.

60. United Kingdom Prospective Diabetes Study Group: Efficacy of atenolol and captopril in reducing risk of macrovascular and microvascular complications in type 2 diabetes: UKPDS 39. Br Med J 317:733, 1998.

61. Curb JD, Pressel SL, Cutler JA et al: Effect of diuretic-based antihypertensive treatment on cardiovascular disease risk in older diabetic patients with isolated systolic hypertension. Systolic Hypertension in the Elderly Program Cooperative Research Group. JAMA 276:1886, 1996.

62. The Heart Outcomes Prevention Evaluation Study Investigators: Effects of an angiotensin-converting-enzyme inhibitor, ramipril, on cariovascular events in high-risk patients. N Engl J Med 342:145, 2000.

63. Heart Outcomes Prevention Evaluation (HOPE) Study Investigators: Effects of ramipril on cardiovascular and microvascular outcomes in people with diabetes mellitus: Results of the HOPE study and MICRO-HOPE substudy. Lancet 355:253, 2000.

64. Estacio RO, Jeffers BW, Hiatt WR et al: The effect of nisoldipine as compared with enalapril on cardiovascular outcomes in patients with non-insulin-dependent diabetes and hypertension (ABCD). N Engl J Med 338:645, 1998.

65. Tatti P, Pahor M, Byington RP et al: Outcome results of the Fosinopril Versus Amlodipine Cardiovascular Events Randomized Trial (FACET) in patients with hypertension and NIDDM. Diabetes Care 21:597, 1998.

66. Tuomilehto J, Rastenyte D, Birkenhager WH et al: Effects of calcium-channel blockade in older patients with diabetes and systolic hypertension. Systolic Hypertension in Europe Trial Investigators. N Engl J Med 340:677, 1999.

67. Hansson L, Zanchetti A, Carruthers SG et al: Effects of intensive blood pressure lowering and low-dose aspirin in patients with hypertension: Principal results of the Hypertension Optimal Treatment (HOT) randomized trial. Lancet 351:1755, 1998.

68. Parving HH, Lehnert H, Brochner-Mortensen J et al: Irbesartan in Patients with Type 2 Diabetes and Microalbuminuria Study Group. The effect of irbesartan on the development of diabetic nephropathy in patients with type 2 diabetes. N Engl J Med 345:870, 2001.

69. Brenner BM, Cooper ME, de Zeeuw D et al: RENAAL Study Investigators Effects of losartan on renal and cardiovascular outcomes in patients with type 2 diabetes and nephropathy. N Engl J Med 345:861, 2001.

70. Bakris GL: A practical approach to achieving recommended blood pressure goals in diabetic patients. Arch Intern Med 161:2661, 2001.

71. American Diabetes Association: Treatment of hypertension in adults with diabetes. Diabetes Care 25:199, 2002.

72. DeFronzo RA, Ferrannini E: Insulin resistance. A multifaceted syndrome responsible for NIDDM, obesity, hypertension, dyslipidemia, and atherosclerotic cardiovascular disease. Diabetes Care 14:173, 1991.

73. Reaven GM, Lithell H, Landsberg L: Hypertension and associated metabolic abnormalities–the role of insulin resistance and the sympathoadrenal system. N Engl J Med 334:374, 1996.

74. Parulkar AA, Pendergrass ML, Granda-Ayala R et al: Nonhypoglycemic effects of thiazolidinediones. Ann Intern Med 134:61, 2001.

75. Walker AB, Chattington PD, Buckingham RE, Williams G: The thiazolidinedione rosiglitazone (BRL-49653) lowers blood pressure and protects against impairment of endothelial function in Zucker fatty rats. Diabetes 48:144, 1999.

76. Buchanan TA, Meehan WP, Jeng YY et al: Blood pressure lowering by pioglitazone. Evidence for a direct vascular effect. J Clin Invest 96:354, 1995.

77. Kaufman LN, Peterson MM, DeGrange LM: Pioglitazone attenuates diet-induced hypertension in rats. Metabolism 44:1105, 1995.

78. United Kingdom Prospective Diabetes Study (UKPDS) Group: Intensive blood-glucose control with sulfonylureas or insulin compared with conventional treatment and risk of complications in patients with type 2 diabetes (UKPDS 33). Lancet 352:837, 1998.

79. Stratton IM, Adler AI, Neil HAW et al, on behalf of the UK Prospective Diabetes Study Group: Association of glycaemia with macrovascular and microvascular complications of type 2 diabetes (UKPDS 35): Prospective observational study. BMJ 321:405, 2000.

80. Malmberg K: Prospective randomised study of intensive insulin treatment on long term survival after acute myocardial infarction in patients with diabetes mellitus. DIGAMI (Diabetes Mellitus, Insulin Glucose Infusion in Acute Myocardial Infarction) Study Group. BMJ 314:1512, 1997.

81. van den Berghe G, Wouters P, Weekers F et al: Intensive insulin therapy in the critically ill patients. N Engl J Med 345:1359, 2001.

82. Malmberg K, Yusef S, Gerstein HC et al: Impact of diabetes on long-term prognosis in patients with unstable angina and non–Q-wave myocardial infarction: Results of the OASIS (Organization to Assess Strategies for Ischemic Syndromes) registry. Circulation 102:1014, 2000.

83. Colwell JA: Aspirin therapy in diabetes. (Technical Review). Diabetes Care 20:1767, 1997.

84. ETDRS investigators: Aspirin effects on mortality and morbidity in patients with diabetes mellitus: Early Treatment Diabetic Retinopathy Study report 14. JAMA 268:1292, 1992.

85. Rolka DB, Fagot Campagna A, Venkat Narayan KM: Aspirin use among adults with diabetes: Estimates from the third national health and nutrition examination survey. Diabetes Care 24:197, 2001.

86. Koshiyama H, Shimono D, Kuwamura N et al: Rapid communication: Inhibitory effect of pioglitazone on carotid arterial wall thickness in type 2 diabetes. J Clin Endocrinol Metab 86:3452, 2001.

87. Bonora E, Kiechl S, Willeit J et al: Prevalence of insulin resistance in metabolic disorders: The Bruneck Study. Diabetes 47:1643, 1998.

88. Festa A, D'Agostino RJ, Howard G et al: Chronic Subclinical Inflammation as Part of the Insulin Resistance Syndrome: The Insulin Resistance Atherosclerosis Study (IRAS). Circulation 102:42, 2000.

89. Huang ES, Meigs JB, Singer DE: The effect of interventions to prevent cardiovascular disease in patients with type 2 diabetes mellitus. Am J Med 111:633, 2001.

90. McFarlane SI, Jacober SJ, Winer N et al: Control of cardiovascular risk factors in patients with diabetes and hypertension at urban academic medical centers. Diabetes Care 25:718, 2002.

OFFICE MANAGEMENT OF THE DIABETIC PATIENT

• WILLIAM HOWELL

The mainstay of the treatment of patients with diabetes occurs in an office setting. More than with most diseases, diabetes care requires an ongoing dialogue between patient and physician, and unlike individuals with other diseases, patients with diabetes themselves make many important decisions about their care. They need appropriate education and guidance from their physician and other health professionals. With the proper interaction between patient and physician, many hospitalizations can be avoided.

No matter how experienced and dedicated a physician is, both patients' knowledge of diabetes and their appropriate judgments in soliciting help from a physician are usually the critical factors that prevent minor problems from becoming major. The education of patients with diabetes is considered in detail in Chapter 12, which was written for patients as well as for the personnel (often nurses) carrying out the teaching. Although most physicians have neither the time nor the inclination to teach patients themselves, it is crucial that diabetic patients understand the material appropriate to their disease, as summarized in Chapter 12. If other professionals are not available to teach the diabetic patients, physicians should read Chapter 12 before carrying out the instructions. Physicians should provide written instructions for patients to take home with them, and patients should be encouraged to keep a list of questions that occur in between appointments. The Internet can be a good resource for patients and physicians should recommend links that would be appropriate for patients. These links include the American Diabetes Association (ADA) (www.diabetes.org) and Juvenile Diabetes Foundation (www.jdrf.org) Web sites, as well as the diabetes Web sites provided by the patient's medication and meter manufacturers.

A team approach to the management of patients with a chronic disease such as diabetes is crucial, and each member of the team serves a fundamental purpose. Although many primary physicians, and indeed many endocrinologists, do not work directly in a setting that allows access to experts in nutrition and education, it is important that they liaison with these services in the community. Referrals for diabetes management, education and nutrition enhance patient care and outcome.

INITIAL EVALUATION AND GENERAL FOLLOW-UP

The recommendations[1] of the ADA regarding history, physical examination, and laboratory evaluation during the initial visit are summarized in Table 9-1. A few comments about some of these elements are in order. For patients taking insulin, it is important to ascertain the frequency, timing (i.e., whether they commonly occur at a specific time of the day), and possible causes of hypoglycemic episodes. Information about unexplained hypoglycemia and especially about severe hypoglycemia (i.e., initiation of treatment by another person is necessary) is critically important to elicit. It is also very

helpful to determine a patient's typical schedule (i.e., time [and dose] of insulin injections, meals, snacks, and exercise) to give more appropriate advice about insulin therapy. It is often helpful to have a patient fill out a questionnaire prior to the office visit that includes questions about timing of meals, work, and exercise. This often facilitates communication with the patient.

Blood pressure should be monitored closely and treated vigorously if elevated. In addition to the well-known detrimental effects of hypertension—macrovascular diseases of the heart and central nervous system—hypertension is also associated with accelerated microvascular damage to the eyes[2-4] and kidneys.[5,6] Because periodontal disease is more common in people with dia-

---

TABLE 9-1 RECOMMENDED ELEMENTS OF THE HISTORY ON THE INITIAL VISIT

Medical history
- Symptoms, results of laboratory tests, and special examination results related to the diagnosis of diabetes
- Prior AIC records
- Eating patterns, nutritional status, and weight history; growth and development in children and adolescents
- Details of previous treatment programs, including nutrition and diabetes self-management education, attitudes, and health beliefs
- Current treatment of diabetes, including medications, meal plan, and results of glucose monitoring and patients' use of data
- Exercise history
- Frequency, severity, and cause of acute complications such as ketoacidosis and hypoglycemia
- Prior or current infections, particularly skin, foot, dental, and genitourinary infections
- Symptoms and treatment of chronic eye; kidney; nerve; genitourinary (including sexual), bladder, and gastrointestinal function (including symptoms of celiac disease in type I diabetic patients); heart; peripheral vascular; foot; and cerebrovascular complications associated with diabetes
- Other medications that may affect blood glucose levels
- Risk factors for atherosclerosis: smoking, hypertension, obesity, dyslipidemia, and family history
- History and treatment of other conditions, including endocrine and eating disorders
- Family history of diabetes and other endocrine disorders
- Lifestyle, cultural, psychosocial, educational, and economic factors that might influence the management of diabetes
- Tobacco, alcohol and/or controlled substance use
- Contraception and reproductive and sexual history

betes,[7] the oral examination should include an evaluation of the gums. Examination of the thyroid gland is important in patients with type 1 diabetes because of the association with Hashimoto's thyroiditis, another autoimmune disease.

Because diabetic patients have an increased susceptibility to macrovascular disease, it is important to carry out baseline recording of pulses and to check for the presence or absence of bruits. These pulses include the carotid, femoral, popliteal (more easily palpated if the leg is slightly bent), posterior tibialis, and dorsalis pedis. The arteries to be examined for bruits are those of the neck (carotid), abdomen (aorta), flanks (renal), and groin (iliac). Because diabetic patients are at risk for neuropathy, a baseline evaluation of the functioning of at least two components of the peripheral nervous system should be performed. Such an evaluation assesses the threshold for vibratory sensation (especially in the lower extremities) and the reflexes. Impairment of one or both of these components is the initial sign of peripheral neuropathy.

Examination of the feet should also determine whether patients able to sense the 5.07 (10-g) monofilament. This simple device, developed to assess patients with leprosy, has been very helpful in delineating which patients are at increased risk for amputation. Patients who are insensate to the 5.07 monofilament are nearly 20 times more likely to develop a foot ulcer that those who can feel it.[8] (The Semes 5.07 [10-g] monofilament can be ordered from Sensory Testing Systems, 1815 Dallas Dr., Suite 11A, Baton Rouge, LA 70806, phone [504] 927-7923, fax [504] 926-9053.)

The rationale for the laboratory evaluation is straightforward. The recommended initial laboratory evaluation is summarized in Table 9-2. Evaluation of the glycemic, lipid, and thyroid status of patients is necessary because, as discussed elsewhere, overwhelming evidence shows that restoring these indices toward normal has a positive

clinical benefit. The rationale for a baseline electrocardiogram is to document baseline abnormalities. Because patients with diabetes are at high risk for macrovascular disease, many need to undergo more dynamic testing to assess their cardiac status.[9,10] Urinalysis is performed to determine the presence of ketones, protein, and sediment. Because a general urinalysis is only sensitive for larger quantities of protein, a test for microalbuminuria should be obtained on patients with a urinalysis with results that are negative for protein.

Finally, diabetic patients should wear some form of medical identification. This is especially important for those taking insulin. If a patient is unable to give a history and a family member or friend is unavailable, he or she may accidentally be given inappropriate and perhaps dangerous therapy unless the medical personnel present are aware of the diabetes. Medic Alert bracelets or necklaces are the best form of identification. The information needed for ordering them is included in the Appendix to Chapter 12.

In addition to the guidelines recommended for initial evaluation of a patient with diabetes, the ADA has also outlined possible areas of referral, which are listed in Table 9-2. As mentioned, these ancillary support services are crucial to maintaining the best possible care for this subgroup of patients.

The elements of the history, physical examination, and management plan on the initial visit recommended by the ADA[1] are listed in Tables 9-1 and 9-2, and are very complete and represent the best possible approach to patients with diabetes. Similar extensive recommendations are suggested for the continuing care of diabetic patients.[1] However, given the current time and financial constraints under which physicians now practice, adhering to these recommendations is often not practical or even possible in some circumstances. Therefore the following guidelines are suggested for the

---

TABLE 9-2 RECOMMENDED ELEMENTS OF THE PHYSICAL EXAMINATION ON THE INITIAL VISIT

Physical Examination

- Height and weight measurement (and comparison to norms in children and adolescents)
- Sexual maturation staging (during pubertal period)
- Blood pressure determination, including orthostatic measurements when indicated, and comparison to age-related norms
- Fundoscopic examination
- Oral examination
- Thyroid palpation
- Cardiac examination
- Abdominal examination (e.g., for hepatomegaly)
- Evaluation of pulses by palpation and with auscultation
- Hand/finger examination
- Foot examination
- Skin examination (for acanthosis nigricans and insulin-injection sites)
- Neurological examination
- Signs of diseases that can cause secondary diabetes (e.g., hemochromatosis, pancreatic disease)

Laboratory evaluation

- A1C
- Fasting lipid profile, including total cholesterol, HDL cholesterol, triglycerides, and LDL cholesterol
- Test for microalbuminuria in type 1 diabetic patients who have had diabetes for at least 5 years and in all patients with type 2 diabetes. Some advocate beginning screening of pubertal children before 5 years of diabetes.
- Serum creatinine in adults (in children if proteinuria is present)
- Thyroid-stimulating hormone (TSH) in all type 1 diabetic patients; in type 2 if clinically indicated
- Electrocardiogram in adults
- Urinalysis for ketones, protein, sediment

Referrals

- Eye exam, if indicated
- Family planning for women of reproductive age
- MNT, as indicated
- Diabetes educator, if not provided by physician or practice staff
- Behavioral specialist, as indicated
- Foot specialist, as indicated
- Other specialties and services as appropriate

---

appropriate care of diabetes-related problems. These are mostly evidence-based outcome or process measures that have been shown to affect the health of patients *directly*. It is important to understand the difference between an outcome and a process measure. An example of a process measure would be a requirement to measure a glycated hemoglobin level four times a year. This *process* measure has not been shown to affect the health of patients with diabetes because A1C values remain fairly constant (and usually high) in an individual patient over many years.[11-15] The outcome measure is a target value to be achieved. This *outcome* measure is associated with markedly reduced risks for retinopathy, nephropathy, and neuropathy in both type 1[16] and type 2[17,18] diabetic patients. Those process measures (e.g., foot examinations) that almost assuredly will lead to improved outcomes (e.g., fewer amputations) are included in the guidelines, although no controlled studies have directly proved the connection.

1. *Self-monitoring of blood glucose (SMBG)*: Because major clinical trials have concluded that glycemic control plays an important role in the reduction of complications, SMBG allows patients and physicians to evaluate their response and assess whether their goals are being met.[19] Results help to adjust medications and lifestyle. Frequency and timing of monitoring is based on each individual's need and should be addressed with each patient at each visit. The results of SMBG should routinely be reviewed and the patients' technique and equipment should be evaluated on occasion.

2. *Glycated hemoglobin levels (now called A1C)*: The target value for A1C levels should be ≤7% (assuming an assay based on A1C levels with a normal range of 4% to 6%). This level is selected because the risks of development and progression of both retinopathy, and nephropathy[16-18,20] markedly increase in patients with diabetes who maintain higher A1C values. If the target level is being met, A1C levels should be measured at least every 6 months (although more frequent measurements identify deterioration of diabetic control sooner). If the target level is not met in patients taking insulin, A1C levels should be measured at least every 3 months.

3. *Low-density lipoprotein (LDL) cholesterol evaluation*; LDL cholesterol concentrations should be measured at least yearly or more often as necessary. The ADA suggests a target LDL cholesterol level of <100 mg/dl control because of the evidence that diabetic patients have a risk of an ischemic event similar to those who have already had a myocardial infarction.[21,22] The current National Cholesterol Education Program guidelines also consider diabetes to be a cardiovascular disease risk equivalent, and echo the same strict lipid control guidelines.[23]

4. *Fasting triglyceride (TG) evaluation*: Fasting TG concentrations should be measured at least yearly or more often as necessary. Target values for diabetic patients should be <200 mg/dl. Hypertriglyceridemia is associated with coronary artery disease in patients with type 2 diabetes, particularly because it is often found in conjunction with low high-density lipoprotein (HDL) cholesterol levels. Furthermore, it is also associated with small, dense LDL particles that are more atherogenic than normally constituted LDL particles. The approach to treating lipid disorders in patients with diabetes is described in Chapter 7.

5. *Renal evaluation*: A test for microalbuminuria should be performed every year. If microalbuminuria is confirmed, the patient should be treated with an angiotensin-converting enzyme inhibitors or an angiotensin receptor blocker unless contraindicated. The rationale for this guideline and the methods for evaluating microalbuminuria are discussed in detail in Chapter 7.

6. *Blood pressure evaluation*: The blood pressure should be measured at every regularly scheduled visit for diabetes or more often as necessary. The target value should be ≤130/80 mm Hg for all patients, although those with nephropathy may benefit from an even lower target of <125/75. To achieve these targets, use of three or more drugs for lower blood pressure may be required.

7. *Scheduling visits*: A regularly scheduled visit for diabetes should occur at least every 6 months as long as target values for A1C levels, lipids, and blood pressure are met. For perspective on how hard this is achieve, less than 5% of all

patients with diabetes seen in an endocrinologist's practice achieve all of these targets.[24] Should any of these exceed target values, patients should be seen at least every 3 months (or more often as necessary to achieve these goals).

8. *Retinal examination*: A dilated funduscopic examination by a health care provider trained in detecting retinopathy should be performed every year in most adults. Patients with new-onset type 1 diabetes who are greater than 10 years of age should have their initial exam within 3 to 5 years of diagnosis, but all patients with type 2 diabetes should have their first examination at the time of diagnosis. Use of nonmydriatic retinal photographs is under study and may replace dilated examinations in certain settings for retinopathy screening.[25] This guideline has been recommended by both the ADA[1] because early detection of diabetic retinopathy leading to laser photocoagulation at the appropriate time can prevent blindness.[26] Detecting and treating diabetic retinopathy is more cost-effective than many other routine health interventions.[27,28]

9. *Foot examination*: The feet should be examined at every regularly scheduled visit for diabetes because at least half of lower extremity amputations in diabetic patients are preventable by early detection and appropriate treatment.[29] It is important, however, to educate patients as to the actual risk for foot ulcers. All patients with diabetes should be aware of the risk and the need to examine their feet. However, young people with normal sensation and perfusion are at low risk for developing an asymptomatic foot ulcer. They should be taught to be aware of their feet, but need not worry excessively about foot care (their focus should be on maintaining normal blood glucose levels to prevent complications from ever developing). Patients with poor circulation, neuropathy, foot deformity, and/or a history of prior foot ulceration should be extremely vigilant about foot care. Their feet should be examined very thoroughly at every visit. They should be told to examine their feet twice a day (assistance by another may be required if the patient has limited vision and/or mobility). These patients may benefit from seeing a podiatrist, as well.

10. *Weight assessment*: Patients should be weighed at every regularly scheduled visit for diabetes. Although long-term dietary success occurs in only a minority of the 80% to 90% of patients with type 2 diabetes who are obese, documentation of current weight with continued encouragement for weight loss is successful in some patients. Conversely, documentation of unexplained weight loss may identify patients whose diabetic control is poor.

11. *Smoking assessment*: Smoking assessment should be carried out yearly, although patients who smoke should be encouraged to stop smoking at every visit. Patients who are current smokers should be counseled or referred to a smoking cessation program. Most patients do not realize that in addition to increasing the risk of cancer, smoking more than doubles the risk of myocardial infarction and peripheral vascular disease (which is already more than doubled by diabetes). Smoking also increases the risks for diabetic retinopathy and nephropathy.

12. *Aspirin*: Patients with diabetes who are older than 40 years should receive low-dose (75 to 325 mg) enteric-coated aspirin each day unless contraindicated. The beneficial effect of low-dose aspirin is clear in patients with established coronary artery disease, regardless of whether they have diabetes.[30] Although caution has been raised about the use of aspirin

in the presence of diabetic retinopathy, no increased risk of retinal or vitreous bleeding, even with relatively high doses of aspirin, was found in patients with established retinopathy enrolled in the Early Treatment Diabetic Retinopathy Study for a median period of 5 years.[31]

Other guidelines recommended by the ADA[1]—for example, those concerned with education and nutritional counseling,[32] are discussed in Chapter 12. Diabetes education and nutritional counseling are integral to helping patients understand and deal with a disease process that requires daily attention and adherence to principles of tight glycemic management.[33]

▼
MONITORING DIABETIC CONTROL

The importance of strict diabetic control was discussed in Chapter 2. The attainment of this goal is critically dependent on the ability to monitor the degree of control achieved. At present, four general methods are used to assess diabetic control, each of which is discussed in detail: (1) semiquantitative testing of urine for glucose and ketone bodies, (2) fasting and/or postprandial whole blood or plasma glucose determinations obtained sporadically at a chemistry laboratory or a physician's office, (3) SMBG, and (4) measurement of A1C levels, or other proteins (serum albumin, serum total protein).

SEMIQUANTITATIVE URINE TESTING

SMBG has made urine testing less attractive. The ADA states that given the ease of SMBG and the limitation of urine testing, SMBG is the better option for monitoring patients with diabetes. SMBG methods have become faster and less painful because they require smaller and smaller amounts of blood, and in the preprandial state can be performed on alternate sites (such as the forearm instead of the fingertips). Most patients will, with some encouragement, learn to measure their blood glucose levels at home, even if infrequently.

At present, urine testing is used in settings in which patients do not want or are unable to use SMBG. It is important that patients realize the limitations of urine testing. The measurement correlates with blood glucose level is not exact and cannot detect hypoglycemia. Also, the urine glucose value is only noted when the blood glucose level is above the renal threshold; this value is known to be approximately 180 mg/dl.

PLASMA GLUCOSE MEASUREMENTS

The role of plasma glucose concentration measured during an office visit has changed with the addition of A1C levels and SMBG to the management of diabetic patients. Indeed, the ADA now states that the assessment of glycemic control should not be made on the basis of a single plasma glucose value. It is recommended by the ADA that providers have the availability to provide immediate blood glucose testing, either a laboratory glucose test or finger-stick. During an office visit this value can determine if, at the time of measurement, the patient is hypoglycemic or severely hyperglycemic. It does not provide information on overall glycemic control. Use of an office glucose measurement can be helpful in calibrating a patient's blood glucose monitoring device. Most meters are now set to measure blood glucose as a plasma sample and can be compared with a plasma blood glucose level obtained in the laboratory (or on an office machine, such as a Hemocue, which is designed for accurate testing).

Self-Monitoring of Blood Glucose

The home management of diabetes has made a significant change in diabetic management. This change was ushered in and validated by the Diabetes Control and Complications Trial (DCCT). There are now many different instruments to measure blood glucose levels. These are relatively easy to use and patients can be quickly taught to do so. The DCCT makes it clear that maintaining blood glucose to a near-normal level is associated with decrease in eye, kidney, and nerve disease. In the DCCT, it was observed that the safest way to achieve near-normal blood sugar is to use SMBG. Thus all patients with type 1 diabetes should perform home glucose measurements. Ideally, this should be performed at multiple times during the day for patients to adjust their insulin doses. This is essentially true for all patients taking insulin injections, whether they have type 1 or type 2 diabetes.[19] In addition, the ADA recommends SMBG for patients on oral agents to monitor for hypoglycemia.[34] As for how often the diabetic patient should monitor blood glucose levels, it is generally agreed that patients on intensive insulin regimens should test their blood glucose levels at least three or four times a day. At this point there is no data to determine definitely how often patients with type 2 diabetes on oral agents should check their blood glucose levels. It is generally felt that patients with type 2 diabetes should be provided with access to SMBG and should test when treatment changes are made and during periods of illness and stress. Pre- and postexercise measurements may be helpful to the patient to become aware of the effects of exercise. Additionally, it is often helpful for patients to periodically test 2 hours after eating to learn the relationship between blood glucose levels and carbohydrate intake. Clearly, testing frequency should be individualized, although as a general rule of thumb, patients test more often initially, while learning, and then perhaps two to three times per week subsequently.

Proper patient education on blood glucose monitoring technique is important. Each meter comes with an instruction manual and many now have useful videos. However, the patient should be shown how to use the meter by a health care provider and subsequently observed using the SMBG instrument. The date and time should be set correctly in the meter so that data can be downloaded accurately from the memory in the future. In addition, the patient should be encouraged to use calibration solutions on a regular basis. If the patient's recorded values appear to be inconsistent with the A1C value, the use of the home monitor should be reassessed (such issues as expiration date and storage of strips can alter glucose readings.)

Many meters have memories. Therefore patients should be told to bring their meters to every office visit. Although patients should be encouraged to log their blood glucose values, food intake, and exercise patterns in a log book, scrolling through the memory in the meter can be very helpful. In addition, simple software programs are provided by the meter companies so that the meters can be downloaded in the office. These printed summaries of data help evaluate trends in glucose levels. Additionally, some meter companies have Web sites so patients can download their meter data from home and send it to the physician. Although this technology is not currently available for everyone, those with access can benefit from more frequent evaluation of their blood glucose monitoring data.

A1C Levels

Measurements of Hgb A_1, Hgb A_{1c}, and glycated hemoglobin[35,36] were introduced into clinical practice approximately 15 years ago as an index of long-term diabetic control, and are now widely used. The newest terminology for describing this measure is *A1C*. This change was made so that patients do not confuse *hemoglobin*, a measure associated with red blood cells (RBCs), and *hemoglobin A_{1c}*, a measure of glycation of RBCs.

In normal individuals, 90% of hemoglobin consists of two alpha chains and two beta chains and is called *Hgb A*. Approximately 2% of hemoglobin contains two alpha chains and two delta chains (Hgb A_2, a normal variant), whereas 1% is fetal hemoglobin (Hgb F), which is composed of two alpha chains and two gamma chains. The remaining 7% of hemoglobin also consists of two alpha chains and two beta chains, with either glucose or a derivative of glucose attached to the beta chain. If glucose is attached, the resulting hemoglobin is called *Hgb A_{1c}*. Hgb A_{1c} is the major component of these hemoglobins and constitutes approximately 5% of total hemoglobins in nondiabetic persons. A number of hemoglobins with glucose derivatives attached have also been isolated. Two of these are Hgb A_{1a} and Hgb A_{1b}, each of which makes up approximately 1% of total hemoglobins in nondiabetic individuals. Because all these hemoglobins contain glucose or one of its derivatives, they are known collectively as *Hgb A_1*.

These additions to the end of the beta chain change the charge characteristics of Hgb A so that the molecules travel faster in certain chromatographic separation techniques, such as ion chromatography, electrophoresis, or high-performance liquid chromatography.

Early longitudinal studies revealed that levels of Hgb A_{1c}[37] and Hgb A_1[38] correlate best with the degree of diabetic control obtained several months earlier. This is expected because of the 120-day life span of the RBC and because the glycation reaction of hemoglobin is mostly irreversible. The lag period before an improvement in diabetic control is reflected in changes in Hgb A_{1c} levels, as shown in Figure 9-1.

Glycation results are influenced by the conditions under which the blood is collected, shipped, and stored; the columns are very sensitive to changes in temperature and buffer pH; falsely high levels may be found in patients with thalassemia (Hgb F coelutes with Hgb A_1), uremia, and lead poisoning; in patients ingesting large doses of aspirin; and in patients with high blood levels of alcohol, TGs, and bilirubin.[38,39] Some hemoglobinopathies invalidate measurements of Hgb A_{1c} and Hgb A_1. In addition to thalassemia, falsely high values are found in

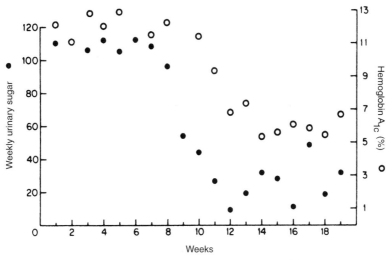

FIGURE 9-1. Temporal relation between weekly urinary glucose levels and hemoglobin A_{1c} in one patient. Urinary glucose was measured semiquantitatively with Clinitest tablets (on a scale of 0 to 4+) four times a day. The results were summed every 7 days to obtain a mean weekly index. *(From Koenig RJ, Peterson CM, Jones RL et al: Correlation of glucose regulation and hemoglobin A_{1c} in diabetes mellitus. N Engl J Med 295:417, 1976.)*

hemoglobinopathies J, K, I, H, Bart's, Raleigh (β_1 ala), Long Island (β_2 pro), and South Florida (β_1 met).[40] Falsely low values are noted in hemoglobinopathies S, D, C, E, G, Lepore, and O-Arab.[40,41] Interference by many of the foregoing factors varies, depending on the assay used,[42] and again, physicians should ascertain the performance of the method used in their laboratory. In such cases, a fructosamine test may be ordered. This test is discussed in detail later in this chapter.

Hgb A_{1c} or Hgb A_1 is not a true measure of glycated hemoglobin.[43] More refined analyses showed that only 60% to 80% of Hgb A_{1c} is glycated. Fortuitously, the values of Hgb A_{1c} and glycated hemoglobin are similar because the amount of nonglycated hemoglobin in Hgb A_{1c} is approximately the same as the amount of glycated hemoglobin in Hgb A that is not measured by the ion chromatography method of separation. Two additional important points must be kept in mind in interpreting the results. Because glycation occurs throughout the life span of the RBC, the presence of conditions that shorten RBC survival (hemolytic anemias, bleeding) produce falsely low values. Conversely, if the life span of the RBC is extended (e.g., by splenectomy), the values are falsely high. Finally, ingestion of large amounts (e.g., >1.0 g/day) of vitamins C[44] and E[45] may lower glycated hemoglobin levels by blocking glycation of proteins.

There seems to be little doubt that levels of total glycated hemoglobin, stable Hgb A_{1c}, and stable Hgb A_1 are an excellent time-integrated measure of overall diabetic control. The National Glycohemoglobin Standardization Program (http://web. missouri.edu/~diabetes/ngsp.html) was designed to help standardize A1C assays to the DCCT reference method. Ideally all A1C values will be certified through this program or one like it to enable comparisons between different physician offices. They are valuable in assessing control, both in diabetic populations and in individual patients.

However, because the lag period before this index reflects changes in diabetic control, it is not as helpful in deciding changes in day-to-day therapy. For instance, a physician would not necessarily know exactly what change to make in the insulin prescription on the basis of a high level of A1C. On the other hand, this measure may be of value in patients whose office test results (or the record they bring to the office) do not coincide with other indices of diabetic control. Glycated hemoglobin levels should be used routinely to monitor diabetic control, because physicians' estimates of control based on historical and laboratory data collected during a routine office visit correlated poorly with the degree of control assessed by A1C levels.[46]

Many patients attempting to achieve near euglycemia measure glucose levels before meals and bedtime, but not postprandially as well. Even though preprandial levels seem satisfactory, glycated hemoglobin values not infrequently are higher than anticipated. This requires further efforts to achieve control, the need for which would not have been evident simply by evaluating the results of SMBG. The relation between fasting and 2-hour postprandial glucose concentrations obtained at clinic visits and stable A1C values in patients with type 1 diabetes is depicted in Figure 9-2. This information furnishes a general context in which to judge diabetic control from a stable A1C value (upper limit of normal is 6.1%). In general, it is believed that a 1% change in A1C values represents a change in the average blood glucose concentration of approximately 30 mg/dl.[38,47]

Glycated Serum Protein

Glycation of proteins is a general phenomenon and enhanced glycation of many proteins occurs in diabetes. Glycated albumin constitutes approximately 80% of the major proteins that are glycated.[48] Because the albumin's half-life is between 17 and 20 days

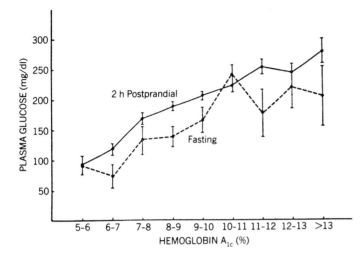

FIGURE 9-2. Relationship between stable hemoglobin A_{1c} and both fasting and 2-hour postprandial plasma glucose concentrations in diabetic youths. Points and vertical lines represent mean ±SEM of a total of 1172 values in 187 patients. *(From Goldstein DE, Parker KM, England JD et al: Clinical application of glycosylated hemoglobin measurements. Diabetes 31 [suppl 3]:70, 1982.)*

as compared with the 120-day half-life of hemoglobin, the changes in glycated serum albumin reflect changes in diabetes control more quickly than glycated hemoglobin.

Glycated albumin is usually measured using affinity chromatography.[49] The glycated serum proteins (GSPs) are separated from the non-GSPs by their difference in chemical reactivity in a fructosamine assay.[50] GSPs have been noted to correlate with glycated hemoglobin values.[51] One place for the use of the glycated proteins is in the setting of hemolytic anemia, in which the A1C levels are noted to be inaccurate. At this point no studies have proven the effectiveness of using the glycated proteins.

MONITORING PATIENTS WHO TAKE INSULIN

Many patients with diabetes require insulin injection. This includes patients with type 1 and type 2 diabetes on multiple injection regimens, patients using an insulin pump, patients with type 2 diabetes on a twice-daily injection regimen, and patients with type 2 diabetes on bedtime insulin plus oral agents. As discussed elsewhere, there are now many types and preparations of insulin, with more

to come. It must be remembered through this maze of treatment options that the ultimate goal is glycemic control as shown in the DCCT and the United Kingdom Prospective Diabetes Study (UKPDS). There are many insulin preparations to choose from, and the choice is at times dictated by the insurance coverage a particular patient does or does not have, patient lifestyle, preferences, and other agents being used for blood glucose control. Glycemic control can be viewed as a mountain peak with many routes to the top. The decision is based on many factors, including physician experience. The physician who is successful using regular insulin and neutral protein hagedorn (NPH) should continue if her or his patients are achieving near-euglycemia. The new preparations may be considered when a patient is not achieving adequate control on a particular regimen.

It is not widely appreciated that sensitivity to exogenous insulin in diabetic patients can vary over time.[52] This can happen in the absence of a recognizable cause (e.g., infection, weight change, emotional stress) and occurs more often in patients with type 1 diabetes. For this reason, it is usually inadequate to assign an insulin regimen to a patient and evaluate it only every 3 to 6 months during an office visit. Insulin doses need to be changed much more frequently, either by the physician, by the diabetic educator, or by the patient with the physician's guidance. This requires that patients collect ongoing information about their degree of diabetic control. SMBG, as discussed previously, is a valuable tool that allows health care providers to review needed information to allow for adjustments of medications to provide optimal control. Even though achieving near-normal glucose levels without undue hypoglycemia is important, factors such as inconvenience, cost, discomfort, and frustration limit SMBG. Providers should be aware of the different resources available, which include systems for obtaining free meters and test strips, and devices on the market that allow for more convenience and less discomfort. This includes meters that allow blood to be collected from sites other than finger tips and lancets that allow patients to dial in the depth that affords the least discomfort.

FASTING HYPERGLYCEMIA

The most difficult test result to bring under control in patients requiring insulin is often the fasting glucose concentration, although achieving success has become easier with the advent of stable, long-acting insulin such as glargine. Assuming that no untoward event has occurred (e.g., large bedtime snack), three reasons for fasting hyperglycemia are possible: waning of insulin action, the dawn phenomenon, and the Somogyi phenomenon. The first situation is due to an inadequate dose of that insulin preparation that is supposed to cover the overnight period.[53] The dawn phenomenon is caused by insensitivity to insulin between approximately 4 AM and 8 AM because of the sleep-induced surge of growth hormone secretion.[54,55] This causes increased lipolysis (i.e., increased free fatty acid release by adipose tissue) during the next several hours, which subsequently

modestly raises glucose concentrations in the period before breakfast,[56] probably via enhanced gluconeogenesis. The Somogyi phenomenon is hyperglycemia caused by the release of counterregulatory hormones after unrecognized hypoglycemia.[55] A great deal of research has led to the following conclusions. First, unrecognized nocturnal hypoglycemia in insulin-requiring diabetic patients is common, especially in type 1 diabetes.[53,57-59] Second, this hypoglycemia rarely causes rebound fasting hyperglycemia.[57–59] Third, although the dawn phenomenon can occur in some patients, the frequency and magnitude are variable.[58] The clinical lessons from these studies are that the Somogyi phenomenon is an unusual cause of fasting hyperglycemia. Waning of insulin action is the most likely reason for fasting hyperglycemia.[53,55] Clinically, it is not important to distinguish between insulin waning and the dawn phenomenon because both situations require provision of more insulin for the overnight period. If relatively large increases seem necessary, it is wise to have the patient perform SMBG at 2 AM to 3 AM to ascertain that hypoglycemia is not occurring at this time. If this is the case, switching the intermediate-acting insulin to bedtime or changing to a long-acting insulin such as glargine helps reduce the fasting hyperglycemia and avoids the dangers of nocturnal hypoglycemia. Alternatively, a patient can be started on an insulin pump, with adjustable overnight basal rates.

MONITORING PATIENTS WHO DO NOT TAKE INSULIN

As described elsewhere in this text, there are now many agents for the management of the patient with type 2 diabetes. From a blood glucose standpoint, the goal is the same as with the insulin user: glycemic control. The recently published Diabetes Prevention Program[60] has shown an unequivocal reduction in risk for developing type 2 diabetes in individuals who are able to adhere to lifestyle recommendations. As stated previously, it is our opinion that SMBG is a valuable tool in patients with diabetes who are not on insulin. It is a useful teaching tool that allows patients to see the consequences of their actions. The immediate feedback furnished by SMBG under different dietary circumstances can teach patients better than any lectures or reading material about which foods to avoid, which ones have the least effect on the blood glucose values, and—the usual problem with these individuals—how meal size affects glucose levels.

Oral medications may be adjusted and changed based on information acquired. For example, with newer oral agents such as repaglinide and nateglinide, dosing before meals may be titrated based on 2-hour postprandial values. In essence, the reason to obtain SMBG information in this group of patients is exactly the same as the reasons listed previously for those patients on insulin. The ultimate goal remains the same—good control—and SMBG is a great tool to help achieve that goal.

GOALS OF THERAPY

Suggested levels of diabetic control for patients requiring insulin who perform SMBG are listed in Table 9-2. The level of control is affected, at least initially, by (1) the age of the patient, (2) the patient's awareness of hypoglycemic symptoms and/or the presence of autonomic neuropathy, and (3) the presence of any comorbidities that may shorten remaining life expectancy. Understanding the hormonal response to hypoglycemia in nondiabetic and diabetic subjects is important for arriving at this decision. In nondiabetic patients and those with type 2 diabetes, four hormones are secreted in response to hypoglycemia. Glucagon and the catecholamines epinephrine and norepinephrine are released rapidly and have an immediate

effect in restoring blood glucose values toward normal. The secretion of growth hormone and cortisol is delayed, and their anti-insulin effect does not occur immediately, but is long lasting. Selective blockade of each of these hormones during hypoglycemia[61] revealed that (1) as long as glucagon was secreted, glucose levels were restored normally; (2) if glucagon was absent but the catecholamines were present, restoration was delayed but eventually occurred; (3) growth hormone and cortisol secretion were unnecessary for return of glucose levels to normal (at least in the short term); and (4) if both glucagon and catecholamines were absent, glucose concentrations remained at the nadir levels. This latter observation becomes extremely important in patients with type 1 diabetes because within a year or two of diagnosis, the glucagon response to hypoglycemia is impaired,[62] even though glucagon is hypersecreted by these patients under other circumstances. By 4 years after the diagnosis, the glucagon response is minimal.[62] Furthermore, the catecholamine response to hypoglycemia also is markedly blunted after 5 years of having developed type 1 diabetes, even in the absence of clinical autonomic neuropathy.[63] Thus in patients with type 1 diabetes who have had their diabetes for more than 5 years, there is a good chance that secretion of both of the critical hormones necessary to respond to hypoglycemia is either absent or markedly impaired. Secretion of the counterregulatory hormones remains either intact or nearly so in patients with type 2 diabetes.

An important factor in achieving tight glucose control has to do with the variability of a patient's lifestyle. If a patient has very constant patterns of eating and activity, a fixed insulin dose regimen works well. However, if a patient has a more varied schedule and meal intake, a flexible multiple injection regimen or insulin pump therapy is preferable. In either situation, a balance must always be achieved between attempting to return glucose concentrations to near euglycemia and the risk of hypoglycemia. Under the present relatively crude system of replacing or supplementing endogenous insulin with exogenous insulin, some episodes of hypoglycemia are almost unavoidable if glucose concentrations are to approach normal most of the time. As is noted in the DCCT, there are likely hypoglycemic events associated with tight control. Insulin analogs, such as lispro, aspart, and glargine all decrease the frequency of hypoglycemic events. More frequent monitoring, education about carbohydrate counting, and adjusting for exercise and prevailing blood glucose levels can also help improve a patient's ability to maintain glucose levels in the near-normal range. If a patient is having severe, recurrent episodes of hypoglycemia, it is important to aim for higher glycemic targets, which will help patients avoid such episodes and may help restore their ability to sense impending hypoglycemia.

The goal of therapy in regard to A1C levels obtained every 2 to 3 months can be simply stated: to achieve normal values. However, the closer patients are to normal, the more hypoglycemia patients requiring insulin experience, especially severe hypoglycemia.[64,65] Therefore a balance must be struck between the two. Because A1C values do not guide day-to-day therapeutic decisions, they are used to help decide whether or not more determined efforts need to be made to optimize control. As discussed earlier, the development and progression of diabetic retinopathy and nephropathy markedly increase at A1C levels >7%. Although a target level below this value is desirable in most patients, higher values might be more appropriate in some (e.g., those who are frail, older, or who have significant coronary artery or cerebrovascular disease, advanced microvascular complications, or hypoglycemia unawareness). Some patients are doing the best they can, and improvement is not possible. Many patients,

however, are able to improve their control (or actually their compliance with the prescribed therapeutic regimen yielding better control), and A1C levels serve as the reminder.

"HONEYMOON PHASE" OF TYPE 1 DIABETES

Shortly after the onset of type 1 diabetes, a *temporary* remission occurs in approximately 20% of patients (even in those who were in profound diabetic ketoacidosis [DKA]). This is termed the *honeymoon phase.* The clinical manifestation of this remission varies from a moderate reduction in insulin requirement to complete normalization of glucose tolerance without therapy. Secretion of endogenous insulin returns, at least in part, during the remission period.[66] The duration of the honeymoon phase usually is short, lasting from a few weeks to several months, although an occasional patient may remain in remission for many years. Although evidence suggests that the earlier and more intensive the initial treatment, the more likely and longer the remission will be, diabetes always returns. Thus it is important to be aware of this phenomenon both to anticipate the possible decrease in insulin requirements and to avoid offering patients false hope that the diabetes has been cured.

WEIGHT REDUCTION IN OBESE PATIENTS WITH DIABETES

Given that weight reduction is a goal in the management, it is advised that the practitioner encourage weight reduction. Moreover, the services of a nutritionist or referral to a weight reduction program should be provided. The recently published Diabetes Prevention Program showed the benefit of weight reduction on glycemia in at risk individuals.[60] Weight control was achieved and maintained with a low-calorie, low-fat diet combined with increased exercise. Further support for a low-calorie, balanced diet combined with exercise can be found in the National Weight Control Registry.[67] This is a registry of patients who have lost weight and maintained their weight loss for more than 1 year. More than 3000 patients are enrolled in this registry, and the most common findings in these patients who have been successful in losing weight and maintaining weight loss is a low-fat, low-calorie (not restricted) diet and significant exercise, totaling more than 2500 calories per week. This amounts to walking 3 to 4 miles a day.

In managing patients with diabetes who are obese, there is the question of whether these patients would benefit from the oral medications available for the reduction of weight. Two agents are available for use in patients who are diabetic: orlistat (Xenical), a fat absorption blocker, and sibutramine hydrochloride monohydrate (Meridia), a centrally acting agent that blocks the neuronal uptake of norepinephrine and, to a lesser extent, serotonin and dopamine. Both agents were associated with a small amount of weight reduction in the diabetic population.[68,69] Only orlistat had a slight decrease in the A1C. At this time, the ADA feels the drugs offer only a small benefit and should only be used in obese patients. The body mass index (BMI) should be greater than 27.0 kg/m^2.[70] In patients without diabetes, hypertension or hyperlipidemia, the recommended BMI for starting sibutramine is greater than 30 kg/m^2. It would appear these agents are best used as a part of a weight loss regimen.

Weight reduction in the morbidly obese population with diabetes is a complex issue. It is clear that if individuals lose a significant amount of weight, their glycemic control will improve. The question that the patients and practitioner must ask is whether the price of surgery is too high for the goal? In any clinical practice in a large urban setting

there are anecdotes that support and refute the use of surgery. Two procedures that have been studied in the diabetic population are gastric bypass and vertical banding gastroplasty. A 3-year study following patients who had the banded gastroplasty procedure had a 32-kg weight loss at 3 years.[71] In addition, a large study using the gastric bypass procedure yielded weight loss of 45 kg at 3 years. They are both of impressive value when read by practitioners that are working to achieve weight control among their patients. The reported mortality rate for the procedures are 1% to 2%. Some of the complications observed are persistent vomiting, vitamin loss, diarrhea, and wound dehiscence. At present, a consensus committee of the ADA would like to have trials performed that compare medical intervention with surgical intervention. The decision to recommend surgery for a patient who trusts the primary provider is certainly a difficult one. The current ADA recommendation is to reserve surgical intervention for patients with BMIs $>35.0 \text{ kg/m}^2$.[70]

HYPOGLYCEMIA

Chapter 6 describes the recognition and treatment of hypoglycemia in a treated patient with diabetes. Hypoglycemia is often the limiting factor in attempting to achieve near-normal blood glucose levels, although newer insulins and monitoring devices (such as sensors) may decrease the frequency of hypoglycemia episodes in intensively treated patients. At each visit patients should be asked about the frequency and severity of their hypoglycemic episodes. Recognition, treatment, and prevention of future episodes should be reviewed. Patients should be queried as to whether or not they are carrying a rapid-acting form of carbohydrate with them. All patients on insulin injections should have rapid-acting carbohydrate with them at all times. It is important to include documentation of the hypoglycemia discussion in the patient's chart. In a patient with hypoglycemia unawareness, this discussion should also include a strategy for safe driving (if a patient drives). Generally this includes testing the blood glucose level immediately before driving and then at intervals thereafter. Just as in other circumstances, patients should carry a supply of rapid-acting carbohydrate with them while driving.

Two studies have attempted to quantitate the response to various treatments for (laboratory-induced) hypoglycemia.[72,73] Their conclusions were that 15 to 20 g of glucose in tablet form or in solution were appropriate for treating these patients. The responses to juices and gels were delayed in both studies. In our experience, patients often have a marked improvement in symptoms with 10 to 15 g of glucose. Our patients are treated just to the point at which they feel better rather than to the point of complete disappearance of symptoms. If the symptoms are not definitely improved in 10 to 15 minutes, another 10 to 15 g of glucose is taken, and this should be repeated every 15 minutes until the symptoms have definitely improved. This conservative approach avoids overtreatment with resultant marked hyperglycemia, an all too common occurrence. If patients perform SMBG at this time, the results can be particularly helpful. Rising values signal a suitable response. Moreover, if the test is performed before

treatment and the symptoms are not associated with a low concentration of glucose, inappropriate therapy is avoided. If, however, the symptoms are severe, a patient cannot test, or past experience has shown that these symptoms are most always the result of hypoglycemia, glucose should be taken without delay. Temporary hyperglycemia is preferable to the risk of severe hypoglycemia.

Table 9-3 lists readily available sources that contain 10 g of glucose. If the next meal is more than 30 to 60 minutes away, the patient should also eat small amounts of complex carbohydrate, equivalent to 1 bread exchange, and 1 to 2 ounces of protein to prevent the recurrence of hypoglycemia. In this manner, hypoglycemic episodes are handled appropriately and are not overtreated.

Hypoglycemia secondary to the use of sulfonylurea agents usually lasts longer than insulin-induced hypoglycemia. Therefore continued treatment for many hours may be necessary to prevent a recurrence. If moderate to marked mentation changes have occurred, hospitalization is advisable, because intravenous glucose therapy is usually necessary for several days.

Finally, it is important to reiterate that if a patient taking acarbose or miglitol experiences hypoglycemia resulting from the concomitant administration of insulin or a sulfonylurea agent, it must be treated with

TABLE 9-3 COMMONLY AVAILABLE SOURCES OF 10 G OF GLUCOSE	
Orange juice	1 cup[*]
Grape juice	½ cup
Table sugar	4 teaspoons[†]
Honey	3 teaspoons
Lifesavers	10
B-D glucose tablets	2
DextroEnergy glucose tablets	3
Dex 4 glucose tablets	2.5
Glutose tablets	2

[*]1 cup = 8 ounces (fluid).

[†]1 tablespoon = 3 teaspoons.

glucose tablets because acarbose blocks the digestion and therefore the absorption of other sources of carbohydrate. Because acarbose does not inhibit lactase, milk might also be an appropriate treatment, although there are no published reports attesting to this.

STARVATION KETOSIS

The mechanism of starvation ketosis is similar to that of diabetic ketosis: increased breakdown of TGs in adipose tissue to free fatty acids, with their subsequent conversion to ketone bodies in the liver (see Chapter 2). In diabetic ketosis, the absence of insulin causes overproduction of free fatty acids; in starvation ketosis, the signal is an underutilization of carbohydrates secondary to decreased carbohydrate intake. The utilization of approximately 80 to 100 g of exogenous carbohydrate per day is required to prevent ketosis. If much less than that amount is available, energy requirements in tissue must be met by increased fat metabolism, which leads to ketosis as described earlier. Although decreased carbohydrate intake is usually associated with diminished ingestion of total calories, ketosis also can occur with eucaloric diets that are low in carbohydrates. Thus the term *starvation ketosis* is not entirely accurate.

There are two ways to distinguish between diabetic and starvation ketosis. The former almost always is associated with marked glucosuria, but the latter is not. However, ketonuria may interfere with the glucose reactions on Keto-Diastix, and patients with type 1 diabetes thus may need an independent check of mild glucosuria occurring in the presence of moderate to large ketonuria by retesting with either Chemstrip uG, Diastix, or Clinitest tablets. Alternatively, glucose levels can be measured by SMBG, although DKA can occur with blood glucose levels less than 200 mg/dl.[74] The most accurate way to distinguish between diabetic and starvation ketosis is to measure plasma ketone bodies. The degree of ketosis is much greater in uncontrolled diabetic patients than in patients whose ketosis is due primarily to inadequate carbohydrate intake. Therefore in diabetic ketosis, results of the nitroprusside test for plasma ketone bodies remain positive when the sample is diluted. In contrast, in starvation ketosis, the results almost invariably are negative after dilution. Clinically, patients with evolving DKA feel sick whereas those with starvation ketosis have relatively few symptoms.

In two situations, differentiation between diabetic and starvation ketosis is important. The first involves obese patients with type 2 diabetes who maintain a hypocaloric diet whose carbohydrate content is low enough to lead to starvation ketosis. This usually is not difficult to distinguish from diabetic ketosis, because the ketosis resistance of patients will already have been established at the time of diagnosis. Furthermore, the urine test results should show little glucosuria. The other circumstance involves patients type 1 diabetes who become ill with gastrointestinal symptoms and are forced to limit their oral intake of food. This can be a difficult situation to resolve. On the one hand, gastrointestinal symptoms can be part of evolving ketoacidosis. Therefore establishing the presence of diabetic ketosis and treating it vigorously is important in preventing hospitalization (see the following section on sick day rules). On the other hand, if the situation is really one of viral gastroenteritis associated with starvation ketosis, overtreatment with insulin may cause hypoglycemia. Although a comparison of the degrees of glucosuria and ketonuria often help in making the decision, patients may need to go to a laboratory facility for measurement of plasma ketone bodies and possibly serum bicarbonate levels.

SICK DAY RULES

In the presence of an infection of any kind, insulin action is impaired by unknown mechanisms. Therefore in such circumstances, diabetic control usually worsens, often quickly and profoundly. Patients with diabetes should alert their care team if they are experiencing an intercurrent illness. Patients with diabetes may become more easily dehydrated and thus more often require hospitalization.[1] Because normal food intake is diminished, patients sometimes decrease their insulin dose or omit it altogether. This is inadvisable for patients with type 1 diabetes. These patients should take the prescribed amount and often even require additional insulin. Patients can take their usual insulin dose and use the regimen shown in Table 9-4 for supplementing it if necessary. One scenario is to use 300 mg/dl as a level at which to add extra insulin. Patients should initially measure their glucose level before each meal. If the value is >300 mg/dl, they should take an additional 4 U of regular or rapid-acting insulin for lean patients and 8 U for obese patients. It is extremely important to ensure that patients with type 1 diabetes also measure ketones in their urine. If, in the presence of these levels of hyperglycemia, the ketone test in the urine is moderate or strong, an additional 4 U of regular or rapid acting insulin should be taken. Glucose measurements should be repeated in 3 to 4 hours to ascertain that a response occurred. For patients with gastrointestinal symptoms, whether resulting from a viral gastroenteritis or possibly secondary to evolving DKA, it is critical to ensure their ability to maintain oral fluid intake. Once the symptoms have progressed to the point at which oral intake is no longer possible, patients must be admitted to a hospital for parenteral fluid therapy. This underscores the importance of frequent testing on days that patients are ill so that this eventuality can be minimized.

Patients who are on a multiple-injection regimen with varying premeal doses of insulin based on carbohydrate counting and correction doses based on the prevailing blood glucose levels may need to alter their ratios when ill. For example, if a patient usually takes 1 U of rapid-acting insulin for every 50 mg/dl above 100 mg/dl, this ratio may need to be changed (doubled) to 1 U for every 25 mg/dl above the target blood glucose level. Another way to talk to patients is to ask what their correction doses are (or sliding scale) for their insulin dose and then suggest doubling it during the period of illness. Sometimes it also helps to increase the basal dose of insulin, although it is important to reduce the dose back to the usual amount as the patient recovers and the insulin resistance abates.

The approach just described for adjusting insulin doses can also be used for patients whose diabetic control deteriorates in association with other kinds of stress (e.g., emotional upsets, trauma). Effective and frequent communication between patient and physician is an important component of care during these periods. Most hospitalizations can be avoided if adjustments in treatment are started early and continued appropriately.

TABLE 9-4 SICK DAY RULES			
1. Take usual insulin dose.			
2. Additional insulin based on results of self-monitoring of blood glucose.			
		Additional Regular or Lispro/Aspart Insulin*	
Blood Glucose	Urine Ketones	Lean	Obese
>300 mg/dl	Negative, trace, small	4	8
>300 mg/dl	Moderate, Large	8	12

*Or double usual compensatory scale

Patients with type 2 diabetes are less of a problem than patients with type 1 diabetes. Their resistance to ketosis most often persists, and they very seldom become ketotic. The increasing hyperglycemia may need treatment, but their metabolic status does not deteriorate to the point at which hospitalization is required. Because these episodes are self-limited, treatment regimens in patients on dietary therapy alone or dietary therapy supplemented with oral antidiabetes medication usually are not altered. The dose of the sulfonylurea agent can be increased temporarily if a patient becomes very symptomatic from uncontrolled diabetes. (Theoretically, one could increase the doses of metformin or acarbose temporarily, but their gastrointestinal side effects make this approach problematic.) However, the benefits of starting either oral hypoglycemic therapy (in those on diet alone) or insulin are outweighed by inconvenience and by the short period for which these new therapies should be necessary. Furthermore, because most patients with type 2 diabetes are obese, the decreased food intake usually associated with illness tends to offset the worsening of control secondary to the infection in these patients.

In addition to adjusting insulin doses, three other modalities of treatment are important in infected diabetic patients: carbohydrate intake, and (in patients with vomiting, diarrhea, or marked polyuria) fluid (sodium) and potassium replacement. Because most of these patients receive insulin, some carbohydrate intake is important. A method for obtaining carbohydrate from more easily digestible foods is described in detail elsewhere in this book. For some patients, this is not feasible because either they are not properly educated in this approach or their gastrointestinal symptoms may prevent them from eating the appropriate amounts of food. These patients should eat foods that they can tolerate from the milk, fruit, bread, and vegetable exchange lists. Liquids and soft foods are easier to digest, and patients are often able to consume six to eight smaller meals more easily than three to four larger ones. Soft drinks (not low-calorie ones) and fruit juices are good sources of carbohydrates.

Fluid losses from the kidneys or gastrointestinal tract are high in sodium. To avoid marked depletion of the intravascular volume (dehydration), replacement must be with fluids that contain relatively large amounts of sodium. As long as enough insulin and fluids can be given, hospitalization can often be avoided. When the severity of the gastrointestinal symptoms precludes oral intake of fluid, patients usually must be hospitalized. Two good sources of sodium are bouillon (1 cup contains ~40 mEq) and tomato juice (1 cup contains ~20 mEq). Other foods high in sodium are canned soups, saltine crackers, and packaged custard pudding mixes. Salt can be added to other juices. Soft drinks contain little sodium.

Sources high in potassium include orange juice, tomato juice, and prune juice (1 cup ~15 mEq). Foods with moderate potassium content (1 cup contains ~10 mEq) include milk, grapefruit juice, and pineapple juice. Apple juice, grape juice, and cranberry juice are low in potassium (1 cup ~5 mEq). A large banana contains ~10 mEq of potassium.

EXERCISE

Exercise is receiving more and more attention as a general health measure to prevent diabetes[60,75,76] as well as a helpful adjunct in managing it.[77-79] It is helpful, however, to put the role of exercise in these patients in its proper perspective. What can realistically be achieved, and by what levels of exercise? Exercise has five main benefits: (1) It leads to a sense of well-being; (2) it aids in weight loss in obese patients; (3) it improves cardiovascular conditioning; in diabetic patients, (4) it improves insulin sensitivity; and (5) it can help prevent the development of type 2 diabetes in conjunction with weight loss.[60,80] Exercise does not need to be done continuously; walking in two 15-minute episodes versus walking continuously for 30 minutes is similarly beneficial.[81] Although performing some form of aerobic exercise for ≥150 minutes per week[60] is beneficial, adding in weight training (resistance exercising) 3 times per week may offer additional metabolic and health benefits.[82]

The level of exercise that provides subjects with a heightened sense of well-being is obviously variable and depends on a person's usual amount of activity. For many of our obese patients, simply walking around the block a few times constitutes increased physical activity and makes patients feel better psychologically.[83–85] More active people need higher levels of exercise to achieve this sense of well-being.

Exercise as the sole method of losing weight is usually unsuccessful without a concomitant reduction of food intake. This is because the amount of extra calories expended in the usual exercise program is not enough to lead to much weight loss. One pound of fat represents approximately 3500 calories. A person running 1 mile uses 100 calories. (Walking a mile also expends 100 calories; it just takes longer.) Two extra cookies cancel out that 100 calories of caloric expenditure. Thus it is apparent why the usual modest exercise programs most patients embark on do not result in much weight loss unless hypocaloric diets are also followed conscientiously. However, as mentioned previously, exercise is very important in maintaining weight loss.

Exercise can be a difficult challenge in the treatment of insulin-requiring patients, especially in those with type 1 diabetes. The reason for this is depicted in Figure 9-3. Normal exercise physiology regarding glucose metabolism is shown in the middle. Four factors can influence glucose levels. Blood flow increases and delivers more glucose to the exercising muscle. Muscle insulin sensitivity also increases. Secretion of the counterregulatory hormones inhibits endogenous insulin secretion and enhances hepatic glucose production. The first two lower glucose levels and are balanced by the second two, which raise them, so that in a normal individual or a patient with diabetes not taking insulin, glucose concentrations remain stable. In underinsulinized patients with diabetes (Figure 9-3, top), increased insulin-mediated glucose utilization in muscle and the restraining effect of insulin on

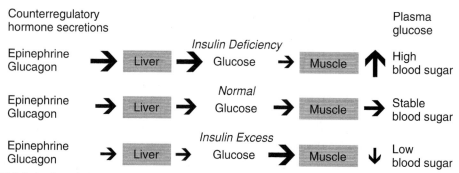

FIGURE 9-3. Insulin and the metabolic response to exercise. *(From Doner K: Exercise and diabetes. A research perspective. JDF International Countdown. Fall, 1989, p. 16. With permission.)*

hepatic glucose production do not occur. Under these circumstances of diminished glucose utilization by muscle and overproduction of glucose by the liver, marked hyperglycemia can occur. In addition, in patients with type 1 diabetes, the increased lipolysis associated with exercise can become excessive because little insulin is available to restrain it. The resultant free fatty acids produced are converted into ketone bodies in the liver (especially because exercise-induced glucagon levels are high and insulin levels are low) and can cause ketosis.

The lower part of Figure 9-3 shows the situation in which excessive insulin is present. Exercise can cause this because the enhanced blood flow to the area in which the insulin has been injected increases its absorption. For this reason, an abdominal rather than an extremity site for injection is recommended before exercise, although if the intensity of the exercise is high enough, rates of absorption from these two areas may differ little. The increased circulating insulin concentrations increase muscle glucose utilization and block the enhanced hepatic glucose production, thus leading to hypoglycemia. Therefore exercise can place insulin-requiring patients at risk for either hyperglycemia (and possibly ketosis in patients with type 1 diabetes) or hypoglycemia.

Because the conditions surrounding exercise cannot be predicted accurately, only general guidelines are offered. In terms of food, it may be beneficial to exercise shortly after eating or, if that is not feasible, to eat a small snack before starting. If the exercise is prolonged and intense, carbohydrate snacking during exercise may be necessary.[86] Patients occasionally become hypoglycemic many hours after exercise, and extra food needs to be eaten at these times. A general approach for balancing the amount of extra food with the anticipated level of exercise is suggested in Chapter 3. However, patients must determine for themselves whether these amounts are applicable to them or whether adjustments are necessary.

Decreasing insulin doses in anticipation of exercise may also be helpful.[87] This is more feasible if regular or rapid-acting insulin can be decreased shortly before exercise. Patients on continuous insulin infusion therapy can temporarily decrease or even stop their basal rate during exercise. For patients on injection, the more time between insulin administration and exercise, the less a repository of subcutaneous insulin is present for enhanced absorption. Thus exercising before breakfast (and before the morning injection of insulin) is an effective way to minimize exercise-induced hypoglycemia.

Some authorities suggest avoiding exercise if glucose levels are high (e.g., >250 mg/dl) or if ketosis is present.[88] Although the principles behind this recommendation are sound (as discussed earlier), often this is not necessary for several reasons. Patients' responses to exercise are variable and depend on, among other things, the intensity and duration of the exercise, as well as the timing of the previous insulin injection. This approach has been vindicated by a study[89] in which only 5 of 74 episodes of exercise in patients with type 1 diabetes begun with blood glucose concentrations exceeding 300 mg/dl resulted in increased levels at the conclusion of the exercise. Most importantly, because exercise often involves other people, canceling plans would have a detrimental effect on the patient's social interactions.

It is very helpful to perform SMBG before, after, and sometimes during exercise (e.g., between sets of tennis) for patients to learn their responses to various levels of exercise, insulin injection schedules, and extra food intake. Patterns that often emerge allow patients (with the help of a physician) to plan an effective and safe approach to exercise. Often it is helpful to have patients decrease the dose of rapid-acting insulin given for the meal immediately preceding the exercise.[87] Table 9-5 provides recommendations for adjusting the pre-meal/preexercise insulin dose. Patients with type 1 diabetes who exercise for more than an hour or two may notice an increase in their blood glucose levels with exercise, particularly if they have suspended their insulin pump or given less insulin in anticipation of exercise. Patients who are more serious athletes need to work closely with their diabetes management team to determine periexercise insulin doses and the need for carbohydrate supplementation. A good resource for patients with diabetes who exercise is *The Diabetic Athlete* by Sheri Colberg.[90] With appropriate guidance, patients with diabetes can run marathons, win gold medals in the Olympics, and perform competitively in virtually all sports.

In conclusion, exercise can be helpful to diabetic patients. Before embarking on a strenuous exercise program, all diabetic patients older than 40 years and those adults with type 1 diabetes who have had diabetes for more than 15 to 20 years should probably undergo a thorough cardiovascular evaluation. Virtually everyone can benefit from increasing their physical activity, particularly those who are sedentary at baseline. It is important for patients to start slowly, increase gradually, and vary their routines over time to keep themselves motivated and interested.

FOOT CARE

Infections of the feet are a major source of morbidity among patients with diabetes and often lead to death. Even though many of these infections are preventable, foot ulcers and gangrene continue to exact a tremendous toll in the diabetic population. Thus physicians must emphasize the importance of proper foot care (see Chapter 7 for a detailed discussion of this topic). The feet of patients who have diabetes should be examined at least yearly, and more often if high risk. The comprehensive examination should include a 10 g monofilament examination. In addition, patients with impairment of blood flow to the feet should have their toenails cut by qualified medical personnel (e.g., podiatrist, nurse, or physician).

Calluses are an important sign of possible future trouble. They represent increased pressure on an area that a patient often cannot feel because of associated sensory neuropathy. Calluses should be shaved routinely (usually by a podiatrist, but other medical personnel can be taught how) and kept to a minimum. Unroofing an innocuous-looking callus sometimes reveals an extensive ulcer, which could have been prevented by treating the callus when it first appeared. The source of the pressure (e.g., ill-fitting shoes, collapsed metatarsal arch, hammertoe) must be identified and corrective measures

TABLE 9-5	GUIDELINES FOR THE REDUCTION IN PREMEAL RAPID ACTING INSULIN DOSE	
Exercise Intensity (% VO$_2$ max)	**% Dose Reduction**	
	30 min. exercise	**60 min. exercise**
25	25	50
50	50	75
75	75	—

(From Rabasa-Lhoret R, Bouque J, Ducros F, Chiasson JL: Guidelines for premeal insulin dose reduction for postprandial exercise of different intensities and durations in type 1 diabetic subjects treated intensively with a basal-bolus insulin regimen (ultralente-lispro). Diabetes Care. 24(4):625-30, 2001.)

taken, if possible. Softer and better-fitting shoes usually are all that is needed, although persuading patients to forgo style simply to prevent calluses is not always easy. Prophylactic surgery to correct or remove a hammertoe is indicated in some patients, because no orthopedic method can reduce the pressure on the offending digit. The evaluation and management of foot problems in patients with diabetes is beyond the scope of this chapter. The important prognostic information obtained by using the 5.07 (10-g) monofilament in the examination[8] has already been mentioned. *Cost-effective* approaches to the diagnosis and treatment of diabetic foot infections and other lesions are available.[91-94]

In summary, *most foot ulcers and other infected lesions of the feet are preventable.* Although examination of the feet and instruction of patients in proper prophylactic foot care seem mundane, probably no other service that the physician performs offers as important a benefit for their patients with diabetes, especially those who are older.

TRAVEL

Patients with diabetes who require insulin who travel should be advised about how to manage their diabetes while on the road. Insulin is stable at room temperature, a feature that facilitates travel for patients. Extra insulin vials and syringes should be taken along, especially for patients going to a foreign country. It is wise for patients to carry their syringes and vials of insulin on their person in case baggage is lost. The timing and occasionally the amount of the insulin dose may need adjustment on the day of travel, especially if patients are flying into a different time zone. Patients should find out from the airline what kind of meal will be served and at what time. The insulin dose is then adjusted to the meal pattern. Traveling from north to south and vice versa is the easiest change to accommodate, because the

time does not change and the eating pattern usually is not too different. Traveling from east to west and vice versa presents more of a problem because the change in time often disrupts both meal and sleeping patterns. A relatively smooth integration of the new eating and activity schedule with the insulin regimen can be accomplished by keeping both schedules geared to the patient's internal clock for the first 12 to 24 hours after arrival before shifting to the changed external time. Patients on long-acting insulin such as glargine, with premeal rapid-acting insulin may not require much in the way of adjustment, except to get on local time as soon as possible—to take the long-acting insulin at nighttime (or breakfast time) in the new time zone. Patients on insulin pump therapy should be sure to change their pump settings to the new time and date upon arrival in the new region.

For patients taking two insulin injections of intermediate-acting and regular (or rapid-acting) insulin per day, an afternoon flight from Los Angeles to New York City might be handled as follows. The flight leaves at 2 PM, and a large meal is served 2 hours later. Patients should start their day approximately 1 hour earlier than usual. They should take the usual insulin dose and eat breakfast and lunch slightly earlier than normal. They should take their second injection of insulin on the plane just before the 4 PM meal (Los Angeles time) is served. Patients arrive in New York City at 11 PM local time (but at 8 PM according to their internal clock) and eat their bedtime snack shortly after arrival. This is necessary because they took their second injection of NPH insulin approximately 4 hours before. They go to sleep at 1 to 2 AM New York time (9 to 10 PM Los Angeles time). On awakening the next day at 8 AM (5 AM Los Angeles time), their fasting glucose level should still be controlled by the NPH insulin, which was taken approximately 12 hours earlier. They now can follow their usual schedule. Although according to their internal clock they are taking their insulin 3 hours earlier than usual, their eating and activity patterns also have shifted by 3 hours, and the relation between the two patterns has not been disrupted seriously.

Traveling from New York City back to Los Angeles requires more of an adjustment. A morning flight leaves the East Coast at 9 AM and arrives on the West Coast at noon (local time). The same patients should take their insulin and a small breakfast several hours before the flight. A large breakfast usually is served shortly after takeoff. Patients could either take a small amount of extra regular insulin to handle these calories or consume only a portion of them as a midmorning snack. Regardless of which they choose, they need to have some food available several hours before landing to serve as a small lunch. After arriving in Los Angeles at noon (3 PM by their internal clock), they should arrange to eat their major meal several hours later. Although this occurs in the middle of the afternoon on the West Coast, it is an appropriate time for their supper according to the peak action of their morning insulin injection. They should delay their second injection of NPH insulin for several more hours (5 PM Los Angeles time, 8 PM New York time). They need to eat their bedtime snack at 8 to 9 PM (local time) to cover this injection, by which time they probably wish to retire (approximately midnight by their internal clock). Although they might arise very early the next morning according to West Coast time, the hour would theoretically be appropriate for the East Coast, and they should delay taking their morning injection and eating until the appropriate Los Angeles time. This delay should not cause much of a problem because their last NPH injection was taken approximately 15 hours previously and should still be effective in controlling their fasting glucose concentration. Their insulin regimen and eating patterns are now adjusted (with respect to time, at least) back to the West Coast schedule.

Although the disruptions encountered by patients taking longer plane trips are greater, the same general approach is used to treat them during the flight and to aid their adjustment after arrival. These examples do not take into account the stress effect of changing time zones ("jet lag"), which may alter endogenous hormonal responses.

In light of September 11, 2001, airport security is much more rigorous. Security personnel require that insulin bottles have their original pharmacy labels on them; likewise for syringes and lancets. Notes written by physicians no longer suffice, because they can easily be forged. The Federal Transportation Safety Administration has a Web site (www.tsa.gov/public/) that provides up-to-date information regarding the requirements for traveling with insulin syringes and lancets. This information can also be found on the ADA Web site (www.diabetes.org) under the section titled "Community Advocacy." Patients on insulin pumps may be required to turn the device on and off. It is recommended that these patients carry a brochure with a picture of the pump on it (supplied by the manufacturer) and a 1-800 contact number for the manufacturer, should an overzealous but underinformed security officer be concerned.

All patients with diabetes on insulin or oral agents that cause hypoglycemia should be encouraged to wear Medic Alert bracelets, particularly when traveling, in case an emergency situation arise.

DENTAL PROCEDURES

Dental infections, especially periodontal disease, are more common in diabetic patients than in nondiabetic individuals.[7] Therefore diabetic patients are more likely to undergo dental procedures that impair food intake. This may be a problem for those taking insulin or sulfonylurea agents unless precautions are taken. Effective communication between the patient's physician and dentist is important so that the extent and timing of the diminished food intake and the severity of the operative stress can be judged.

If a patient taking sulfonylurea agents will miss more than one meal because of a dental procedure, the drugs should be omitted that morning and resumed when normal food intake occurs.

Hypoglycemia is more likely to occur secondary to insulin therapy than to oral hypoglycemic agents. In these patients, dental procedures should be performed in the morning, if possible, because the effects of intermediate-acting insulins injected before breakfast peak late in the afternoon and because an insulin reaction may occur if the supper calories are decreased. If the lunch calories are diminished, regular and rapid-acting insulin should be omitted from the morning dose. In addition, NPH insulin and breakfast might be taken a little later than usual to minimize the risk of early afternoon hypoglycemia. If the amount of food intake at supper will be decreased, the dose of morning intermediate-acting insulin should be reduced. However, patients with type 1 diabetes must have some insulin to avoid ketosis and possibly ketoacidosis. Therefore a balance must be achieved between the decreased insulin requirements caused by decreased food intake and the need for insulin caused by the stress of the dental procedure and possibly by the infection that led do it. It is important that patients monitor their control closely after the procedure and communicate with their physician. If extensive dental work that impairs food intake is necessary for ketosis-prone diabetic patients, hospitalization sometimes is advisable.

SURGICAL AND POSTOPERATIVE MANAGEMENT

Traditionally, the therapeutic goals during surgery in patients with diabetes are to minimize fluid and electrolyte losses secondary to osmotic diuresis by limiting hyperglycemia, to prevent diabetic ketosis in patients with type 1 diabetes, and to avoid hypoglycemia while patients are anesthetized. New data have emerged revealing the benefits of insulin use during hospitalization for myocardial infarction[95] as well as the improvements in morbidity and mortality when insulin is used to treat stress-related hyperglycemia in critically ill patients.[96] While it is beyond the scope of this book to review the literature in this field, it is increasingly clear that reductions in glucose levels during cardiovascular events and cardiac surgery have a positive impact on outcomes.[97,98] Many hospitals are implementing detailed flowsheets for the use of insulin drips in ICU and CCU settings, and studies are underway to determine optimal blood glucose levels for hospitalized patients both with and without diabetes. The use of insulin and glucose described in the following section should be considered in all perioperative and critically ill patients who are hyperglycemic.

During operative procedures, some anesthesiologists (and patients) fear that hypoglycemia will occur during surgery if insulin is given preoperatively, but this rarely happens. The stress of surgery for patients usually receiving intravenous glucose almost always leads to hyperglycemia. Indeed, in a prospective study of 58 patients receiving NPH insulin on the morning of surgery with glucose infusions begun at the time of the insulin injection and continuing throughout surgery, hypoglycemia only occurred *before* the operation when surgery was delayed until the afternoon.[99] The average glucose level at the end of surgery was 258 mg/dl, excluding three patients who were treated intraoperatively when their glucose concentrations exceeded 400 mg/dl.[99]

Although several insulin regimens have been proposed, one is clearly superior. This involves continuous insulin and glucose infusions given through separate sets of tubing. Patients receive their usual insulin regimen until the morning of surgery. At this time, 5% dextrose in water is infused at 125 ml/hr and insulin is piggy-backed onto the glucose line through an infusion pump. Suggested insulin infusion rates are shown in Table 9-6. Capillary blood glucose levels are measured by a bedside glucose meter every hour or two before surgery, and the insulin infusion rate is adjusted accordingly. During surgery, the anesthesiologist must be able to measure glucose concentrations *hourly* and infuse insulin appropriately. This approach requires that the intravenous line infusing glucose and insulin be under the control of the anesthesiologist and a separate intravenous line be used to give saline, plasma, blood, and so on as required by the surgeon. Although the insulin infusion rates in Table 9-6 may need to be changed accord-

ing to an individual patient's response, they seem to work very well in most types of operations except for kidney transplants and open heart surgery, during which higher rates are required.[100] This glucose–insulin infusion method is also ideal for the perioperative period until patients can eat. However, it requires nurses able to use a bedside glucose meter accurately (on the ward, in the recovery room, and in the intensive care unit) and a cooperative anesthesiologist or anesthesia assistant who can use a glucose meter in the operating room. If a pump to infuse insulin is not available, insulin can be added to the glucose solution.[101] This latter modification has two drawbacks. It does not allow for separate adjustments of the infusion rates for insulin and glucose. Moreover, every time an adjust-

---

TABLE 9-6 ALGORITHM FOR INTRAVENOUS INSULIN INFUSION ADJUSTMENT BEFORE, DURING, AND AFTER SURGERY

A. Stop feeding and usual treatment with insulin or oral hypoglycemic agents 12 hours before surgery.

B. Start infusion of a solution containing 5% dextrose at a rate of 125 ml/hr.

C. Start intravenous insulin infusion as follows:

Whole Blood Glucose (mg/dl)	Insulin Infusion Rate (U/hr)
≤100	None
101–150	1
151–250	2
251–350	3
>350	4 (Dextrose infusion is held until blood glucose level ≤250 mg/dl.)

1. Measure blood glucose level with a glucose meter every 2 hours before and after surgery and hourly during surgery.
   a. Do not change insulin infusion rate if blood glucose level ranges between 100 and 180 mg/dl.
   b. Increase insulin infusion rate by 0.5 U/hr if blood glucose level is >180 mg/dl.
   c. Hold dextrose infusion if blood glucose level >350 mg/dl. Restart once blood glucose level ≤250 mg/dl.
   d. Decrease insulin infusion rate by 0.5 U/hr if blood glucose level is <100 mg/dl, and increase dextrose infusion rate by 50 ml/hr.
      1) Once blood glucose level increases to >100 mg/dl, decrease dextrose infusion rate back to 125 ml/hr.
2. Measure blood glucose level 1 hour after an adjustment is made to assess response, and readjust if indicated.
3. If glucose level stable postoperatively, blood glucose determinations can be carried out every 4 hours.

ment is made, a new solution must be made up. Even so, this method is superior to the two methods discussed next.

If monitoring glucose levels by bedside meters is not feasible, the following two approaches are recommended for insulin-requiring diabetic patients. In one, patients receive half of their total daily insulin dose (i.e., half of the entire amount of intermediate- and short-acting insulin taken normally) as NPH insulin on the morning of surgery, or if on long-acting insulin such as glargine, patients maintain their usual dosing schedule. An infusion of 5% dextrose in water is administered at a rate of 125 ml/h. If surgery must be delayed for more than 4 hours after the insulin is given, the glucose concentration should be measured. If this value is <150 mg/dl, the rate of glucose infusion should be increased to 200 ml/h.

The second approach is to withhold insulin before surgery and not give patients dextrose-containing fluids until the postoperative period. This requires communication with and the cooperation of the anesthesiologist. In patients with type 1 diabetes, this method should largely be avoided. However, this approach often works well for patients with type 2 diabetes, in whom glucose concentrations will not rise in the preoperative period because they are not eating or receiving glucose. One must ensure, however, that both patients with type 1 and type 2 diabetes are not hypoglycemic on the morning of surgery in response to the previous evening's insulin dose. If this is the case, a dextrose infusion must be started and one of the alternate methods used (i.e., either giving half of the total insulin requirement as NPH insulin or starting an insulin infusion or using glargine insulin). If both insulin and glucose are withheld until after surgery, the postoperative blood glucose level is usually similar to the preoperative level.[102]

Insulin treatment after surgery depends on two factors: which insulin regimen was used and whether a patient will resume eating that day (arbitrarily defined here as *minor* surgery) or not (defined as *major* surgery). Thus there are six possible situations, which involve four insulin regimens (intravenous insulin, half of the usual total dose given as intermediate-acting insulin, giving the usual dose of long-acting glargine insulin or withholding insulin [and the glucose infusion] until after surgery), in patients undergoing either minor or major surgery.

Patients given an insulin infusion are the easiest to treat postoperatively irrespective of which kind of surgery they undergo. The same approach, with sampling for glucose measurements and adjustments of the insulin infusion rate every 2 to 4 hours, is used until they eat. To disrupt the usual time course of insulin for patients as little as possible, subcutaneous administration should be started at the same times as before surgery, usually before breakfast and before supper (or bedtime for the evening intermediate- or long-acting insulin preparation). If lunch is eaten on the day of surgery, the insulin infusion can be stopped at that time and subcutaneous regular insulin given to carry patients to the evening meal. If the insulin infusion is used instead, the rate can be increased arbitrarily for the 2-hour period after the meal is started in anticipation of the postprandial rise of glucose concentrations. The usual amounts of regular or rapid-acting insulin may need to be adjusted downward if caloric intake will be less than usual, but upward because of postoperative discomfort. These possible changes in insulin doses need to be considered for patients undergoing minor surgery managed by the other insulin regimens as well. (The one exception to this is the dose of the evening intermediate- or long-acting insulin in patients who receive their usual morning insulin prescription, albeit delayed, after a short minor surgical procedure.)

Patients receiving half of their total insulin dose as NPH or their usual glargine insulin on the morning of surgery along with a dextrose infusion should be treated postoperatively as follows. In those undergoing *minor* surgery, the glucose infusion is stopped when they eat. If the first meal is lunch, subcutaneous regular or rapid-acting insulin is given to control the blood glucose level until supper. If patients do not eat until supper on the day of surgery, subcutaneous regular or rapid-acting insulin is still given postoperatively (every 4 hours) to control the blood glucose level until the dextrose infusion is discontinued and patients eat. In both situations, glucose should be measured as soon as patients enter the recovery room, because not only is the glucose concentration usually elevated immediately postoperatively when this insulin regimen is used[99] but the glucose infusion is usually being continued. Therefore these factors must be taken into consideration when determining the dose of regular or rapid-acting insulin at this time. The submaximal amount of the preoperative NPH insulin has only a minor role after surgery and should not be relied on to have a large effect on postoperative patients receiving intravenous glucose. The same principles apply in those patients who are treated with this regimen and who undergo *major* surgery—that is, their glucose concentrations are managed by subcutaneous regular insulin every 4 hours until the evening. Longer-term treatment of surgical patients unable to eat is discussed later.

Those patients who are undergoing minor surgery and in whom both a glucose infusion and insulin are withheld fall into two categories. If the procedure is short (~2 hours or less) and general anesthesia is not necessary, their usual insulin dose can be given postoperatively. This approach applies to those patients who will be able to eat soon after receiving their insulin. The usual eating and insulin administration schedule for the rest of the day should be delayed as well to minimize disruption of the relationship between the two. This method of insulin management works very well for patients undergoing minor outpatient procedures, especially

those with type 2 diabetes. One needs to be certain that the delay before insulin administration will not be more than several hours for type 1 patients, who may develop hyperglycemia and possibly ketosis after a (painful) surgical procedure when the effect of the previous evening's insulin wanes. If patients will be unable to eat until supper (whether inpatient or outpatient), regular or rapid-acting insulin should be given every 3 to 4 hours to control the blood glucose level until supper. If patients are in the hospital, a concomitant glucose infusion is preferred to lessen the chances of hypoglycemia. If patients return home after an outpatient procedure, the physician must be certain that they (or a family member) will be able to measure the blood glucose reliably and respond appropriately by giving the suggested insulin doses.

Patients undergoing major surgery, especially abdominal operations, will not be able to eat for various lengths of time postoperatively. Their parenteral nutrition should include at least 100 g of glucose (2 L of 5% dextrose in water) over each 24-hour period to avoid starvation ketosis. It is important that the physician managing the insulin regimen also write the orders concerning the glucose infusion (or for any other source of carbohydrate administration). There is a potential danger if the rate of glucose administration is changed or possibly even reduced to zero once insulin has been given on the basis of a presumed different rate of glucose infusion. This may entail two intravenous lines, but this additional safeguard against a mismatch between insulin and glucose administration is well worth it.

The principle underlying the postoperative insulin management of diabetic patients is to provide continuous insulin coverage because patients are receiving a constant amount of glucose per unit of time. Four insulin regimens conveniently accomplish this. Although labor-intensive, an insulin infusion with bedside glucose monitoring and insulin rate adjustments every 2 to 3 hours leads to the least variation in glucose levels (see Table 9-6). A second approach is to administer subcutaneous regular or rapid-acting insulin every 4 or 6 hours on the basis of the results of bedside glucose monitoring. NPH insulin can be given every 12 hours with additional regular or rapid-acting insulin at that time if necessary. This approach does not require bedside monitoring or a particularly rapid response from the laboratory. The glucose concentration obtained before each administration of NPH insulin reflects the effectiveness of the previous injection (i.e., that given 12 hours before). As long as patients are receiving dextrose continuously (i.e., by infusion or nasogastric tube), high values should be treated with extra regular insulin as soon as they become available—for example, for glucose concentrations between 150 and 250 mg/dl, 2 to 4 U is given; between 250 and 350 mg/dl, 6 to 8 U; and for >350 mg/dl, 8 to 10 U. Similar considerations can be applied to the even more simplified approach of giving long-acting insulin at 10 PM and regular or rapid-acting insulin every 4 to 6 hours.

As a general rule of thumb, lean patients are started on 10 U of NPH every 12 hours, and obese patients (i.e., those at >120% of desirable body weight are begun on 16 U of NPH insulin at both times. (These initial amounts of insulin may be changed if patients' sensitivity to insulin, as reflected in their usual insulin regimen, suggests that different doses would be more effective.) Each dose of NPH insulin is increased by 4 to 6 U if the appropriate glucose concentration is >180 mg/dl. If the glucose level is >150 mg/dl, extra regular or rapid-acting insulin is given. The dose of evening glargine insulin should be 15 U in lean patients and 20 units in obese patients, with regular or rapid-acting insulin given every 6 to 4 hours, respectively. As patients begin to eat, increasing amounts of insulin can be added to the morning injection if on NPH insulin. When intravenous glucose is no longer infused overnight (which should occur after oral caloric intake improves considerably), some of the evening dose of NPH insulin also can be shifted to the morning or the dose of glargine insulin decreased. In

this manner, the transition from total parenteral nutrition through partial oral supplementation to normal food intake can be accomplished smoothly without large fluctuations in diabetic control. The following case should serve to illustrate this approach.

CASE 9-1

The patient is a 37-year-old woman who has had type 1 diabetes for 17 years. She is 5 feet 5 inches tall and weighs 142 pounds. Her insulin regimen consists of 24 U of NPH and 4 U of rapid-acting insulin in the morning, 10 U of rapid-acting insulin before supper and 10 U of NPH insulin before bedtime. She was admitted to the hospital for an elective cholecystectomy after intermittent episodes of colicky pain in the right upper quadrant associated with mild postprandial nausea. (Several previous abdominal operations for appendicitis and gynecologic problems precluded a laparoscopic cholecystectomy.) On the morning of surgery, July 23, she received 24 U of NPH insulin; the appropriate glucose infusion was started, and she went to the operating room at 0900. Her postoperative course is summarized in Table 9-7.

A blood sample for glucose determination was made at 1300 when she arrived in the recovery room. The value of 384 mg/dl was recorded, for which she was given 10 U of regular insulin. Another blood sample was sent at 1800, which was 227 mg/dl, for which she received 4 U of regular insulin. At 2200, another blood sample was sent and she was given 10 U of NPH insulin because she is not obese. She received 6 U of regular insulin at 2200.

Unfortunately, the response to this injection of regular insulin was not evaluated and she probably remained markedly hyperglycemic throughout the night. Her morning glucose level on July 24, the first day after surgery, revealed an inadequate response to the insulin given the previous evening, and she was given 10 U of regular insulin when the value was reported.

If the morning or evening glucose concentration exceeds 250 mg/dl, the response to the regular insulin administered should be checked 3 to 4 hours later. This ensures that marked hyperglycemia is not present throughout the 12-hour period until the sampling before the next NPH insulin injection. If glucose levels continue to exceed 250 mg/dl at these subsequent times,

TABLE 9-7	POSTOPERATIVE COURSE OF A TYPE 1 DIABETIC PATIENT AFTER CHOLECYSTECTOMY			

Date	Time	Plasma Glucose (mg/dl)	Amount (U) of Insulin (Type)	Remarks
7/23	1300	384	10 (Reg)*	Enters recovery room; receives 5% dextrose solution at 125 ml/h
	1400			
	1800	227	4 (Reg)*	
	1900		10 (NPH)	
	2200	289	6 (Reg)*	
	2330		10 (NPH)	
7/24	0800	397		
	1000		10 (Reg)*	
	1400	241	14 (NPH)	
	2000	283	8 (Reg)*	
	2200			
7/25	0200	206	14 (NPH)	
	0800	313	10 (Reg)*	
	1000			
	1400	190	18 (NPH)	
	2000	275	6 (Reg)*	
	2200			
7/26	0200	187	18 (NPH)	Bowel sounds present
	0800	225	4 (Reg)*	
	1000			
	1400	168	18 (NPH)	
	2000	210	3 (Reg)*	
	2130			
7/27	0130	163	18 (NPH)	Liquid diet started but patient vomited
	0800	178	18 (NPH)	
	2000	164	18 (NPH)	
7/28	0800	172	18 (NPH)	Liquid diet tolerated
	2000	154	18 (NPH)	
7/29	0800	163	18 (NPH)	Soft diet started
	2000	143	18 (NPH)	
7/30	0800	174	12 (NPH)	Glucose infusion stopped; soft diet continued
	1600	265	22 (NPH)	
7/31	0800	143		
	1130	258	12 (NPH)	
	1600	225	26 (NPH) 2 Lispro	Normal diet tolerated
8/1	0800	158		
	1130	227	12 (NPH)	
	1600	179		
	2200	284	26 (NPH) 4 Lispro	
8/2	0800	138		Patient ambulatory
	1130	198		
	1600	183	12 (NPH) 4 Lispro	
	2200	217	26 (NPH) 6 Lispro	
8/3	0800	147		
	1130	156		
	1600	163	12 (NPH) 6 Lispro	
	2200	172	26 (NPH) 6 Lispro	
8/4	0800	153		Patient discharged after breakfast

*Regular insulin given according to glucose value measured several hours previously.

appropriate amounts of regular insulin can be given again. Although both the previous NPH insulin and the subsequent regular insulin doses will have their maximal effects during the same period, hypoglycemia is very unlikely to occur given the fact that the blood glucose level exceeded 250 mg/dl when the regular insulin was received and that glucose is being infused. On the other hand, it is not necessary to measure the blood glucose level during the 12-hour period between NPH insulin administration if the last value was <250 mg/dl because marked hyperglycemia is unlikely to occur during this time. In the case under discussion (see Table 9-7), the glucose concentration 4 hours after 10 U of regular insulin was 241 mg/dl and no further regular insulin was given.

That evening, the amount of NPH insulin was increased to 14 U because the dose on the previous evening was inadequate. Because the glucose concentration that evening was 283 mg/dl, she was given 8 extra U of regular insulin at 2200, and the response to it was adequate. The morning dose of NPH insulin was increased the following day. The amounts of NPH insulin were increased gradually on July 25 and 26. Decreasing amounts of regular insulin also had to be given during this period. Strict control during the immediate postoperative period, when a patient is experiencing pain and receiving infusions of glucose, can be difficult to attain.

Although the patient began a liquid diet on July 27, the insulin doses were not changed because the glucose infusions were maintained and the initial oral intake was limited. Extra regular insulin was withheld because glucose values were mostly <200 mg/dl. On July 30, when she could tolerate a soft diet and the intravenous dextrose was discontinued, the effect of the morning dose of NPH insulin was evaluated before supper (at 1600 instead of 2000) and the evening dose of insulin was reduced.

The following approach is recommended for patients who do not require insulin. Those whose diabetes is controlled by dietary therapy alone can be treated in the same way as nondiabetic patients. Monitoring of glucose concentrations is important, however, because hyperglycemia can occur secondary to the stress of surgery and postoperative discom-fort. Although deterioration of diabetic control usually is temporary, glucose concentrations persistently elevated at >250 mg/dl should be treated with small doses of NPH insulin. Sulfonylurea agents and thiazolidinediones should be held on the day of surgery. Metformin should also be discontinued 48 hours before surgery, and alpha-glucosidase inhibitors (AGIs) and rapid-acting insulin secretagogues can simply be omitted when patients stop eating. With minor surgery, oral medication should be resumed when patients resume eating. Major surgical procedures often cause marked elevations in glucose concentration in patients who required oral antidiabetes medication before surgery. Therefore lean individuals should receive 10 U of NPH insulin and obese individuals (>120% desirable body weight) should receive 16 U of NPH insulin on the morning of surgery. All patients should then be monitored in the manner described for insulin-requiring diabetic patients. When patients start eating again, the insulin should be withdrawn gradually and the oral antidiabetes agent resumed. Metformin and AGIs can also be resumed but may cause gastrointestinal symptoms and need to be retitrated if they have been withheld for a week or more. Patients' responses in this situation will vary. In the stable recovering postoperative patient, it is reasonable to restart metformin as long as renal function is normal. Thiazolidinediones can be restarted as soon as the patient can eat, as long as liver function remains normal. Insulin secretagogues, both long- and short-acting, can be restarted once a patient is eating.

INFECTIONS IN PATIENTS WITH DIABETES

Certain specific infections are more common in patients with diabetes, and some occur almost exclusively in this set of patients. In addition, the incidence and severity of some infections are exaggerated in the diabetic population (Table 9-8).

TABLE 9-8 CLINICAL FEATURES, DIAGNOSIS, AND CAUSATIVE ORGANISMS OF SELECTED INFECTIONS IN PATIENTS WITH DIABETES.

Infection	Clinical Features	Diagnostic Procedure	Organisms	Comments
Respiratory tract				
Community-acquired pneumonia	Cough, fever	Chest radiography	Streptococcus pneumoniae, Staphylococcus aureus, Haemophilus influenzae, other gram-negative bacilli, atypical pathogens	Pneumococcal infection carries a higher risk of death in diabetic than in nondiabetic patients
Urinary tract				
Acute bacterial cystitis	Increased urinary frequency, dysuria, suprapubic pain	Urine culture	Escherichia coli, proteus species	Bacteriuria more common in diabetic than in nondiabetic women
Acute pyelonephritis	Fever, flank pain	Urine culture	E. coli, proteus species	Emphysematous infection should be considered
Emphysematous pyelonephritis	Fever, flank pain, poor response to antibiotics	Radiography or CT scanning	E. coli, other gram-negative bacilli	Emergency nephrectomy often required
Perinephric abscess	Fever, flank pain, poor response to antibiotics	Ultrasonography or CT scanning	E. coli, other gram-negative bacilli	Surgical drainage usually required
Fungal cystitis	Same as for acute bacterial cystitis	Urine culture	Candida species	Difficult to distinguish colonization from infection
Soft tissue				
Necrotizing fasciitis	Local pain, redness, crepitus, bullous skin lesions	Radiography or CT scanning	Gram-negative bacilli, anaerobes (type I), or group A streptococci (type II)	High mortality; emergency surgery required
Other				
Invasive otitis externa	Ear pain, otorrhea, hearing loss, cellulitis	Clinical examination, magnetic resonance imaging	Pseudomonas aeruginosa	Prompt otolaryngologic consultation recommended

Rhinocerebral mucormycosis	Facial or ocular pain, fever, lethargy, black nasal eschar	Clinical examination, magnetic resonance imaging, pathologic findings	Mucor and rhizopus species	Strong association with ketoacidosis; emergency surgery required
Abdomen Emphysematous cholecystitis	Fever, right-upper-quadrant abdominal pain, systemic toxicity	Radiography	Gram-negative bacilli, anaerobes	High mortality; gallstones in 50%; emergency cholecystectomy required

CT, Computed tomography.

(From Joshi N, Caputo GM, Weitekamp MR, Karchmer AW: Infections in patients with diabetes mellitus. New Engl J Med 341:1906, 1999.)

Possible reasons for this increase of infection include poor glycemic control and acidemia, and other associated factors such as age, renal disease, and cardiovascular disease may also play a role.

There is a known increase in bacteriuria in women with diabetes compared with a normal cohort.[103] This increase of 2 to 4 times may be directly related to the diabetes, or to other factors such as more frequent catheterizations during hospitalizations. In patients with diabetes, there is a role for chronic prophylactic treatment if a history of recurrent urinary tract infections (UTIs) is obtained. UTIs are more likely to involve the upper urinary tract[104] and lead to complications in patients with diabetes. For example, pyelonephritis is seen with the usual presentation, except that bilateral renal involvement is more common.[104] The severe sequelae of emphysematous pyelonephritis is still unusual, but is seen much more often (90% of cases) in those with diabetes.[105] These patients present with fever, chills, nausea, flank pain, and often an abdominal mass. Failure to resolve the fever with 72 hours of intravenous (IV) antibiotics should clue the physician that emphysematous pyelonephritis may be present. Papillary necrosis and perinephric abscesses are also seen with increasing frequency.[106] In these cases surgical intervention may be required. The usual pathogens for UTIs include *Escherichia coli* and other gram-negative organisms. *Candida* may be implicated in fungal cystitis. When isolated to the bladder, irrigation of the bladder with amphotericin B[107] or a single IV dose of amphotericin B[108] are viable options for treatment, as is a course of oral fluconazole.[109] The latter is treatment of choice because it results in less toxicity.

The importance of regular foot examinations has been stressed earlier in this chapter. Shallow ulcers with less than 2 cm cellulitis and with no evidence of osteomyelitis, fascitis, or osteomyelitis may be treated in the outpatient setting with oral antibiotics and wound care.[110] Anything more severe than mentioned should involve hospitalization with work-ups completed for osteomyelitis and a surgical opinion. Intravenous antibiotics should be started and wound care ordered. In addition to foot infections, the other extremely important soft tissue infection is necrotizing factitis.[111] Mortality is more than 40% and the infection spreads quickly along fascial planes, most commonly occurring in the limbs and the abdominal wall. The hallmark clinical finding in these patients is a degree of pain much higher than the severity of clinical finding. In the later stages, bullous lesions may form on the skin, and crepitus may be heard as a result of bacterial gas formation. Any suspicion of necrotizing fascitis warrants urgent and immediate hospitalization and broad-spectrum antibiotic coverage.

Respiratory tract infections are common in patients with diabetes, and the causative organisms are the usual pathogens suspected. In the case of community-acquired pneumonia, morbidity and mortality are not significantly increased in the diabetic population.[112] However, *Streptococcus pneumoniae* and influenza do carry a higher risk in patients with diabetes. The incidence of *Staphylococcus pneumoniae* is increased because of a reduction of pulmonary ciliary function during influenza infection and a higher nasal carriage rate of *S. aureus* in this population.

Certain infections have a predisposition for patients with diabetes. Invasive otitis externa most commonly caused by *Pseudomonas aeruginosa* may actually become severe enough to involve the skull. Patients present with severe pain and possibly hearing loss. Fever is absent. Treatment may include ear, nose, and throat (ENT) evaluation with biopsy to confirm the diagnosis and debridement, along with topical and systemic antibiotic therapy for 4 to 6 weeks. Rhinocerebral mucormycosis tends to occur after episodes of DKA, presumably because the acidosis results in an inability to inhibit the causative organism, *Rhizopus oryzae.* Facial pain and nasal congestion occur first, followed by chemosis and black necrotic lesions on the oral and nasal mucosa and turbinates. Diagnosis is made by biopsy and culture, and treatment involves debridement, sinus drainage, and antifungal therapy (fluconazole or itraconazole).

Emphysematous cholecystitis occurs more commonly in diabetes. The clinical presentation is similar to that of acute cholecystitis, but the sequelae of gallbladder gangrene and perforation are much higher, as are the mortality rates. There is an increased association with male patients. Only 50% of patients actually have gallstones. The presentation is similar to acute cholecystitis, and although peritoneal signs may not be present, crepitus in the abdominal wall may be noted. Gram-negative organisms are usually to blame, and antibiotic coverage must be started immediately. Cholecystectomy is necessary.

INFLUENZA AND PNEUMOCOCCAL VACCINES

Because of the increase in morbidity and mortality associated with pneumococcal respiratory infections in diabetes,[113] vaccination is recommended. As for influenza, it is associated with an increased number of hospitalizations and deaths for a variety of conditions, including diabetes. Patients with diabetes have actually been shown to have a delayed response to influenza immunization, perhaps because of impaired T cell function. Because immune response to pneumococcus is not T cell–dependent, this is not a factor in pneumococcal vaccinations.

Pneumococcal vaccination is indicated to reduce invasive disease from pneumococcus in people with diabetes.[114,115] A one-time revaccination is recommended for individuals older than 64 years of age if the prior vaccination was administered more than 5 years earlier. In addition, those with nephrotic syndrome, chronic renal failure, and those

who have had organ transplantation or are in other immunocompromised states should be revaccinated.[114] Mild local side effects usually last less than 48 hours and severe systemic reactions are rare.

Influenza vaccination is recommended for patients with diabetes older than the age of 6 months, and should be given in the early fall season annually.[116] Because of its easy transmission, vaccination of health care workers and their family members may be justified. Patients traveling to the southern hemisphere between April and September should consider vaccination before travel. Patients may experience mild local pain after injection. Those with an allergy to chicken eggs should not be given the vaccine. In these patients, chemoprophylaxis with anitidine can be used, or an immunization protocol developed by Murphy et al.[117] should be followed. There may be an increased risk of developing Guillain Barré syndrome within 6 weeks of immunization.

FUTURE DIRECTIONS/CONCLUSIONS

Treatment of patients with diabetes is a task usually done by primary care providers in the office setting. Although non–diabetes-related complaints may often be more acute and immediately troubling for the patient, it is the long-term maintenance of normal blood glucose, lipid, and blood pressure levels that will prevent complications in the years to come. The benefits of more normal glucose control were well documented by the DCCT[16] and UKPDS[18] studies, along with a significant benefit from blood pressure seen in the latter trial. Increasingly, research is looking at reducing the high cardiovascular risk in diabetes. The STENO-2 study[118] showed that a multifactorial intervention to treat hyperglycemia, hypertension, dyslipidemia, and microalbuminuria produced a reduction in the risk of cardiovascular disease, nephropathy, retinopathy, and autonomic neuropathy.

These results are encouraging, and the much larger ACCORD trial (n = 10,000), underway in the United States, is addressing multiple questions about the role of hyperglycemia, dyslipidemia, and hypertension. These results will not be available until after 2010, however, and in the interim each of us must strive to provide our patients with high-quality health care, lowering risks for micro- and macrovascular complications as thoroughly as possible.

REFERENCES

1. American diabetes Association: Standards of medical care for patients with diabetes mellitus. Diabetes Care 26 (suppl 1): S33, 2003.
2. Ishihara M, Yukimura Y, Aiza T et al: High blood pressure as risk factor in diabetic retinopathy development in NIDDM patients. Diabetes Care 10:20, 1987.
3. van Leiden HA, Dekker JM, Moll AC, Nijpels G, Heine RJ, Bouter LM, Stehouwer CD, Polak BC: Blood pressure, lipids, and obesity are associated with retinopathy: The hoorn study. Diabetes Care. 25(8):1320, 2002.
4. Stratton IM, Kohner EM, Aldington SJ, Turner RC, Holman RR, Manley SE, Matthews DR: UKPDS 50: Risk factors for incidence and progression of retinopathy in Type II diabetes over 6 years from diagnosis. Diabetologia. 44(2):156–63, 2001.
5. Adler AI, Stratton IM, Neil HA, Yudkin JS, Matthews DR, Cull CA et al: Association of systolic blood pressure with macrovascular and microvascular complications of type 2 diabetes (UKPDS 36): Prospective observational study. BMJ 321:412, 2000.
6. Raptis AE, Viberti G: Pathogenesis of diabetic nephropathy. Experimental & Clinical Endocrinology & Diabetes. 109 Suppl 2:2424, 2001.
7. Mealey BL, Rethman MP: Periodontal disease and diabetes mellitus: Bidirectional relationship. Dentistry Today. 22(4):107–13, 2003.
8. McNeely MY, Boyko EJ, Ahroni JH et al: The independent contributions of diabetic neuropathy and vasculopathy in foot ulceration. Diabetes Care 18:216, 1995.
9. Inzucchi SE: Noninvasive assessment of the diabetic patient for coronary artery disease. Diabetes Care 24:1519–1521, 2001.
10. Nesto RW: Screening for asymptomatic coronary artery disease in diabetes. Diabetes Care 22:1393-1395, 1999.
11. Daneman D, Wolfson DH, Becker DJ et al: Factors affecting glycosylated hemoglobin values in children with insulin-dependent diabetes. J Pediatr 99:847, 1981.
12. Drash AL, Kingsley LA, Doft B et al: Observations on the effects of changing therapeutic strategies on metabolic status and microvascular complications in IDDM. Pediatr Adolesc Endocrinol 17:206, 1988.
13. Peter Chase H, Jackson WE, Hoops SL et al: Glucose control and the renal and retinal complications of insulin-dependent diabetes. JAMA 261:1155, 1989.
14. Larsen ML, Horder M, Mogensen EF: Effect of long-term monitoring of glycosylated hemoglobin levels in insulin-dependent diabetes mellitus. N Engl J Med 329:977, 1993.
15. Daneman D: Glycated hemoglobin in the assessment of diabetes control. Endocrinologist 4:33, 1994.
16. The Diabetes Control and Complications Trail Research Group: The effect of intensive treatment of diabetes on the development and progression of long-term complications in insulin-dependent diabetes mellitus. N Engl J Med 329:977, 1993.
17. Ohkubo Y, Kishikawa H, Araki E et al: Intensive insulin therapy prevents the progression of diabetic microvascular complications in Japanese patients with non-insulin-dependent diabetes mellitus: A randomized prospective 6-year study. Diabetes Res Clin Pract 28:103, 1995.
18. UK Prospective Diabetes Study Group: Effect of intensive blood-glucose control with metformin on complications in overweight patients with type 2 diabetes (UKPDS 34). Lancet 352:854, 1998.
19. Karter AJ, Ackerson LM, Darbinian JA, D'Agostino RB Jr., Ferrara A, Liu J, Selby JV: Self-monitoring of blood glucose levels and glycemic control: The Northern California Kaiser Permanente Diabetes registry. Am J Med. 111(1): 1–9, 2001.
20. Krolewski AS, Laffel LMB, Krolewski M et al: Glycosylated hemoglobin and the risk of microalbuminuria in patients with insulin-dependent diabetes mellitus. N Engl J Med 332:1251, 1995.
21. Haffner SM, Lehto S, Ronnemaa T, Pyorala K, Laakso M: Mortality from coronary heart disease in subjects with type 2 diabetes and in nondiabetic subjects with and without prior myocardial infarction. N Engl J Med. 339:229–234, 1998.
22. Stamler J, Vaccaro O, Neaton JD, Wentworth D: Diabetes, other risk factors, and 12-yr cardiovascular mortality for men screened in the Multiple Risk Factor Intervention Trial. Diabetes Care. 16:434–44, 1993.
23. Expert Panel on Detection, Evaluation, and Treatment of High Blood Cholesterol in Adults (Adult Treatment Panel III): Executive summary of the third report of the National Cholesterol Education Program (NCEP) Expert Panel on Detection, Evaluation, and Treatment of High Blood Cholesterol in Adults (Adult Treatment Panel III). JAMA 285:2486, 2001.
24. Beckles GL, Engelau MM, Narayan KM et al: Population-based assessment of the level of care among adults with diabetes in the U.S. Diabetes Care 21:1432–1438, 1998.
25. Lin DY, Blumenkranz MS, Brothers RJ, Grosvenor DM: The sensitivity and specificity of single-field nonmydriatic monochromatic digital fundus photography with remote image interpretation for

diabetic retinopathy screening: A comparison with ophthalmoscopy and standardized mydriatic color photography. Am J of Ophthalmology. 134(2): 204–13, 2002

26. Fong, Donald S, Lloyd Aiello, Thomas W. Gardner, George L. King, George Blankenship, Jerry D. Cavallerano, Fredrick L. Ferris, III, Ronald Klein: Diabetic Retinopathy. Diabetes Care 26:S99–102, 2003.

27. Norris SL, Nichols PJ, Casperson CJ, Glasgow RE, Engelgau MM, Jack L, Isham G, Snyder SR, Carande-Kulis VG, Garfield S, Briss P, McCulloch D: The effectiveness of disease and case management for people with diabetes: A systematic review. Am J Prev Med. 22(4 Suppl): 15–38, 2002.

28. Bjorvig S, Johansen MA, Fossen K: An economic analysis of screening for diabetic retinopathy. Journal of Telemedicine & Telecare. 8(1):32–5, 2002.

29. Edmonds ME, Blundell MP, Morris HE et al: The diabetic foot: Impact of a foot clinic. Q J Med 232:763, 1986.

30. Colwell JA: Aspirin therapy in diabetes. Diabetes Care. 20:1767–1771, 1997.

31. EDTRS Investigators: Aspirin effects on mortality and morbidity in patients with diabetes mellitus: early treatment diabetic retinopathy study report 14. JAMA 268:1292, 1992.

32. Mensing C, Boucher J, Cypress M, Weinger K, Mulcahy K, Barta P, Hosey G, Kopher W, Lasichak A, Lamb B, Mangan M, Norman J, Tanja J, Yauk L, Wisdom K, Adams C: National standards for diabetes self-management education. Diabetes Care 26 Suppl 1:S149–56, 2003.

33. Norris SL, Lau J, Smith SJ, Schmid CH, Engelgau MM: Self-management education for adults with type 2 diabetes: A meta-analysis of the effect on glycemic control. Diabetes Care. 25(7): 1159–71, 2002.

34. American Diabetes Association: Tests of Glycemia in Diabetes. Diabetes Care (Suppl 1) 2 26:S106–S117, 2003.

35. Baynes JW, Bunn HF, Goldstein D et al: National Diabetes Data Group: Report of the expert committee on glucosylated hemoglobin. Diabetes Care 7:602, 1984.

36. Goldstein DE, Little RR, Wiedmeyer HM et al: Glycated hemoglobin: Methodologies and clinical applications. Clin Chem 32:B64, 1986.

37. Koenig RJ, Peterson CM, Jones RL et al: Correlation of glucose regulation and hemoglobin A_{1c} in diabetes mellitus. N Engl J Med 295:417, 1976.

38. Gabbay KH, Hasty K, Breslow JL et al: Glycosylated hemoglobins and long-term blood glucose control in diabetes mellitus. J Clin Endocrinol Metab 44:859, 1977.

39. Bunn HF: Evaluation of glycosylated hemoglobin in diabetic patients. Diabetes 30:613, 1981.

40. Fairbanks V: The incidence of hemoglobin variants and their effect on glycated hemoglobin assay results. In Service FJ, Sheehan J (eds): Symposium Proceedings, Isolab, Akron, OH, 1988, p. 28.

41. Eberentz-Lhomme C, Ducrocq R, Intrator S et al: Haemoglobinopathies: A pitfall in the assessment of glycosylated haemoglobin by ion-exchange chromatography. Diabetologia 27:569, 1984.

42. Goldstein DE, Little RR, Lorenz RA et al: Tests of glycemia in diabetes. Diabetes Care 18:896, 1995.

43. Garlick RI, Mazer JS, Higgins PJ, Bunn HF: Characterization of glycosylated hemoglobins. Relevance to monitoring of diabetic control and analysis of other proteins. J Clin Invest 71:1062, 1983.

44. Davie SJ, Gould BJ, Yudkin JS: Effect of vitamin C on glycosylation of proteins. Diabetes 41:167, 1992.

45. Ceriello A, Giugliano D, Quatraro A et al: Vitamin E reduction of protein glucosylation in diabetes: New prospect for prevention of diabetic complications? Diabetes Care 14:68, 1991.

46. Nathan DM, Singer DE, Hurxthal K, Goodson JD: The clinical information value of the glycosylated hemoglobin assay. N Engl J Med 310:341, 1984.

47. Santiago JV: Perspectives in diabetes: Lessons from the Diabetes Control and Complications Trial. Diabetes 42:1549, 1993.

48. McFarland KF, Catalano EW, Day JF et al: Nonenzymatic glycosylation of serum proteins in diabetes mellitus. Diabetes 28:1011, 1979.

49. Rendell M, Kao G, Mecherikunnel P et al: Use of aminophenylboronic acid affinity chromatography to measure glycosylated albumin levels. J Lab Clin Med 105:63, 1985.

50. Goldstein DE, Little RR, Lorenz RA et al: Test of glycemia in diabetes (Technical Review). Diabetes Care 18:896, 1995.

51. Benjamin RJ, Sacks DB: Glycated protein update: Implications of recent studies including Diabetes Control and Complications Trial. Clin Chem 40:683, 1994.

52. Pirart J: Diabetes mellitus and its degenerative complications: A prospective study of 4.400 patients observed between 1947 and 1973. Diabetes Care 1:168, 1978.

53. Gale EA, Kurtz AB, Tattersall RB: In search of the Somogyi effect. Lancet 2:279, 1980.

54. Gerich JE: Dawn phenomenon: Pathophysiology, diagnosis, and treatment. Clin Diabetes 6:1, 1988.

55. De Feo P, Perriello G, Bolli GB: Somogyi and dawn phenomena: Mechanisms. Diabetes Metab Rev 4:31, 1988.

56. Davidson MB, Harris MD, Ziel FH et al: Suppression of sleep-induced growth hormone secretion by anticholinergic agent abolishes dawn phenomenon. Diabetes 37:166, 1988.

57. Lerman IG, Wolfsdorf JI: Relationship of nocturnal hypoglycemia to daytime glycemia in IDDM. Diabetes Care 111:636, 1988.

58. Stephenson JM, Schernthaner G: Dawn phenomenon and Somogyi effect in IDDM. Diabetes Care 12:245, 1989.

59. Hirsch IB, Smith IJ, Havlin CE et al: Failure of nocturnal hypoglycemia to cause daytime hyperglycemia in patients with IDDM. Diabetes Care 13:133, 1990.

60. Diabetes Prevention Program Research Group: Reduction in the incidence of type 2 diabetes with lifestyle intervention or metformin. N Engl J Med 346:393, 2002.

61. Cryer PE: Glucose counterregulation in man. Diabetes 30:261, 1981.

62. Bolli G, De Feo P, Compagnucci P et al: Abnormal glucose counterregulation in insulin-dependent diabetes mellitus: Interaction of anti-insulin antibodies and impaired glucagon and epinephrine secretion. Diabetes 32:134, 1983.

63. Kleinbaum J, Shamoon H: Impaired counterregulation of hypoglycemia in insulin-dependent diabetes mellitus. Diabetes 32:493, 1983.

64. Goldstein DE, Parker KM, England JD et al: Clinical application of glycosylated hemoglobin measurements. Diabetes 31(suppl 3):70, 1982.

65. Lorenz RA, Santiago JV, Siebert C et al: Epidemiology of severe hypoglycemia in the Diabetes Control and Complications Trial. Am J Med 90:450, 1991.

66. Park BN, Soeldner JS, Gleason RE: Diabetes in remission. Insulin secretory dynamics. Diabetes 23:616, 1974.

67. Wing RR, Hill JO: Successful weight loss maintenance. Annu Rev Nutr 21:323, 2001.

68. Fujioka K, Seaton TB, Rowe E et al., for the Sibutramine/Diabetes Clinical Study Group: Weight loss with sibutramine improves glycaemic control and other metabolic parameters in obese patients with type 2 diabetes mellitus. Diabetes Obes Metab 2:175, 2000.

69. Hollander PA, Elbein SC, Hirsch IB et al: Role of orlistat in the treatment of obese patients with type 2 diabetes: A randomized double-blind study. Diabetes Care 21:1288, 1998.

70. Franz MJ, Bantle JP, Beebe CA et al: Evidence-based nutrition principles and recommendations for the treatment and prevention of diabetes and related complications. Diabetes Care 25:148, 2002.

71. Nightengale ML, Sarr MG, Kelly KA et al: Prospective evaluation of vertical banded gastroplasty as the primary operation for morbid obesity. Mayo Clin Proc 66:773, 1991.

72. Brodows RG, Williams C, Amatruda JM: Treatment of insulin reactions in diabetics. JAMA 252:3378, 1984.

73. Slama G, Traynard P-Y, Desplanque N et al: The search for an optimized treatment of hypoglycemia: Carbohydrates in tables, solution, or gel for the correction of insulin reactions. Arch Intern Med. 150:589, 1990.

74. Munro JF, Campbell IW, McCuish AC, Duncan IJP: Euglycaemic diabetic ketoacidosis. BMJ 2:578, 1973.

75. Lynch J, Helmrich SP, Kakha TA, et al: Moderately intense physical activities and high levels of cardiorespiratory fitness reduce risk of non-insulin-dependent diabetes mellitus in middle-aged men. Arch Intern Med. 156:1307–1314, 1996.

76. Wei M, Gibbons LW, Mitchell TL, Kampert JB, Lee CD, Blair SN: The association between cardiorespiratory fitness and impaired fasting glucose and type 2 diabetes mellitus in men. Ann Intern Med. 130(2):89–96, 1999.

77. Schneider SH, Ruderman NB: Exercise and NIDDM. Diabetes Care 13:785, 1990.

78. Wasserman DH, Zinman B: Exercise in individuals with IDDM. Diabetes Care 17:924, 1994.

79. Schneider SH, Morgado A: Effects of fitness and physical training on carbohydrate metabolism and associated cardiovascular risk factors in patients with diabetes. Diabetes Rev 3:378, 1995.

80. Tuomilehto J, Lindstrom J, Eriksson JG, et al: Prevention of type 2 diabetes mellitus by changes in lifestyle among subjects with impaired glucose tolerance. N Engl J Med. 344:1343–1350, 2001.

81. Jakcic JM, Wing RR, Butler BA, Robertson RJ: Prescribing exercise in multiple short bouts versus one continuous bout: Effects on adherence, cardiorespiratory fitness, and weight loss in overweight women. Int J Obes 19:893–901, 1995.

82. Castaneda C, Layne JE, Munoz-Orians L, Gordon PL, Walsmith J, Foldvari M, Roubenoff R, Tucker KL, Nelson ME: A randomized controlled trial of resistance exercise training to improve glycemic control in older adults with type 2 diabetes. Diabetes Care. 25(12):2335–41, 2002.

83. Hu FB, Sigal RJ, Rich-Edwards JW, et al: Walking compared with vigorous physical activity and risk of type 2 diabetes in women. JAMA. 282:1433–1439, 1999.

84. Trost SG, Owen N, Bauman AE, Sallis JF, Brown W, Correlates of adults' participation in physical activity: Review and update. Medicine & Science in Sports & Exercise. 34(12):1996–2001, 2002 Dec.

85. Gregg EW, Gerzoff RB, Caspersen CJ, Williamson DF, Narayan KM: Relationship of walking to mortality among US adults with diabetes. Archives of Internal Medicine. 163(12):1440–7, 2003.

86. Hernandez JM, Moccia T, Fluckey JD, Ulbrecht JS, Farrell PA: Fluid snacks to help persons with type 1 diabetes avoid late onset postexercise hypoglycemia. Medicine & Science in Sports & Exercise. 32(5): 904–10, 2000.

87. Rabasa-Lhoret R, Bouque J, Ducros F, Chiasson JL: Guidelines for premeal insulin dose reduction for postprandial exercise of different intensities and durations in type 1 diabetic subjects treated intensively with a basal-bolus insulin regimen (ultralente-lispro). Diabetes Care. 24(4):625–30, 2001.

88. Schneider SH, Khachadurian AK, Amorosa LF et al: Ten-year experience with an exercise-based outpatient life-style modification program in the treatment of diabetes mellitus. Diabetes Care 15(suppl 4):1800, 1992.

89. Hanisch R, Snyder A: Exercise in insulin dependent diabetes (IDDM) may be safe with starting glucose < 16.7 mM. Diabetes 45(suppl 2):107A, 1996.

90. Colberg Sheri: "The Diabetic Athlete." Champaign, IL: Human Kinetics, March 2001.

91. Young MJ, Veves A, Boulton AJM: The diabetic foot: Aetiopathogenesis and management. Diabetes Metab Rev 9:109, 1993.

92. Caputo GM, Cavanagh PR, Ulbrecht JS et al: Assessment and management of foot disease in patients with diabetes. N Engl J Med 331:854, 1994.

93. Grayson ML, Gibbons GW, Balogh K et al: Probing to bone in infected pedal ulcers: A clinical sign of underlying osteomyelitis in diabetic patients. JAMA 273:721, 1995.

94. Eckman MH, Greenfield S, Mackey WC et al: Foot infections in diabetic patients: Decision and cost-effectiveness analysis. JAMA 273:712, 1995.

95. Malmberg K, Norhammar A, Wedel H, Ryden L: Glycometabolic state at admission: Important risk marker of mortality in conventionally treated patients with diabetes mellitus and acute myocardial infarction: Long-term results from the Diabetes and Insulin-Glucose Infusion in Acute Myocardial Infarction (DIGAMI) study. Circulation. 99:2626–32, 1999.

96. van den Berghe G, Wouters P, Weekers F, et al: Intensive insulin therapy in critically ill patients. N Engl J Med. 345:1359–67, 2001.

97. Hirsch IB, Paauw DS, Brunzell J: Inpatient management of adults with diabetes. Diabetes Care. 18(6):870–8, 1995.

98. Levetan CS, Magee MF: Hospital management of diabetes. Endocrinol & Metab Clin North Am. 29(4):745–70, 2000.

99. Walts LF, Miller J, Davidson MB, Brown J: Perioperative management of diabetes mellitus. Anesthesiology 55:104, 1981.

100. Rosenstock J, Raskin P: Surgery! Practical guidelines for diabetes management. Clin Diabetes 5:62, 1987

101. Alberti KG, Gill GV, Elliott MJ: Insulin delivery during surgery in the diabetic patient. Diabetes Care 5(suppl 1):65, 1982.

102. Fletcher J, Langman MJS, Kellock TD: Effect of surgery on blood-sugar levels in diabetes mellitus. Lancet 2:52, 1965.

103. Vejlsgaard R: Studies on urinary tract infection in diabetes I: Bacteriuria in patients with diabetes mellitus and in control subjects. Acta Med Scand 179:173, 1966.

104. Ellenbogen PH, Talner LB: Uroradiology of diabetes mellitus. Urology 8:413, 1976.

105. Smitherman KN, Peacock JE Jr: Infectious emergencies in patients with diabetes mellitus. Med Clin North Am 67:118, 1988.

106. Michaeli J, Mogle P, Perlberg S et al: Emphysematous pyelonephritis. J Urol 131:203, 1984.

107. Wise GJ, Kozinn PJ, Goldberg P: Amphotericin B as a urologic irrigant n the management of non invasive candiduria. J Urol 128:82, 1982.

108. Patrick AW, Gill GV, MacFarlane IA et al: Home glucose monitoring in type 2 diabetes: Is it a waste of time? Diabetic Med 11:62, 1994.

109. Leu HS, Huang CT. Clearance of funguria with short course antifungal regiments: A prospective, randomized, controlled study. Clin Infect Dis 20:1152, 1995.

110. Joshi N, Caputo GM, Weitekamp MR, Karchmer AW: Infections in patients with diabetes mellitus. New Engl J Med 341:1906, 1999.

111. Sentochnik DE: Deep soft-tissue infections in diabetic patients. Infect Dis Clin North Am 9:53, 1995.

112. Fine MJ, Smith MA, Carson CA et al: Prognosis and outcomes of patients with community acquired pneumonia: A meta-analysis. JAMA 275:143, 1996.

113a. Smith SA, Poland GA: Use of influenza and pneumococcal vaccines in people with diabetes (Technical Review). Diabetes Care 23:95–108, 2000.

114. Advisory Committee on Immunization Practices (ACIP): Prevention of pneumococcal disease: Recommendations of the Advisory Committee on Immunization Practices (ACIP) MMWR 46:1, 1997.

115. Smith SA, Poland GA: Use of influenza and pneumococcal vaccines in people with diabetes (Technical Review). Diabetes Care 23:95–108, 2000.

116. Advisory Committee on Immunization Practices (ACIP): Prevention and control of influenza: Recommendations of the Advisory Committee on Immunization Practices (ACIP). MMWR 46:1, 1997.

117. Murphy KR, Strunk RC: Safe administration of influenza vaccine in asthmatic children hypersensitive to egg proteins. J Pediatr 106:931, 1985.

118. Gaede P, Vedel P, Larsen N, Jensen GV, Parving HH, Pedersen O: Multifactorial intervention and cardiovascular disease in patients with type 2 diabetes. N Engl J Med. 348(5):383–93,2003.

DIABETES MANAGEMENT IN CHILDREN AND ADOLESCENTS

• FRANCINE RATNER KAUFMAN

Diabetes mellitus in children and adolescents results from an impairment of insulin secretion, insulin action, or both. Approximately 80% of pediatric patients have type 1 diabetes resulting from complete or near-complete destruction of the pancreatic β cell mass on an immune or idiopathic basis. Type 2 diabetes, resulting from insulin resistance and impairment of compensatory insulin secretion, is rapidly increasing in incidence and has been labeled a new epidemic in the pediatric population.[1] In addition, children have secondary diabetes caused by a variety of other disease processes such as cystic fibrosis and genetic syndromes and as a side effect of certain medications. Rarely, adolescent females develop gestational diabetes.

There are many common features to the different forms of diabetes in children, particularly between types 1 and 2 diabetes. These are outlined in Table 10-1. For example, there are genetic and environmental factors that are involved in the pathogenesis of both type 1 and type 2 diabetes. For type 1 diabetes, multiple loci in the major histocompatability leukocyte antigen region, such as the class II DR and DQ alleles, confer diabetes susceptibility.[2,3] Environmental factors include infectious agents such as

viruses, components of the diet, and toxins.[4] For type 2 diabetes, genetic predisposition is proven by the fact that >85% of affected children have a family member with type 2 diabetes. The environmental factors include the dietary intake of excess total and fat calories and sedentary life style that promotes obesity. There is a prodromal period for the different types of diabetes during which the patient is essentially asymptomatic despite progressive insulin deficiency, insulin resistance, or both. This prodromal time may allow for interventions that will preserve some element of β cell function or improve insulin resistance to ameliorate the disease state. The clinical disease onset involves the same set of symptoms that result from hyperglycemia. Chronic disease management requires both alteration of life style and pharmacologic interventions. There are an ever-increasing number of potential pharmacologic agents that can be used, and disease management requires that the patient and family integrate complex treatment plans into their daily lives. Finally, there are similar chronic complications resulting from recurrent, persistent hyperglycemia that involve the microcirculation (retinopathy, nephropathy, neuropathy) and macrocirculation (cardiovascular disease

TABLE 10-1	COMMON FEATURES OF TYPE 1, TYPE 2, AND SECONDARY DIABETES IN CHILDREN	
Pathogenesis	Genetic and environmental factors • Lead to the disease process	
Prodromal period	Variable asymptomatic period • Resulting from progressive insulin deficiency, insulin resistance or both	
Clinical disease onset	Symptoms resulting from hyperglycemia • Polyuria, polydipsia, polyphagia, weight loss, fatigue, genitourinary infection	
Chronic disease management	Dual management approach • Lifestyle and pharmacologic interventions	
Chronic complications	Recurrent, persistent hyperglycemia • Microcirculatory and macrocirculatory complications	

and stroke), and there is the risk of hypoglycemia.

Major advances have been made in type 1 and type 2 diabetes disease management. Advances have come forth from a number of large clinical trials, such as the Diabetes Control and Complications Trial (DCCT)[5-7] for type 1 and the United Kingdom Prospective Diabetes Study[8] for type 2 diabetes. Both of these trials illustrated that intensive diabetes regimens have a major impact on improving short- and long-term diabetes outcome. Although neither trial was primarily pediatric in focus, it appears that the results can be generalized to conclude that children and youth should follow intensive management protocols similar to those for adults. These intensive diabetes regimens mandate that glucose levels be monitored throughout the day. Glucose lowering agents, insulin, and/or oral hypoglycemic agents need to be given per complex algorithms, and food and activity need to be balanced to facilitate glycemic control. With appropriate glucose control, children with both type 1 and type 2 diabetes should be expected to experience a reduction in short- and long-term diabetes complications, to have normalization of growth and pubertal development, and to optimize physical and psychosocial

well-being. The systems of diabetes management that are advocated must be carefully taught and reinforced to patients and families. School and day care personnel and other caregivers must be informed of diabetes treatment goals and given the tools to enable the child to be safe and well while under their care. To accomplish this, a team of diabetes specialists and primary care providers need to work together to promote the physical and emotional health of patients and their families.

This chapter reviews the multiple components of diabetes management for type 1 and type 2 diabetes in children and youth. The focus is on intensive regimens that require patients and families to measure glucose levels; set glycemic targets; take glucose lowering medications per complex algorithms; and balance food, activity, and the effects of illness. The psychosocial issues surrounding the impact that these comprehensive, intensive diabetes management protocols have on daily life is addressed. The emphasis is placed on that fact that affected children still need to reach the normal developmental milestones of infancy, childhood, and adolescence; strive to succeed in school and in extracurricular activities; and develop eventual independence and autonomy.

TYPE I DIABETES

PRINCIPLES OF DIABETES MANAGEMENT

Insulin

Type 1 diabetes in children and youth is treated with insulin, either by giving multiple injections each day, with continuous subcutaneous insulin infusion (CSII) via an insulin pump, or with inhaled insulin, which is presently being evaluated in children in clinical trials.

At present, virtually all insulin-treated children should use human insulin preparations. Compared to animal insulin, human insulin has a more predictable time course, lower anti-insulin antibody titers indicative of reduced antigenicity and decreased immunogenicity.[9,10] There are five categories of human insulin preparations: rapid-acting insulin (lispro [Humalog], aspart [NovoLog]), short-acting insulin (regular, semilente), intermediate-acting insulin (NPH, lente), long-acting insulin (ultralente), and basal insulin (glargine [Lantus]). There are some unique qualities that these insulin preparations have in pediatric subjects. Rapid-acting insulin preparations have been shown to have an important role, particularly in young children. Because these preparations have an onset of action within 15 to 30 minutes, a peak action at 1 to 2 hours, and duration of action of 3 to 5 hours, rapid-acting insulin can be given either 10 to 15 minutes before the meal, or just after the meal. Because of the unpredictable food intake pattern of young children, immediate postmeal administration of rapid-acting insulin has been shown to be effective[11,12] in reducing hypoglycemia. Rapid-acting insulin has also been shown to lead to less hyperglycemia after eating and less hypoglycemia in the late postprandial period and at nighttime when children are particularly susceptible to hypoglycemia.[13] Although this reduction in glycemic excursion exists, for the most part rapid-acting insulin has been shown to have a negligible or minimal effect on reducing hemoglobin A_{1c} (A1C) in clinical trials.[13,14] Children often have a more unpredictable duration of action with intermediate- and long-acting insulin preparations. Because of this unpredictability, the older long-acting insulin preparations never gained wide-spread acceptance. Initial studies of insulin glargine (Lantus) in children are presently underway. Insulin glargine has been shown to result in less hypoglycemia in adults[15] and lower free insulin levels compared with NPH insulin.[16-19] As of this writing, there is insufficient data concerning this long-acting basal insulin preparation with regard to clinical efficacy in children. Other new long-acting basal analogues (NN304, manufactured by Novo Nordisk) are also being developed with potentially unique properties and durations of action.[20] The use of premixed insulin has minimal benefit in children and youth. Although premixed insulin has been shown to improve adherence with the medical regimen in adults with diabetes, particularly type 2, it has more limited value in children resulting from the inability to alter insulin dosages in concert with glucose levels and carbohydrate intake.[21]

Insulin delivery with devices other than the insulin syringe appears to have a role in pediatric diabetes.[22] The pen devices are appealing to children and youth for three reasons: (1) They obviate the need for accurately drawing insulin from a vial, (2) they are easy to use, and (3) they can deliver insulin at half-unit increments. The pen devices have a unique role in the school setting, where there is concern about the accuracy and safety of insulin delivery with a syringe. Pen devices can be used by children taking multiple daily injections or by those who only intermittently need to correct an abnormal blood glucose level. Automatic injection devices used to hide the needle of the insulin syringe and jet injectors have a place in diminishing needle phobia.

Subcutaneous insulin can be delivered in a number of sites on the body, even in infants and toddlers. Insulin can be injected in the lateral aspect of the arm, the abdomen, the front of the thigh, and the lateral thigh. Children and youth should be encouraged to rotate injection sites, but to use the same part of the body at a particular time of the day, such as the arms for bedtime or abdomen for breakfast. They should be advised not to inject into the exact same location. However, young children often will agree to be injected in only one body area. As long as there is no local adverse effect, it may be important to acquiesce for the psychologic benefit of the young child who needs some control over the diabetes regimen. In general, insulin absorption is faster in children because they have better circulation, less adipose, and take a smaller dosage of insulin. They also have undesired local reactions as the result of insulin administration.[23] These include lipohypertrophy and lipoatrophy, and only rarely local insulin allergy. Lipoatrophy is due to a local reaction from impurities and can be minimized by injecting around the periphery of the lesions. Lipohypertrophy occurs in areas of chronic insulin injections or at the sites of pump catheter insertion. Because hypertrophic areas have diminished pain sensation, areas of lipohypertrophy are popular sites for repeated injection.

Children as young as 6 years of age have been enrolled in inhaled insulin trials. To date, there has been good efficacy and little toxicity in adult trials with inhaled insulin.[24] Higher titers of insulin antibodies have been recognized in those receiving inhaled insulin. The significance of these antibodies is presently unknown. In the future, it may be possible to deliver insulin orally or transdermally. These novel ways to deliver insulin may have a particular benefit in pediatrics because some children have needle phobia, because some perceive that insulin injections are painful, and because delivery of insulin via a needle and a syringe requires cognitive and developmental skills that young children do not possess.

Initiation of Insulin Therapy

Daily subcutaneous insulin injections are begun at the time of the diagnosis of type 1 diabetes. Two or three insulin injections per day are given.[14,25-28] The total amount of insulin is variable, depending on the severity of illness and the age of the subject at presentation. Table 10-2 gives the dosage and the distribution of insulin for patients with new-onset diabetes.[29] For those subjects who present in diabetic ketoacidosis (DKA), a high total dose of insulin is required (1 to 2 U/kg per day), whereas those less ill but symptomatic (½ to 1 U/kg per day) and those asymptomatic (½ U/kg per day) require a lesser total dosage of insulin. The total insulin dosage is initially split; two thirds of the dose is administered in the morning, one third in the evening. For two injections, the morning dose is usually split: one third is short- or rapid-acting insulin and two thirds is intermediate-acting. The dinner dose is divided equally between short- or rapid-acting and intermediate-acting insulin. For three injections, the morning injection is the same as noted for two injections and the evening dose is split. Half is given as short-or rapid-acting insulin before dinner and half as intermediate-acting insulin before bed. Thereafter, dosage adjustment becomes individualized according to blood glucose levels, carbohydrate intake, and specific glycemic patterns.[29,30] For example, if prebreakfast glucose levels are above the target range, the evening intermediate-acting insulin is adjusted until fasting levels improve. Or if prelunch glucose levels are below the target range, the morning short- or rapid-acting insulin is decreased. To optimize glucose control, most patients with new-onset diabetes and their families have frequent if not daily contact with the health care team. At that time, the health care team advises the patient and family how to alter the

TABLE 10-2	DISTRIBUTION OF INSULIN AT DIABETES DIAGNOSIS		
Total Dosage	**After DKA**	**Symptomatic**	**Asymptomatic**
	1–2 U/kg/day	½–1 U/kg/day	½ U/kg/day
	Morning	*Dinner*	*Bedtime*
	⅔ *Total Dose*	⅓ *Total Dose*	
2 injections	⅓ Rapid or short ⅔ Intermediate	½ Rapid or short ½ Intermediate	
	⅔ *Total Dose*	⅙ *Total Dose*	⅙ *Total Dose*
3 injections	⅓ Rapid or short ⅔ Intermediate	Rapid or short	Intermediate or long

DKA, diabetic ketoacidosis.

Adapted from Kaufman FR, Halvorson M: New trends in managing type I diabetes. Contemp Pediatr 16:112, 1999.

insulin regimen with the goal that they will eventually learn dosage adjustment skills themselves.

Within weeks to months of the diagnosis of diabetes, most patients enter a remission or "honeymoon" phase of diabetes. The remission phase is characterized by excellent glycemic control with a minimum of hyperglycemic and hypoglycemic episodes. This is due to the resurgence of endogenous insulin secretion as the result of the recovery of β-cells that have not yet been destroyed by the autoimmune type 1 process. Because of endogenous insulin secretion, the dosage of exogenous insulin can be decreased, often to total insulin doses lower than ⅓ U/kg per day. In the past, patients were weaned off one or another insulin injections or off insulin altogether during this period. However, this is no longer recommended. It not only appears advantageous to continue multiple injections so that subjects remain accustomed to them, but meticulous glycemic control itself appears to prolong the remission period.[1,31] Despite this, the duration of the remission rarely persists more than 6 to 12 months. The end of the remission phase is characterized by an increase in the variability of blood glucose concentrations, A1C levels, and exogenous insulin requirements. At this time, diabetes management becomes more difficult.

Because it is challenging to control glycemia, the patient and family must advance their knowledge and skills and develop the appropriate attitudes so that they will succeed in integrating the diabetes regimen, which may change over time, into their lives.

Insulin Regimens

The goal of diabetes management is to achieve optimal glycemia with as great a reduction in short- and long-term complications as is possible. Over the long term, some pediatric patients, particularly very young children, may do extremely well on two or three insulin injections per day. However, other children, particularly older children, adolescents, and those with a long diabetes duration, may not be able to control glycemia with two or three injections because it offers less flexibility in matching insulin with food and activity. This has led to more and more subjects eventually being placed on intensive or flexible regimens that utilize basal-bolus therapy. The basal insulin component must have a sufficient effect throughout the 24-hour period to cover basal requirements. Bolus insulin is delivered in a flexible manner to match carbohydrate and food intake, changes in activity level, and insulin. Basal-bolus therapy can be achieved with multiple daily injections (MDIs) of insulin combining an intermediate-, long-acting insulin or basal with a rapid-acting insulin bolus given before meals.[29] Basal-bolus can also be achieved with CSII with an insulin pump.[32] These methods are compared in Table 10-3. Insulin pump therapy has been shown to be ideal for patients wishing to optimize glycemia, improve life style, reduce hypoglycemia, and prevent recurrent ketoacidosis or progression of diabetes complications.[32-35] Flexible or intensive treatment regimens require that specific glycemic targets be set with regard to preprandial and postprandial glucose and A1C levels and that dosage adjustment algorithms are utilized. In young children, insulin pump therapy at nighttime only has been shown to be beneficial.[33] It has become clearly evident that children and youth, including young children, can use these intensive, flexible insulin regimens when

coupled with education, motivation, and support.[36–38]

In our center, patients on CSII have been followed longitudinally from 1994 to 2000 to determine short- and long-term outcomes. We have tracked multiple measures that have all shown improvement. The mean A1C has decreased from $8.4 \pm 1.8\%$ to $7.8 \pm 1.2\%$ ($p < 0.01$). The severe hypoglycemia event rate decreased from 0.09 to 0.04 events per patient per year ($p < 0.05$), and the DKA rate was decreased from 0.15 to 0.09 events per patient per year ($p < 0.05$).[33,37] In school-aged children, the mean number of pump basal rates was 4.1 ± 1.8 and the mean insulin dosage was 0.62 ± 0.17 U/kg per day. Scores on tests of knowledge (82 ± 10 versus 92 ± 6, $p < 0.001$), integration (79 ± 12 versus 90 ± 6, $p < 0.01$) and quality of life (3.9 ± 0.4 versus 4.2 ± 0.3, $p < 0.005$) were higher the year following initiation of CSII compared with the year prior.

TABLE 10-3 COMPARISONS OF REGIMENS OF MDI AND CSII

	MDI		CSII	
	Basal	**Bolus**	**Basal**	**Bolus**
Insulin Type	Intermediate (NPH, lente) or long-acting (ultralente, glargine)	Rapid-acting (aspart [NovoLog], lispro [Humalog])	Rapid-acting (aspart [NovoLog], lispro [Humalog])	Rapid-acting (aspart [Novolog], lispro [Humalog])
Percent of Total	50%	50%	50%	50%
Formula to Determine Dosage for Carbohydrate Intake		Total daily insulin dose ÷ 450 = g of CHO covered by 1 unit		Total daily insulin dose ÷ 450 = g of CHO covered by 1 unit
Formula to Determine Dosage for Correction of Blood Glucose > Target Range		1800 ÷ total daily insulin dose = the amount 1 U will lower theblood glucose level		1800 ÷ total daily insulin dose = the amount 1 U will lower the blood glucose level

CHO, carbohydrate; CSII, continuous subcutaneous insulin infusion; MDI, multiple daily injections; NPH, neutral protein hagedorn.

To use pump treatment successfully, patients and families must have sufficient knowledge and skills and the appropriate attitudes to manage the technology, as outlined in Table 10-4.[33,37] In preschool- and early school-aged children, the tasks required are done by the parent or guardian. As the child progresses, more and more pump management is gradually assumed by the patient, so that by late adolescence, teens can assume responsibility for CSII.

Blood Glucose and Ketone Monitoring

Measurement of the blood glucose level multiple times during the day and intermittently during the night is imperative if glycemic targets are to be met. In a number of studies, glycemic control was associated with the frequency of blood glucose monitoring.[39-44] In a large cohort of youth 7 to 16 years of age, it was the sole modifiable predictor of A1C levels.[45] Blood glucose should be measured according to the schema given in Table 10-5.

It is likely also important to determine blood glucose levels in the postprandial period.[46] Because it is unknown how significant peak glucose levels after meals are in adding to the glycemic burden of diabetes, it might be of value to obtain some 2-hour postmeal glucose levels. These glucose levels are of particular relevance to those on basal-bolus regimens because postmeal levels help determine how to dose bolus insulin.

There have been many advances that have made home glucose monitoring easier, faster, less painful, and more relevant. Glucose measurements can be done on very small blood samples. Preprandial samples can be taken from the forearms. Forearm

TABLE 10-4	SKILLS, KNOWLEDGE, AND ATTITUDES REQUIRED FOR INSULIN PUMP BY AGE	
Specific Skills	**Knowledge/Attitudes**	
School-Age Children (6–10 Yr of Age)		
Insert pump catheter, wear pump with help Unhook and rehook with assistance Activate bolus with supervision		
School-Age Children (10–12 Yr of Age)		
Protect pump during activities Unhook and rehook without assistance Activate bolus without supervision	Carbohydrate count Understand role of exercise Start to calculate correction dose	
Young Adolescents (12–14 Yr of Age)		
Suspend basal dose Program basal rates with assistance	Calculate and deliver bolus Understand temporary basal changes	
Older Adolescents (15–18 Yr of Age)		
Program basal rate change	Determine what affects basal/bolus rates Use algorithms Understand sick days	

Adapted from Kaufman FR, Halvorson M, Miller D et al: Insulin pump therapy in type I pediatric patients: Now and into the year 2000. Diabetes Metab Res Rev 15:338, 1999; Kaufman FR, Halvorson M, Carpenter S, Devoe D: Insulin pump in young children with diabetes. Diabetes Spectrum 14:84, 2001; Kaufman FR, Halvorson M, Fisher LK, Pitukcheewanont P: Insulin pump therapy in type I pediatric patients. J Pediatr Endocrinol Metab 12:759, 1999.

TABLE 10-5	SCHEMA FOR BLOOD GLUCOSE MONITORING
Routinely	
A minimum of four values per day before meals and bedtime To confirm hypoglycemia	
Intermittently	
At midnight and/or 0200–0300 After strenuous exercise During illness When traveling Midmorning and afternoon snack times When the routine is altered	

sampling may not be as reliable in the nonsteady, postmeal state or at times of hypoglycemia. Results are available in 5 to 45 seconds; glucose meters are small enough to fit in a pocket. Glucose meters store glucose values that can be displayed in a variety of forms and graphs either directly on the meter or on a home computer. Although this enables patients and their families to better identify undesired patterns and trends, keeping a logbook is still important to determine how to alter the regimen. Review of stored glucose values can also detect periods in which the patient may not be testing despite reporting glucose values. If this is found, it is an indication that acceptance and integration of diabetes may not have occurred.

Recently, semi-invasive, continuous, or frequent glucose monitoring devices have been developed. In the research setting, these glucose monitoring systems, such as the MiniMed CGMS (Medtronic, Inc, Northridge, CA) and the Cygnus GlucoWatch Automatic Glucose Biographer (Cygnus, Inc, Redwood City, CA), have been shown to facilitate identification of glycemic patterns and trends and lead to improvement in glycemic control.[22,47-50] These systems appear to be accepted by children with only some minor local reactions at the site of skin penetration or insertion. When continuous systems can be used in the clinical arena to give patients and families real-time continuous glucose levels, it is likely that a marked improvement in short- and long-term diabetes outcome will be appreciated. Eventually, it is anticipated that these will be linked to insulin infusion devices creating a near-artificial pancreas.

Measuring urine or blood ketones during times of severe or sustained hyperglycemia, stress, fever, or intercurrent illness is important. Blood ketones can now be measured with a home device that has a combined glucose and ketone sensor (Medisense/ Abbott Laboratories, Abington, U.K.).[51] Any child who has vomiting or evidence of dehydration should determine whether ketonuria or ketonemia is present. Urine and blood tests measure different metabolites: (1) Urine ketone tests measure acetoacetate, and (2) blood ketone tests measure β-hydroxybutyrate. Because β-hydroxybutyrate is the predominant ketone body in DKA, urine measurement may give false negative results.[52] Because ketoacidosis can develop with failure of insulin delivery in patients using CSII, patients on insulin pump therapy need to be able to assess for the presence of ketonuria or ketonemia. The presence of ketones should lead to immediate evaluation and intervention because DKA requiring hospitalization can be avoided if recognized early and treated appropriately.

Glycemic Targets

The management goal for infants, children, and teens with type 1 diabetes is to have blood glucose and A1C levels fall within an age-specific target range that takes into account the developmental, cognitive, and communicative abilities of the child and the abilities and resources of the family.[14,29] Because it appears that young children are more susceptible to severe hypoglycemia, the target ranges for blood glucose and A1C levels are generally higher. However, as children age, the primary concern shifts from avoidance of excessive hypoglycemia to avoidance of hyperglycemia as a means to decrease long-term diabetes complications. Table 10-6 outlines glycemic and A1C targets for children by age.

Multiple studies, including the DCCT with its adolescent cohort, a multicenter, multinational report by Danne et al.,[53] and a recent study by Levine et al.[45] from an academic center in the United States, have shown that it is difficult to achieve optimal A1C outcome in children and adolescents with type 1 diabetes.

Insulin Dosage Adjustment

Insulin doses need to be adjusted to correct for blood glucose levels outside of the target range (correction algorithm). The insulin sensitivity factor that illustrates how much a unit of rapid-acting insulin will decrease the blood glucose level (in mg/dl) is given in Table 10-3 and is derived by dividing 1800 by the total daily insulin dosage. For short-acting insulin, the amount is derived by dividing 1500 by the total daily insulin dosage. These amounts can then be divided in half to determine the amount of insulin required for every 50 mg/dl that the blood glucose level is increased above the target range. In addition to this calculation, there are other formulas, given in Table 10-7, that can be used to determine how much insulin is required to correct a blood glucose level that is above the target range. These insulin dosage algorithms can be taught to the patient and family by several methods. The algorithm can be written on a piece of paper, algorithms are available on plastic cards,[54] or they can be found in computerized devices.

Adjustments are often required for physical activity. Increases in activity not only cause fluctuations at the time, but can result in delayed or nocturnal hypoglycemia. In general, for an isolated period of activity lasting ½ to 2 hours, a child will likely need to take 10 to 15 g of carbohydrate for every ½ to 1 hour. This depends on the starting blood glucose concentration, the level of activity, and prior experience with similar exercise. Occasionally, activity can cause elevation of blood glucose levels. This usually occurs in the afternoon for children taking two or three insulin injections per day or if CSII is disconnected for greater than 1½ to 2 hours. With repeated strenuous physical activity, the total daily insulin dose may need to be decreased by 10% to 20%.

TABLE 10-6	GLYCEMIC AND A1C TARGETS			
Blood Glucose	**0–2 yr**	**3–6 yr**	**7–12 yr**	**>13 yr**
Premeal mg/dl	100–180	70–150	70–150	70–150
2–3 Hour postprandial mg/dl	<200	<200	<180	<180
Before bed mg/dl	100–200	100–180	90–160	80–150
2–4 AM mg/dl	>100	>100	>90	>80
A1C %	<8.5	<8.0	<7.5	<7.0

Adapted from Buckingham BA, Bluck B, Wilson DM: Intensive diabetes management in pediatric patients. Curr Diabetes Rep 1:18, 2001.

| TABLE 10-7 | EXAMPLES OF HOW TO DETERMINE THE AMOUNT OF INSULIN TO BE GIVEN TO CORRECT AN ABNORMAL BLOOD GLUCOSE LEVEL, BY TOTAL INSULIN DOSAGE OR BY AGE |

Insulin Dosage	Age	Amount/50 mg/dl that Blood Glucose Is Elevated
<5 U	<5 yr	¼ U
5–10 U	6–9 yr	½ U
10–20 U	10–12 yr	I U
>20 U	Teens	2 U

For immediate correction of an abnormal blood glucose level, add insulin according to the algorithm following if blood glucose is above the target range.

Add insulin before meals, snacks, and at bedtime (at bedtime, give 50% of the dosage and check blood glucose in 2-3 hours).

Adapted from Kaufman FR, Halvorson M: New trends in managing type I diabetes. Contemp Pediatr 16:112, 1999; Kaufman FR, Halvorson M, Carpenter S: Use of a plastic insulin dosage guide to correct blood glucose levels of the target range and for carbohydrate counting in subjects with type I diabetes. Diabetes Care 22:1252, 1999.

Adjustments in the basic or set dose of insulin can be made in response to a pattern of glycemia that has been determined over a number of days.[30] Table 10-8 gives guidelines used in my center as to how to make adjustments in the base or set dose of insulin.

TYPE 2 DIABETES

PRINCIPLES OF MANAGEMENT

Presentation of Type 2 Diabetes in Children and Youth

Type 2 diabetes is almost exclusively diagnosed in older children and youth who present with subtle symptoms of diabetes.[55-60] These mildly symptomatic youth have characteristics that are outlined in Table 10-9. Rarely, patients present more ill with ketoacidosis, particularly African American children, and occasionally there can be extreme elevation of the blood glucose level with hyperosmolar coma.

Asymptomatic children and youth are diagnosed as the result of routine screening or by investigating a variety of complaints such as vaginal moniliasis, infections, morbid obesity, sleep apnea, hyperlipidemia, hypertension, and hirsutism or irregular periods associated with polycystic ovarian syndrome. The American Diabetes Association consensus statement[60] for type 2 diabetes in children and adolescents, which was endorsed by the American Academy of Pediatrics, recommended that overweight children and teens with two or more risk factors for type 2 diabetes be tested for asymptomatic type 2 diabetes every 2 years beginning at 10 years of age or at the onset of puberty. The criteria for screening for type 2 diabetes in asymptomatic children and youth are given in Table 10-10.

Type 2 diabetes is preceded by a period in which insulin resistance is found. Factors associated with insulin resistance are given in Table 10-11.[61-68] As this progresses and becomes coupled with a defect of insulin secretion, patients develop impaired fasting glucose or impaired glucose tolerance (IGT), conditions referred to as *prediabetes*.[69,70,71] Prediabetes is common in children and youth, as well as in adults. Evaluation of obese children and adolescents by Sinha et al.[69] with oral glucose tolerance testing showed that IGT or predi-

TABLE 10-8	PRINCIPLES USED FOR ADJUSTMENTS IN BASIC OR SET INSULIN DOSE

Rapid-, short-, intermediate-long-acting or basal insulin is adjusted after a pattern has been identified over 3-7 days.

Increase or decrease by 0.5, 1.0, 1.5 or 2.0 U (10% of the dose)

Two or Three Insulin Injections

Time of Abnormal Test	Change this Insulin
Before breakfast	Evening intermediate- or long-acting
Before lunch	Morning rapid- or short-acting
Before dinner	Morning intermediate- or long-acting
Before bedtime	Evening rapid- or short-acting
In the night	Evening intermediate- or long-acting

Multiple Insulin Injections

Fasting, night	Evening intermediate-, long-acting, or basal
Before lunch, dinner	Morning intermediate-, long-acting, or basal
2 hours after meal	Change bolus

Insulin Pump

2 hours after meal	Change bolus
>3 hours after meal, night, fasting	Change basal

Recheck to be sure the changes made return BG levels to the target range.

BG, blood glucose.

Adapted from Kaufman FR, Halvorson M: New trends in managing type 1 diabetes. Contemp Pediatr 16:112, 1999.

abetes was detected in 25% of obese children 4 to 10 years of age and 21% of obese adolescents 11 to 18 years of age, and that the best predictor of IGT was insulin resistance. In this limited study of 167 subjects, IGT was found in all ethnic groups and overt type 2 diabetes was predicted by determining that there was an element of β cell failure as assessed by a reduced ratio of the 30-minute change in the insulin concentration compared with the 30-minute change in the glucose level. Whether these findings imply that obese children should have an oral glucose tolerance test performed to predict

TABLE 10-9	CHARACTERISTICS OF CHILDREN AND YOUTH WITH TYPE 2 DIABETES

>90% are overweight or obese (BMI >85th percentile, normal 15-27 kg/m^2)

Majority are ethnic/racial minorities

More girls than boys are affected

Glycosuria and weight loss are present for weeks to months

33% have ketonuria and 5%–10% have ketoacidosis, with even higher rates described in African American youth

50%–75% have a parent and 85%–90% have at least one first- or second-degree relative with type 2 disease

60%–90% have acanthosis nigricans

BMI, body mass index.

TABLE 10-10   CRITERIA FOR SCREENING FOR TYPE 2 DIABETES IN CHILDREN AND YOUTH

Criteria:

Overweight (BMI > 85th percentile for age and sex, weight for height > 85th percentile or weight > 120% ideal for height)
Plus
Any two of the following risk factors:
   Family history of type 2 diabetes in first- or second-degree relative
   Race/ethnicity (Native American, African American, Hispanic, Asian/Pacific Islander)
   Signs of insulin resistance or condition associated with insulin resistance (acanthosis nigricans, hypertension, dyslipidemia, PCOS)

Age of initiation:

Age 10 yr or at onset of puberty if puberty occurs at a younger age

Frequency:

Every 2 yr

Test:

Fasting plasma glucose preferred

BMI, body mass index; PCOS, polycystic ovarian syndrome.

Adapted from the American Diabetes Association: Type 2 diabetes in children and adolescents. Consensus statement. Diabetes Care 23:381, 2000.

IGT is undetermined as of the time of this writing. However, with numerous studies indicating the benefit of life style intervention in adults to prevent the progression of prediabetes to frank diabetes, it is likely that at-risk children should be tested for IGT and put into prevention protocols that affect food intake and exercise patterns.[70-72] Use of

TABLE 10-11   FACTORS ASSOCIATED WITH INSULIN RESISTANCE

Puberty	Female Gender	Obesity	Familial/ Ethnicity	Maternal Diabetes
2-3 fold ↑ in insulin response to glucose challenge during puberty	1.7:1 female preponderance of type 2 diabetes in youth	Obesity accounts for 55% variance in insulin sensitivity	Youth with family history of type 2 diabetes have lower insulin-stimulated glucose disposal	Type 2 diabetes associated with increased birth weight
30% ↓ insulin mediated glucose disposal during puberty	PCOS and premature adrenarche associated with 40% ↓ glucose disposal	Associated with hyperinsulinism 40% ↓ in glucose disposal	Decreased insulin sensitivity in African American youth	19% of infants exposed to maternal diabetes have IGT by age 16

IGT, impaired glucose tolerance; PCOS, polycystic ovarian syndrome.

pharmacologic agents, on the other hand, should be reserved for clinical trials.[72]

Glucose Lowering Agents

There are many agents available to improve the metabolic abnormalities seen in subjects with type 2 diabetes.[73–76] Presently there is little primary data on the use of many of these agents in pediatric and adolescent patients. The available agents and the potential advantages and disadvantages are given in Table 10-12.

The schema for the treatment of type 2 diabetes in pediatric subjects includes diabetes education for both the patient and family, with emphasis on increasing exercise and following an appropriate nutrition plan.[76,77] Glycemic targets should be set and

the patients and families taught how to use the tools of diabetes management. The goal to have the A1C less than 7.0% and fasting glucose levels less than 130 mg/dl, as set for adults with type 2 diabetes, may be difficult to achieve in children and adolescents. It is more realistic to use the age-specific targets for type 1 subjects as shown in Table 10-6.

Appropriate exercise and nutrition therapy are important components of the type 2 regimen. It is often difficult to convince adolescents to adapt life style behaviors that are healthy and that promote weight loss. Effective programs need to be developed that are attractive to teens, involve the entire family, and promote peer support.[77] Overall, less than 10% of pediatric subjects diagnosed with type 2 diabetes can achieve glycemic targets by following life style inter-

TABLE 10-12 AGENTS FOR TYPE 2 DIABETES—ADVANTAGES AND DISADVANTAGES

Class	Advantages	Disadvantages
Insulin	Overcomes glucotoxicity	Hypoglycemia
	Will control all patients	Weight gain
	Flexibility of dosing	Need for injections
	Data in pediatric patients available	
Sulfonylureas	Rapid acting	Weight gain
	Well tolerated	Hypoglycemia
	Broad range of dosing	
Meglitinides	Improves insulin secretion	Hypoglycemia
	Used with meals	Weight gain
	No lag period	Unknown long-term effects
	Flexibility of life style	
	Low risk of hypoglycemia	
Biguanides	Improves insulin resistance	GI side effects
	High initial response rate	Risk of lactic acidosis
	Less weight gain or weight loss	Risk with impaired renal, hepatic, and cardiac function
	Advantageous lipid profile	
	Good for PCOS	
α-Glucosidase Inhibitors	Good safety profile	Needs high-carbohydrate diet
	No weight gain or weight loss	Flatulence, GI pain
	Dose coupled with meals	Treat hypoglycemia with dextrose or milk
Thiazolidinediones	Corrects insulin resistance	Delayed action
	Once daily dosing	Weight gain
	May improve lipids	

GI, gastrointestinal; PCOS, polycystic ovarian syndrome.

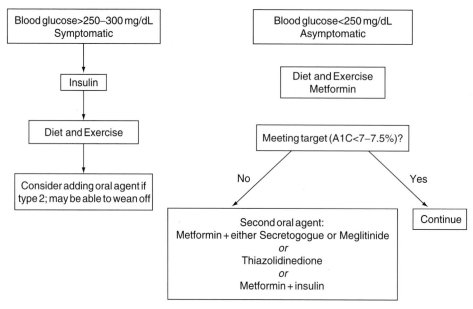

FIGURE 10-1. Schema for type 2 diabetes management.

ventions alone. Figure 10-1 outlines the schema for management. If it is unclear whether the patient has type 1 or 2 diabetes at presentation, insulin should be used while waiting for antibody and c-peptide level results. Comorbidities, such as hypertension and hyperlipidemia, require treatment.

OUTPATIENT DIABETES MANAGEMENT

OUTPATIENT VISITS

Pediatric patients with type 1 or type 2 diabetes should have comprehensive, multidisciplinary outpatient visits at frequent intervals, optimally quarterly. It has been shown that there is an increase in ketoacidosis, poor glycemic control, and the incidence of long-term complications when outpatient follow-up is infrequent and interrupted.[78] We reported that visits as infrequent as one to two times per year were

associated with significantly higher A1C levels than when visits occurred three to four times per year[79]. The purpose of these multidisciplinary visits is to assess overall health and diabetes-related health status, alter the diabetes regimen, advance diabetes knowledge and competency, and motivate patients and families to follow the regimen to improve short- and long-term outcome.

During outpatient visits, it is important to obtain (1) a comprehensive interval history, and (2) a diabetes-related physical examination.[21,80] As outlined in the American Diabetes Association Clinical Practice Recommendations for 2001,[27] and modified for pediatric patients, Table 10-13 gives the basics of a comprehensive outpatient visit.

A comprehensive physical examination should be done. Growth parameters such as height, weight, and body mass index should be plotted on standardized, age-adjusted curves. Head circumference should be plotted until age 3 years. Tanner staging should be done to assess pubertal development. Important goals of diabetes manage-

TABLE 10-13 OUTLINE FOR DIABETES OUTPATIENT VISITS

Assess During History at Each Visit

Frequency, causes, and severity of hypoglycemia or hyperglycemia
Results of home glucose monitoring from logbooks and blood glucose meter downloads
Self-adjustments made to diabetes regimen
Integration of home care management behavior, understanding of diabetes management plan and goals
Education assessment and needs
Review of systems for intercurrent problems or diabetes complications
Current medications
Psychosocial issues
Changes in life situations
School performance, after-school, weekend, and sports activities
Risk-taking behavior, particularly for adolescents

Physical Examination	Frequency/ Recommendations
Weight, height, BMI	Every 3 mo assess changes in percentile
Tanner stage	Every 3 mo note pubertal progression
Blood pressure	Every 3 mo target <90th percentile for age
Eye	Dilated funduscopic examination every 12 mo after 5 yr of diabetes
Thyroid	Every 3 mo assess presence of goiter, signs of thyroid dysfunction
Abdomen	Every 3 mo assess presence of hepatomegaly, fullness, signs of malabsorption, inflammation
Foot, peripheral pulses	Every 3 mo inspection after age 12 yr, thorough examination for sensation, pulses, vibration yearly
Skin, joints, injections sites	Every 3 mo injection sites, joint mobility, lesions associated with diabetes
Neurologic	Every 12 mo signs of autonomic changes, pain, neuropathy

Laboratory Examination	Frequency
A1C	Every 3 mo
Microalbuminuria	Every 12 mo after puberty or after 5 yr with diabetes
U/A, creatinine	At presentation and with signs or renal problems
Lipid profile	At diagnosis and every 12 mo
Thyroid function tests	Every 12 mo for type 1 patients
Celiac screen	At time of diagnosis, if symptoms, at puberty in type 1 patients
Islet and other antibodies	
Consider fasting c-peptide	At diagnosis to distinguish type 1 from type 2

BMI, body mass index; U/A, urinalysis.

ment are normalization of growth parameters and normal pubertal entrance and development. Weight stabilization is an important goal for those with type 2 diabetes. Blood pressure should be assessed at each visit with an appropriate cuff for the patient's size. Blood pressure results should be <85th percentile for age compared to age-specific norms. Elevation of the blood pressure can accelerate diabetes complications and may be the first sign of diabetic nephropathy.

Laboratory monitoring is important to complete the assessment of children and youth with type 1 and type 2 diabetes. A1C levels should be obtained at quarterly visits. Preferably, A1C values are available at the time of the clinic visit so the health care practitioner can determine whether glycemic targets are being met. A face-to-face discussion at the time of the visit, rather than a phone call at a later date, is the optimal way to deal with A1C levels that are not in the target range for age. Thyroid function tests should be obtained in subjects with type 1 diabetes at yearly intervals.[81] Of pediatric patients with type 1 diabetes, 20% to 30% have thyroid autoantibodies; however, overt hypothyroidism occurs in only 1% to 5% and compensated hypothyroidism in 5% to 10%. A fasting lipid profile that includes total cholesterol, high-density lipoprotein cholesterol, low-density lipoprotein cholesterol, and triglyceride levels should be obtained in children and adolescents after glucose control has been established, particularly in those with type 2 diabetes and those with a family history of cardiovascular disease. If values fall within age-adjusted norms, they should be repeated at yearly intervals. If not, nutrition counseling should focus on reducing lipid levels and the values should be repeated. There is little data as of the time of this writing to know at what lipid levels children and teens should be considered for antilipid therapy. Urine microalbumin should be obtained beginning at puberty or 5 years after diagnosis and then yearly. In patients with type 2 diabetes, urine assessment should be done at the time of diabetes diagnosis. Microalbumin levels can be measured using the following: (1) A random microalbumin-to-creatinine ratio, (2) timed overnight microalbumin assay-to-albumin excretion rate assessment, or (3) 24-hour timed urinary microalbumin-to-albumin excretion rate measurement. Celiac disease has been reported to occur 10 to 50 times more often in children with type

1 diabetes when compared with the general population; therefore patients should be screened for this disorder with an antibody panel that includes antiendomysial immunoglobulin A antibody quantitation.[82,83] Celiac disease has been reported to be present in 1% to 10% of children and adolescents with type 1 diabetes. At the time of diagnosis, patients should have liver function tests and a creatinine and urinalysis. To determine whether a patient has type 1 or type 2 diabetes, assessment of islet autoimmunity should be made by obtaining specific antibodies to islet antigens and fasting c-peptide should be obtained.

Sick Day Management

It is important to alter the diabetes regimen during intercurrent illness. Although children with diabetes are generally not more susceptible to illness or infection, once contracted, such processes can markedly deteriorate glycemic control. Hypoglycemia can occur, particularly in young children, as the result of illnesses associated with vomiting and diarrhea. Hyperglycemia can result from febrile illnesses because of the elevation of the counterregulatory hormones that lead to insulin resistance and gluconeogenesis. Ketogenesis may result from either. To reduce the frequency and severity of glycemic aberrations associated with intercurrent illness, patients and families must be taught about sick day management and the diabetes health care team must be available 24 hours a day to provide guidance so that dehydration, DKA, and hypoglycemia and hyperglycemia can be avoided. In patients with type 2 diabetes, oral hypoglycemic agents should be held until advice from the health care provider can be obtained. Metformin can lead to lactic acidosis, the sulfonylureas to hypoglycemia, and the thiazolidinediones have not been studied in the pediatric population, making them all potentially contraindicated during intercurrent illness. Sick day management guidelines are given in Table 10-14.[29]

TABLE 10-14	SICK DAY MANAGEMENT GUIDELINES

1. **Warning Signs**: Call the health team in the event of:
   a. Vomiting (more than two times or >4 hours)
   b. Elevated blood sugar level (two or more readings outside of the target range or >250 mg/dl)
   c. Presence of blood or large urinary ketones
   d. Weakness, dry mouth, or signs of dehydration, excessive thirst
   e. Heavy breathing, shortness of breath
   f. Abdominal pain, diarrheal stools
   g. Evidence of bacterial infection
   h. Altered level of consciousness or change in mental status
2. **Never Stop Insulin. Do not take oral glucose lowering agents until you talk to the health care team**
3. **Phone Numbers:**   Pediatrician_____
   Diabetes Team_____
   Emergency #_____
4. **Log Sheet**

	1st Hour	2nd Hour	3rd Hour	4th Hour	5th Hour	6th Hour	7th Hour
Blood Sugar							
Ketone Level							
Temperature							
Fluid Input							
Output Urine							
Insulin Dose							

5. **Principles for High Blood Sugar:**
   a. Give extra rapid-acting (or short-acting) insulin every 2 hours
   b. Add extra insulin for each 50 mg/dl above target (200 mg/dl)
      i. For children <5 years   = 0.25 U for each 50 mg/dl
      ii. For grade-school age   = 0.5–1.0 U for each 50 mg/dl
      iii. For adolescents   = 1–2 U for each 50 mg/dl
   c. Non–glucose-containing fluids should be given until the blood glucose level reaches 250 mg/dl
   d. Fluids containing sodium and potassium should be used if there is excessive fluid loss
   e. Replacement of fluids is more important than food
6. **Principles for Low Blood Sugar:**
   a. Glucose-containing fluids should be given in small quantities
   b. Insulin should be decreased by 20%–50%
   c. If persistent hypoglycemia occurs and patients are not able to retain glucose-containing solutions, consider a minidose of glucagon (for children ≤2 years, 20 μg or 2 "units" on the insulin syringe; for children >2 years, 150 μg or 15 "units")

The Multidisciplinary Diabetes Team

The multidisciplinary team consists of a pediatrician specializing in diabetes and endocrinology (or a physician with special interest in childhood and adolescent diabetes), a nurse who is a diabetes specialist and/or diabetes educator (preferably certified), and a dietitian. These essential members of the team also need access to a psychologist, psychiatrist, or counselor knowledgeable about diabetes, and a social worker. The team members work together to provide expert practical guidance and skill training, education, advice, and support for the psychological needs of the patient and family.[21]

Active collaboration between the diabetes team and the primary care provider, who is a pediatrician or family practitioner, is essential for optimal outcome. The diabetes team must give the primary care provider the following information: (1) changes in the diabetes regimen, (2) findings on quarterly evaluations and A1C results, (3) records of intercurrent illnesses, (4) issues surrounding the psychosocial adaptation of the patient and family, and problems with school, and (5) information about adverse events and diabetes-related complications. The primary care provider in turn gives routine pediatric care, assesses developmental and behavioral issues, ensures adjustment to chronic illness, offers age- and gender-appropriate anticipatory guidance, facilitates obtaining diabetes supplies, assesses the appropriateness of clinical trials, and arranges subspecialty care visits. Most importantly, the pediatrician should serve as the patient's advocate with the parents, other caregivers, school personnel, coaches, and the diabetes team.

Diabetes Care in School and Day Care Settings

Appropriate diabetes management must occur during school, in after-school programs, and in day care settings.[84,85] Personnel responsible for children with diabetes must receive the necessary information and training to help effectively manage type 1 or type 2 diabetes. For school and day care personnel to understand and provide for the needs of the individual child, an individualized Diabetes Health Care Plan (Table 10-15) must be developed. Federal laws protect children with diabetes against discrimination. These laws include the Rehabilitation Act of 1973, Section 504; the Individuals with Disabilities Education Act of 1991, and the Americans with Disabilities Act of 1992.[86] Families can ask to develop a formal 504 Plan, in addition to the Diabetes Health Care Plan, to obtain the necessary accommodations with as little disruption to the routine as possible.

The Diabetes Health Care Plan outlines how diabetes is to be managed during school hours, after school, and on field trips. Personnel must train to comply with the Health Care Plan, and to guarantee privacy. Children must be allowed access to the restroom and fluids, and be given permission to miss school without consequences for medical reasons and appointments. There are specific responsibilities for each of the parties involved: (1) The parents or guardians must give the school or day care center all diabetes supplies and emergency information, (2) the child must participate in diabetes-related tasks as allowed by his or her developmental stage, and (3) the health

---

TABLE 10-15 WHAT SHOULD BE INCLUDED IN THE DIABETES HEALTH CARE PLAN

Emergency numbers, including for the health care team
Blood glucose monitoring, including when and where testing should be done
Insulin administration, if necessary, including doses and who can administer injections or oral hypoglycemic agents
Meals and snacks, including amounts and timing
Symptoms and treatment of hypoglycemia, including the use of glucagon
Symptoms and treatment of hyperglycemia
Ketone testing if indicated
Management tasks the child can perform, those requiring supervision

care team must be available for questions and emergency situations. In this way, children and youth can participate in day care, school, and after-school activities without compromising diabetes outcomes.

PSYCHOSOCIAL ASPECTS OF DIABETES IN CHILDREN AND YOUTH

The rigors of the diabetes regimen, the fear of short- and long-term diabetes complications, the loss of normalcy and the financial burden of diabetes care can cause a number of psychological issues for patients and their families. The psychological impact of diabetes is usually seen at the time of diagnosis, when the majority of patients exhibit mild depression, anxiety, and somatic complaints.[87,88] This initial adjustment to diabetes often predicts how patients will cope over the long term. Although in most cases the mild depression seen at diagnosis is self-limited and usually resolves within 6 to 9 months, in some subjects, depressive symptoms and anxiety continue to increase over time.[89] It is important to assess the patient and family at the time of diabetes diagnosis to ensure that coping strategies are appropriate, that detrimental psychodevelopmental issues that might have been present prior to the diagnosis do not re-emerge, and that the patient and family are able to manage diabetes with a normal amount of support from the health care team. The psychosocial factors affecting initial diabetes management and the important factors in overall management as outlined by Schiffrin[87] are given in Table 10-16.

A number of coping mechanisms at the time of diagnosis can be employed by patients and their families.[90] Intellectualization and denial are often employed to decrease anxiety and realistically begin to plan for the future of life with diabetes. Many children develop familiar rituals concerning their diabetes management that enables them to feel in control. It is important to help children and their families mourn after diagnosis and to learn to express and take ownership for their feelings, because children with expressive and cohesive families appear to have better metabolic control.[91] The health care team should involve the entire family in education sessions, teach problem-solving skills, and give realistic goals and clear roles and responsibilities to the family members while they remain sensitive to the family's beliefs, culture, and life style.

The goal of diabetes management is to gradually have the child assume more and more responsibility within the context of parental support and involvement. The goal is not to have teens assume totally responsibility devoid of parental involvement.

TABLE 10-16	THE PSYCHOSOCIAL FACTORS AFFECTING INITIAL DIABETES MANAGEMENT
Patient's and family's adjustment to losses and uncertainties inherent in diagnosis	
Cultural and health beliefs competing with treatment requirements	
Emotional reactions to diabetes-specific tasks and complications (fear of injections, blood glucose monitoring, responses to hypoglycemia and hyperglycemia, long-term complications)	
Psychiatric and social problems preceding diagnosis	
Community and social support surrounding the family	
Relationship and communication with health care team	
Financial resources for treatment and access to good caretakers	

Adapted from Schiffrin A: Psychosocial issues in pediatric diabetes. Curr Diabetes Reports 1:33, 2001.

A number of studies support this approach. Anderson et al.[92] showed that a teamwork approach between parents and teens allows for reduced family conflict. This, coupled with research that shows that parental involvement is the single most important predictor of adolescent outcome,[93,94] validates helping families learn how to remain a team in diabetes management.

Many psychological issues come in to play over the long term for patients and their families. Studies have shown that it is difficult to chronically adhere to the diabetes regimen and that understanding how to change the regimen to respond to unexpected alterations of glycemia is very hard for children and youth.[95] Having a demanding daily routine and still being expected to deal with unanticipated episodes of hypoglycemia and hyperglycemia leads to depression and feelings of hopelessness and helplessness and to burnout. Children and youth who experience burnout skip injections and blood tests and have deterioration of glycemic control. To resolve this problem, patients must be allowed to regularly express their negative feelings and their frustrations. Only with a consolidated effort between the diabetes team and skilled mental health professionals and with psychological assessment and intervention as early as possible can it be expected that patients and their families will achieve optimal glycemic control without impairment in quality of life.

CONCLUSIONS

Many advances have been made for both type 1 and type 2 diabetes management over the last 1 to 2 decades. These include new insulin preparations, new insulin delivery devices, increasing numbers of oral hypoglycemic agents, and technologically more advanced glucose monitoring systems. Further advances are anticipated over the next years while research progresses toward understanding and preventing the consequences of gluco-

toxicity, and preventing and curing diabetes altogether. In the interim, the importance of effectively managing diabetes on a day-to-day basis cannot be overstated. Patients and families must understand how to use diabetes tools of management, and be given education and support so that they may gain the knowledge, attitudes, and skills to meet glycemic goals. To ensure optimal physical and psychosocial outcome, health care visits with a multidisciplinary team must occur at set intervals. The patient, parents, family members, school and day care personnel, the diabetes team, and the primary care provider must develop a partnership so that there is the appropriate commitment to a multicomponent diabetes regimen that is intensive and safe.

REFERENCES

1. Kaufman FR: Diabetes mellitus. Pediatr Res 18;383, 1997.
2. She JX: Genetic factors in type 1 diabetes: A complex disease. J Clin Ligand Assay 21:272, 1998.
3. Morales AE, She JX, Schatz DA: Prediction and prevention of type 1 diabetes. Current Diab Rep 1:28, 2001.
4. Leslie RDG, Elliot RB: Early environmental events as a cause of IDDM: Evidence and implications. Diabetes 43:843, 1994.
5. Diabetes Control and Complications Trial Research Group: The effect of intensive treatment of diabetes on the long-term development and progression of long-term complications in insulin-dependent diabetes mellitus. N Engl J Med 329:977, 1993.
6. Diabetes Control and Complications Trial Research Group: Effect of intensive diabetes treatment on the development of long-term complications in adolescents with insulin-dependent diabetes mellitus: Diabetes Control and Complications Trial. J Pediatr 125:177, 1994.
7. Diabetes Control and Complications Trial Research Group: Implementation of treatment protocols in the diabetes control and complications trial. Diabetes Care 18:361, 1995.
8. United Kingdom Prospective Diabetes Study Group: Intensive blood glucose control with sulphonylureas or insulin compared with conventional treatment and risk of complications in patients with type 2 diabetes. Lancet 352:837, 1998.
9. Hirsch IB, Farkas-Hirsch R, Skyler JS: Intensive insulin therapy for treatment of type 1 diabetes. Diabetes Care 13:1265, 1990.
10. Hirsch IB: Intensive treatment of type 1 diabetes. Med Clin North Am 82:689, 1998.

11. Chase HP, Lockspeiser T, Perry B et al: The impact of the diabetes control and complications trial and Humalog insulin on glycohemoglobin levels and severe hypoglycemia in type 1 diabetes. Diabetes Care 24:430, 2001.

12. Brunner GA, Hirschberger S, Sendhofer G et al: Post-prandial administration of the insulin analogue insulin aspart in patients with type 1 diabetes mellitus. Diabetic Medicine 17:371, 2000.

13. Hedman CA, Lindstrom T, Arnqvist HJ: Direct comparison of insulin lispro and aspart shows small differences in plasma insulin profiles after subcutaneous injection in type 1 diabetes. Diabetes Care 24:1120, 2001.

14. Buckingham BA, Bluck B, Wilson DM: Intensive diabetes management in pediatric patients. Current Diabetes Reports 1:11, 2001.

15. Ratner RE, Hirsch IB, Neifing JL et al: Less hypoglycemia with insulin glargine in intensive insulin therapy for type 1 diabetes. U.S. Study Group of Insulin Glargine in Type 1 Diabetes. Diabetes Care 23:639, 2000.

16. Rosenstock J, Park G, Zimmerman J for U.S. Insulin Glargine (HOE 901) Diabetes Investigator Group: Basal insulin glargine (HOE 901) versus NPH insulin in patients with type 1 diabetes on multiple daily insulin regimens. Diabetes Care 23:1137, 2000.

17. Mohn A, Strang S, Lang AM et al: Nocturnal glucose control and free insulin levels in children with type 1 diabetes by use of the long-acting insulin HOE 901 as part of a three-injection regimen. Diabetes Care 23:557, 2000.

18. Rosskamp R, Park G: Long-acting insulin analogs. Diabetes Care 22(Suppl. 2):B109, 1999.

19. Owens DR, Coates PA, Luzio SD et al: Pharmacokinetics of 125I-labeled insulin glargine (HOE 901) in healthy men: Comparison with NPH insulin and the influence of different subcutaneous injection sites. Diabetes Care 23:813, 2000.

20. Brunner GA, Sendlhofer G, Wutte A et al: Pharmacokinetic and pharmacodynamic properties of long-acting insulin analogue NN304 in comparison to NPH insulin in humans. Exp Clin Endocrinol Diabetes 108:100, 2000.

21. ISPAD: Consensus Guidelines 2000, International Society for Pediatric and Adolescent Diabetes, Medical Forum International, Zeist, Netherlands, 2000.

22. Lawlor MT, Laffel LMB: New technologies and therapeutic approaches for the management of pediatric diabetes. Curr Diab Rep 1:56, 2001.

23. Galloway JA, Spradlin CT, Nelson RL et al: Factors influencing the absorption, serum insulin concentration, and blood glucose responses after injections of regular insulin and various insulin mixtures. Diabetes Care 4:366, 1981.

24. Skyler JS, Gelfand RA, Kourides IA, for the Inhaled Insulin Phase II Study Group: Treatment of type 1 diabetes mellitus with inhaled human insulin: A 3-month, multicenter trial. Diabetes 47:A61, 1998.

25. Wilson DM: Diabetes mellitus in children and adolescents. In Behrman RE, Kleigman RM, Arvin AM (eds): Nelson Textbook of Pediatrics, 15th ed. WB Saunders, Philadelphia, 1995.

26. American Diabetes Association: Medical Management of Type 1 Diabetes, 3rd ed. American Diabetes Association, Alexandria, VA, 1998.

27. American Diabetes Association: Clinical practice recommendation 2001. Diabetes Care 24(Suppl. 1):S33–50, 2003.

28. American Diabetes Association: Standards of medical care for patients with diabetes mellitus. Diabetes Care 20(Suppl 1):S5, 1997.

29. Kaufman FR, Halvorson M: New trends in managing type 1 diabetes. Contemp Pediatr 16:112, 1999.

30. Skyler JS, Skyler DL, Seigler DE: Algorithms for adjustment of insulin dosage by patients who monitor blood glucose. Diabetes Care 4:311, 1981.

31. Plotnick L: Insulin-dependent diabetes mellitus. Pediatr Rev 15:137, 1994.

32. Kaufman FR, Halvorson M, Miller D et al: Insulin pump therapy in type 1 pediatric patients: Now and into the year 2000. Diabetes Metab Res Rev 15:338, 1999.

33. Kaufman FR, Halvorson M, Carpenter S, Devoe D: Insulin pump in young children with diabetes. Diabetes Spectrum 14:84, 2001.

34. Steindel BS, Roe TF, Costin G et al: Continuous subcutaneous insulin infusion (CSII) in children and adolescents with chronic poorly controlled type 1 diabetes mellitus. Diabetes Res Clin Pract 27:199, 1995.

35. Boland EA, Grey M, Oesterle A et al: Continuous subcutaneous insulin infusion. Diabetes Care 22:1779, 1999.

36. Kaufman FR: Diabetes in children and adolescents: Areas of controversy. Med Clin North Am 82:721, 1998.

37. Kaufman FR, Halvorson M, Fisher LK, Pitukcheewanont P: Insulin pump therapy in type 1 pediatric patients. J Pediatr Endocrinol Metab 12:759, 1999.

38. Kaufman FR, Fisher LK, Gibson LC et al: A pilot study of the continuous glucose monitoring system: Clinical decisions and glycemic control after its use in pediatric type 1 diabetic subjects. Diabetes Care 24:2030, 2001.

39. Mortensen HB, Hartling SG, Petersen KE, for the Danise Study Group of Diabetes in Childhood: A nation-wide cross-sectional study of glycosylated hemoglobin in Danish children with type 1 diabetes. Diabet Med 5:871, 1988.

40. Mortensen HB, Villumsen J, Volund A et al, for the Danish Study Group of Diabetes in Childhood: Relationship between insulin injection regimen and metabolic control in young Danish type 1 diabetic patients. Diabetic Med 9:834, 1992.

41. Mortensen HB Hougaard P (1997). Comparison of metabolic control in a cross-sectional study of 1,873 children and adolescents with IDDM from 18 countries. Diabetes Care 20, 714–720.

42. Anderson B, Ho J, Brackett J et al: Parental involvement in diabetes management tasks: Relationships to blood glucose monitoring

adherence and metabolic control in young adolescents with insulin-dependent diabetes mellitus. J Pediatr 130:257, 1997.

43. Kaufman FR: Searching for glycemic control in pediatric type 1 diabetes: A long way to go. J Pediatr 139:174, 2001.

44. Nathan DM, McKitrick C, Larkin M et al: (1996). Glycemic control in diabetes mellitus: Have changes in therapy made a difference? Am J Med 100:157, 1996.

45. Levine B-S, Anderson BJ, Butler DA et al: Predictors of glycemic control and short-term adverse outcomes in youth with type 1 diabetes. J Pediatr 139:197, 2001.

46. American Diabetes Association: Postprandial blood glucose. Diabetes Care 24:775, 2001.

47. Bode BW, Gross TM, Thornton KR, Mastrototoro JM: Continuous glucose monitoring used to adjust diabetes therapy improves glycosylated hemoglobin: A pilot study. Diabetes Res Clin Pract 46:183, 1999.

48. Chase HP, Kim LM, Owen SL et al: Continuous subcutaneous glucose monitoring in children with type 1 diabetes. Pediatrics 107:222, 2001.

49. Garg SK, Potts RO, Ackerman NR et al: Correlation of finger stick blood glucose measurements with GlucoWatch Biographer glucose results in young subjects with type 1 diabetes. Diabetes Care 22:1708, 1999.

50. Pitzer KR, Desai S, Dunn T et al: Detection of hypoglycemia with the GlucoWatch Biographer. Diabetes Care 24:881, 2001.

51. Byrne HA, Tieszen KL, Hollis S et al: Evaluation of an electrochemical sensor for measuring blood ketones. Diabetes Care 23:500, 2000.

52. Fulop M, Murphy V, Michilli A et al: Serum B-hydroxybutyrate measurement in patients with uncontrolled diabetes mellitus. Arch Intern Med 159:381, 1999.

53. Danne T, Mortensen HB, Hougaard P et al: Persistent differences among centers over 3 years in glycemic control and hypoglycemia in a study of 3,805 children and adolescents with type 1 diabetes from the Hvidore study group. Diabetes Care 24:1342, 2001.

54. Kaufman FR, Halvorson M, Carpenter S: Use of a plastic insulin dosage guide to correct blood glucose levels of the target range and for carbohydrate counting in subjects with type 1 diabetes. Diabetes Care 22:1252, 1999.

55. Pihoker C, Scott CR, Lensing SY et al: Non-insulin dependent diabetes mellitus in African American youths of Arkansas. Clin Pediatr 37:97, 1998.

56. Glaser NS, Jones KL. (1998) Non-insulin-dependent diabetes mellitus in Mexican-American children. West J Med 168:11–16.

57. Savage PJ, Bennett PH, Senter G, Miller M: High prevalence of diabetes in young Pima Indians. Evidence of phenotypic variation and in a genetically isolated population. Diabetes 28:837, 1979.

58. The Expert Committee on the Diagnosis and Classification of Diabetes Mellitus: Report of the Expert Committee on the Diagnosis and Classification Diabetes Mellitus. Diabetes Care 22(Suppl 1):S5, 1999.

59. Kaufman FR: Type 2 diabetes in children and youth: A new epidemic. J Pediatr Endocrinol Metab 15(suppl 2):737, 2002.

60. American Diabetes Association: Type 2 diabetes in children and adolescents. Consensus statement. Diabetes Care 23:381, 2000.

61. Legro RS, Kunselman AR, Dodson WC, Dunaif A: Prevalence and predictors of risk for type 2 diabetes mellitus and impaired glucose tolerance in polycystic ovary syndrome: A prospective, controlled study in 254 affected women. J Clin Endocrinal Metab. 84:165, 1999.

62. Arslanian SA, Kalhan SC: Correlations between fatty acid and glucose metabolism: Potential explanation of insulin resistance of puberty. Diabetes 43:908, 1994.

63. Saad RJ, Keenan BS, Danadian K et al: Dihydrotestosterone treatment in adolescents with delayed puberty: Does it explain insulin resistance of puberty? J Clin Endocrinol Metab. 86:4881, 2000.

64. Fagot-Campagna A, Pettitt DJ, Engelgau MM et al: Type 2 diabetes among North American children and adolescents: An epidemiological review and a public health perspective. J Pediatr 136:664, 2000

65. Wong WW, Butte NF, Ellis KJ et al: Pubertal African-American girls expend less energy at rest and during physical activity than Caucasian girls. J Clin Endocrinol Metab 84:906, 1999.

66. Danadian K, Balasekaran G, Lewy V et al: Insulin sensitivity in African-American children with and without family history of type 2 diabetes. Diabetes Care 22:1325, 1999.

67. Cho NH, Silverman BL, Rizzo TA, Metzker BE: Correlations between the intrauterine metabolic environment and blood pressure in adolescent offspring of diabetic mothers. J Pediatr 136:587, 2000.

68. Silverman BL, Metzker BE, Cho NH, Loeb CA: Fetal hyperinsulinism and impaired glucose tolerance in adolescent offspring of diabetic mothers. Diabetes Care 18:611, 1995.

69. Sinha R, Fisch G, Teague B et al: Prevalence of impaired glucose tolerance among children and adolescents with marked obesity. N Engl J Med 346:802, 2002.

70. Tuomilehto J, Lindstrom J, Eriksson JG et al, for the Finnish Diabetes Prevention Study Group: Prevention of type 2 diabetes mellitus by changes in lifestyle among subjects with impaired glucose tolerance. N Engl J Med 344:1343, 2001.

71. The Diabetes Prevention Program Research Group: Reduction in the incidence of type 2 diabetes with life-style intervention or metformin. N Engl J Med 346:393, 2002.

72. Freemark M, Bursey D: The effects of metformin on body mass index and glucose tolerance in obese adolescents with fasting hyperinsulinemia and a family history of type 2 diabetes. Pediatrics 104:E55, 2001.

73. DeFronzo RA: Pharmacologic therapy for type 2 diabetes mellitus. Ann Intern Med 131:281, 1999.

74. Mahler RJ, Adler ML: Clinical review 102 type 2 diabetes mellitus: Update on diagnosis, pathophysiology and treatment. J Clin Endocrinol Metab 84:1165, 1999.

75. The American Association of Clinical Endocrinologists: The American Association of Clinical Endocrinologists medical guidelines for the management of diabetes mellitus: The AACE system of intensive diabetes self-management. Endocr Pract 6:43, 2000.

76. Rosenbloom AL, Joe JR, Young RS, Winter WE: The emerging epidemic of type 2 diabetes mellitus in youth. Diabetes Care 22:345, 1999.

77. Mackenzie M, Halvorson M, Kaufman FR et al: Effect of a Kids N Fitness weight management program on obesity and other pediatric health factors. Diabetes 50(Suppl 1):A22, 2001.

78. Jacobson AM, Hauser ST, Willett J et al: Consequences of irregular versus continuous medical follow-up in children and adolescents with insulin-dependent diabetes mellitus. J Pediatr 131:727, 1997.

79. Kaufman FR, Halvorson M, Carpenter S: Association between diabetes control and visits to a multidisciplinary pediatric diabetes clinic. Pediatrics 103:948, 1999.

80. Brink SJ: Complications of pediatric and adolescent type 1 diabetes mellitus. Curr Diabetes Rep 1:47, 2001.

81. Brink SJ: Thyroid dysfunction in youngsters with IDDM. J Pediatr Endocrinol 1:181, 1983.

82. Carlsson A, Axelsson IE, Borulf SK et al: Prevalence of IgA-antiendomysium and IgA-antigliadin autoantibodies at diagnosis of insulin-dependent diabetes mellitus in Swedish children and adolescents. Pediatrics 103:1248, 1999.

83. Pocecco M, Ventura A: Coeliac disease and insulin dependent diabetes mellitus: A causal association? Acta Pediatr 84:1432, 1995.

84. American Diabetes Association: Care of children with diabetes in the school and day care setting. Diabetes Care 23(Suppl 1):S100, 2000.

85. American Diabetes Association: Care of children with diabetes in the school and day care setting. Diabetes Care 36(Suppl 1):S131–135, 2003.

86. Kaufman FR: Special report: Diabetes at school: What a child's health care team needs to know about federal disability law. Diabetes Spectrum 15:63, 2002.

87. Schiffrin A: Psychosocial issues in pediatric diabetes. Curr Diabetes Rep 1:33, 2001.

88. Kovacs M, Finkelstein R, Feinberg TL et al: Initial psychologic responses of parents to the diagnosis of insulin-dependent diabetes in their children. Diabetes Care 8:568, 1985.

89. Jacobson AM, Hauser ST, Wertleib D et al: Psychological adjustment of children with recently diagnosed diabetes mellitus. Diabetes 9:323, 1989.

90. Grey M, Cameron ME, Thurber FW: Coping and adaptation in children with diabetes. Nurs Res 40:144, 1991.

91. Jacobson AM, Hauser S, Lavori P et al: Family environment and glycemic control: A four-year prospective study of children and adolescents with insulin-dependent diabetes mellitus. Psychosom Med 56:401, 1994.

92. Anderson BJ, Miller P, Auslander WF, Santiago JV: Family characteristics of diabetic adolescents: Relationships to metabolic control. Diabetes Care 4:586, 1981.

93. Wysocki T: Parents, teens, and diabetes. Diabetes Spectrum 15:6, 2002.

94. Rubin R: Working with diabetic adolescents. In Anderson BJ, Rubin R (eds): Practical Psychology for Diabetes Clinicians. American Diabetes Association, Alexandria, VA, 1996.

95. Bennet-Johnson S, Perwein A, Silverstein J: Response to hypo-hyperglycemia in adolescents with type 1 diabetes. J Pediatr Psychol 25:171, 2000.

CHAPTER II

DIABETES AND PREGNANCY*

In this chapter, we address concerns regarding preconception, conception, pregnancy, delivery, and the postpartum state in women with prepregnancy diabetes. Screening for and treatment of gestational diabetes is also discussed, along with strategies for the prevention of subsequent type 2 diabetes in the woman with a history of gestational diabetes. Pregnant women with abnormalities of glucose metabolism need to be carefully and rigorously managed during pregnancy. If this is done, the odds for a healthy outcome for both mother and child can be markedly increased.

CONTRACEPTION

Because only approximately two thirds of pregnancies in women with diabetes are planned, information on contraception is a vital part of prepregnancy counseling.[1] Sexual activity with no protection leads to an 85% chance of pregnancy within 1 year. Table 11-1 lists available methods of contraception. There is no evidence that the failure rate or adverse effects of any method are different between women with and without dia-

betes. The choice depends on a couple's preference; the presence of diabetes does not dictate one method over another. Because contraception is necessary only until near euglycemia is achieved, a readily reversible, highly effective method should be chosen in a woman contemplating pregnancy. The choice usually is between an oral contraceptive or a barrier method.

Although high-dose estrogen preparations have been associated with increased vascular sequelae, including deep vein thrombosis, stroke, and hypertension, large prospective studies using low-dose estrogen preparations have a much looser association. Therefore, except for older women who smoke, oral contraceptives with doses of estrogen ≤35 μg of ethinyl estradiol or its methylated derivative, mestranol, and low doses of a progestin offer a safe, very effective, and usually readily reversible contraceptive. An attractive alternative is a low dose of a progestin only. The "mini pill," a progestin-only oral contraceptive, provides an option if a woman cannot take estrogen. The currently available progestin preparations have lower doses of progestin than in the combination oral contraceptives.

In women with diabetes who are at risk for dyslipidemia and dysregulation of glucose metabolism, it should be noted that the progesterone component of oral contraceptives

---

*Material for this chapter provided by John L. Kitzmiller, M.D., Director, Maternal–Fetal Medicine, Good Samaritan Hospital, San Jose, California.

TABLE 11-1 CONTRACEPTIVE METHODS

Type	Effectiveness (%)	Comments
Barrier methods		
Spermicides	70%–90%	Depends on the amount of spermicide used, and timing prior to intercourse; no STD protection
Male condom	87%–90%	No STD protection; not for use in latex allergies
Female condom	79%	May cause irritation and allergic reactions to the polyurethane
Contraceptive sponge	64%–82%	Cannot remain in place for longer than 30 hr because of risk of toxic shock syndrome
Diaphragm	82%	No STD protection; may be associated with increased urinary infections
Cervical cap	80%	May interfere with Pap results; no STD protection
Mechanical Methods		
IUDs	98%–99%	No protection against STDs; may worsen menstrual cramping and bleeding
Hormonal Methods		
Oral hormones—"the pill"	97%–99%	Increased risk of thromboembolism and stroke especially in smokers and with older preparations; no STD protection
Injections—Depo Provera	99%	Not for use in women with a history of breast cancer, liver disease, blood clots, or unexplained vaginal bleeding
Norplant	99%	Menstrual irregularities
Patch	97%–99%	Once a week application
"Natural" Methods		
Calendar rhythm	Can be up to 80%	Considered outdated; more than one ovulation can occur per cycle
Basal body temperature	Can be up to 80%	
Mucus inspections	Can be up to 80%	
Withdrawal	75%–85%	Not reliable
Lactation infertility	N/A	Not reliable
		Ovulation may begin prior to menstruation resumes.
Permanent Methods of Contraception		
Vasectomy	99%	No STD protection; can usually be reversed
Tubal ligation	98%	
Selective tubal occlusion procedure	N/A	Nonsurgical form of birth control; not yet FDA approved
Hysterectomy	100%	

FDA, Food and Drug Administration; IUD, intrauterine device; Pap, Papanicolaou; STD, sexually transmitted disease.

may play a role in aggravating these factors. Progestins have been shown to decrease glucose tolerance by increasing insulin resistance and secretion.[2] Subsequent data revealed a dose dependent relationship.[3] As a result, the lowest dose of progestin containing oral contraceptive that is tolerated should be advocated. Studies done looking directly at the effect of low-dose combination therapy in patients with type 1 diabetes have found little effect on glycemic control, although others did note a small increase in insulin dose requirements.[4] There is a direct relationship between an increase in low-density lipoprotein (LDL) and decrease in high-density lipoprotein levels and the dose of progestins along with their androgenicity.[5] This is another reason to advocate the lowest dose possible.

Barrier methods have a higher failure rate than oral contraceptive agents (see Table 11-1). They are most effective when combined with a spermicide or foam. If conception occurs, it is almost always the result of user failure rather than inadequacy of the method itself. A condom is the only method that protects against sexually transmitted diseases.

After pregnancy, longer-term contraception may be a consideration. One approach is the use of an intrauterine device (IUD). In general, these are safe; however, one of them, the Dalkon shield (which is no longer on the market) was associated with increased risks of pelvic infection. There is no evidence to show that the currently available IUDs are associated with increased rates of infection in women with diabetes compared with women without diabetes.[6] The greatest risk for pelvic infection in all women occurs in the first 4 months of insertion, and this incidence has been quoted at 1.6 per 1000 women-years, with a sixfold increase in pelvic inflammatory disease occurring during the first 20 days after insertion compared with later dates The costs of the Norplant system and 5 years of oral contraceptives are similar. The Norplant system

is a reversible, 5-year, low-dose, progestin-only contraceptive. The Norplant system consists of six very small matchstick size capsules (made of silastic tubing) that are placed just under the skin of the upper arm. Because the cost of the former is borne all at once at the time of insertion of the silastic capsules, it appears to be more expensive. Some method of contraception should also be instituted postpartum because breast-feeding (if carried out) is a relatively ineffective method of protection against pregnancy. Tubal ligation is a feasible option in women desiring a permanent form of contraception. Similarly, in men with diabetes, vasectomy may be performed with little (if any) increased risk compared with men without diabetes.

Women who have polycystic ovarian syndrome (PCOS) may have impaired fertility. This may be a comorbid condition in women with type 2 diabetes. Women may need to be aware that even though ovulation may not be regular, pregnancy may still occur, and as a result, contraception should be used until glycemic control is optimal. Patients who are treated for insulin resistance with drugs such as thiazolidinediones or biguanides may experience a return to normal ovulatory patterns and perhaps an increase in fertility as they become more insulin sensitive. They should be advised about this possibility, and in those who do not desire pregnancy, contraception should be used.[7,8]

PREPREGNANCY COUNSELING

Any discussion of diabetes and pregnancy must begin with prepregnancy counseling. Ideally, any woman who is of childbearing age and who has diabetes should be informed of the risks of pregnancy to both her and her fetus. Effective contraception should be practiced until a woman and her partner are ready for pregnancy. At this point, more detailed prepregnancy counseling and care should take place. This information should be provided by the woman's primary care physician, obstetrician, and diabetes health care team (if such a team is available). Many high-risk obstetricians that follow women with diabetes during the second and third trimesters of pregnancy do not take care of the patient early in pregnancy. Therefore it is important that the woman's existing health care team assist with the preconception and first trimester care.[9]

The purpose of preconception care is specifically to minimize congenital malformations and thereby reduce the subsequent health care costs and burden. Such a program should ideally be multidisciplinary and involve some or all of the following: primary care provider, obstetrician, diabetologist, diabetes nurse educator, dietitian with a special knowledge of diabetes, ophthalmologist, and social worker. Preconception glycemic goals (A1C <7%) should be stated early in the process of planning a pregnancy and women should learn how to test and interpret both preprandial and postprandial blood glucose (BG) levels. Ultimately, the woman with diabetes should be empowered with tools to allow her to achieve a healthy pregnancy and a healthy baby. Depending on the patient's ability, practical self-management skills should be reviewed, including self-monitoring of blood glucose (SMBG), meal planning, insulin adjustments, hypoglycemia treatment, and lifestyle modifications. Often it is helpful to include the woman's partner in these discussions, so he or she can learn what to expect and understand the risks to mother and baby. Additionally, instruction in the use of glucagon may be needed if strict blood glucose control leads to an increase in episodes of hypoglycemia.

For the provider, it is important to note that the only true acceptable goal prior to conception is euglycemia, and this applies to women with both type 1 and type 2 diabetes. Any alteration that results in changes in maternal metabolism results in changes in the intrauterine environment. The types of abnormalities that may occur depend on the timing of metabolic dysregulation. Prepregnancy counseling is specifically important to avoid negative impact on the fetus during the first 6 weeks of development.[10] Also, there is evidence that enrollment in a preconception diabetes care program can reduce the excess congenital anomalies and spontaneous abortions that occur in this group.[11]

Special focus should be given to certain groups of women with diabetes during this stage of pregnancy consideration. Although these are mentioned in detail later in the text, they warrant a quick reference here. Those who have significant hypoglycemia need particularly close follow-up and supervision. The risks of hypoglycemia are greater to the mother than to the fetus, and are similar to the risks of hypoglycemia in nonpregnant individuals). Women with a history of retinopathy should be told that eye disease may accelerate during pregnancy; women should be advised that an ophthalmologic evaluation should be made prior to pregnancy and regularly during pregnancy. In general, pregnancy does not accelerate the progression of diabetic nephropathy if the disease is mild, but with moderate renal disease (defined as a creatinine from 1.7 to 2.7 mg/dl), there may be an accelerated decline in renal function.[12] Although not an absolute contraindication to pregnancy, an informed decision regarding conception should be made. Women with a history of coronary artery disease and diabetes have an increased mortality rate during pregnancy. Women with a history of heart disease prior to conception should have a through cardiac evaluation to ensure they can tolerate the increased cardiovascular demands of pregnancy. Symptomatic ischemic heart disease and congestive heart failure are contraindications to pregnancy because of the high risk of maternal mortality.

General measures for preconception health should also be discussed. This includes starting folic acid supplementation prior to conception to reduce the risk for neural tube defects. Women who are attempting to become pregnant should be counseled about the effects of alcohol and smoking during pregnancy, and should be encouraged to avoid both during pregnancy. In conjunction with the health care team, medications such as angiotensin-converting enzyme inhibitors (ACEIs), statins, antidepressants, and other agents may need to be stopped or changed to a medication approved for use in pregnancy. A general checklist to help a woman with diabetes prepare for pregnancy is shown in Table 11-2.

IMPACT OF MATERNAL DIABETES ON THE FETUS AND CHILD

Diabetes in a pregnant woman can be detrimental to her fetus for four reasons. First, women with diabetes have an increased spontaneous abortion rate compared with the rate in nondiabetic pregnant women. This increase, however, can be eliminated if near euglycemia is achieved at the time of conception[13,14] and during the first trimester.[15,16] Second, infants of women with pregestational type 1 diabetes were found to have 6.4 times the reported risk of congenital malformations and 5.1 times the reported risk of perinatal mortality than infants in the general population.[17] As related to A1C results, adverse outcomes increase as glycemic control worsens. Compared with fair control, there is a reported fourfold increase in adverse outcome and spontaneous abortion, and a ninefold increase in major congenital malformations in the infants of women with type 1 diabetes and glycated hemoglobin concentrations higher than 7.5%.[18] The risk of congenital anomalies in the nondiabetic population has a rate of approximately 2%.[19,20] The usual major malformations involve neural tube defects and cardiac anomalies; affected tissues are formed during the early part of the first trimester during the period of organogenesis (Table 11-3). Fortunately, the rate of major congenital anomalies can be returned to the nondiabetic rate if near euglycemia can be achieved at the time of conception.[11,19,21,22] The severity of maternal

TABLE 11-2 CHECKLIST FOR PREPARING FOR PREGNANCY		
Type of Diabetes	**Issue**	**Action**
All	A1C	✓ <7%
Type 1	Insulin	✓ Glargine not approved in pregnancy; stabilize on the regimen that will be used in pregnancy
Type 2	Medication	✓ Stop oral agents; switch to insulin
All	Monitoring	✓ To monitor pre- and postprandial blood glucose values; lower targets as needed to bring A1C to <7%
All	Neural Tube Defects	✓ Start folic acid replacement
All	Retinopathy	✓ Dilated retinal examination prior to conception
All	Other medications	✓ Stop or change in conjunction with health care team
All	Renal Function	✓ Address implications if abnormal
All	Smoking; alcohol and illicit drug use	✓ Counsel cessation

TABLE 11-3 MALFORMATIONS IN INFANTS OF MOTHERS WITH PREGESTATIONAL DIABETES	
Type of Malformation	**Gestational Week of Development**
Caudal regression (skeletal)	3
Neural tube defects	4
Hydrocephalus	4
Cardiac anomalies (e.g., AV transposition, septal defects)	5–6
Renal agenesis	5

AV, arteriovenous.

vasculopathy and nephropathy may also independently affect the fetus, resulting in intrauterine growth restriction.[23] Although the actual cause of intrauterine growth retardation is not known, animal studies have shown that in rats with streptozotocin-induced diabetes, placental pathology and alterations in placental function early on in pregnancy were thought to contribute to the defective growth in the offspring.[24] The prepregnancy target for conception is an A1C level (based on a Diabetes Control and Complications Trial standardized method) of less than 7%.

The other negative consequences that maternal type 1 diabetes may have on a fetus are certain neonatal morbidities, such as respiratory distress syndrome (RDS), hypoglycemia, hyperbilirubinemia, and hypocalcemia. Lung maturation in infants born of mothers with diabetes does not appear to be delayed in those with good glycemic control, and RDS is rare in this population,[25] but fetal pulmonary maturation, as evidenced by the onset of phosphatidylglycerol production in the amniotic fluid can be delayed in diabetic pregnancies by 1 to 1.5 weeks.[26] In women with poorly controlled diabetes who cannot confirm gestational age, amniotic fluid analysis for lung maturity prior to delivery may be warranted. In women with type 2 diabetes or gestational diabetes, macrosomia can make delivery more difficult and thus can lead to increased rates of cesarean sections or shoulder dystocias during vaginal deliveries. In one series, the incidence of macrosomia ranged from 20% in gestational diabetes to 35% in pre-existing diabetes.[27] Both macrosomia[28–30] and neonatal morbidity[28] are associated with maternal hyperglycemia, and near euglycemia needs to be achieved during the second and third trimesters to reduce these outcomes rather than at the time of conception and during the first trimester. These potential complications should be discussed with women who have type 1 and type 2 diabetes and are contemplating pregnancy, to prepare them for the possible challenges ahead.

Regarding long-term sequelae, there is some evidence to suggest that in addition to the previously mentioned sequelae, abnormalities were found more often in the offspring of mothers with poorly controlled diabetes during pregnancy that resulted in speech difficulties, eye-movement incoordination, and socialization problems.[31] There is also recent data showing that among 231 women with gestational diabetes, chromosomal defects are twice as prevalent as defects seen in the offspring of women without diabetes. Put in other terms, there is a 7.7 times increase in chromosome defects in these offspring. The clinical significance of this remains unclear.[32]

The risk of developing type 2 diabetes is significantly higher in children who have a mother with type 2 diabetes then those with nondiabetic mothers.[33] It is also higher in children of mothers who had gestational diabetes. Children of mothers with diabetes also have an increased risk of developing impaired glucose tolerance, and this rate actually doubles if the mother had diabetes during her pregnancy compared with development of diabetes after her pregnancy (33% versus 14%),[34] In comparison, in children who have a father with diabetes, the incidence of gestational diabetes is only 7%.[35]

There is evidence that the intrauterine environment has long-term implications later in life. Although this topic requires a chapter in itself, there are a few interesting examples to point out. Numerous cross-sectional studies have demonstrated the relationship between birth weight of term infants and their disease development as adults. Type 2 diabetes, insulin resistance, hypertension, and coronary heart disease have all been shown to have a relationship with birth weight.[36] In one study, children of mothers with type 1 diabetes had higher LDL cholesterol levels, total cholesterol levels, and plasminogen activator inhibitor-1 levels at ages 5 to 11 years than did children whose mothers did not have diabetes.[37] Westbom et al.[38] looked at 4380 children born from women with pregestational diabetes. They found the odds ratio for having childhood cancer in these children was 2.25 compared with children born from mothers without diabetes. Compared with mothers with other autoimmune diseases such as lupus, rheumatoid arthritis, Crohn's disease, thyroiditis, and multiple sclerosis, there was still an increase, suggesting that the autoimmunity of mothers with pregestational diabetes is not the factor implicated in the increase of cancer in their offspring. Much more work needs to be done on the area of intrauterine environment and subsequent disease sequelae.

IMPACT OF DIABETES ON THE PREGNANT WOMAN

In addition to emphasizing the importance of achieving near euglycemia before concep-

tion and throughout pregnancy, prepregnancy counseling should include a frank discussion of how pregnancy will affect the complications of diabetes in both the near term and long term. As mentioned, background retinopathy can worsen, possibly because of the rapid imposition of near euglycemia in patients who have poor control prior to preparing for pregnancy.[39,40] The other postulated mechanism is an increase in circulating growth factors during pregnancy. Progression of retinopathy in pregnancy depends on a variety of factors, including severity of retinopathy at conception, duration of diabetes, metabolic control before pregnancy, and the presence of hypertension.[41] Reported rates of new cases or progression of diabetic retinopathy during pregnancy range from 10% to 70%.[42] Although background retinopathy may progress during pregnancy, it usually regresses to the prepregnant baseline status after delivery.[20] If the vision-threatening changes of proliferative retinopathy or macular edema are treated with laser before or during pregnancy, the eyes remain quiescent without further deterioration.[20] For these reasons, it is extremely important that a patient be evaluated by an ophthalmologist as soon as pregnancy is established and her eyes monitored periodically until delivery.

The situation regarding diabetic nephropathy is similar to that of retinopathy. For the most part, pregnancy does not affect the typical progression of renal disease, particularly if kidney function is well preserved at the time of pregnancy.[43] Fortunately, less than 5% of diabetic women who become pregnant have overt nephropathy (i.e., dipstick positive or clinical proteinuria).[20] Because total protein excretion increases by 50% to 100% during normal pregnancy up to 200 mg per day,[44] evaluation of nephropathy during pregnancy in women with diabetes mellitus is difficult. Total protein excretion less than 190 mg/day but below the level of overt nephropathy (500 mg/day) is associated with the same increased prevalence of preeclampsia as in women with clinical proteinuria.[45] It is likely that some of the women with this level of protein excretion have incipient nephropathy. In patients who have had renal transplantation, retrospective data on 44 pregnancies in 26 women revealed 32 live-born infants and 12 stillborn/abortuses; of those born live, there was an increase in preterm delivery and low birth weight. The authors of this study also noted that these offspring had normal postnatal growth and development.[46]

Clinical proteinuria usually increases during pregnancy but returns to prepregnancy levels after delivery in most cases.[20,47] Hypertension often becomes more of a problem, and stringent efforts must be made to control it because it may lead to preeclampsia and hydramnios. In contrast to clinical proteinuria with normal renal function, if a woman has azotemia (almost always accompanied by hypertension) before pregnancy, she may have further loss of renal function during pregnancy, and this may not regress after delivery.[20] Although ACEIs are particularly suited to treat hypertension in diabetic patients (see Chapter 7), they *must* be avoided in pregnancy because of their association with fetal renal damage, oligohydramnios, and congenital anomalies.[20] Fortunately, no increased fetal problems were found in pregnant women inadvertently treated with ACEIs in the first trimester.[20]

Peripheral neuropathy has no bearing on the outcome of pregnancy. However, symptomatic autonomic neuropathy involving the stomach (i.e., gastroparesis diabeticorum) can cause intractable vomiting, with its attendant risks to metabolic control and nutrition.

Macrovascular disease per se presents no risk to a fetus, but has led to the death of pregnant diabetic women who have it.[48] Therefore a careful cardiac evaluation is recommended for such women contemplating pregnancy. Although rare, coronary artery bypass surgery may be required to ensure a successful outcome.[48]

HORMONAL AND METABOLIC ALTERATIONS DURING PREGNANCY

HORMONAL CHANGES

Concentrations of circulating hormones during pregnancy (which are produced by the placenta) are depicted in Figure 11-1. Placental production of human chorionic gonadotropin peaks early in pregnancy and plateaus at low levels after the first trimester. Its action is similar to that of the gonadotropins of pituitary origin, which have little direct effect on carbohydrate metabolism. The rise in the other three hormones—estrogen, progesterone, and human chorionic somatomammotropin (hCS) (also known as *human placental lactogen* [*hPL*]) occurs gradually, paralleling the growth of the placenta. All of these antagonize the action of insulin, especially hPL, which has many of the properties of pituitary growth hormone. Thus increasing insulin resistance characterizes the second and third trimesters of pregnancy. Therefore the pattern of insulin secretion (Figure 11-2) is expected to parallel the changes of hormone secretion during pregnancy. Increased concentrations of insulin are necessary to overcome the hormonally induced state of insulin resistance. Failure of the pancreatic β cells to meet this increased demand is responsible for the development of gestational diabetes mellitus (GDM) (discussed later).

METABOLIC CHANGES

To compare the metabolic changes in pregnancy with the nongravid state, it is helpful to consider separately the normal fed and fasted states. After an overnight fast, plasma glucose concentrations are maintained fairly constantly by an equilibrium between glucose utilization and hepatic glucose production, occurring mainly via the pathways

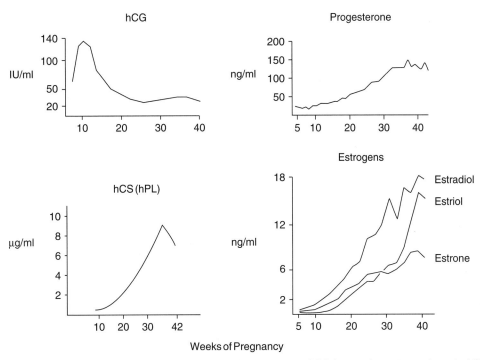

FIGURE 11-1. Circulating levels of "pregnancy" hormones during gestation. hCG, human chorionic gonadotropin; hCS, human chorionic somatomammotropin; hPL, human placental lactogen. *(From Freinkel N: Of pregnancy and progeny, Diabetes 29:1023, 1980.)*

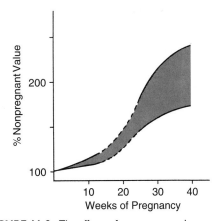

FIGURE 11-2. The effects of pregnancy on glucose-stimulated insulin secretion. The increments above fasting values of insulin concentrations after a glucose challenge have been summated to derive an index of the secretory response. The figure compares the range of published values during pregnancy and in nongravid women. *(From Freinkel N: Of pregnancy and progeny. Diabetes 29:1023, 1980.)*

of gluconeogenesis (synthesis of glucose from noncarbohydrate precursors [i.e., amino acids, lactate, and glycerol]). The majority of glucose utilization in the fasting state occurs in tissues that are not insulin sensitive, and therefore insulin levels are low. After food consumption, glucose and amino acid concentrations rise, triggering increased insulin secretion. This results in storage of ingested glucose and amino acids in muscle and liver and cessation of hepatic glucose production.

Both maternal glucose and amino acids enter the fetus through the placenta. Glucose is transported via facilitated diffusion, the same process that occurs in the insulin-sensitive tissues of muscle and fat. Although this process is not influenced by insulin (insulin is destroyed by the placenta), the ability of the placenta to transport glucose by facilitated diffusion results in greater entrance of glucose into the fetus than would be the case if glucose uptake simply occurred down its concentration gradient as it does in most other tissues (e.g., brain, liver). Amino acids are transported across the placenta *against* their concentration gradient. In this manner, the fetus serves as a trap for maternal glucose and amino acids. A normal fasting glucose concentration cannot be maintained for two reasons. More glucose is siphoned off to serve the fetus (causing increased glucose utilization), and an important gluconeogenic precursor, the amino acid alanine, is not as available (causing decreased hepatic glucose production). This results in a lowering of the fasting glucose concentration in normal pregnancy.

Other changes occur in the fasting state as well. These are termed *accelerated starvation*. In addition to the lower concentrations of glucose and alanine mentioned earlier, higher levels of free fatty acids and ketone bodies are found in pregnant women than in nongravid controls after extending an overnight fast by several hours. These changes are caused, in part, by the lipolytic action (i.e., the hydrolysis of adipose tissue triglycerides) of hPL. The increased tendency to develop ketosis in pregnancy has some implications for the subsequent intellectual development of the child (discussed later).

Changes also occur in the fed state owing to the increasing insulin resistance during the second and third trimesters. Although insulin secretion increases markedly (Figure 11-3), glucose concentrations are often increased (albeit still in the normal range) compared with the nongravid state. If insulin secretion cannot meet this increased demand, the resulting hyperglycemia of GDM can have important detrimental effects on the fetus (discussed later).

PREGNANCY IN WOMEN WITH PREGESTATIONAL DIABETES—TYPE I OR TYPE 2

CLASSIFICATION

Diabetic pregnant women were classified on the basis of duration and severity of diabetes (Table 11-4) by Priscilla White,[49] a pioneer in the management of diabetes in pregnancy who worked for 50 years at the Joslin Clinic in Boston. Her classification system was originally used to estimate prognosis for perinatal outcome and to determine some aspects of obstetric management, such as timing of delivery. The system is no longer used for that purpose because perinatal outcome has improved for many reasons in women of all White classes. It is now recognized that the major determinants of outcome are the degree of glycemic control and the presence of hypertension and/or impaired renal function that exist before and during pregnancy.

NONMETABOLIC COMPLICATIONS IN WOMEN WITH PREGESTATIONAL DIABETES

The hormonal changes of early pregnancy stimulate nausea and vomiting in many pregnancies. Although mild symptoms are common, rarely hyperemesis occurs. Severe hyperemesis can be quite problematic in nondiabetic women, but it can be particularly devastating in diabetic women, particularly in those with autonomic neuropathy and gastroparesis diabeticorum.[50] Weight loss and ketonemia are common indications for hospitalization and intravenous hydration. Occasionally, diabetic women continue to be unable to retain oral feedings, and placement of a postpyloric feeding tube may be necessary. As a last resort, parenteral nutrition via a central line may be necessary

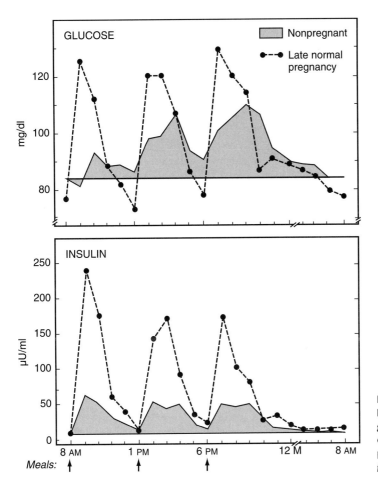

FIGURE 11-3. The effect of normal late pregnancy (weeks 33 to 39 of gestation) on glucose and insulin concentrations throughout a 24-hour period. *(From Freinkel N: Of pregnancy and progeny. Diabetes 29:1023, 1980.)*

to provide adequate substrates for normal fetal growth and development.

Clinically detected *polyhydramnios* was formerly quite common (15% to 30%) in women with poorly controlled diabetes.[51] In these series, the diagnosis was based on dramatically increased maternal abdominal girth resulting from excess amniotic fluid. This was sometimes associated with maternal dyspnea or preterm labor (PTL) caused by overdistention of the uterus. Using ultrasonography, the diagnosis of polyhydramnios has been defined as a four-quadrant amniotic fluid index of more than 20 cm, but most cases defined this way are not clinically significant.

Studies of the cause of polyhydramnios in diabetic women, in the absence of fetal anomalies such as open neural tube defects or tracheoesophageal fistulas, are inconclusive. The concentration of solutes is not greater in the amniotic fluid in cases of polyhydramnios. The hypothesis that the polyhydramnios is due to fetal glucosuria and excess urine output is not supported by ultrasonographic studies of fetal bladder emptying in diabetic women with and without excessive amniotic fluid volume.[52] However, polyhydramnios is clearly associated with maternal hyperglycemia and fetal macrosomia, but the primary causal mechanisms remain unclear.

TABLE 11-4 CLASSIFICATION OF DIABETES DURING PREGNANCY

Class	Characteristics	Implications
A	Impaired glucose tolerance diagnosed before pregnancy (as compared with GDM diagnosed during pregnancy); any age at onset	Treated with diet to produce euglycemia and optimal weight gain; if insulin is needed, manage as in classes B, C, and D
B	Onset age ≥20 years; duration <10 years	Can be type 1 or 2 diabetes mellitus; maternal insulin secretion may persist, but exogenous insulin prescription is usually necessary for euglycemia to reduce fetal and neonatal risks
C	Onset age 10–19 years or duration 10–19 years	Usually type 1 insulin-deficient diabetes, but MODY is possible; glycemic control is major focus
D	Onset before age 10, or duration >20 years, or chronic hypertension, or background retinopathy	Fetal growth depends on balance of diabetic microvascular disease and glycemic control; retinal microaneurysms, dot hemorrhages, and exudates may progress during pregnancy, then regress after delivery
F	Diabetic nephropathy with clinical proteinuria	With control of glycemia, hypertension, and anemia, renal function is usually stable, but proteinuria increases and then declines after delivery; fetal growth restriction, superimposed preeclampsia common; perinatal survival can exceed 90%
H	Coronary artery disease	Serious maternal risk
R	Proliferative retinopathy	Neovascularization, with risk of vitreous hemorrhage or retinal detachment; laser photocoagulation needed

GDM, gestational diabetes mellitus; MODY, maturity-onset diabetes of the young (see Chapter 1 for description). From Hare JW, White P: Gestational diabetes and the White classification. Diabetes Care 3:394, 1980.

Treatment of severe polyhydramnios by transabdominal drainage is usually not successful for more than a short time owing to reaccumulation of amniotic fluid. The role of maternal indomethacin therapy, which reduces fetal urine output and amnionic fluid volume, has not been evaluated in diabetic women. Because treatment is difficult, it is fortunate that prevention is possible by intensified maternal glycemic control, which is shown to reduce the frequency of polyhydramnios to approximately 12%.

Some evidence shows that PTL may be more common in women with diabetes than in those without, even without polyhydramnios, but the causes are obscure.[51] Various frequencies of PTL or of tocolytic treatment (5% to 30%) in different studies of diabetes and pregnancy may be due to the use of different criteria for diagnosis.[53] PTL should be diagnosed on the basis of changes in the cervix: effacement or shortening, with or without dilatation, in response to uterine contractions, which may be subtle. Many factors predict an increased risk of PTL, including more than five uterine contractions per hour, cervical length less than 3 cm or funneling seen on ultrasound studies, and fetal fibronectin measured in cervical secretions as a response to inflammatory changes in the amniotic membranes.

Because the degree of preterm birth (by gestational age) is a major determinant of mortality, morbidity, and cost of care of infants of diabetic mothers, effective identification and treatment of PTL is essential. The first-choice uterine tocolytic agent should be magnesium sulfate given intravenously to avoid the hyperglycemic effects of β-adrenergic agents such as ritodrine and terbutaline. Total intravenous fluid volume should be carefully controlled to 100 to 125 ml/hr to avoid iatrogenic pulmonary edema. The dosage of tocolytic drug is titrated to keep the frequency of uterine contractions under the threshold that causes cervical change. This amount seems specific for each patient. If additional tocolytic effect is needed in the acute management of an episode of PTL at less than 30 weeks' gestation, oral indomethacin is effective and does not impair glycemic control. Its effectiveness must be balanced against a possible association with intracranial bleeding or bowel perforation in very low-birth-weight infants born to indomethacin-treated mothers. Beyond 30 weeks' gestation, maternal use of indomethacin can result in significant narrowing of the fetal ductus arteriosus.

Limited evidence suggests that continued long-term tocolytic treatment, in addition to bed rest, can reduce the likelihood of recurrent episodes of PTL. Oral nifedipine (10 to 20 mg every 4 hours) may be successful in controlling contractions and may allow a patient to be monitored at home. Long-term oral terbutaline (2 to 5 mg every 4 to 6 hours) may induce desensitization of uterine adrenergic responses with failed tocolytic effect. However, low-dose subcutaneous terbutaline pump therapy (0.5 to 1.0 mg/hr, with boluses of 0.25 mg/hr every 4 to 6 hours) probably avoids down-regulation of the uterine β-adrenergic receptors. The moderate hyperglycemic side effects can be counteracted with increased insulin doses.

For cases of possible preterm birth before 34 weeks' gestation in women with diabetes, it is presumed that the corticosteroid betamethasone given intramuscularly to gravidas stimulates fetal surfactant production and decreases neonatal mortality and morbidity resulting from RDS. However, betamethasone also stimulates marked maternal hyperglycemia, which can lead to ketoacidosis. To prevent this, the insulin dose should be doubled by 4 hours after the initial injection of betamethasone for a duration of 48 to 72 hours. This also prevents the possible harmful result of fetal hyperglycemia and fetal hyperinsulinemia, which may block the hoped-for effect of the corticosteroid on the surfactant system in the fetal alveolar type II cells.[54,55] Another potentially harmful result of fetal hyperglycemia and hyperinsulinemia is fetal hypoxia and acidosis.[56] Therefore be vigilant in preventing maternal hyperglycemia while managing PTL or preterm ruptured membranes in women with diabetes.

Hypertension in pregnancy occurs with similar incidence in patients with type 1 and type 2 diabetes (41% versus 45%) but the characteristics are different.[57] Women with type 2 diabetes were noted to have more chronic hypertension and less preeclampsia than women with type 1 diabetes, and perhaps as a result, adverse outcomes associated with hypertension were noted as being less prevalent in women with type 2 diabetes.[57] A prospective study looking at 196 women with pregestational diabetes and 428 patients with gestational diabetes found that women with pregestational diabetes were at increased risk for caesarean delivery, shoulder dystocia or cephalopelvic disproportion, gestational hypertension, and toxemia compared with those with gestational diabetes.[58] Infants of these mothers also had a higher likelihood of requiring neonatal intensive care unit care. Maternal obesity and to a lesser degree excessive weight gain were factors influencing many of these outcomes.

The *pre-eclamptic toxemic (PET)* syndrome of acute hypertension, proteinuria, variable edema, but reduced plasma volume and potential end-organ damage caused by vasospasm and intravascular coagulation in liver, brain, and kidneys is a frequent and serious complication of pregnancy in women with diabetes. The prevalence of PET ranges from 8% to 14% in women with gestational or established diabetes without microalbuminuria, to 30% to 40% in women with diabetic microalbuminuria, and up to 50% to 60% in women who have diabetes with overt nephropathy (e.g., those with clinical proteinuria) or renal transplants.[45] The causes of preeclampsia are still obscure, but probably relate to uteroplacental vascular insufficiency, perhaps secondary to diabetic vasculopathy, although the placenta-related "toxins" that damage the peripheral maternal vasculature remain to be identified.[59] Some evidence suggests that the risk of developing PET is greater with poor glycemic control.[60] Peterson et al.[61] showed in the Diabetes in Early Pregnancy Project that systolic blood pressure increased throughout pregnancy in women with diabetes compared with controls, and that diastolic blood pressures were also higher throughout pregnancy. Diagnosis of PET in diabetic women with prior hypertension and proteinuria is difficult, but the rapid acceleration of hypertension and proteinuria in the third trimester with or without laboratory evidence of end-organ damage should be managed as superimposed preeclampsia to protect the gravida and fetus.

The dangerous effects of preeclampsia are related to reversible ischemia of regional vascular beds. Decreased glomerular filtration and tubular dysfunction are marked by rising serum creatinine and uric acid levels and falling creatinine clearance and urine output. Hematuria is possible, and renal cortical necrosis is an avoidable end-stage result. Ischemia of hepatocytes is marked by rising serum transaminase values. Periportal microhemorrhages can lead to epigastric and right upper quadrant pain caused by distention of the liver capsule. Here spontaneous rupture of the liver is the avoidable end-stage result. Foci of ischemia and perivascular hemorrhage in the brain are associated with generalized convulsions (eclampsia) or coma. Pulmonary endothelial changes, fluid retention, and left-sided heart failure resulting from increased afterload can lead to acute pulmonary edema. Finally, decreased uteroplacental blood flow in diabetic gravidas with PET is associated with placental infarction, fetal growth restriction, and fetal asphyxia, with the possible end result of stillbirth.

The objective of management of PET in women with diabetes is to recognize and prevent progression of the maternal or placental vascular damage. The only known cure for severe preeclampsia is to deliver the placenta, which is the reason PET is a leading cause of premature birth in diabetic women. Short of that, sequential monitoring of blood pressure, proteinuria, creatinine clearance, platelet counts, and transaminase levels, and estimation of fetal growth and hypoxia are used to determine how long a preterm pregnancy can safely be continued. Intravenous infusions of magnesium sulfate have been shown to be the most effective therapy to prevent convulsions and improve maternal and fetal outcomes,[62] and magnesium sulfate may have beneficial hemodynamic effects as well.[63] In women with diabetes, blood pressure should be kept below 140/90 to minimize retinal and renal damage, and long-term antihypertensive therapy with methyldopa, diltiazem, prazosin, and clonidine is usually effective and safe for a woman and her fetus. ACEIs should not be used in pregnancy because they cause fetal renal damage and malformation. For severe acute hypertension (>160/110) in the peripartum situation, epidural anesthesia, intravenous labetalol, or nitroglycerin infusions can be quite effective.

Symptomatic generalized maternal edema has been reported in up to 22% of pregnancies in patients with pre-existing diabetes.[64] This can be severe enough to require bed rest. The cause remains unclear. Hypoalbuminemia may play a role in severe cases associated with nephropathy, but there are many others with normal renal function that exhibit significant edema as well.

Pyelonephritis is also seen in associated with diabetes.[65] Treatment during pregnancy may required hospitalization for administration of intravenous antibiotics.

METABOLIC COMPLICATIONS IN WOMEN WITH PREGESTATIONAL (TYPE 1) DIABETES

The metabolic complications of diabetes in pregnant women are the same as in the nongravid state—that is, hyperglycemia, diabetic ketoacidosis (DKA), and hypoglycemia. As opposed to the acute symptoms of marked hyperglycemia (i.e., polyuria, polydipsia, blurred vision, and fungal infections), the consequences of hyperglycemia (i.e., retinopathy, nephropathy, and neuropathy) are not evident for years. In pregnancy, the long-term consequences of maternal hyperglycemia involve the fetus (e.g., congenital anomalies, stillbirths, macrosomia, RDS, and neonatal hypoglycemia) and obviously occur in months, not years. Thus pregnant diabetic women do not have the luxury of gradually achieving near euglycemia; they must do it quickly and sustain it.

The diagnosis and treatment of DKA are discussed in detail elsewhere in this book and are the same whether a patient is pregnant or not. An urgent concern, however, is either prompt recognition of impending DKA or, if it develops, rapid treatment of the pregnant woman because fetal demise commonly follows the episode. Prevention, of course, is preferred and is maximized by frequent communication between the patient and the health care provider, especially when the

woman is feeling ill. Particularly challenging is the situation (usually in the first trimester) of nausea and sometimes vomiting in association with ketonuria. This could either be morning sickness with "starvation" ketosis secondary to decreased carbohydrate intake or mild DKA. Unfortunately, the BG concentration may not be entirely helpful to distinguish between the two because near normal or even normal levels are sometimes found in patients in DKA.[66] This seems to be more common in those who are vomiting. Because the consequences of delaying the treatment of DKA can be so dire to a fetus, it is better to err on the side of caution and measure a serum bicarbonate level whenever the distinction between these two diagnoses is in doubt. Even if the diagnosis is hyperemesis, a patient with type 1 diabetes who has protracted vomiting often requires hospitalization to receive appropriate fluids and to balance the administration of glucose and insulin.

Considerations regarding hypoglycemia are similar in the gravid and nongravid states, with one potential difference. One of the causes of hypoglycemia unawareness is lowered thresholds for both the symptoms and the release of counterregulatory hormones. The brain accommodates to the prevailing level of BG to which it is exposed. Thus patients who are chronically hyperglycemic (e.g., average BG concentrations of 250 mg/dl) experience symptoms of hypoglycemia at BG levels that are not low (e.g., 125 mg/dl). Conversely, in patients whose average BG levels are lower than usual (e.g., in pregnancy and/or those achieving very strict control), hypoglycemic symptoms and counterregulatory hormones do not appear at the usual BG concentrations (50 to 60 mg/dl) but do so at lower values (30 to 40 mg/dl). Thus the possibility that a patient may experience the consequences of severe hypoglycemia (e.g., confusion, seizures, or coma) is enhanced because the milder signs and symptoms did not warn the patient to initiate actions to avoid this outcome. (See elsewhere in this book for a detailed discussion of hypoglycemia and hypoglycemia unawareness.) This is another reason why frequent SMBG is necessary in pregnancy, so that asymptomatic hypoglycemia can be recognized and appropriate adjustments made. A recent study evaluated the frequency of severe hypoglycemia in women with type 1 diabetes during their first trimester of pregnancy and in the 4 months prior to conception to try to identify predictors of hypoglycemia.[67] The authors studied 278 women and noted an increase in the incidence of hypoglycemia from 0.9 ± 2.4 episodes per 4 months prior to pregnancy to 2.6 ± 6.3 episodes during the first trimester. There was also an increase in incidence of hypoglycemic coma. The authors noted that in these women with type 1 diabetes, the risk of severe hypoglycemia was associated with a history of severe hypoglycemia prior to pregnancy, duration of diabetes, and an A1C level of less than 6.5%. Also, patients on a higher daily dose of insulin were at higher risk. It is obvious that a delicate balance must be reached between tight control and minimal hypoglycemia in this population.

TREATMENT TO PREVENT COMPLICATIONS OF PREGNANCY IN WOMEN WITH PREGESTATIONAL (TYPE 1) DIABETES

Diet

The goal of appropriate dietary management for a pregnant diabetic woman is to provide adequate nutrition for both the woman and fetus and to achieve near euglycemia. Pregnancy imposes certain nutritional demands that necessitate alterations in the diet.

Calories

To determine the appropriate caloric intake during pregnancy, one must estimate the desirable body weight (DBW) of the woman. The DBW for women is based on height, weight, and frame size. This can be calculated using the following formula: 100 pounds for the first 5 feet of height, and 5 pounds for each inch over 5 feet.

For large-framed individuals, 10% is added and 10% is subtracted for small-framed subjects. Frame size can be grossly estimated by having the patient's predominant hand grasp the other wrist and oppose the thumb and middle finger. If these two fingers meet, the patient has a medium frame. If they overlap appreciably, the patient is small framed. If they fail to meet, the patient is large framed. Appropriate adjustments are made to the DBW in the latter two circumstances.

Women within 90% to 120% of DBW before becoming pregnant should gain between 25 and 30 pounds to minimize obstetric complications and premature births. Women who are less than 90% of DBW prepregnancy should gain between 28 and 40 pounds to ensure delivery of an infant of appropriate size. Overweight women do not need to gain as much weight to ensure delivery of a healthy baby. Recommended weight gain for those between 120% and 150% of DBW before pregnancy should be between 15 and 25 pounds. Appropriate weight gain for women less than 150% of DBW is approximately 15 pounds. Any indicated weight loss should be deferred until the postpartum period.

The normal pattern of weight gain is a gradual one. A 2- to 5-pound increase in the first trimester represents the growth of the uterus and expansion of the maternal blood volume. Appropriate weight gain during the second and third trimesters is 0.5 to 1 pound per week. In the second trimester, the weight gain represents mostly maternal changes to support the pregnancy. During the third trimester, the weight gain is mainly due to the growth of the placenta and fetus. On average, a nonpregnant woman of normal weight ingests approximately 2200 kcal per day. To support the necessary weight gain of pregnancy, an additional 300 kcal per day is required (Table 11-5). However, these additional calories are necessary during only the latter two trimesters. Caloric recommendations are summarized in Table 11-6.

Protein

Pregnant women need approximately 60 g of protein every day. This is about 10 extra g of protein each day. The additional protein is required for growth of the fetus and the increased size of the maternal blood volume, uterus, and breasts. Proteins in the placenta and fetus are synthesized from amino acids supplied by the mother (see Table 11-6).

Carbohydrate

Postprandial glucose concentrations depend mainly on the carbohydrate content of the preceding meal. Because achieving maternal euglycemia is so important in avoiding fetal complications and macrosomia, the carbohydrate content of the diet in a pregnant diabetic women is often less than in the prepregnant state—for instance, 40% to 50% instead of 50% to 60%. This is the recommendation of the California Diabetes and Pregnancy Sweet Success Program.[68] However, carbohydrate intake must be enough to avoid "starvation" ketosis (i.e., ketosis resulting from insufficient carbohydrate intake) because maternal ketosis, especially during the third trimester, is associated with a small but statistically significant decrease in the subsequent intelligence quotient of the child measured between 2 and 5 years after birth.[69] Although the principle of adjusting the timing and number of meals to accommodate the life style and physical activity of the patient applies, three daily meals and three snacks during pregnancy seem to be optimal. Distributing the carbohydrate intake throughout the day not only blunts the higher postprandial rise that occurs if the carbohydrate is ingested in only three meals and a bedtime snack, but also prevents hypoglycemia. Because the postprandial rise of glucose is often greater in the morning than during other times of the day, carbohydrate intake is usually restricted at breakfast. One example of the distribution of calories during the day is as follows:

10% of calories at breakfast
20% to 30% of calories at lunch
30% to 40% of calories at supper
30% of calories as snacks

TABLE 11-5	DIETARY ALLOWANCES FOR WOMEN 25 TO 50 YEARS OF AGE		
Constituent	**Nonpregnant**	**Pregnant**	**Increase**
Protein (g)	50	60	10
Average kcal*	2200	2500	300
Vitamin C (mg)	60	70	10
Vitamin B$_6$ (mg)	1.6	2.2	0.6
Folate (μg)	180	400	220
Calcium (mg)	800	1200	400
Magnesium (mg)	280	320	40
Iron (mg)	15	30	15
Zinc (mg)	12	15	3

*Additional calories are needed during the second and third trimesters only.

Adapted from American Diabetes Association: Nutritional management during pregnancy in preexisting diabetes. In Jova-novic-Peterson L (ed): Medical Management of Pregnancy Complicated by Diabetes. American Diabetes Association, Alexandria, VA, 1993, pp. 47-56.

TABLE 11-6	RECOMMENDED DAILY CALORIC INTAKE DURING THE SECOND AND THIRD TRIMESTERS OF PREGNANCY		
Prepregnancy Weight	**Kilocalories/kg/day**	**Kilocalories/pound/day**	
90% to 120% DBW	30	14	
>120% DBW	24	11	
<90% DBW	36–40	16–18	

DBW, desirable body weight.

Adapted from American Diabetes Association: Nutritional management during pregnancy in preexisting diabetes. In Jovanovic-Peterson L (ed): Medical Management of Pregnancy Complicated by Diabetes. American Diabetes Association, Alexandria, VA, 1993, pp. 47-56.

Fat

Decreasing the carbohydrate content of the diet to achieve normoglycemia results in increased fat intake, sometimes to as much as 40%. Whatever the final amount of dietary fat, less than one third should be saturated fat, no more than one third should be polyunsaturated fat, and the remainder should be monounsaturated fat.

Fiber

Soluble fibers form gels that delay the absorption of carbohydrate from the gastrointestinal tract. This tends to blunt the postprandial rise of glucose. Therefore consumption of foods high in soluble fibers, such as fruit, beans, and oat bran, should be encouraged. Insoluble fibers, such as wheat bran, are not digested and thereby increase fecal bulk, which contributes to regularity, also a favorable outcome.

Vitamins and Minerals

The extra requirements of certain vitamins and minerals imposed by pregnancy are summarized in Table 11-5. Additional calcium is necessary for calcification of fetal bones and teeth, especially during the third trimester, when most of the calcium is deposited. If this extra amount is not supplied by the diet, maternal demineralization occurs. Additional iron is needed for the development of erythrocytes, to supply iron to the fetus, and to replace blood loss during delivery. Most of the additional require-

ments are necessary during the second and third trimesters because the conservation of iron stores caused by the cessation of menstruation balances the smaller increased need during the first trimester. The extra 15 mg of iron per day cannot be supplied by the typical American diet, and one daily 30-mg tablet of ferrous sulfate is recommended. The folate requirement during pregnancy more than doubles. Folate supplementation (prenatal vitamins by prescription contain 100 to 400 μg of folate) markedly decreases neural tube defects and the rate of small-for-date neonates. Women eating a well-balanced, nutritious diet need only iron and folate supplementation. A multivitamin-mineral preparation containing vitamins B_6, C, D, folate, and the minerals iron, zinc, copper, and calcium is often given, however, especially to women with inadequate dietary intakes or with special problems.

Exercise

In general, pregnant women with diabetes should be encouraged to be active. Strenuous activity is not advocated, but simple activities such as swimming, walking, and jogging should be encouraged. With the progression of pregnancy, activity should be assessed frequently to prevent hyperglycemia. The same precautions apply for activity, as in the patient with diabetes who is not pregnant. If extremes of glucose levels (i.e., <60 mg/dl or >200 mg/dl) are seen, activity should be avoided. A Medic Alert bracelet should be worn, and of course a source of rapid-acting glucose should be carried at all times, which is especially important when exercising. Exercise is discussed in more detail in the gestational diabetes section.

Insulin and Glucose Monitoring

As stated, the goal in pregnancy is to maintain a BG level as close to normal as possible without causing hypoglycemia. Optimal therapy is as close to physiologic as possible. If the prepregnancy insulin regimen incorporates two or more insulin injections a day, it may be suitable to achieve the near euglycemia necessary for a successful outcome of the pregnancy. Indeed, if appropriate prepregnancy counseling has occurred and near euglycemia had been achieved before conception, the physician and patient will have arrived at an insulin regimen that has the potential of meeting the target levels during the initial stages of pregnancy (Table 11-7). (Note that these BG goals are lower than ones in the nongravid state because they reflect the changes in carbohydrate metabolism that occur during pregnancy, as discussed earlier.) Several caveats should be recognized in choosing an insulin regimen, however. A regimen combining an intermediate-acting basal insulin (such as NPH) with a short-(regular insulin) or rapid-acting (lispro or aspart) premeal insulin is pre-

ferred. When NPH insulin is used as a basal insulin and is given before supper, it has the likelihood of producing overnight hypoglycemia because the dose is increased to control the next morning's fasting value (even though the patient eats a bedtime snack). This happens because the peak action of the intermediate-acting insulin occurs during the middle of the night. Moving the injection of the evening NPH insulin to bedtime shifts the time of peak action toward breakfast and minimizes the possibility of overnight hypoglycemia. Given the duration of action of NPH, it is often given twice a day to achieve 24-hour control of basal insulin rates.

Controlling the morning fasting BG concentration requires adjustments in the evening NPH insulin. During the second and third trimesters, gradual increases in insulin doses are usually necessary (because of the increasing insulin resistance discussed earlier). This necessitates frequent follow up (at least weekly) with analysis of blood glucose levels and insulin dose adjustments. Ultralente insulin and glargine insulin (Lantus) are longer-acting preparations that may be given once a day as basal insulins. Glargine has not yet been approved for use in pregnancy, although recent animal studies have shown that reproductive toxicity (such as increased risk of miscarriage and intrauterine death) is directly related to incidence of hypoglycemia, and not the insulin compound itself when compared with NPH insulin.[70] Long-acting preparations such as

TABLE 11-7	BLOOD GLUCOSE TARGET LEVELS DURING PREGNANCY IN WOMEN WITH PREPREGNANCY DIABETES	
Time	**Target**
Fasting	60–90 mg/dl
1-hr postprandial	100–130 mg/dl
2-hr postprandial	90–120 mg/dl
Preprandial	60–105 mg/dl
0200–0600 AM	70–120 mg/dl

ultralente may be given as a single shot either at bedtime or first thing in the morning. The morning injections may be of greater benefit in reducing nocturnal hypoglycemia.

Regarding premeal rapid-acting insulins, using three injections of short or rapid-acting (lispro or aspart) insulin before each meal gives a patient more flexibility in regard to eating and exercise. For instance, if lunch is delayed, the short- or rapid-acting insulin taken before breakfast will have mostly been expended and preprandial hypoglycemia is unlikely, particularly if the patient is not on a concomitant shot of AM NPH. If a patient had taken NPH insulin before breakfast, it would be starting to work before lunch and the delayed meal might precipitate a hypoglycemic reaction. Conversely, in patients with type 1 diabetes, the rapid-acting insulin may wear off and the patient may become hyperglycemic before supper. Preprandial short- or rapid-acting insulin can be particularly helpful during the first trimester, when nausea and anorexia (morning sickness) are common. The benefit of rapid-acting insulin is its short duration of action. It peaks quickly and usually lasts less than 4 hours. It matches well with carbohydrate absorption and can be given 15 minutes before to 15 minutes after a meal, allowing for increased flexibility of lifestyle. In a study of 33 pregnant patients with diabetes on lispro, and 27 on regular insulin, there were 4 babies born with malformation in the lispro group and 1 in the regular insulin group.[71] Although the authors stated that the risk differences for malformations were not higher in the lispro group, they did note that a case control study was needed to get a precise risk estimate. Other studies have concluded that the use of insulin lispro in pregnant women with type 1 diabetes results in outcomes comparable with other large studies of diabetic pregnancies.[72,73] Although many pregnant patients do well on lispro, at this time the American Diabetes Association recommends that human nonanalogue insulins should be used in pregnancy and states that insulin analogues have not been adequately tested.[74]

Some patients have been treated with continuous subcutaneous insulin infusion (CSII) therapy during pregnancy. Although there are some data to suggest that CSII therapy can be used in pregnancy,[75] patients must be very careful to test frequently and avoid the development of ketoacidosis. Rates of DKA can be higher on insulin pump therapy, because of the lack of a subcutaneous depot of insulin. Therefore pregnant patients on CSII therapy need to be expert at troubleshooting the pump and reacting appropriately (e.g., with infusion set change and insulin injection by syringe) if hyperglycemia develops. In addition to use in patients with type 1 diabetes, CSII therapy may also be safe and effective for maintaining glycemic control in patients with GDM and those with type 2 diabetes.[76]

SMBG eight times a day is considered ideal during pregnancy.[77] This should occur before and between 1 and 2 hours after each meal and before the bedtime snack. It should also be performed in the middle of the night whenever nocturnal hypoglycemia is suspected or during the second and third trimesters when insulin doses are being increased frequently. How to adjust insulin doses based on the results of both preprandial and postprandial SMBG values is not always obvious. This is because the same component of the insulin regimen affects both the postprandial BG level of a meal and the preprandial value of the subsequent one. These two results can sometimes dictate contradictory actions. Table 11-8 lists the combination of possible values and suggested actions in each case. In addition to adjusting doses of insulin, if a patient is taking short-acting insulin, changing the timing of injections before meals can be helpful. This is because regular insulin is usually given ½ hour before a meal because it does not start to work until approximately 30 minutes after injection. The timing of injection is often used in intensive insulin management protocols to help achieve near euglycemia. For instance, if the BG concentration is high before eating, delaying the start of the meal beyond ½ hour allows the short-acting insulin to achieve a lower, more appropriate BG level before starting to eat so that the height of the postprandial rise is attenuated. In this case, the action of the preprandial regular insulin may wane before the next meal. This may be helpful if those values were below target. Alternatively, if the preprandial BG concentration is low, eating immediately after the injection prevents a further lowering and a possible hypoglycemic reaction. Changing the timing in this direction allows more of an effect before the next meal, and this may be helpful if those values were high. In the case of rapid-acting insulin, adjustments of this sort are not as necessary, because the onset is sooner (15 to 20 minutes) and the duration of action is shorter (3 to 4 hours).

Adjusting insulin doses probably is easier than changing the timing between injection and eating. However, if dose adjustments to ameliorate one problem (e.g., too high a postprandial value) cause unacceptable BG levels at another time (e.g., too low a preprandial value before the next meal), changing the timing between injection and eating may be helpful. In instances in which contradictory changes in the dose of insulin would seem indicated (e.g., postprandial values above target levels with preprandial values before the next meal too low or vice versa), changes in the timing of injection relative to eating should be tried (see Table 11-8).

During the first trimester, fluctuations of glucose concentrations often increase. Hypoglycemia may be more common, especially overnight. Insulin requirements commonly decrease at the end of the first trimester. The insulin resistance that characterizes pregnancy becomes apparent by 18 to 24 weeks, and insulin requirements start to increase gradually. As long as the physician realizes that insulin requirements need to be progressively increased, controlling glycemia is usually easier during the final two trimesters. Final doses may be up to twice the prepregnancy requirement. At approximately 36 weeks, placental growth ceases and contrainsulin hormone production plateaus. Thus insulin requirements increase very little and may even decline. At this point in the pregnancy, a decrease in the insulin dose does not necessarily mean that the fetoplacental unit is failing.

If a patient has not been on insulin prior to pregnancy (e.g., a patient with type 2 diabetes managed on oral agents), the amount of starting insulin dose can be estimated. In general, the recommendation for starting doses of insulin in the first trimester is 0.5 U/kg daily. This requirement changes in the second trimester to a higher dose of approximately 0.75 U/kg daily, and 1.0 U/kg daily in the third trimester. The model of two thirds of the daily dose in the morning and one third of the daily dose in the evening is a reasonable guideline to follow. In general, two thirds of this morning dose is given as an intermediate-acting insulin and in the evening, half the dose is given as an intermediate-acting insulin. These are general guidelines and need to be tailored to the patient's lifestyle and glycemic profile and choice of insulin used.

The insulin dose is adjusted if a consistent pattern is observed at the same time (e.g., before lunch) during a 3-day period. If no consistent pattern develops over 3 days, 7 days of results are evaluated. If the majority of values (i.e., at least four of seven at the same time of day) fail to meet the target level, the appropriate adjustment is made. Motivated patients can be taught to self-adjust their own doses, especially using the 3-day rule. The principles of intensively managing diabetes in pregnant women are no different from the ones used in nonpregnant patients.

TABLE 11-8 SUGGESTED RESPONSES TO VARIOUS PATTERNS OF BLOOD GLUCOSE CONCENTRATIONS

TEST	TYPE OF INSULIN			
	Premeal Rapid-Acting	Premeal Short-Acting	Prebreakfast/Prebed Intermediate-Acting Insulin	CSII
Fasting glucose above or below target	No change	No change	Adjust prebed insulin	Adjust basal rate; may require measurement of 3 AM BG
Postbreakfast BG above target	Increase prebreakfast dose	Increase prebreakfast dose and/or increase time interval between injection and ingestion of carbohydrate[a]	No change	Increase prebreakfast bolus dose; if prelunch BG remains high, basal rate may need to be increased
Postbreakfast BG below target	Decrease prebreakfast dose	Decrease prebreakfast dose and/or decrease time interval between injection and ingestion of carbohydrate	No change	Decrease prebreakfast bolus dose; if prelunch BG remains low, basal rate may need to be decreased
Postlunch BG above target	Increase prelunch dose	Increase prelunch dose and/or increase time interval between injection and ingestion of carbohydrate[a]	Increase prebreakfast dose	Increase prelunch bolus dose; if presupper BG remains high, basal rate may need to be increased
Postlunch BG below target	Decrease prelunch dose	Decrease prelunch dose and/or decrease time interval between injection and ingestion of carbohydrate	Decrease prebreakfast dose	Decrease prelunch bolus dose; if predinner BG remains low, basal rate may need to be decreased
Postsupper BG above target	Increase presupper dose	Increase presupper dose and/or increase time interval between injection and ingestion of carbohydrate[a]	No change	Increase presupper bolus dose; if prebed BG remains high, basal rate may need to be increased

Postsupper BG below target	Decrease presupper dose	Decrease presupper dose and/or decrease time interval between injection and ingestion of carbohydrate	No change	Decrease presupper bolus dose; if prebed BG remains low, basal rate may need to be decreased
Overnight hypoglycemia	May need an increase in prebedtime snack	May need decrease in presupper insulin dose and/or increase in prebedtime snack	May need decrease in prebedtime NPH dose and/or increase in prebedtime snack	May need adjustment in nocturnal basal rate(s)

BG, blood glucose; CSII, continuous subcutaneous insulin infusion; NPH.

aChanging the timing of meals and the short-acting insulin dose should be considered if postprandial glucose levels above target but the BG before the next meal falls below target.

In general, hyperglycemia is more of a concern than hypoglycemia during pregnancy, especially for the fetus. Several clinical studies did not establish as association between maternal hypoglycemia and diabetic embryopathy. However, animal studies clearly show a teratogenic effect of hypoglycemia during organogenesis.[78] Whether this translates to clinically significant outcomes in humans is unclear. Regardless, efforts should be made to avoid hypoglycemia during pregnancy for the sake of the mother.

Oral Antidiabetes Drugs

Patients with type 2 diabetes at the time of (unplanned) conception are often taking one or more oral antidiabetic agents. Although some believe that sulfonylurea agents, at least, are associated with increased congenital malformations,[79] others have not found this to be the case.[80-84] Coetzee and Jackson[84] have not noted increased congenital anomalies in pregnant women with type 2 diabetes treated with metformin. Nevertheless, these drugs are not recommended during the first trimester of pregnancy. They should be discontinued during prepregnancy counseling, and insulin should be used. The role of oral agents for the treatment of diabetes in the second and third trimesters is addressed in the section on gestational diabetes.

GESTATIONAL DIABETES

SCREENING AND DIAGNOSIS

The definition of gestational diabetes is glucose intolerance with initial onset or recognition during pregnancy.[85] The initial impetus to test for glucose intolerance during pregnancy was the recognition that women who developed diabetes many years after childbearing had excessive fetal loss and large babies in their prior pregnancies.

The "prediabetes" was then studied prospectively during pregnancy, and O'Sullivan et al.[86] and others[87] found that women in the top 2.5% of BG levels after being given 100 g of oral glucose had increased perinatal mortality and morbidity (often related to fetal islet hyperplasia and macrosomia) compared with women with normal glucose tolerance. The pregnant women with glucose intolerance also had an increased likelihood of developing clinical diabetes during 5 to 15 years of follow-up after pregnancy,[88,89] and thus the potential prediabetic state during pregnancy was termed *GDM*.

Approximately 7% of all pregnancies are complicated by gestational diabetes. Pregnant women at highest risk for glucose intolerance include those with glucosuria (especially in the fasting state), obesity, a family history of diabetes in first-degree relatives, or any prior fetal macrosomia, stillbirth, or diagnosis of GDM. However, it is not sufficient to screen only high-risk women because these factors are not present in 40% to 50% of pregnant women who have glucose intolerance and who do have risks of perinatal morbidity if undiagnosed and untreated.[90] Pregnant women with high-risk factors for GDM should be screened at 12 to 14 weeks' gestation, and if the screening test result is negative, the test should be repeated at 24 to 28 weeks' gestation because insulin resistance induced by placental hormones increases the diagnostic yield in the third trimester. All other pregnant women should be screened routinely at 24 to 28 weeks except those who meet *all* of the following criteria: less than 25 years of age, normal body weight, no first-degree relative with diabetes, not of Hispanic, Native American, Asian American, or African American origin, no history of abnormal glucose tolerance, and no history of poor obstetrical outcome.[74]

To avoid giving a 3-hour oral glucose tolerance test (OGTT) to most pregnant women, O'Sullivan et al.[90] and others[91] suggested a screening test of plasma glucose measured 1 hour after a 50-g glucose load. Even simpler fasting or random glucose measurements lack sensitivity, and assays for glycated hemoglobin are almost always in the normal range. If the screening test is performed in the morning after an overnight fast, a 1-hour plasma glucose value above 140 mg/dl (7.8 mM) is a sensitive threshold, predicting over 90% of women with GDM. If the screening test is performed in the fed state, the screening threshold should be reduced to greater than 130 mg/dl (7.2 mM) to retain adequate sensitivity.[92] If the appropriate screening values exceed these thresholds, then the diagnostic test that should be performed is the 3-hour, 100-g OGTT. However, if the 1-hour screening value is over 200 mg/dl (11.1 mM), the diagnosis of GDM (or type 2 diabetes) is so probable that it is not necessary to perform the full OGTT. In this situation, it is wise to obtain a glycated hemoglobin level to determine whether hyperglycemia has been prolonged and to start treatment promptly.

In North America (in contrast to other areas of the world), the standard diagnostic test for GDM is the 3-hour, 100-g OGTT, studied extensively by O'Sullivan and Mahan[93] and others.[94] The diagnosis of GDM is made if two or more values exceed the set limits (see Table 11-9). O'Sullivan's et al. criteria (two standard deviations above the mean for a large population of pregnant subjects) identified women at risk of stillbirth, fetal macrosomia, and subsequent diabetes.[95,96] Their original criteria were based on measurements of reducing substances in whole blood by the Somogyi-Nelson technique. The National Diabetes Data Group (NDDG) adjusted the values upward by 14% to account for the higher glucose concentration in plasma samples in which glucose-poor red blood cells are excluded.[97] However, they did not consider the effect of the more specific glucokinase or hexokinase assays for glucose measurements in current use. Carpenter and Coustan[91] calculated a conversion of O'Sullivan's criteria based on

hexokinase measurements of glucose in plasma or serum. The validity of these modified criteria was confirmed experimentally by Sacks et al.,[98] who compared both types of measurements in paired whole blood and plasma samples from 995 pregnant women. Thus the modified criteria most accurately reflect the values originally determined by O'Sullivan and Mahan.[93] Support for this view comes from the study by Magee et al.,[99] who compared the effect of using the two different OGTT criteria on predicting fetal hyperinsulinemia, macrosomia, and perinatal morbidities in a large group of pregnant women. In this study, pregnancies with OGTT values above the diagnostic levels of the modified criteria but below the NDDG levels had perinatal morbidity equivalent to that predicted by using the traditional criteria. Kaufmann et al.[100] also found that OGTT values similar to the criteria of Carpenter and Coustan,[91] but lower than the NDDG[97] were more efficient at identifying pregnant women who would develop diabetes observed 7 years after pregnancy. Therefore we believe that the modified 3-hour OGTT criteria (Table 11-9) should be used for the diagnosis of GDM.

METABOLIC AND NONMETABOLIC COMPLICATIONS IN WOMEN WITH GESTATIONAL DIABETES MELLITUS

The nonmetabolic complications are similar to those occurring in women with pregestational diabetes and were discussed earlier. The metabolic complications are also similar, except that DKA is not a problem and hypoglycemia occurs only in those women treated with insulin. Of interest are new data showing a relationship between C-peptide and insulin levels at 24 to 30 weeks, and increased risk for the development of hypertension in later pregnancy.[101] There are also data looking beyond pregnancy, showing that 27% of

TABLE 11-9	DIAGNOSIS OF GESTATIONAL DIABETES MELLITUS USING 3-HOUR 100-G ORAL GLUCOSE TOLERANCE TEST*

Indication: Positive results of screening test (see text for discussion, generally 1-hour value after a 50 g glucose challenge of ≥140 mg/dl [7.8 mmol/L]).

Procedure: After 3 days with carbohydrate intake of at least 150 g per day, in the fasting state, measure fasting serum glucose and give 100 g of glucose by mouth. (Capillary blood should not be used for screening tests unless the precision of the meter is known; it has been correlated with simultaneously obtained venous samples, and has met the federal standards for laboratory testing.) If two or more values exceed the following criteria, diagnose GDM and start treatment. If one value is met or exceeded, the OGTT should be repeated in 4 weeks.

Time of Test	Serum Glucose Concentration (must exceed two or more values for diagnosis)†
Fasting	>95 mg/dl (5.3 mmol/L)
One hour	>180 mg/dl (10 mmol/L)
Two hour	>155 mg/dl (8.6 mmol/L)
Three hour	>140 mg/dl (7.8 mmol/L)

ADA, American Diabetes Association; GDM, gestational diabetes mellitus; GTT, glucose tolerance test; NDDG, National Diabetes Data Group; WHO, World Health Organization.

*Based on recommendations from the Fourth International Workshop Conference on Gestational Diabetes.

†NDDG criteria are somewhat less stringent, with higher cutpoints. The ADA currently recommends these values, with the knowledge that this approach will diagnose more patients with GDM.) A 2-hr 75-g GTT has also been suggested by the ADA and WHO, but has not been as well validated as the 100-g test.

women with a history of gestational diabetes developed the insulin resistance syndrome within 11 years of delivery versus 8% of controls.[102] Although it is already known that gestational diabetes is a predictor for the development of type 2 diabetes, specific predictors are not yet clear. In one study, subanalysis 1 year after pregnancy showed that body mass index (BMI), fasting and postprandial plasma glucose, plasma glucose at each point of OGTT, and plasma insulin levels at 30 minutes OGTT were predictive of the development of type 2 diabetes.[103] In another study, 1636 women with gestational diabetes underwent an OGTT 1 to 4 months after delivery. Diabetes mellitus was diagnosed in 230 women (14%), with the highest independent predictor being highest fasting glucose level during pregnancy.[104] Finally, 315 women with gestational diabetes were given an OGTT 1 year postpartum and were compared with a control group of 153 women without a history of gestational diabetes. The OGTT was abnormal in 31% of women with a history of gestational diabetes compared with 60% in the control group. Maternal age older than 40, high 2-hour OGTT value during pregnancy, and insulin treatment during pregnancy are identified as predictive factors for developing type 2 diabetes.[105] As the literature shows, the actual predictive value of factors evaluated in the subanalysis is still not clear, but what remains important is the increased risk these women with gestational diabetes have of manifesting overt diabetes in the course of their postpartum years, and the metabolic sequelae.

As an interesting aside, a woman's risk of developing gestational diabetes correlates with her own birth weight. The highest risks are U-shaped, and are associated with the low and high ends of birth weight.[106] So the development of gestational diabetes and its subsequent metabolic complications in a woman may actually be related to her own mother's gestational health while pregnant.

Treatment

Diet

Although the nutritional principles discussed earlier for pregestational diabetes apply in general for GDM, more controversy surrounds the dietary approach to the latter. This is probably because these women are often obese, sometimes markedly so, and only if diet alone fails is insulin required. Because insulin therapy represents such a marked change in life style, a more varied approach to diet has been tried to avoid insulin. The areas of controversy include the relative amounts of carbohydrate and fat in the diet, the distribution of calories throughout the day, and the use of calorie-restricted diets for obese patients.

The disagreement about the carbohydrate and fat content in the diet mirrors a similar controversy in the nutritional approach in type 2 diabetes. The higher the carbohydrate content, the greater is the postprandial rise of BG concentrations. This has specifically been demonstrated in GDM.[107] To maintain a 1-hour postprandial BG level less than 140 mg/dl, the percent of carbohydrate in meals needs to be approximately 50% or less. To achieve a 1-hour postprandial BG level lower than 120 mg/dl, the carbohydrate content should be approximately 40% or less. This is especially important at breakfast because of the increased insulin resistance at that time.[107] On the other hand, because fat is more than twice as calorically dense as carbohydrate, to achieve a similar calorie level with a high-fat diet, less food is required. This might lead to less satiety and increased hunger as well as the possibility of starvation ketosis because of the lowered carbohydrate intake. Controlling weight gain in these (often already obese) women with a diet high in fat might also pose a problem. In practice, recommendations concerning the carbohydrate content of the diet in women with GDM have been less than 40%,[108] 40% to 50%,[109] to 55%.[110] Conversely, recommendations for the fat content range from 20% to 40%.

The second controversy concerns the distribution of calories throughout the day.[109] Many advocate three meals and three snacks a day to spread out the carbohydrate intake and lessen postprandial hyperglycemia. Others believe that obese patients with GDM are better served regarding glycemic control and weight gain by ingesting only three meals and a bedtime snack (to limit ketone body production overnight). In obese women with gestational diabetes, snacks are often eliminated to lower BG concentrations.[111] In general, the breakfast meal must be small (approximately 10% of total calories), to prevent morning postprandial BG levels from rising.

The third controversy concerns the safety of calorie restriction in obese patients with GDM. Limiting calories would be helpful in terms of maternal obesity but might be detrimental to fetal development because of impaired nutrient flow across the placenta and/or starvation ketosis. Although a 50% reduction in caloric intake in obese women with GDM resulted in ketonemia and ketonuria, a 33% reduction did not.[112] A clinical study in which calorie intake in women with GDM was 30% less than their prepregnancy diet resulted in a frequency of macrosomia in their infants similar to that of normal women.[113] Furthermore, none of the infants of the mothers with GDM were below the 10th percentile for weight even though the mean maternal weight gain after the 28th week of gestation was less than 4 pounds. A 30% to 33% calorie reduction from their prepregnancy diet in women with a BMI above 30 kg/m^2 appears to be the safest restriction level.

Because no clear-cut evidence favors one particular regimen over another, we have selected the following approach to nutritional therapy for women with GDM. Those whose pregestational weight was 80% to 120% of DBW are prescribed 30 kcal/kg of their present (pregnant) weight. If their pregestational weight had been 120% to 150% of DBW, 24 kcal/kg of present weight is recommended. If their pregestational weight exceeded 150% of DBW, only 12 kcal/kg of present weight is given. Diet composition consists of 35% to 45% carbohydrate, 30% to 40% fat, and the remainder (20% to 25%) protein. The majority of the fat intake should be monounsaturated and polyunsaturated fat. Calories are distributed in three meals and three snacks. The results of postprandial SMBG are used to adjust the foods containing carbohydrate so that insulin therapy can be avoided if possible. Approximately 75% of women with GDM achieve acceptable levels of glycemia with this dietary regimen.[109,114] More liberal intake of carbohydrate results in approximately 50% of patients' requiring insulin.[115] Restriction of carbohydrate to 35% to 46% has been shown to decrease maternal glucose levels and improve postpartum outcome for both mother and baby.[116] As a general guideline, a nonobese woman requires a daily caloric intake of 32 kcal/kg ideal body weight in the first trimester, and this increases to 36 to 38 kcal/kg ideal body weight for the remainder of pregnancy. In the obese woman, 25 kcal/kg ideal body weight is approximately what is needed through the course of pregnancy. In general, pregnant women, regardless of size, should not consume less than 1800 calories per day in the second and third trimester.

Exercise

Several small studies have evaluated exercise in the treatment of women with GDM. Potential drawbacks to exercise in pregnancy include increased uterine contractions, fetal distress, small-for-gestational-age (SGA) infants, and maternal hypertension.[109] Exercise that uses lower body muscles and puts stress on the trunk region does increase uterine contractions, whereas exercises that use either upper extremity muscles or lower extremity muscles while recumbent do not.[117,118] A 6-week exercise program using upper extremity muscles in women

with GDM treated with diet lowered the fasting plasma glucose (FPG) concentration modestly and the plasma glucose concentration markedly 1 hour after a 50-g glucose challenge.[117] In a second study,[118] patients with GDM who had failed diet therapy were randomized either to receive insulin or to enroll in an exercise program that used a recumbent bicycle. The glycemic and clinical outcomes were similar in the two groups, suggesting that appropriate exercise for patients who fail diet therapy may prevent insulin therapy. More recently, it has been shown that light postprandial exercise decreases postprandial BG excursions in women with gestational diabetes. Light exercise in this case was simply an elevation in heart rate of 9 beats per minute over baseline, and no adverse outcomes of such modest activity were observed.[119]

Insulin and Glucose Monitoring

Approximately 20% to 25% of women with gestational diabetes require insulin therapy. The treatment of GDM with insulin requires several decisions. What criteria should be used to add insulin to the dietary regimen? Related to this, what pattern of monitoring should be recommended? If a woman is started on insulin, what should the glycemic goals be? In a normal (nondiabetic) pregnancy, the FPG concentration ranges between 55 and 70 mg/dl, the 1-hour postprandial glucose level is less than 120 mg/dl, and A1C values are less than normal (e.g., an A1C level of 3.8% to 4.5% in an assay in which the normal nonpregnant range is 4.3% to 6.1%).[120] (The A1C level is less than the normal nonpregnant range because not only are glucose concentrations lowered in pregnancy, but red blood cell turnover is increased; see Chapter 9 for reasons why this leads to decreased A1C levels.)

Various criteria have been proposed for the initiation of insulin therapy (Table 11-10). The simplest way to monitor women with GDM is to perform SMBG. If the fasting BG exceeds 90 mg/dl or the 1-hour

TABLE 11-10	AMERICAN DIABETES ASSOCIATION CRITERIA RECOMMENDED FOR THE INITIATION OF INSULIN THERAPY IN WOMEN WITH GESTATIONAL DIABETES	
Fasting*	**1 hr Postprandial**	**2 hr Postprandial**
>95	>140 mg/dl	>120

*Recommendations for starting insulin vary among various experts. Additionally, prior recommendations were based on meters that measured capillary blood glucose; now many meters are calibrated to plasma glucose, which gives a slightly higher reading. It is very important to assess glucose trends—if the fasting and/or postprandial values are generally trending upward above these targets over the course of a week, insulin should be started.

postprandial is greater than 120 mg/dl on multiple occasions within a 2-week interval despite nutritional intervention, we feel insulin therapy should be instituted. The American Diabetes Association recommends institution of insulin therapy if the fasting BG is above 95 mg/dl, 1-hour postprandial BG is above 140 mg/dl, or the 2-hour postprandial BG is above 120 mg/dl.[121] No consensus has been reached regarding the optimal timing of postprandial measurements (1 hour versus 2 hours).

Measuring postprandial rather than preprandial glucose concentrations by SMBG in women who did require insulin resulted in significant decreases in A1C levels, cesarean sections for cephalopelvic disproportion, macrosomia, large-for-gestational-age babies, and neonatal hypoglycemia.[122]

In our view, performing SMBG before breakfast and postprandially maximizes the chance for a successful outcome. If the FPG concentration on the OGTT is 120 mg/dl or above, the patient is started on insulin imme-diately. Others are seen by a dietitian within 3 days and are also taught SMBG to be performed before breakfast and 1 and/or 2 hours after each meal. Insulin is started within 1 to 2 weeks if the majority (i.e., at least four of seven per week) of fasting BG values exceed 90 mg/dl. Similarly, if the majority of postprandial values after a particular meal exceed 120 mg/dl, insulin is started. Either a split/mixed regimen or preprandial short or rapid-acting insulin with evening NPH insulin is appropriate (see Chapter 5), with the decision being left up to the patient after a thorough discussion. See Table 11-11 for recommended timing of insulin doses. Depending on which regimen is selected and which glucose concentration needs to be lowered, the principles outlined earlier in this chapter may be employed. Each regimen should be individually tailored. Also, given the fact that patients with gestational diabetes are likely to be heavier in general than those with type 1 diabetes, insulin requirements may be higher. The patient should contact the physician or

TABLE 11-11	STARTING INSULIN IN GDM
Time BG Elevated	**Insulin to Start**
Fasting	Bedtime NPH insulin
After breakfast	Prebreakfast short-/rapid-acting insulin
After lunch	Prelunch short-/rapid-acting insulin
After dinner	Predinner short-/rapid-acting insulin

BG, blood glucose; GDM, gestational diabetes mellitus; NPH.

program frequently (daily or every other day if possible) during the first week and then once or twice a week subsequently for insulin dose adjustments. The goals of therapy are to keep the glucose concentrations below the levels used to initiate insulin therapy. In contrast to pregnant women with type 1 diabetes, in whom insulin requirements often decrease during the last month of pregnancy, the need for insulin in insulin-requiring women with GDM continually increases.

Oral Agents

Oral glucose-lowering medications are generally not recommended in pregnancy. Studies from Coetzee and Jackson[123] did not reveal any adverse perinatal outcomes when oral agents were used in gestational diabetes. Glyburide does not cross the placenta and was studied by Langer et al.[124] In their randomized unblinded clinical trial, women treated with insulin therapy and women treated with glyburide both had similar outcomes. All patients in this study were beyond the first trimester when these interventions were added to medical nutritional therapy.

In another study, Glueck et al.[125] assessed whether metformin safely reduced development of gestational diabetes in women with PCOS. Among the women receiving metformin at the time of conception, gestational diabetes developed in 1 of 33 (3%) pregnancies. Among women not treated with metformin, 14 of 60 (23%) pregnancies were complicated by gestational diabetes. At this time, the Food and Drug Administration has not approved the use of oral glucose lowering medications in gestational diabetes.

FETAL MONITORING AND TIMING OF DELIVERY

Many decades ago, clinicians recognized a threat of fetal demise late in pregnancies complicated by diabetes.[126] The risk was 50% in the presence of ketoacidosis, 7% to 14% in women with type 1 or type 2 diabetes, and 3% to 6% in women with GDM (versus 1% to 2% in nondiabetic women in that era). Because the risk increased as gestation approached full term, pioneer investigators such as White[49] and Pedersen and Molsted-Pedersen[127] recommended that women with diabetes be delivered at 35 to 37 weeks to prevent stillbirth. Unfortunately, this policy contributed to neonatal morbidity and mortality resulting from hyaline membrane disease (also termed RDS), which was also much more common in near-term infants of diabetic mothers than in control infants. Thus the risk of stillbirth and neonatal death was frightening to patients with type 1 diabetes and daunting to their clinicians.

In the present day, women with well-controlled diabetes and no other pregnancy complications are not at an increased risk for antepartum fetal death.[128] However, poor metabolic control increases neonatal morbidity. This morbidity may be reduced by fetal monitoring in the third trimester.[129]

To prevent unnecessary preterm births in infants of diabetic mothers, investigators developed techniques to estimate fetal well-being and to predict risk of stillbirth, so that only those babies at high risk would be delivered early. The first tests were the measurement of maternal urinary or plasma estriol levels, which usually reflected fetoplacental function, based on fetal adrenal production of an androgen that was sulfated in the fetal liver and converted to estrogen in the placenta. Sensitivity was good but specificity was not, so the biochemical assays were supplanted by biophysical methods to predict acute changes in fetal well-being.[130] Because uterine contractions transiently decrease placental oxygen transfer to the fetus and fetal heart rate (FHR) *decelerations* following the peak of the contractions reflect the degree of fetal hypoxia, a stress test was developed in which contractions were produced by infusion of oxytocin or by maternal nipple stimulation. Fetuses at risk of demise in utero (to be considered for delivery) were those with late decelerations, and the remainder of pregnancies were allowed to continue. Greater diagnostic specificity was attained by assessment of FHR *accelerations* and variability between (or in the absence of) contractions, which reflect a normoxic brain and a nonacidotic fetus. This led to the application of nonstress tests to diabetic pregnant women. Finally, *real-time ultrasonography* was used to measure fetal body and limb movements and chest wall motion ("fetal breathing"), as well as amniotic fluid volume, all of which indicate normal fetal oxygenation. Combined with antepartum FHR monitoring (nonstress tests), this schema of testing became known as the fetal *biophysical profile,* which was shown to be valuable in the management of diabetic and other high-risk pregnancies.[130] Indeed, many medical centers demonstrated that frequent systematic use of these measures of fetal well-being in various combinations, independent of maternal glycemic control, reduced the risk of stillbirth to less than 2% in pregnancies complicated by diabetes.[126]

During the period that fetal monitoring was developed, clinical studies of pregnant diabetic women demonstrated that the risk of fetal distress and stillbirth was clearly associated with the degree of maternal hyperglycemia and that the risk was very low when euglycemia was attained.[126] Experimental studies demonstrated that infusions of glucose into pregnant animals or their fetuses decreased the fetal blood oxygen content and pH, which could explain the association of fetal distress and hyperglycemia. These studies provide the basis for the modern management of diabetes and pregnancy (Table 11-12), in which intensive fetal monitoring and consideration of early delivery are applied to cases with persistent hyperglycemia or other possible maternal causes of fetal hypoxia, such as hypertension, severe stress, uterine vascular lesions, or illicit drug use. On the other hand, uncom-plicated cases with verified euglycemia can be managed as normal pregnancies and allowed to continue to full term.

In cases with persistent maternal hyperglycemia (>20% of postprandial values >130 mg/dl), another possible reason for early delivery is fetal macrosomia. The hypothesis that excessive fetal growth and fat deposition are due to the causal chain of maternal hyperglycemia → fetal hyperglycemia → fetal hyperinsulinemia is amply supported by experimental and clinical studies. Because a macrosomic infant of a diabetic mother is at extra risk for birth trauma because of increased shoulder dimensions, ultrasonography is widely used to estimate fetal weight, with only fair accuracy demonstrated.[126] If the estimated fetal weight is 3800 to 4100 g at 37 to 38 weeks' gestation, it may be best to induce labor, using intravaginal prostaglandins to ripen the cervix as needed. If the estimated fetal weight is above 4200 g and the maternal pelvis is untested for a large baby, it is best to perform a primary cesarean section at 39 weeks' gestation owing to the high risk of shoulder dystocia in these cases.[131]

If maternal hyperglycemia has been present in the third trimester, another possible result of fetal hyperinsulinemia is delay in the production of components of the fetal alveolar surfactant system. This helps to explain the previous high risk of RDS in infants of diabetic mothers delivered before 39 weeks' gestation. The measurement of surfactant in amniotic fluid obtained by amniocentesis is a major advance in the perinatal management of pregnancies complicated by diabetes.[132] A low risk of RDS is predicted by an amniotic fluid lecithin-to-sphingomyelin ratio of greater than 3.4 (supranormal ratio required in diabetes, probably because of low surfactant apoprotein with ratios of 2.2 to 3.4),[133] or positive phosphatidylglycerol content, or a mature fluorescence polarization test result. In cases of verified maternal euglycemia, amniocentesis is not necessary for delivery at 37 to 38 weeks' gestation because the risk of RDS is quite low.

TABLE 11-12	VALUATION DURING PREGNANCY FOR WOMEN WITH TYPE 1 AND TYPE 2 DIABETES		
Time of Gestation	**Low Risk**	**High Risk***	
Baseline	A1C, CBC count, TSH, urine culture, 24-hr urine test for microalbumin and creatine clearance, retinal examination (if retinopathy present, may need more frequent follow-up)	Same plus ECG	
Every 4–12 wk	A1C or fructosamine	A1C Same	
16 wk	Expanded serum α-fetoprotein	Same	
20–22 wk	Targeted fetal US survey for anomalies, including echocardiogram	Same	
25–26 wk		Fetal growth and umbilical Doppler flow by US every 3–4 wk; NST/CST or BPP weekly	
28–32 weeks	Fetal growth by US retinal examination	Retinal examination	
34–36 weeks	NST/CST or BPP weekly		
Before delivery at term	Fetal size by US study, amniocentesis	Same	

BPP, biophysical profile (fetal motion and amniotic fluid volume by US); CBC, complete blood cell; CST, contraction stress test; ECG, electrocardiogram; NST, nonstress test of fetal heart rate pattern; TSH, thyroid-stimulating hormone; US, ultrasound..

*Definition of high-risk categories:

Baseline—women at risk for coronary artery disease or those with microalbuminuria or clinical proteinuria.

25–26 weeks—women with hypertension or nephropathy.

Before delivery at <39 weeks—need for amniocentesis determined by fetal development and maternal status. Necessary in most cases.

The management of labor in diabetic women is based on standard obstetric principles, with an emphasis on prevention of maternal-fetal hyperglycemia or hypoglycemia by intravenous infusions of insulin and dextrose and careful FHR monitoring to detect signs of fetal hypoxia.[134] To decrease the chance of shoulder dystocia and birth trauma in term pregnancies, it is wise not to attempt operative vaginal deliveries in cases of failure of descent in the second stage of labor.

Special postpartum concerns for diabetic women include prevention of plasma glucose excursions of more than 200 mg/dl to decrease the risk of problems with infections or wound healing and recognition that insulin requirements are usually substantially lower after deliver (discussed later). As with women without diabetes, diabetic women are encouraged to breast-feed their babies. The breast milk is normal both in production and content in well-controlled diabetes.

INSULIN TREATMENT DURING DELIVERY

Metabolic studies of nondiabetic pregnant women during labor revealed that glucose turnover increased fourfold with little change in insulin levels.[135] This strongly suggests that muscle contractions (probably both uterine and skeletal) independent of insulin are the predominant determinant of glucose utilization during labor. These data are consistent with the results obtained in pregnant women with type 1 diabetes in labor attached to an artificial endocrine pancreas (Biostator), which delivers appropriate amounts of insulin and glucose to maintain the glucose concentration at a preset level. During active labor, the insulin requirement was zero while glucose requirements were relatively constant at 2.6 mg/kg/min or approximately 10 g/hr in a 60-kg woman.[136]

Based on these considerations, the following approach (modified from that of Jovanovic and Peterson[136]) is suggested for treating an insulin-requiring woman with *pregestational* diabetes as she progresses through labor and delivery. If labor is to be induced, induction should start in the morning. The usual dose of evening NPH insulin is taken, but no morning insulin is given. The goal is to maintain the glucose concentration between 70 and 100 mg/dl. Most labor and delivery units have the ability to measure finger-stick glucose concentrations, and this should be done every hour. If labor is to be induced, intravenous saline is infused until active labor begins unless the initial glucose concentration is less than 70 mg/dl. If this should be the case, 5% dextrose is infused at 100 ml/hr until the glucose level is in the appropriate range. If the initial BG concentration is between 100 and 150 mg/dl, insulin at a rate of 1 U/hr is infused. If the initial glucose concentration is greater than 150 mg/dl, insulin is infused at a rate of 2 U/hr. In case the glucose concentration remains greater than 100 mg/dl 2 hours after starting an insulin infusion, the rate should be increased by 0.5 U/hr. This should be repeated every 2 hours as long as the glucose concentration remains greater than 100 mg/dl. Insulin is discontinued when the glucose concentration decreases to less than 100 mg/dl. When active labor begins, 5% dex-

trose is infused at a rate of 200 ml/hr (or 10% dextrose at 100 ml/hr). If the glucose level falls to less than 60 mg/dl during active labor, the glucose infusion is doubled during the subsequent hour. No insulin is usually required during active labor, but the same insulin infusion rate described earlier is used, depending on the glucose concentration at this time as well. A similar approach should be used for spontaneous labor.

In contrast, a woman with GDM or pregestational type 2 diabetes does not require insulin once labor begins. If labor is to be induced, the usual evening NPH insulin should be taken the night before, but no subcutaneous insulin is given the following morning when induction begins. The same approach described earlier regarding dextrose and insulin infusions can be used if the glucose concentrations are not between 70 and 100 mg/dl until active labor ensues. Women scheduled for an elective cesarean section can be treated as any other insulin-requiring patient undergoing major surgery.

NEONATAL MORBIDITIES

Table 11-13 lists the neonatal morbidities that are possible in both pregestational and gestational diabetes. The pathogenesis of many (but not all) of them are shown in Figure 11-4. Maternal insulin is degraded by the placenta and never reaches the fetus, and under euglycemic conditions, fetal insulin concentrations are low. The β cells typically start to respond to glucose several days after birth. The Pedersen hypothesis[127] holds that maternal hyperglycemia leads to fetal hyperglycemia, which in turn causes fetal β cell hyperplasia and increased insulin secretion. Freinkel[137] later extended this hypothesis to include other maternal substrates reaching the fetus (especially amino acids, which also stimulate fetal insulin secretion) because of inadequate maternal insulin levels. This surfeit of mixed nutrients

TABLE 11-13	NEONATAL COMPLICATIONS
Macrosomia	Polycythemia/hyperviscosity
Hypoglycemia	Hyperbilirubinemia
Respiratory distress syndrome	Cardiomyopathy
Hypocalcemia	Small for gestational age
	Congenital anomalies

in the presence of elevated fetal insulin concentrations is responsible for *macrosomia.* The carryover of fetal hyperinsulinemia after birth and the hyperresponsiveness of the β cells in newborns cause *hypoglycemia.* Hyperinsulinemia decreases hepatic glucose production, increases glucose utilization by the insulin-sensitive (mostly muscle) tissues, and blunts the rise of the rapid-acting counterregulatory hormones, glucagon and catecholamines. Neonatal hypoglycemia, defined as a plasma glucose concentration of less than 40 mg/dl, occurs within the first 4 to 6 hours of life in at least 20% to 25% of infants of poorly treated diabetic mothers.

Fetal hyperinsulinemia is also responsible for RDS by inhibiting the synthesis of various phospholipids that are components of surfactant. This feared neonatal complication is much less common today because of the emphasis on maintaining near euglycemia during pregnancy and the enhanced ability to monitor a fetus accurately to forestall early delivery. Fetal hyperinsulinemia probably also causes neonatal *polycythemia* by stimulating erythropoietin production. This can lead to *hyperviscosity* (red blood cell sludging), which can damage any organ. Finally, fetal hyperinsulinemia may underlie neonatal *cardiomyopathy.*

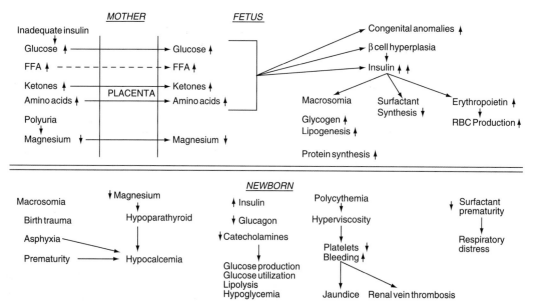

FIGURE 11-4. Proposed mechanisms of the abnormalities in infants of diabetic mothers. (See text for discussion.) FFA, free fatty acid; RBC, red blood cell. *(From Sperling MA: Diabetes mellitus. In Kaplan SA [ed]: Clinical Pediatric Endocrinology. WB Saunders, Philadelphia, 1990, p. 127.)*

Thickened heart muscle is found in many infants of diabetic mothers. Although most of them are asymptomatic, a few may develop congestive heart failure as a result of left ventricular outflow obstruction. Because insulin stimulates the growth of cardiac muscle, it is believed that increased insulin levels late in pregnancy may be responsible for this lesion.

The remaining neonatal complications are not secondary to fetal hyperinsulinemia. *Hypocalcemia* is probably related to the blunted secretion of parathyroid hormone during the first 4 days of life in infants of diabetic mothers compared with infants of nondiabetic mothers. Impaired secretion of parathyroid hormone may be due to neonatal hypomagnesemia that is secondary to maternal hypomagnesemia. This is thought to occur because of urinary magnesium loss associated with maternal hyperglycemia and resultant polyuria. (The renal threshold for glucose is lowered in pregnancy, and therefore even mild hyperglycemia causes a diuresis.) Hyperbilirubinemia may be a result of increased catabolism of red blood cell membranes. Why this should occur is not clear. Bruising of a macrosomic infant at delivery as well as possible bleeding in the hyperviscosity syndrome could also contribute. As discussed earlier, congenital anomalies are two to four times more common in infants of diabetic mothers, especially if hyperglycemia is present during the first 2 months after conception. In vitro studies show that the anomalies are related to the increased availability of fetal fuels (glucose and probably other substrates), the presence of which in vivo is nicely explained by the Pedersen-Freinkel hypothesis. SGA infants of diabetic mothers are much less common today than in the past. If growth retardation occurs early within the first trimester, it is termed *early growth delay,* and some of these fetuses have congenital anomalies.[138] Subsequent growth seems normal. Growth retardation in the third trimester is theorized to be the result of uteroplacental vascular insufficiency, although it also occurs in women whose postprandial glucose concentrations are controlled too tightly.[30,139]

Table 11-14 shows the outcomes of pregnancies in women with type 1 diabetes

TABLE 11-14	OUTCOMES OF PREGNANCY IN WOMEN WITH TYPE 1 DIABETES ACCORDING TO GLYCEMIC CONTROL UPON PRESENTATION TO CLINIC		
Outcome	Fair Control (AIC <7.5%)	Poor Control (AIC ≥7.5%)	P Value
Number of women	110	48	
Mean (SD) age (years)	29 (4.4)	26.2 (6.1)	0.007
Mean (SD) weight at booking (kg)	67.3 (10.3)	68.5 (10.4)	NS
Mean (range) duration of diabetes (years)	12 (1-28)	12.5 (1-32)	NS
Mean (SD) time of booking (weeks)	7.6 (2.4)	8.2 (2.5)	NS
Microvascular complications	13 (12%)	10 (21%)	NS
Pregnancy Outcome			
Spontaneous abortion	4 (4%)	7 (15%)	0.019
Major congenital malformation	1 (1%)	4 (8%)	0.03
Stillbirth	1 (1%)	1 (2%)	NS
Neonatal death	1 (1%)	1 (2%)	NS
Total pregnancy loss	7 (6%)	13 (27%)	<0.0001

NS, not significant; SD, standard deviation.

From Temple R, Aldridge V, Greenwood R et al: Association between outcome of pregnancy and glycaemic control in early pregnancy in type 1 diabetes: Population based study. BMJ 325:1275, 2002.

according to glycemic control. The incidence of spontaneous abortion and major congenital malformations increase with poor glycemic control.

POSTPARTUM

WOMEN WITH PREGESTATIONAL DIABETES

An immediate and profound decrease in insulin requirements follows delivery. One obvious reason is that the insulin-antagonistic hormones produced by the placenta are suddenly removed, reversing the insulin resistance that characterizes pregnancy. This is probably not the entire explanation because the lowered insulin requirement during the immediate postpartum period is far less than the pregestational insulin dose. Some women may not even need insulin for several days. Two explanations have been offered to account for this consistently noted phenomenon. Some of the large amounts of insulin administered during the third trimester became bound to circulating insulin antibodies and are now leaking off to supply free insulin. With the introduction of purified insulins (which include all human insulin preparations), titers of insulin antibodies are extremely low, making this explanation untenable. During pregnancy, the placental production of human chorionic somatomammotropin (which has growth hormone–like actions) suppresses pituitary secretion of growth hormone. After delivery, a lag period intervenes before growth hormone release by the pituitary returns to normal. Growth hormone is a potent insulin antagonist, and patients lacking it (e.g., type 1 diabetic patients after hypophysectomy, an older treatment for proliferative diabetic retinopathy) are extremely sensitive to insulin. This seems more likely than the first explanation, but whether it can account for near euglycemia for several days without any insulin in some women with type 1 diabetes is not certain.

It may be better not to attempt to achieve near euglycemia in the immediate postpartum period because too many factors are changing (e.g., insulin sensitivity, food intake, sleep patterns if the new mother is nursing, and so on). If the delivery was vaginal and the woman can soon eat, the simplest approach is to measure her BG concentration before each meal and at bedtime and return to the prepregnancy insulin regimen. Many patients have an increased sensitivity to insulin in the first 1 to 2 weeks postpartum, so the basal insulin dose should be started at 50% to 75% of the prepregnancy insulin dose and premeal insulin bolus doses should similarly be reduced. As glucose levels begin to rise and the insulin requirements return to prepregnancy needs, the dose of insulin can be adjusted upward. It is important to note that many new mothers wake up frequently in the middle of the night, eat at erratic hours and breast-feed their infants. All of these factors make diabetes more difficult to manage, and it is wise to aim for slightly higher glucose targets than in the preconception and pregnant state to avoid hypoglycemia.

If delivery is by cesarean section and the patient is unable to eat for several days, the management is similar to that described for patients undergoing major surgery. Bear in mind, however, the increased insulin sensitivity in the immediate postpartum period, and select and adjust the insulin doses accordingly.

If a new mother breast-feeds, which should be encouraged because diabetes itself is not a contraindication, she should ingest an additional 500 kcal/day per child.[140] The effect of breast-feeding on insulin requirements is variable, and some patients experience a more erratic pattern of SMBG values and more hypoglycemia. These episodes seem to occur overnight (necessitating periodic measurements of BG concentrations during that period) and an hour or so after breast-feeding. Decreasing the evening dose of intermediate-acting insulin is appropriate for the former, and a snack before breast-feeding prevents the latter.

WOMEN WITH GESTATIONAL DIABETES MELLITUS

Insulin-requiring women with GDM do not need insulin after delivery. The issue for these patients is the increased possibility that they will develop type 2 diabetes in the future. Within 5 to 15 years, approximately half of them do so.[141,142] Pregnancy acts as stress on the pancreatic β cells, via the increased insulin resistance, and those women who cannot respond because of impaired insulin secretion develop GDM.[143] Therefore it is to be expected that these individuals would be susceptible to the subsequent development of type 2 diabetes. Not surprisingly, predictive factors for this outcome include pregestational weight, maternal hyperglycemia, insulin secretion both during and shortly after pregnancy, and the gestational age at which GDM was diagnosed.[141-144] A few Caucasian[145] but not African American[146] women with GDM have a defect in the pancreatic β cell glucokinase gene that codes for an important enzyme involved in insulin secretion (see Chapter 1 for discussion of maturity-onset diabetes of the young). Therefore more than 95% of the diabetes that subsequently develops in women with GDM is the usual type 2 diabetes.

To ascertain their carbohydrate status after pregnancy, women with GDM should have a 75-g OGTT 6 weeks after delivery. They should be fasting, and only two samples need to be drawn, before and 2 hours after the glucose load. The 2-hour glucose concentration identifies a woman as being either normal (<140 mg/dl), having impaired glucose tolerance (140 to 199 mg/dl), or having diabetes (≥200 mg/dl). As stated earlier, the higher this glucose concentration, the more likely type 2 diabetes is to develop in the future. For instance, 80% of Latina women with impaired glucose tolerance 6 weeks after delivery develop type 2 diabetes within 5 years.[142] Women with a history of GDM should be monitored yearly and counseled strongly to achieve DBW. As discussed previously, lean women with a history of GDM developed type 2 diabetes at only half the rate of their obese counterparts.[147]

REFERENCES

1. American Diabetes Association: Preconception care of women with diabetes. Diabetes Care 25(suppl 1):S82, 2002.
2. Spellacy W: Carbohydrate metabolism during treatment with estrogen, progestogen and low dose oral contraceptive preparations on carbohydrate metabolism. Am J Obstet Gynecol 142: 732, 1982.
3. Perlman JA, Russell-Briefel R, Ezzati T et al: Oral glucose tolerance and the potency of contraceptive progestins. J Chron Dis 338:857, 1985.
4. Radberg T, Gustason A, Skryten A et al: Oral contraception in diabetic women: Diabetes control, serum and high density lipoprotein lipids during low dose progestogen, combination oestrogen/progestogen and non-hormonal contraception. Acta Endocrinol 98:246, 1981.
5. Wabi P, Walden C, Knopp R et al: Effect of estrogen/progestin potency on lipid/lipoprotein cholesterol. N Engl J Med 308:862, 1981.
6. Kjos SL: Contraception in diabetic women. Obstet Glynecol Clin North Am 23:243, 1996.
7. Heard MJ, Pierce A, Carson SA, Buster JE: Pregnancies following use of metformin for ovulation induction inpatients with polycystic ovary syndrome. Fertil Steril 77:669, 2002.
8. Hasegawa I, Murakawa H, Suzuki M et al: Effect of troglitazone on endocrine and ovulatory performance in women with insulin resistance related to polycystic ovary syndrome. Fertil Steril 71:323, 1999.
9. American Diabetes Association: Position statement. Preconception care of women with diabetes. Diabetes Care 20 (suppl 1):S40, 1997.
10. Mills JL, Baker L, Goldman AS: Malformations in infants of diabetic mothers occur before the seventh gestational week: Implications for treatment. Diabetes 28:292, 1979.
11. Kitzmiller JL, Gavin LA, Gin GD et al: Preconception care of diabetes. Glycemic control prevents congenital malformations. JAMA 265:731, 1991.
12. Buchanan TA, Coustan DR: Diabetes mellitus. In Burrow GN, Ferris TF (eds): Medical Complications During Pregnancy, 4th ed. WB Saunders, Philadelphia, PA, 1995, pp. 29–61.
13. Dicker D, Feldberg D, Samuel N et al: Spontaneous abortion in patients with insulin-dependent diabetes mellitus: The effect of

preconceptional diabetic control. Am J Obstet Gynecol 158:1161, 1988.

14. Mills JL, Simpson JL, Driscoll SG et al: Incidence of spontaneous abortion among normal women and insulin-dependent diabetic women whose pregnancies were identified within 21 days of conception. N Engl J Med 319:1617, 1988.

15. Key TC, Giuffrida R, Moore TR: Predictive value of early pregnancy glycohemoglobin in the insulin-treated diabetic patient. Am J Obstet Gynecol 16:1096, 1987.

16. Hanson U, Persson B, Thunell S: Relationship between haemoglobin A_{1c} in early type I (insulin-dependent) diabetic pregnancy and the occurrence of spontaneous abortion and fetal malformation in Sweden. Diabetologia 33:100, 1990.

17. Platt MJ, Stanisstreet M, Casson IF et al. St. Vincent's Declaration 10 years on: Outcomes of diabetic pregnancies. Diabet Med 19:216, 2002.

18. Temple R, Aldridge V, Greenwood R et al: Association between outcome of pregnancy and glycaemic control in early pregnancy in type 1 diabetes: Population based study. BMJ 325:1275, 2002.

19. Kitzmiller JL, Buchanan TA, Kjos S et al: Pre-conception care of diabetes, congenital malformations, and spontaneous abortions. Diabetes Care 19:514, 1996.

20. Lowy C: Management of diabetes in pregnancy. Diabetes Metab Rev 9:147, 1993.

21. Goldman JA, Dicker D, Feldber D et al: Pregnancy outcome in patients with insulin-dependent diabetes mellitus with preconceptional diabetic control: A comparative study. Am J Obstet Gynecol 155:293, 1986.

22. Steel JM, Johnstone FD, Hepburn DA et al: Can pregnancy care of diabetic women reduce the risk of abnormal babies? BMJ 301:1070, 1990.

23. Van Assche FA, Holemans K, Aerts L: Long-term consequences for offspring of diabetes during pregnancy. Br Med Bull 60:173, 2001.

24. Padmanabhan R, Shafiullah M: Intrauterine growth retardation in experimental diabetes: Possible role of the placenta. Arch Physiol Biochem 109:260, 2001.

25. Piper JM: Lung maturation in diabetes in pregnancy: If and when to test. Semin Perinatol 26:206, 2002.

26. Moore TR: A comparison of amniotic fluid fetal pulmonary phospholipids in normal and diabetes pregnancy. Am J Obstet Gynecol 186:641, 2002.

27. Carrapato MR, Marcelino F: The infant of the diabetic mother: The critical developmental windows. Early Pregnancy 5:57, 2001.

28. Landon MB, Gabbe SG, Piana R et al: Neonatal morbidity in pregnancy complicated by diabetes mellitus: Predictive value of maternal glycemic profiles. Am J Obstet Gynecol 156:1089, 1987.

29. Jovanovic-Peterson L, Peterson C, Reed GF et al: Maternal postprandial glucose levels and infant birth weight: The diabetes in early pregnancy study. Am J Obstet Gynecol 164:103, 1991.

30. Combs CA, Gunderson E, Kitzmiller JL et al: Relationship of fetal macrosomia to maternal postprandial glucose control during pregnancy. Diabetes Care 15:1251, 1992.

31. Kowalczyk M, Ircha G, Zawodniak-Szalapska M et al: Psychomotor development in the children of mothers with type 1 diabetes mellitus of gestational diabetes mellitus. J Pediatr Endocrinol Metab 15:277, 2002.

32. Moore LL, Bradlee ML, Singer MR et al: Chromosomal anomalies among offspring of women with gestational diabetes. Am J Epidemiol 155:719, 2002.

33. Knowler W, Pettitt DJ, Kunzelman CL, Everhart J: Genetic and environment determinants of non-insulin dependent diabetes mellitus. Diabetes Res Clin Pract Suppl 1:S309, 1985.

34. Martin AO, Simpson JL, Ober C, Freinkel N: Frequency of diabetes mellitus in mothers of probands with gestational diabetes: Possible maternal influence on the predisposition to gestational diabetes. Am J Obstet Gynecol 151:471, 1985.

35. Phenekos C: Influence of fetal body weight on metabolic complications in adult life: Review of the evidence. J Pediatr Endocrinol Metab 15(Suppl 5):1361, 2001.

36. Pettitt DJ, Aleck KA, Baird HR et al: Congenital susceptibility to NIDDM. Role of intrauterine environment. Diabetes 37:622, 1988.

37. Manderson JG, Mullan B, Patterson CC et al: Cardiovascular and metabolic abnormalities in the offspring of diabetic pregnancy. Diabetologia 45:991, 2002.

38. Westbom L, Aberg A, Kallen B: Childhood malignancy and maternal diabetes or other autoimmune disease during pregnancy. Br J Cancer 86:1078, 2002.

39. Phelps RL, Sakol P, Metzger BE et al: Changes in diabetic retinopathy during pregnancy: Correlations with regulation of hyperglycemia. Arch Opthalmol 104:1806, 1986.

40. Klein BEK, Moss SE, Klein R: Effect of pregnancy on progression of diabetic retinopathy. Diabetes Care 13:34, 1990.

41. Oguz H: Diabetic retinopathy in pregnancy: Effects on the natural course. Semin Ophthalmol 14:249, 1999.

42. Massin P, Ben Mehidi A, Paques M, Gaudric A: Management of diabetic complications during pregnancy using diabetic retinopathy as an example. Diabetes Metab 27:S48, 2001.

43. Rossing K, Jacobsen P, Hommel E et al: Pregnancy and progression of diabetic nephropathy. Diabetologia 45:36, 2002.

44. Davison JM: The effect of pregnancy on kidney function in renal allograft recipients. Kidney Int 27:74, 1985.

45. Combs CA, Rosenn B, Kitzmiller JL et al: Early-pregnancy proteinuria in diabetes related to preeclampsia. Obstet Gynecol 82:802, 1993.

46. Sgro MD, Barozzino T, Mirghani HM et al: Pregnancy outcome post renal transplantation. Teratology 65:5, 2002.

47. Reece EA, Coustan DR, Hayslett JP et al: Diabetic nephropathy: Pregnancy performance and fetomaternal outcome. Am J Obstet Gynecol 159:56, 1988.

48. Reece EA, Egan JFX, Coustan DR et al: Coronary artery disease in diabetic pregnancies. Am J Obstet Gynecol 154:150, 1986.

49. Hare JW, White P: Gestational diabetes and the White classification. Diabetes Care 3:394, 1980.

50. Maceold AF, Smith SA, Sonksen PH et al: The problem of autonomic neuropathy in diabetic pregnancy. Diabetic Med 7:80, 1990.

51. Cousins LM: Pregnancy complications among diabetic women: Review 1965–1985. Obstet Gynecol Surv 42:140, 1987.

52. VanOtterlo I, Wladimiroff J, Wallenberg H: Relationship between fetal urine production and amniotic fluid volume in normal pregnancy and pregnancy complicated by diabetes. Br J Obstet Gynaecol 84:205, 1977.

53. Mimouni F, Miodovnik M, Siddiqi TA et al: High spontaneous premature labor rate in insulin-dependent diabetic pregnant women: An association with poor glycemic control and urogenital infection. Obstet Gynecol 175:1988, 1972.

54. Smith BT, Giroud CJP, Robert M et al: Insulin antagonism of cortisol action on lecithin synthesis by cultured fetal lung cells. J Pediatr 87:983, 1975.

55. Snyder JM, Mendelson CR: Insulin inhibits the accumulation of the major lung surfactant apoprotein in human fetal lung explants maintained in vitro. Endocrinology 120:1250, 1987.

56. Carson BS, Phillips AF, Simmons MA et al: Effects of a sustained insulin infusion upon glucose uptake and oxygenation in the ovine fetus. Pediatr Res 14:147, 1980.

57. Cundy T, Slee F, Gamble G, Neale L: Hypertensive disorders of pregnancy in women with type 1 and type 2 diabetes. Diabet Med 19:482, 2002.

58. Ray JG, Vermeulen MJ, Sapiro JL, Kenshole AB: Maternal and neonatal outcomes in pregestational and gestational diabetes mellitus and the influence of maternal obesity and weight gain: The DEPOSIT study. Diabetes Endocrine Pregnancy Outcome Study in Toronto. QJM. 94:347, 2001.

59. Rosenn B, Miodovnik M, Combs CA et al: Poor glycemic control and antepartum obstetric complication in women with insulin-dependent diabetes. Int J Gynaecol Obstet 43:21, 1993.

60. Combs CA, Katz MA, Kitzmiller JL et al: Experimental preeclampsia produced by chronic constriction of the lower aorta: Validation with longitudinal blood pressure measurements in conscious rhesus monkeys. Am J Obstet Gynecol 169:215, 1993.

61. Peterson CM, Jovanovic-Peterson L, Mills JL et al: The Diabetes in Early Pregnancy Study: Changes in cholesterol, triglycerides, body weight and blood pressure. Am J Obstet Gynecol. 166:513, 1992.

62. Lucas MJ, Leveno KJ, Cunningham FG: A comparison of magnesium sulfate with phenytoin for the prevention of eclampsia. N Engl J Med 333:201, 1995.

63. Scardo JA, Hogg BB, Newman RB: Favorable hemodynamic effects of magnesium sulfate in preeclampsia. Am J Obstet Gynecol 173:1249, 1995.

64. Coustan DR, Berkowitz RL, Hobbins JC et al: Tight metabolic control of overt diabetes in pregnancy. Am J Med 68:845, 1980.

65. Cousins L: Obstetric complications. In Reece EA, Coustan DR (eds): Diabetes Mellitus in Pregnancy: Principles and Practice. Churchill Livingstone, New York, 1988, pp. 455–468.

66. Munro JF, Campbell IW, McCuish AC et al: Euglycaemic diabetic ketoacidosis. BMJ 2:578, 1973.

67. Evers IM, ter Braak EW, de Valk HW et al: Risk indicators predictive for severe hypoglycemia during the first trimester of type 1 diabetic pregnancy. Diabetes Care 25:554, 2002.

68. State of California, Department of Health Services, Maternal and Child Health Branch: Sweet Success, California Diabetes and Pregnancy Program Guidelines for Care. State Printing Office, Sacramento, CA, 1992.

69. Rizzo T, Metzger BE, Burns WJ et al: Correlation between antepartum maternal metabolism and intelligence of offspring. N Engl J Med 325:911, 1991.

70. Hofmann T, Horstmann, G, Stammberger I: Evaluation of the reproductive toxicity and embryotoxicity on insulin glargine (Lantus) in rats and rabbits. Int J Toxicol 21:181, 2002.

71. Scherbaum WA, Lankisch MR, Pawlowski B, Somville T: Insulin Lispro in pregnancy—Retrospective analysis of 33 cases and matched controls. Exp Clin Endocrinol Diabetes 110:6, 2002.

72. Masson EA, Patmore JE, Brash PD et al: Pregnancy outcome in type 1 diabetes mellitus treated with insulin lispro (Humalog). Diabet Med 20:46, 2003.

73. Buchbinder A, Miodovnik M, Khoury J, Sibai, BM: Is the use of insulin lispro safe in pregnancy? J Matern Fetal Neonatal Med 11:232, 2002.

74. American Diabetes Association. Gestational diabetes mellitus. Clinical practice recommendations 2003. Diabetes Care Supplement 1:S106, 2003.

75. Lenhard MJ, Reeves GD: Continuous subcutaneous insulin infusion: A comprehensive review of insulin pump therapy. Arch Intern Med 161:2293, 2001.

76. Simmons D, Thompson CF, Conroy C, Scott DJ: Use of insulin pumps in pregnancies complicated by type 2 diabetes and gestational diabetes in a multiethnic community. Diabetes Care 24:2078, 2001.

77. American Diabetes Association: Monitoring. In Jovanovic-Peterson L (ed): Medical Management of Pregnancy Complicated by Diabetes. American Diabetes Association, Alexandria, VA, 1993, pp. 31–38.

78. Ter Braak EW, Evers IM, Willem Erkelens, D, Visser GH: Maternal hypoglycemia during

pregnancy in type 1 diabetes: Maternal and fetal consequences. Diabetes Metab Res Rev 18:96, 2002.

79. Piacquadio K, Hollingsworth DR, Murphy H: Effects of in-utero exposure to oral hypoglycaemic drugs. Lancet 338:866, 1991.

80. Jackson WPU, Campbell GD, Notelovitz M et al: Tolbutamide and chlorpropamide during pregnancy in human diabetes. Diabetes 2(suppl):98, 1962.

81. Dolger H, Bookman JJ, Nechemias C: The diagnostic and therapeutic value of tolbutamide in pregnant diabetes. Diabetes 2(suppl):97, 1962.

82. Douglas CP, Richards R: Use of chlorpropamide in the treatment of diabetes in pregnancy. Diabetes 16:60, 1967.

83. Sutherland HW, Bewsher PD, Cormack JD et al: Effect of moderate dosage of chlorpropamide in pregnancy on fetal outcome. Arch Dis Child 49:283, 1974.

84. Coetzee EJ, Jackson WPU: The management of non-insulin-dependent diabetes during pregnancy. Diabetes Res Clin Pract 1:281, 1986.

85. Metzger BE, Coustan DR (eds): Proceedings of the Fourth International Workshop Conference on Gestational Diabetes Mellitus. Diabetes Care 21(Suppl 2):B1, 1998.

86. O'Sullivan JB, Charles D, Mahan CM et al: Gestational diabetes and perinatal mortality rate. Am J Obstet Gynecol 116:901, 1973.

87. Carrington ER, Reardon HS, Shuman CR: Recognition and management of problems associated with prediabetes during pregnancy. JAMA 166:245, 1958.

88. O'Sullivan JB: Body weight and subsequent diabetes mellitus. JAMA 248:949, 1982.

89. Gregory KD, Kjos SL, Peters RK: Cost of non-insulin-dependent diabetes in women with a history of gestational diabetes: Implications for prevention. Obstet Gynecol 81:782, 1993.

90. O'Sullivan JB, Mahan CM, Charles D et al: Screening criteria for high-risk gestational diabetic patients. Am J Obstet Gynecol 116:895, 1973.

91. Carpenter MW, Coustan DR: Criteria for screening tests for gestational diabetes. Am J Obstet Gynecol 144:768, 1982.

92. Coustan DR, Widness JA, Carpenter MW et al: Should the fifty-gram, one-hour plasma glucose screening test for gestational diabetes be administered in the fasting or fed state? Am J Obstet Gynecol 154:1031, 1986.

93. O'Sullivan JB, Mahan CM: Criteria for the oral glucose tolerance test in pregnancy. Diabetes 13:278, 1964.

94. Mestman JH: Outcome of diabetes screening in pregnancy and perinatal morbidity in infants of mothers with mild impairment in glucose tolerance. Diabetes Care 3:447, 1980.

95. O'Sullivan JB, Gellis SS, Dandrow RV et al: The potential diabetic and her treatment in pregnancy. Obstet Gynecol 27:683, 1966.

96. O'Sullivan JB, Mahan CM, Charles D: Medical treatment of the gestational diabetic. Obstet Gynecol 43:817, 1974.

97. National Diabetes Data Group: Classification and diagnosis of diabetes mellitus and other categories of glucose intolerance. Diabetes 28:1039, 1979.

98. Sacks DA, Abu-Fadil S, Greenspoon JS et al: Do the current standards for glucose tolerance testing in pregnancy represent a valid conversion of O'Sullivan's original criteria? Am J Obstet Gynecol 161:638, 1989.

99. Magee MS, Walden CE, Benedetti TJ et al: Influence of diagnostic criteria on the incidence of gestational diabetes and perinatal morbidity. JAMA 269:609, 1993.

100. Kaufmann RC, Schleyhahn FT, Huffman DG et al: Gestational diabetes diagnostic criteria: Long-term maternal follow-up. Am J Obstet Gynecol 172:621, 1995.

101. Valensise H, Larciprete G, Vasapollo B et al: C-peptide and insulin levels at 24-30 weeks gestation: An increased risk of adverse pregnancy outcomes? Eur J Obstet Glynecol Reprod Biol 103:130, 2002.

102. Verma A, Boney CM, Tucker R, Vohr BR: Insulin resistance syndrome in women with prior history of gestational diabetes mellitus. J Clin Endocrinol Metab 87:3227, 2002.

103. Dalfra MG, Lapolla A, Masin M et al: Antepartum and early postpartum predictors of type 2 diabetes development in women with gestational diabetes mellitus. Diabetes Metab 27:675, 2001.

104. Schaefer-Graf UM, Buchanan TA, Xiang AH et al: Clinical predictors for a high risk for the development of diabetes mellitus in the early puerperium in women with recent gestational diabetes mellitus. Am J Obstet Gynecol 186:751, 2002.

105. Aberg AE, Jonsson EK, Eskilsson I et al: Predictive factors of developing diabetes mellitus in women with gestational diabetes. Acta Obstet Gynecol Scand 81:11, 2002.

106. Innes KE, Byers TE, Marshall JA et al: Association of a woman's own birth weight with subsequent risk for gestational diabetes. JAMA 287(24):3212, 2002.

107. Peterson CM, Jovanovic-Peterson L: Percentage of carbohydrate and glycemic response to breakfast, lunch, and dinner in women with gestational diabetes. Diabetes 40(suppl 2):172, 1991.

108. Jovanovic-Peterson L, Peterson CM: Dietary manipulation as a primary treatment strategy for pregnancies complicated by diabetes. J Am Coll Nutr 9:320, 1990.

109. Gestational diabetes. In Jovanovic-Peterson L (ed): Medical Management of Pregnancy Complicated by Diabetes. American Diabetes Association, Alexandria, VA, 1993, pp. 79–90.

110. Langer O: Gestational diabetes: A contemporary management approach. Endocrinologist 5:180, 1995.

111. Jovanovic-Peterson L, Peterson CM: Dietary manipulation as a primary treatment strategy for

pregnancies complicated by diabetes. J Am Coll Nutr 9:320, 1990.

112. Knopp RH, Magee MS, Raisys V et al: Metabolic effects of hypocaloric diets in management of gestational diabetes. Diabetes 40(suppl 2):165, 1991.

113. Dornhorst A, Nicholls JSD, Probst F et al: Calorie restriction for treatment of gestational diabetes. Diabetes 40(suppl 2):161, 1991.

114. Ramus RM, Kitzmiller JL: Diagnosis and management of gestational diabetes. Diabetes Rev 2:43, 1994.

115. Langer O, Berkus M, Brustman L et al: Rationale for insulin management in gestational diabetes mellitus. Diabetes 40(suppl 2):186, 1991.

116. Major CA, Henry MJ, De Veciana M, Morgan MA: The effects of carbohydrate restriction in patients with diet controlled gestational diabetes. Obstet Gynecol 91:600, 1998.

117. Jovanovic-Peterson L, Peterson CM: Is exercise safe or useful for gestational diabetic women? Diabetes 40(suppl 2):179, 1991.

118. Bung P, Artal R, Khodiguian N et al: Exercise in gestational diabetes: An optional therapeutic approach? Diabetes 40(suppl 2):182, 1991.

119. Garcia Patterson A, Martin E, Ubeda J et al: Evaluation of light exercise in the treatment of gestational diabetes (letters: observations). Diabetes Care 24:2006, 2001.

120. Jovanovic-Peterson L: The diagnosis and management of gestational diabetes mellitus. Clin Diabetes 13:32, 1995.

121. American Diabetes Association: Gestational diabetes mellitus. Diabetes Care 26(suppl 1):S103, 2003.

122. De Veciana M, Major CA, Morgan MA et al: Postprandial versus preprandial blood glucose monitoring in women with gestational diabetes mellitus requiring insulin therapy. N Engl J Med 33:1237, 1995.

123. Coetzee EJ, Jackson WPU: The management of noninsulin dependent diabetes during pregnancy. Diabetes Res Clin Pract 1:281, 1986.

124. Langer L, Conway DL, Berkus MD et al: A comparison of glyburide and insulin in women with gestational diabetes mellitus. N Engl J Med 343:1134, 2000.

125. Glueck CJ, Wang P, Kobayashi S et al: Metformin therapy throughout pregnancy reduces the development of gestational diabetes in women with polycystic ovary syndrome. Fertil Steril 77:520, 2002.

126. Kitzmiller JL: Sweet success with diabetes. The development of insulin therapy and glycemic control for pregnancy. Diabetes Care 16(suppl 3):107, 1993.

127. Pedersen J, Molsted-Pedersen L: Prognosis of the outcome of pregnancies in diabetes. A new classification. Acta Endocrinol 50:70, 1965.

128. Landon MB, Gabbe SG: Antipartum fetal surveillance in gestational diabetes mellitus. Diabetes 34:50, 1985.

129. Bracero LA, Schulman H: Methods of fetal surveillance in pregnancies complicated by

diabetes. In Jovanovic-Petersen L: Controversies in Diabetes and Pregnancy, Endocrinology and Metabolism 2:115, 1988.

130. Landon MB, Gabbe SG: Fetal surveillance and timing of delivery in pregnancy complicated by diabetes mellitus. Obstet Gynecol Clin North Am 23:109, 1996.

131. Langer O, Berkus MD, Huff R et al: Shoulder dystocia: Should the fetus weighing ?4000 grams be delivered by cesarean section? Am J Obstet Gynecol 165:831, 1991.

132. Mueller-Heuach E, Caritis SN, Edelestone DI et al: Lecithin/sphingomyelin ratio in amniotic fluid and its value for the prediction of neonatal respiratory distress syndrome in pregnant diabetic women. Am J Obstet Gynecol 30:28, 1978.

133. Kaytal SL, Amenta JS, Singh G et al: Deficient lung surfactant apoproteins in amniotic fluid with mature phospholipid profile from diabetic pregnancies. Am J Obstet Gynecol 148:48, 1984.

134. Mimouni F, Miodovnik M, Siddiqi TA et al: Glycemic control and prevention of perinatal asphyxia. J Pediatr 113:345, 1988.

135. Maheux PC, Bonin B, Dizazo A et al: Glucose homeostasis during spontaneous labor in normal human pregnancy. J Clin Endocrinol Metab 81:209, 1996.

136. Jovanovic L, Peterson CM: Optimal insulin delivery for the pregnant diabetic patient. Diabetes Care 5(suppl 1):24, 1982.

137. Freinkel N: Of pregnancy and progeny. Diabetes 29:1023, 1980.

138. Pedersen JF, Molsted-Pedersen L: Early fetal growth delay detected by ultrasound marks increased risk of congenital malformation in diabetic pregnancy. BMJ 283:269, 1981.

139. Langer O, Brustman L, Anyaegbunam A et al: Glycemic control in gestational diabetes—How tight is tight enough: Small for gestational age versus large for gestational age? Am J Obstet Gynecol 161:646, 1989.

140. American Diabetes Association: Nutritional management during pregnancy in preexisting diabetes. In Jovanovic-Petersen L (ed): Medical Management of Pregnancy Complicated by Diabetes. American Diabetes Association, Alexandria, VA, 1993, pp. 47–56.

141. Metzger BE, Cho NH, Roston SM et al: Prepregnancy weight and antepartum insulin secretion predict glucose tolerance five years after gestational diabetes mellitus. Diabetes Care 16:1598, 1993.

142. Kjos SL, Peters RK, Xiang A et al: Predicting future diabetes in Latino women with gestational diabetes: Utility of early postpartum glucose tolerance testing. Diabetes 44:586, 1995.

143. Catalano PM, Tyzbir ED, Wolfe RR et al: Carbohydrate metabolism during pregnancy in control subjects and women with gestational diabetes. Am J Physiol 264:E60, 1993.

144. Damm P, Kuhl C, Hornnes P et al: A longitudinal study of plasma insulin and glucagon in women

with previous gestational diabetes. Diabetes Care 18:654, 1995.

145. Stoffel M, Bell KL, Blackburn CL et al: Identification of glucokinase mutations in subjects with gestational diabetes mellitus. Diabetes 42:937, 1993.

146. Chiu KC, Go RCP, Aoki M et al: Glucokinase gene in gestational diabetes mellitus: Population association study and molecular scanning. Diabetologia 37:104, 1994.

147. O'Sullivan JB: Body weight and subsequent diabetes mellitus. JAMA 248:949, 1982.

CHAPTER 12

DIABETES SELF-MANAGEMENT EDUCATION

Diabetes care is a complex balancing act. Its lifelong management requires a partnership between patient and health care professionals. Because individuals with diabetes must assume much of their care, they must be provided the opportunity to have the tools necessary to successfully manage their condition. Diabetes self-management education (DSME) must be an integral component of care for all patients to achieve successful diabetes and health-related outcomes. The purpose of this chapter is to provide information that can be useful to diabetes educators and other health care professionals who care for patients with diabetes.

CHAPTER OBJECTIVES

After reading this chapter, the provider will be able to:

- Explain the goals of DSME.
- Discuss possible impact of the educator's philosophy on self-management education.
- Describe the six components of the teaching/learning process.
- Discuss the 10 key content areas for DSME.

The self-management education strategies discussed in this chapter are divided into two levels—a basic information section labeled "Basic Self-Management Education" and an in-depth information section identified as "Advanced Self-Management Education." The advanced sections may be useful for patients who have mastered basic information, and are interested in and capable of learning more detailed self-management information. More in-depth information for health care professionals can be found in other chapters of this book.

GOALS OF DIABETES SELF-MANAGEMENT EDUCATION

DSME can be defined as an interactive, collaborative, and ongoing process involving the individual with diabetes and the educator. The ultimate goal of DSME is to help the individual with diabetes make the necessary changes in their health management behavior to achieve successful health outcome.

Strategies to help the educator achieve this goal include the following:

1. Providing the individual with diabetes (and their significant others) with the

365

knowledge and skills necessary for successful diabetes self-management with minimum adverse effects of treatment

2. Empowering the individual with diabetes to be an active participant and to make informed decisions regarding his or her health management
3. Helping to prepare the individual with diabetes to assume responsibility for his or her self-care and make important and complex decisions about daily management
4. Assisting the individual with diabetes in developing sound health maintenance behaviors to achieve positive health outcome
5. Supporting the individual with diabetes and families in developing positive coping mechanisms to deal with the psychosocial challenges of diabetes management

EDUCATOR SELF-ASSESSMENT

Each educator has his or her own unique beliefs, values, and experiences that influence the teaching approach. A lack of clarity about differences between the patient and the educator can sometimes impair communication and learning. Following are some examples of areas in which differences in style or approach may hinder the teaching/learning process.

TEACHING PHILOSOPHY

The basis of this chapter is to stress that the underlying approach to teaching needs to be *flexible, practical,* and *realistic.* Dogmatic and rigid approaches to teaching are not appropriate, especially when attempting to teach patients and their families to deal with many details and responsibilities within the context of continually changing life challenges.

Having a detailed, organized approach to diabetes teaching sessions is very helpful, but can be limiting. Although it is very efficient to have prepackaged educational materials to be used in a specific order, a mismatch between the educator's approach and the patient's or family's interest and abilities can seriously hamper the quality of learning. The educator may consider using a mixture of these two approaches to education as appropriate to the patient's situation.

The two major approaches to DMSE are compliance based or empowerment based; the latter approach is currently preferred.

Compliance-Based Philosophy

In this philosophy, the goal is to improve patient adherence to diabetes regimen as defined by the expert health care professionals. DSME means to influence the patient to follow diabetes management recommendations. When providers adopt this philosophy, they tend to be dogmatic, blame the patient, and label them as noncompliant if things do not go as planned.

Empowerment-Based Approach

The goal of the empowerment philosophy is to prepare patients to take responsibility for making important and complex decisions about their daily management. Self-management education aims to prepare patients to make informed decisions about their own care. To facilitate a successful teaching/learning process within this philosophy, the diabetes educator can do the following:

- Facilitate a positive relationship between the patient and the rest of the health care team.
- Foster the patient's active participation in designing the learning process and setting realistic diabetes management goals and modalities.
- Address the patient's concerns and questions at each visit.

- Recognize and promote patient responsibility in self-care.
- Encourage participation by family and significant others in the educational process when possible.
- Set realistic and specific learning objectives and behavior change goals with patient's participation.
- Provide information and teach skills gradually using a stepwise and flexible approach, taking into consideration the patient's specific needs, interest, abilities, preferences, and willingness to learn.
- Present information with simplicity and clarity and periodically check patient understanding.
- Acknowledge and consider other factors that may affect diabetes care and the teaching/learning process such as cultural and religious beliefs, lifestyle issues, and financial concerns.
- Adopt an open and nonjudgmental attitude.
- Make use of community and other support resources such as the internet.

A flexible, practical, and realistic approach to DSME demands balancing a number of different variables and being willing to make compromises between competing demands. A physician may request self-management training on certain topics, but the preteaching assessment of a patient or other factors such as available teaching time or patient's lifestyle may dictate a different plan for self-management training. Certain situations may afford more latitude in allowing a patient to select the order of topics covered, but other situations may present pressing medical concerns that require immediate attention to certain aspects of DSME regardless of a patient's desire.

PERSONAL TEACHING AND LEARNING STYLE

Our own learning style may at times influence the way we teach our patients. For example, if we find detailed written instructions or analogies helpful, we may tend to use the same type of materials in teaching. If we find learning easiest through a particular medium (e.g., visual, auditory, or hands-on instruction), we tend to favor that approach in teaching. We need to be open to adapting our teaching methods to a particular patient's learning ability. As mentioned previously, questioning a patient at frequent intervals throughout the teaching session helps the educator assess comprehension. If problems arise, changes in the teaching approach may improve patients' comprehension.

PERSONAL LIFE STYLE

We each have our own personal approach toward issues such as time management, eating habits, timing of meals, work habits, exercise habits, role of family, and so on. We need to avoid assuming that patients have a similar approach or should have a similar view of life style issues. A classic example in diabetes care is the patient who is started on insulin injections with the assumption that mealtimes and snack times will be at approximately 7 to 8 AM, 12 to 1 PM, 5 to 6 PM, and 9 to 10 PM. Patients may feel unduly forced into completely changing their normal schedule because of feelings of guilt or embarrassment about certain habits such as eating or sleeping late. Another example is a patient who feels strongly that taking care of basic family needs (child care, food preparation, and so on) takes precedence over certain health-related behaviors that the educator views as priorities (e.g., keeping all appointments or buying health care supplies).

A nonjudgmental approach by the educator is crucial in negotiating a treatment plan that is acceptable to all involved. Having an awareness and acceptance of differences in life style approach helps keep communication open.

PERSONAL HEALTH MANAGEMENT PHILOSOPHY

Many health care professionals receive training from the perspective of a methodic, scientific approach to solving health problems. We may have personal experience demonstrating the success of combining knowledge with self-discipline in adapting certain health behaviors in our own lives. We may firmly believe that self-care and independence represent the appropriate approach to managing health issues. We may feel strongly that patients must learn to function independently in terms of health care behaviors such as insulin injections, glucose monitoring, or food planning, but a patient's background may focus on the role of other family members in taking over these tasks. Educators need to learn to avoid promoting their own personal approach to health care without knowing what will work best for a patient.

NATIONAL STANDARDS FOR DIABETES SELF-MANAGEMENT EDUCATION

The national standards for DSME were designed to define criteria for quality DSME that can be implemented in diverse settings to facilitate improvement in diabetes and health care outcomes.[1] The educator is encouraged to use these standards as a guide for developing the self-management education. Meeting these standards and achieving education recognition will not only help to develop a quality education experience for the patients, but also help to obtain reimbursement for DSME. These standards are published yearly in Diabetes Care, Supplement 1, and can be found at the American Diabetes Association (ADA), Web site at *www.diabetes.org*. The details of the structure and process for DSME as well as measurement of outcomes can be found on the ADA website.

TEACHING/LEARNING PROCESS

The teaching/learning process refers to the sequence or flow of the educational experience. This process includes the following:

- Preteaching assessment of the individual's specific educational needs and identification of the individual's specific diabetes self-management goals
- Teaching/learning plan based on needs assessment
- Implementation of self-management education strategies and behavioral intervention directed toward helping the individual achieve identified self-management goals
- Evaluation of individual's knowledge and skills acquisition and attainment of identified self-management goals and behavior change
- Feedback, review, reteaching, and resetting of education strategies and self-management goals as needed
- Documentation

PRETEACHING ASSESSMENT AND IDENTIFICATION OF THE INDIVIDUAL'S SPECIFIC DIABETES SELF-MANAGEMENT GOALS

Each participant and significant other living with diabetes brings with them unique life experiences and preferences that affect the teaching/learning process. Preteaching assessment is an important first step in the teaching/learning process. It entails collecting information about patients' medical, nutritional, psychosocial, and educational history, and health beliefs and readiness to learn. The assessment can be performed through chart review or use of formal written questionnaires. A brief guided conversation at the beginning of the teaching session can also reveal helpful information. In addition, frequent questioning of patients during the course of a session helps the educator to identify previously undiscovered issues and barriers to learning or adherence.

MEDICAL HISTORY

Medical issues most relevant to the diabetes educator include the type and duration of diabetes, current treatment regimen, medications (including adherence to prescribed medications, vitamins, herbal, and complementary medicines used—it is helpful to have patients bring all medications and herbs taken for better assessment), current level of blood glucose control, hypoglycemia and hyperglycemia history (hypoglycemia history for patients already taking oral insulin secretagogues, and/or insulin), concurrent health problems, presence of chronic diabetic complications, and goal and motivation for control. In addition, assessing the current self-care practices helps evaluate the patient's attitude and level of responsibility in diabetes and self-management.

This information may be obtained through chart review, discussion with the referring health care provider, and/or questioning of the patient.

NUTRITIONAL HISTORY

Because nutrition is one of the cornerstones of blood glucose control and is tied to several other issues such as lifestyle, cultural beliefs, and coping style, a thorough nutritional assessment is very important in helping to set learning needs and behavioral change goals needed for optimal diabetes control and health outcome. This assessment includes the following:

- Attitude toward nutrition
- Past dieting history related to diabetes and weight management
- Food preferences
- Knowledge of the impact of food on blood glucose, lipids, and weight
- Composition and timing of meals (this can be accomplished by asking the patient to provide a 2- to 3-day food diary)
- Frequency of eating out and types of restaurant
- Food habits related to stress and cultural and social situations
- Alcohol and caffeine intake

SOCIAL HISTORY

Information about the social situation of patients helps to identify household members, neighbors, or coworkers who may be able to assist with diabetes management or who need to learn such skills as recognition and treatment of hypoglycemia. It is also important to find out the general lifestyle and typical daily schedule of patients, including the times of meals and snacks, work schedule, activity level at work (i.e., sedentary versus physically demanding work), activity level at home (e.g., housework, exercise, shopping), and variations in the daily schedule on days off. Information about unusual schedules (e.g., night shift work) or erratic schedules needs to be communicated to the physician and dietitian so that the diabetes treatment plan can be adapted accordingly. Financial and insurance issues should also be discussed. This information is used in helping patients and families purchase equipment needed for diabetes care, obtain tools for ongoing education (e.g., books, journal subscriptions), and register for health education classes and exercise programs.

CURRENT LEVEL OF KNOWLEDGE

A patient's current level of knowledge and skills in diabetes management can be assessed through use of a pretest, a questionnaire, a brief interview, and/or observation of techniques of any procedures that patients or their families already perform at home. (Relying on observation rather than simple verbal description of technique, especially for glucose monitoring and insulin injection, is critical in evaluating patients' skill level.) Other important knowledge assessment areas include educational background, barriers to learning (cognitive, psychomotor psychosocial), readiness and willingness to learn, and preferred learning style (reading, listening, discussion, or audiovisual mean such as video).

EMOTIONAL/COPING ISSUES, HEALTH BELIEFS, AND READINESS TO LEARN

Asking patients and family members a few broad, open-ended questions can help open dialogue or allow them to admit uncomfortable feelings. Examples of this type of questioning include, "What concerns you most about the diabetes?" Patients who do not believe that they have diabetes or have a mild case or "touch of diabetes" will have difficulty learning and assuming self-care. "How do your family, friends, and coworkers react to the diabetes? Do you feel supported by them?" Negative experience with diabetes and other health problems through family, friends, or social environment may affect a patient's health care and self-care beliefs (belief that control and recommended behaviors can influence health outcome), attitude about learning, and readiness to change behavior. For patients uncomfortable about expressing these types of feelings, an educator may help by giving examples such as, "Diabetes can be really overwhelming (or scary, or depressing, or can make you feel angry). Are you having any of these feelings?"

Engaging in this line of questioning and discussion may be difficult for some educators. They may fear opening up a whole line of dialogue that they are not prepared to handle. Nevertheless, such discussions are an important part of assessing patients' and families' responses to DSME and to identifying potential barriers to successful learning and coping. Some educators may be able to refer patients and families as needed for professional mental health intervention. In other situations, the only opportunity a patient may have to discuss emotions and coping issues may be with a diabetes educator.

CULTURAL AND RELIGIOUS ISSUES

In the broadest sense, the cultural and religious background of a patient (and of a diabetes educator) provides the context in which the patient develops certain values, beliefs, behaviors, attitude, self-care habits, and relationships with family and health care providers. If an educator works with a large population of patients who belong to a unique group (e.g., based on country of origin, language, or religion), these patients may have some common beliefs or behaviors that influence the health-related behaviors. However, caution is advised in assuming that certain beliefs or behaviors apply to all members of a particular group, because this could lead to inappropriate stereotyping of patients. In addition, an educator needs to appreciate that a simple translation of information (e.g., diet information and food choices) into a patient's native language does not necessarily represent a culturally sensitive approach to DSME.

The best method for determining how patients' cultural background is affecting health-related behaviors is simply to ask general questions that allow patients to voice their unique beliefs and behaviors. The general line of questioning mentioned in the previous preteaching assessment sections would contribute to a cultural assessment of patients. An educator should make note of any comments relative to a patient's or family's beliefs about the causes of diabetes and its complications, the effect that diabetes treatments may have on the patient's life, the use of certain foods or herbs for perceived health benefits, the role of certain family members regarding health care decisions and responsibilities, and the importance of certain customs or observances that may influence the diabetes treatment plan.

It is important to remain nonjudgmental when exploring the beliefs of patients and families. Educators' attempts to correct what they believe to be erroneous beliefs can hinder establishment of rapport. Instead, an educator and the diabetes team can use this information when negotiating a treatment plan or when trying to discover why a certain plan of care has not been effective.

GENERAL LEARNING ABILITIES (VISUAL, READING, MOTOR, COMPREHENSION ABILITIES)

An informal assessment of a patient's visual and reading abilities can be performed at the beginning of the teaching session by having the patient read from readily available printed material (e.g., lines from a diabetes information pamphlet, numbers on a syringe, or instructions on a vial of visual strips for glucose testing). Further information on working with a visually impaired patient is presented later.

Fine motor skills and depth perception may be quickly assessed by watching patients insert the insulin needle through the tip of the insulin bottle or apply a control solution or a drop of blood to a strip for blood glucose testing.

Range of motion and other motor abilities required for foot inspection may be assessed by having patients attempt to visualize the bottoms of their feet (with a mirror) and touch all aspects of their feet as if washing or applying lotion.

Comprehension of information (and ability to apply the information) should be assessed at frequent intervals throughout the teaching session. The diabetes team may be quite surprised to discover, for example, that some patients lack understanding of basic mathematic concepts (e.g., addition required for mixing insulins or comparing a blood glucose result with a desired goal range). Other patients may be able to repeat information given but may not be able to apply it to practical situations. Examples of questions and explanations tailored to assessment of patients' comprehension (and adjustment of teaching as needed) are given in several sections of this chapter.

A diabetes educator's assessment of a patient provides important input into formulating the actual plan of care. For example, a patient's medical situation may indicate the need for starting two injections of mixed insulin per day. However, an educator's assessment of the patient may indicate that the regimen prescribed is simply not practical or realistic and that a less intensive insulin regimen be used initially. Challenging the status quo, questioning routine practices, and advocating on behalf of patients with diabetes are important roles for diabetes educators. The 10 content areas recommended by the ADA should be offered by any education program that wants to achieve recognition. However, the content must be tailored to the individual patient needs.

IMPLEMENTATION OF SELF-MANAGEMENT EDUCATION STRATEGIES AND BEHAVIORAL INTERVENTION DIRECTED TOWARD HELPING THE INDIVIDUAL ACHIEVE IDENTIFIED SELF-MANAGEMENT GOALS

Implementation of self-management education strategies and behavioral intervention should be directed toward helping the individual achieve identified self-management goals. The following strategies may assist the educator in promoting learning and behavior change:

- Use culturally appropriate educational materials in the language and at the reading level of the patients and be mindful of cultural learning habits, interaction styles, rules, and preferences.

- Whenever possible include relevant significant others in the educational process and decision-making. If possible, encourage the participation of the entire family in both the dietary modification and exercise program.
- Discuss food significance and preferences and provide appropriate and individualized nutritional counseling, which should include discussion of how to include and/or modify ethnic food in the meal plan and integrate consideration of cultural eating habits. Encourage discussion about cultural norms and preferences regarding weight and diet.
- If unable to speak the patient's language, obtain the assistance of an interpreter.
- Encourage verbalization and open discussion of perceptions of and misconceptions about diabetes and its management.
- Provide information in a stepwise manner, building on knowledge and skills already mastered.
- Promote patients' self confidence by reinforcing their successful experiences in self-management.
- Provide ample opportunity to practice skills.

TEACHING TOOLS

Various teaching tools are available to help patients master new information and skills. Drug companies and diabetes organizations provide a wide selection of teaching materials. Videotapes, samples, and models of equipment are useful supplements to individual or group teaching sessions. Written instructions that reinforce information covered in teaching sessions are helpful for many patients. Some patients prefer comprehensive booklets that cover a wide variety of topics. Other patients may become overwhelmed

with excessive written materials and should be given simple handouts that cover the basic information on topics addressed.

Individualizing the written information as much as possible helps with comprehension and application of skills in the home setting. An educator may want to consider having some patients write down in their own words the steps to be followed.

The Appendix at the end of the chapter provides some resources that educators can use in collecting a wide array of teaching materials. Mixing different materials from different sources may provide the best personalized DSME packet for patients. In addition, educators should encourage patients to pursue ongoing DSME through referral to a specialized DSME center, encourage them to join the ADA and other local diabetes organizations, refer them to diabetes support groups or camps, and encourage them to subscribe to diabetes magazines published for lay people. Patients can also access information on the internet, either at home or at their local library. Because of the possible misinformation on the internet, the educator can encourage patients to go to the ADA Web site or other Web sites listed in appendix, which have links to other reliable diabetes information.

EVALUATION OF INDIVIDUAL'S KNOWLEDGE/SKILLS ACQUISITION AND ATTAINMENT OF IDENTIFIED SELF-MANAGEMENT GOALS AND BEHAVIOR CHANGE

Conventional educational theory suggests that learners may retain only a small percentage of what is taught to them. Retention can be increased by using several teaching modalities, providing ample opportunity for practical application, and allowing learners to guide the teaching session as much as possible. Repetition, reassessment, and evaluation of a patient's knowledge of diabetes information and skills are crucial. This is often not practical, but it must be built into the practice of every diabetes educator as much as possible. Other members of the team dealing with patients with diabetes need to be made aware that simply attending a diabetes teaching class or individual session does not usually translate into immediate changes in behavior or a knowledge base of a patient. Because patients may change only certain aspects of their health behaviors, behavior changes need to be evaluated and goals need to be reinforced at each medical visit. Specific feedback should be given for accomplishments and progress. In addition, constant review and reinforcement of knowledge and skills helps with retention and behavior change.

One theory that has gained attention in the last decade in the area of behavior change is the transtheoretical model, more commonly referred to as the *stage of change model*.[2] This model originally developed at the University of Rhode Island can be very useful in helping the educator develop specific strategies to help patients change their health-related behaviors. In this model, people are believed to go through the following five stages when making permanent health behavior change:

1. **Precontemplation:** The patient reports no intention to change a target behavior within the next 6 months. The patient may be in denial, may not be aware that a change needs to be made, or may not be aware of the potential impact of current behavior on his or her health. In some cases, the patient may have tried to change behavior unsuccessfully in the past, and may lack self-efficacy and self-confidence. In the patient's decisional balance, the negatives outweigh the positives, and the patient may see more barriers than benefits to the change. The educator's intervention should be focused in helping the patient to become aware of the need to change

by providing information and assisting the patient to see the potential benefits of the proposed change.

2. **Contemplation:** The patient is aware of the need to change a specific behavior, and is thinking about making a change in the near future. The pros and cons are almost equal, with the balance slightly toward the negatives. The role of the educator is to emphasize the benefits of the change, and help the patient gain confidence in his or her abilities through establishment of a trusting relationship. It is important at this stage to discuss interpersonal, social or other factors that may be influencing the patient attitude and behavior.

3. **Preparation:** The patient intends to make a change in the target behavior within the next month. Often, some small steps have already been taken. For example, the patient may have obtained a blood glucose monitor in the process toward beginning blood glucose monitoring. The educator can help by reinforcing the change already made and negotiate some specific and achievable behavior change goals such as testing three times a week before and after a meal of patient choice.

4. **Action:** Patients who are in the action stage have implemented the behavior change process in the target area within the last 6 month and are trying to resist temptations. At this stage, the goal of the educator is to stabilize the behavior change. Strategies such as reinforcing the action plan, providing problem solving skills training, and emphasizing the importance of social support can be very helpful.

5. **Maintenance:** Patients in the maintenance stage have maintained the targeted behavior change for at least 6 months and are working at preventing relapse into the previous

behavior. Although patients in this stage are more confident in their capacity to maintain the target behavior, the educator must pay special attention to providing praise and positive reinforcement. Self-reliance can be promoted by discussing preventive planning for challenging situations.

It is important to note that the stage of change is specific to one health-related behavior. The educator must be aware that a patient may be ready to start testing his or her blood glucose levels, but not necessarily to begin an exercise program. Consequently, different behavioral change strategies should be developed for a patient depending on where she or he is in the stage of change.

FEEDBACK/REVIEW/ RETEACHING AND RESETTING OF EDUCATION STRATEGIES AND SELF-MANAGEMENT GOALS AS NEEDED

Because learning is enhanced when patients know how well they are doing, the educator must pay special attention to providing regular and specific feedback to patients. Poor knowledge and skills and lack of outcome achievement can be used as an opportunity to discuss understanding, review skills, and reevaluate appropriateness of teaching approach, treatment goals and/or modalities.

DOCUMENTATION

The educator must develop a mechanism to document the self-management education process. Key components of documentation include the following:

1. Maintenance of an accurate record of patient care
2. Fulfillment of billing requirements
3. Fulfillment of documentation requirements consistent with national standards for recognition

A form such as the one shown in Figure 12-1 may help educators to organize the initial diabetes management information. The form shown in Figure 12-2 may be used to organize and document the teaching/learning and evaluation process.

DIABETES CONTENT SELF-MANAGEMENT EDUCATION CURRICULUM

A written curriculum, with criteria for successful learning outcomes, should be available at any site where diabetes education occurs. A variety of published curriculums exist, which can be purchased through the ADA (among other organizations). The content provided to each individual patient depends on his or her assessed needs. The next portion of this chapter goes through a basic curriculum with advice on how to present it to patients, both at a basic level as well as at a more advanced level. This can be supplemented with reading from other chapters in this book, as well as through other references that are targeted toward diabetes education.

DESCRIBING THE DIABETES DISEASE PROCESS AND TREATMENT OPTIONS

Definition

Diabetes mellitus is a metabolic syndrome characterized by hyperglycemia (elevated blood glucose levels). The two general types of diabetes, type 1 and type 2, differ greatly in their pathophysiology, but both produce hyperglycemia and the complications associated with it. These complications include microvascular, neuropathic, and macrovascular problems. Microvascular complications are abnormalities of small blood vessels that are manifested in diabetic retinopathy (diabetic eye disease) and nephropathy (diabetic kidney disease). The neuropathic complications cause loss of function of both peripheral and autonomic nerves, and the macrovascular (large blood

Social History

Name _____ Age _____ Height/Weight _____

Occupation _____ Lives with _____

Daily schedule (usual meal/work/exercise times) _____

_____

_____

Past diabetes education _____

Medical History

Type of diabetes: Type 1 _____ Type 2 _____ Duration _____

Other illnesses/infections _____

Hyperglycemia symptoms _____

Hypoglycemia symptoms/frequency _____

Medications taken at home _____

Insulin (type/doses/usual times) _____

Insulin sites used _____ Syringe size _____

Frequency of missed or altered dosages _____

Lab glucose /A1C/SMBG results _____

_____

Complications of Diabetes

1. Cardiovascular: MI _____ Angina _____ HTN _____ CHF _____

                 Hyperlipidemia _____ CABG _____

2. Cerebrovascular: CVA _____ TIA _____ Bruits _____

3. Peripheral vascular: Leg pain (on exercising/at rest) _____

                 Ulcer _____ Amputations _____

                 Bypass surgery _____

4. Retinopathy: Yes/no   Vision affected _____ Laser tx _____

5. Other eye problems: Cataracts _____ Glaucoma _____

6. Nephropathy: Protein in urine _____ Dialysis _____ Other _____

7. Neuropathy:

     a. Peripheral: Numbness _____ Tingling _____ Burning sensations _____

     b. Autonomic: Bladder problems _____

                Feeting full after eating small amounts _____

                Nausea after eating _____

                Intermittent diarrhea _____

                Impotence _____

                Orthostatic hypotension (dizzy on rising) _____

FIGURE 12-1. Patient assessment form. CABG, coronary artery bypass graft; CHF, congestive heart failure; CVA, cerebrovascular accident (stroke); HTN, hypertension; MI, myocardial infarction; SMBG, self-monitoring blood glucose; TIA, transient ischemic attack (prestroke); tx, treatment.

vessel) complications include myocardial infarction (heart attack), peripheral vascular disease, and stroke. Hypertension is commonly associated with diabetes, especially with type 2.

The microvascular and neuropathic complications of diabetes occur because of prolonged exposure to hyperglycemia for many years. The Diabetes Control and Complications Trial[3] and the United

Kingdom Diabetes Prospective Diabetes Study,[4] in addition to numerous other studies, proved that maintaining near euglycemia (near normal blood glucose levels) for many years considerably reduces the risk of developing these complications of diabetes. The macrovascular complications are not as clearly linked to the levels of blood glucose control, but controlling blood glucose levels in addition to treat-

ing lipid abnormalities and hypertension and assisting patients in smoking cessation lower the risk of these complications as well.

Diagnosis

Diabetes is diagnosed either in a patient who has symptoms of diabetes (such as polyuria, polydipsia, nocturia, blurring of vision, invol-

Note: Enter code and Initial for each entry		Assessment		Education-*Commants on Back*							
I = **INSTRUCTED** **RA** = **REQUIRES ASSISTANCE** **C** = **COMPETENT**		Initial									
		Date									
	Patient can verbalize/demonstrate:	Yes	No								
General Info	1. Defenition of DM and normal blood sugar values										
	2. Effect of food on blood sugar										
	3. Effect of insulin/oral agents on blood sugar										
	4. Effect of physical activity on blood sugar										
	5. Effect of illness on blood sugar										
Insulin	1. Action of insulin										
	2. Differentiation of types of insulin										
	3. Medication schedule—amounts and times taken										

	4. Correct technique for insulin prep—one type:
	  a. Rotates bottle to mix (cloudy insulin)
	  b. Withdraws proper amount of insulin										

	5. Correct technique for insulin prep—two types:
	  a. Rotates bottle to mix (cloudy) insulin
	  b. Withdraws proper amount of first insulin
	  c. Adds proper amount of second insulin										

	6. Correct technique for insulin administration:
	  a. Cleans site with alcohol
	  b. Pinches skin and inserts needle all the way
	  c. Injects insulin, holding needle steady
	  d. Rotates injection site: abdomen, arm, leg
	    (list site demonstrated)*										

Orals	1. Action of oral medication										
	2. Name of medication and schedule										
Hypoglycemia	1. Definition and causes of hypoglycemia										
	2. Symptoms of hypoglycemia										
	3. Treatment of hypoglycemia/Medic Alert I.D.										

*Focus instruction on rotation of injections within *one* area, preferably the abdomen.

FIGURE 12-2. Diabetes assessment and education record. DM, diabetes mellitus.

Note: Enter code and Initial for each entry	Assessment		Education—*Comments on Back*									
I = INSTRUCTED RA = REQUIRES ASSISTANCE C = COMPETENT	Initial												
	Date												
Patient can verbalize/demonstrate:	Yes	No										
Hyperglycemia 1. Definition and causes of hyperglycemia												
2. Symptoms of hyperglycemia												
3. Illness and "sick day" rules a. Need for taking insulin when ill b. When and how to test urine ketones c. When to call doctor d. Sick day diet												
Monitoring 1. Capillary blood glucose monitoring: a. Loads and operates lancing device b. Obtains large hanging drop of blood c. Places blood on strip properly d. Appropriately removes blood (if applicable) e. Reads visually and records results f. Uses meter correctly to obtain result g. Changes meter code h. Cleans meter i. Compares meter result to lab												
Complications 1. Reasons for foot care												
2. Daily cleansing of feet												
3. Inspection of feel												
4. Do's and don'ts for protection of feet												
5. Reasons for yearly eye examination												
6. Need for yearly urine testing												
7. Role of blood sugar and blood pressure control a. Knows normal glycated hemoglobion b. Knows own glycated hemoglobin c. Knows normal blood pressure d. Knows own blood pressure												
8. Role of control of other cardiac risk factors a. Weight control b. Lipid control c. Exercise												
9. Skin and dental care												
Follow-up 1. Community resources for information and support												

FIGURE 12-2.—CONT'D

untary weight loss, and vaginal infections in women, or more severe manifestations such as diabetic ketoacidosis [DKA]) or in an asymptomatic person. In asymptomatic individuals, diabetes is usually diagnosed by measuring a fasting plasma glucose (FPG) concentration (Table 12-1). If a patient has an FPG concentration 126 mg/dl or higher, or a random blood glucose concentration 200 mg/dl or higher, with symptoms of hyperglycemia, the diagnosis of diabetes is established.

Although not officially recommended, in some patients, hemoglobin A_{1c} (A1C) level is measured to diagnose diabetes. An A1C level is a measure of a patient's overall glucose concentration throughout the preceding 2 to 3

TABLE 12-1	OFFICIAL CRITERIA FOR THE DIAGNOSIS OF DIABETES MELLITUS

1. Symptoms of diabetes plus casual plasma glucose concentrations ≥200 mg/dl (11.1 mmol/L). (Casual = any time of day without regard to time since last meal. The classic symptoms of diabetes include polyuria, polydipsia, and unexplained weight loss.)

or

2. Fasting plasma glucose (FPG) ≥126 mg/dl (7.0 mmol/L). Fasting is defined as no caloric intake for at least 8 hours.

or

3. Two-hour plasma glucose (2hPG) >200 mg/dl during a 75 g oral glucose tolerance test (OGTT).

In the absence of unequivocal hyperglycemia with acute metabolic decompensation, these criteria should be confirmed by repeat testing on a different day.
The third measure (OGTT) is not recommended for routine clinical use.

Adapted from Report of the Expert Committee on the Diagnosis and Classification of Diabetes Mellitus. Diabetes Care, 20:1, 1997.

months. It is the best measure of a patient's diabetic control over time. Although A1C levels correlate poorly with results from oral glucose tolerance tests (OGTTs), if the A1C is 7.0% or more it is likely that the patient has diabetes and particularly indicates that the patient has treatment-requiring diabetes (diet and exercise with or without medication, depending on the clinical circumstances).

Classification

Diabetes mellitus can be divided into several different types. One kind is called *type 1 diabetes*. This type is defined by the presence of serum (blood) ketones in the absence of exogenous insulin. This almost complete lack of effective insulin means that without insulin therapy, these patients usually develop DKA and die. Although most of these patients are children and young adults (i.e., <30 years of age), the older terminology, *juvenile-onset diabetes*, was not entirely accurate because some lean adult and elderly patients can also have ketosis-prone diabetes. Of the 6% of the total population, or approximately 6 million Americans who have diabetes, only 10% or approximately 1 million have type 1 diabetes.

The second kind of diabetes is called *type 2 diabetes*. The important metabolic characteristic of this type of diabetes is the absence of ketosis. Older terms were *adult-onset, maturity-onset,* or *ketosis-resistant diabetes*. The fact that these patients do not develop DKA signifies that they have at least some effective insulin. Of patients with type 2 diabetes, 80% to 90% are obese. *Non–insulin-dependent diabetes* is a confusing designation because approximately 25% of these patients receive insulin. The difference is that they do not need insulin to sustain life as patients with type 1 diabetes do. Obesity and older age are two independent risk factors for this kind of diabetes. It is estimated that the chance of developing type 2 diabetes doubles for every 20% increase over desirable body weight and for each decade after the fourth, regardless of weight. The prevalence of diabetes mellitus in persons age 65 to 74 years is nearly 20%. It is likely that a higher percentage of people in the 9th and 10th decades of life have diabetes mellitus.

A third kind of diabetes is termed *other specific types*. It was formerly called *secondary diabetes* and included (1) diseases of the pancreas that destroyed the β cells (e.g., hemochromatosis, pancreatitis, cystic fibrosis), (2) hormonal syndromes (e.g., acromegaly, Cushing's syndrome, pheochromocytoma) that interfere with insulin secretion and/or inhibit insulin action, (3) disease caused by drugs that may interfere with insulin secretion (e.g., phenytoin [Dilantin]) or that may inhibit insulin action (e.g., glucocorticoids, estrogens), (4) rare conditions involving abnormalities of the insulin receptor, (5) various rare genetic syndromes in which diabetes mellitus inexplicably occurs more frequently than in normal persons, and (6) diabetes in very rare families that inherit an inability to make normal insulin but make an abnormal insulin molecule that is ineffective.

The results of OGTTs that are higher than normal but fail to meet the criteria for diabetes mellitus (see Table 1-2) are classified as *impaired glucose tolerance (IGT)* or *impaired fasting glucose*. Of the population over 65 years of age, 10% to 30% have IGT (in addition to the 15% to 20% with diabetes mellitus). Former terminology included *chemical, latent, subclinical, borderline,* and *asymptomatic diabetes*. When the subjects are retested with an OGTT, even after many years, approximately 30% have reverted to normal, 50% continue to show IGT, and the remaining 20% are diabetic. Progression to overt diabetes in this latter population occurs at 5% to 7% per year. Conversely, patients with type 2 diabetes can revert to IGT (especially obese patients who lose weight). Patients with IGT are unlikely to develop the neuropathic and microvascular complications of diabetes. However, these patients are especially prone to the macrovascular complications: coronary artery disease, peripheral vascular disease, and cerebrovascular disease.

Gestational diabetes is really IGT that occurs in pregnancy (see Chapter 11). Thus patients with diabetes who subsequently become pregnant are not included in this class. In normal pregnancy, hormones that are produced by the placenta interfere with the action of insulin. In 2% to 5% of pregnant women, the increased demands on the pancreatic β-cells to produce more insulin cannot be met and abnormal carbohydrate metabolism develops. Gestational diabetes is associated with increased perinatal risks to the offspring and an increased risk to the mother for progression to type 2 diabetes mellitus within the next 10 to 15 years.

Pathogenesis (Cause)

The onset of type 1 diabetes is associated with a combination of genetic, immunologic, and in some cases viral factors. The genes involved produce certain human leukocyte antigens, whereas the immunologic abnormality involves autoimmunity (i.e., the production of antibodies against one's own tissue). It is believed that patients with a particular genetic predisposition (i.e., type 1) have some sort of environmental stress (e.g., virus, toxin, or other) that causes their immune system to make antibodies against their own insulin-producing cells in the pancreas (the β cells). Once the β cells are destroyed, patients can no longer make insulin and type 1 diabetes develops.

Less is known about the causes of type 2 diabetes, although heredity is a strong influence and both obesity and aging increase the risk of developing it. The factors that are involved in causing hyperglycemia in patients with type 2 diabetes include peripheral insulin resistance (i.e., the inability of insulin to exert its normal effect on the tissues that should respond to it), a relative decrease in the secretion of insulin from the pancreas, and increased glucose production by the liver. A more detailed discussion of the pathogenesis of types 1 and 2 diabetes can be found in Chapter 2.

Basic Self-Management Education

For patients who have limited learning capacity, who are very anxious, or who do not believe that they actually have diabetes, try the following approach:

Having diabetes means that your blood sugar is too high. The normal blood sugar is about 100. Your blood sugar is _____. Having high blood sugar can make you feel tired and thirsty and can give you other problems such as blurry vision, excess urination, and infections, but it's also possible for you to feel fine when your blood sugar is too high. Our biggest concern is that if your blood sugar stays high for a while, it can cause permanent damage to your eyes, kidneys, feet, and sexual function.

Intermediate Self-Management Education

For patients who demonstrate readiness to advance their basic knowledge:

Normal Physiology

It is normal for your blood sugar to go up and down all day long. It usually goes up about 50 points after you eat—even when you eat healthy food. Insulin is a substance that your body is supposed to make to help process the food you eat. Food makes the blood sugar go up. Insulin makes the blood sugar go (back) down.

Diabetes Physiology

When someone has diabetes, it means that something is wrong with their insulin. So when a person with diabetes eats, the blood sugar goes up (that is normal) but it doesn't come back down properly.

In type 1 diabetes, the insulin is missing completely. The body just stops making insulin. This is most common in children and thin young adults. The main treatment for this type of diabetes is to give insulin shots.

In type 2 diabetes, there is still insulin in the body but the body doesn't make enough insulin (or strong enough insulin). This is most common in older adults and in people who are overweight. The treatments for type 2 diabetes are supposed to help the body make more insulin and use it better. The most important treatments for type 2 diabetes are weight loss and exercise. Pills that help the body to make and use its own insulin are started if diet and exercise fail, and insulin shots are added if the pills do not work.

Symptoms of Diabetes

When the blood sugar goes up and stays up, the extra sugar goes into the urine and you urinate more. When your body makes extra urine, you can become very thirsty. Your vision can also become temporarily blurry. The loss of sugar can make you lose weight and feel very hungry, and it can make you very tired (Figure 12-3).

When you are first found to have diabetes, you may feel all of these symptoms, just one or two of the symptoms, or no symptoms at all. It depends how high your blood sugar has been and how long it's been high. If you had very few or no symptoms of diabetes when it was first diagnosed, it does not mean that you just have mild or borderline diabetes. No matter how or when your diabetes was discovered, it is important to learn to control your blood sugar as much as possible even if you feel fine. If the blood sugar level runs too high, it can damage the blood vessels and nerves, causing problems with the eyes, kidneys, legs, and sexual functions.

Questions to Test Knowledge/Stimulate Thoughts

The purpose of this line of questioning is to ascertain a patient's very basic understanding of diabetes and to make sure a patient (especially an asymptomatic patient) is aware that diabetes treatment measures might not seem related to any immediate symptoms or problems but are for prevention of future problems. In addition, it is hoped that questions will encourage patients to express some concerns about which they may feel some embarrassment or anxiety, such as questions about diabetic complications that they may have seen in relatives or acquaintances. Some patients may harbor guilt or may be accused by family members of bringing on the diabetes by eating too much sugar, and the hope is that this discussion will clarify any misconcep-

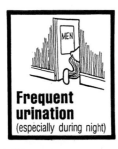

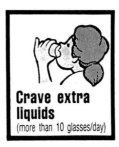

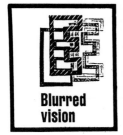

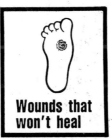

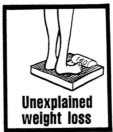

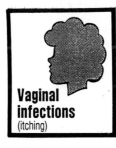

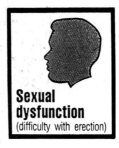

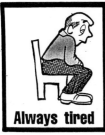

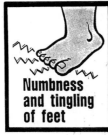

FIGURE 12-3. Symptoms of marked hyperglycemia.

tions regarding the causes and treatment of diabetes.

Does having diabetes mean that your blood sugar level is too high or too low?

What would happen if you ignored the diabetes and decided not to treat it?
Is diabetes caused by eating too much sugar?

What is your biggest fear or concern about having diabetes?
Why does high blood sugar sometimes cause problems like thirst and frequent urination?
If you just stop eating sweets, would that be enough to take care of the diabetes?

Table 12-2 presents some common misconceptions that patients may have about

TABLE 12-2 MISCONCEPTIONS RELATED TO DIABETES OR ITS TREATMENT

Misconception	Educator's Response
Diabetes is caused by eating too much sugar.	Diabetes happens because you have a problem with the insulin in your body, not because you are eating too much sugar.
	For patients with type 1 diabetes or lean patients with type 2 diabetes: The pancreas is the organ in your body that is supposed to make insulin, but the part of your pancreas that's supposed to make the insulin stopped working properly. We're not exactly sure why the pancreas stopped making insulin—it may be a combination of a problem inherited from your family and something that harmed the pancreas, like a virus (for type 1 diabetes). Eating sugar did not harm your pancreas. However, once diabetes develops, eating too much sugar can make your blood sugar level go too high.
	For overweight patients with type 2 diabetes: Diabetes was not caused by eating too much sugar per se, but because you ate too many calories and gained too much weight. Eating foods that contain a lot of fat causes more of a problem with weight gain than eating sugar. In addition to the genes for developing diabetes, being overweight helped cause you to develop diabetes. If you learn to follow a lower-calorie diet, start to exercise, and begin to lose weight, your diabetes will improve.
The only diet change needed in the treatment of diabetes is just to stop eating sugar.	First it's important to know that sugar and desserts are not the only foods that can cause your blood sugar to go up. Many nutritious foods like starch (bread, pasta, corn), fruit, and milk also make your blood sugar rise. You don't need to completely *stop* eating any one type of food—try to have smaller servings of the foods that make blood sugar go up. It also helps your blood sugar stay more balanced if you eat a variety of foods including vegetables and low-fat or no-fat protein foods. If you take medication to treat your diabetes, it is important to try to eat meals or snacks on a regular basis without skipping meals. If you need to lose weight, the most important diet change is to eat less fat. It is acceptable for people with diabetes to eat foods that contain sugar as long as you have been taught how to balance sugar foods with the rest of your diet and your medication.
If I only have to watch my diet or take pills then I just have "mild" or "borderline" diabetes.	The diagnosis of diabetes is based on results of a blood sugar test. No matter what you have to do to treat the diabetes and to control your blood sugar, you still have actual diabetes. People who just have to watch their diet or take pills can have the same problems from diabetes as people who take insulin shots. No matter how you feel or what you have to do to treat your diabetes, it's important to see your medical team regularly so that you can

TABLE 12-2	MISCONCEPTIONS RELATED TO DIABETES OR ITS TREATMENT—Cont'd	
Misconception	**Educator's Response**	
	be tested for any problems with your heart, circulation, feet, kidneys, and eyes. (Sometimes people who do *not* take insulin shots can have more problems with their diabetes because they may think it's not a serious problem and may ignore it for many years).	
Blood sugar levels remain the same throughout the day.	Blood sugar levels normally swing up and down during the day. They are usually the lowest before meals and the highest 1 to 2 hours after eating. The goal of the diabetes treatment plan is to prevent the sugar from going too high or low, not to stop the normal up-and-down swings in sugar. You and/or your doctor should be testing your blood sugar at different times and should do a special blood test in the laboratory (AIC level) to make sure the average amount of sugar in your blood is not too high.	

diabetes and offers some suggested responses. Later in the chapter, common misconceptions and concerns about insulin treatment are addressed.

Treatment Options for Diabetes

Although specific goals may vary from patient to patient, the main goal is to lower blood glucose levels safely to as near normal as possible and to keep blood glucose levels in a desirable range throughout a patient's lifetime. This takes persistent follow-up and reinforcement of the principles of diabetes management. The following are the five components of the management of diabetes:

- Self-management education
- Meal planning
- Exercise and physical activity
- Glucose monitoring
- Medication

Because of the increased risk for long-term complications, effective diabetes management involves more than blood glucose control. Patients with diabetes need to have meticulous control of hypertension and elevated lipid levels because these are conditions commonly found in patients with type 2 diabetes. Other health concerns, such as smoking cessation, compliance with vaccinations, and stress management, should also be emphasized, in addition to the recommendation to take one aspirin a day.

Because diabetes is a progressive disease, treatment needs may change throughout the course of the disease, with changes in a patient's life style and physical status. In addition, advances in therapy resulting from research necessitate periodic updating of the treatment regimen. The diabetes management plan therefore involves frequent assessment and modification by health professionals as well as daily adjustments in therapy by patients themselves. For these reasons, education (including repeated assessment of patients' knowledge and provision of ongoing, in-depth diabetes teaching) is listed as an essential component of treatment for all patients with diabetes.

INCORPORATING APPROPRIATE NUTRITIONAL MANAGEMENT

Regulating food intake is essential to successful management of diabetes. This does not mean that patients must eat the same food every day or must never vary their mealtimes. Rather, patients should be encouraged to learn as much as possible about the nutritional content of the foods they eat and the affect that foods have on their blood glucose levels. Generally, the more that patients know about diet, the more flexible their meal plan can be (see Chapter 3 for more details).

To increase the chances of dietary adherence, individualizing the meal plan and incorporating as many current eating habits as is safe and practical are important. If at all possible, patients should be referred to a nutritionist (preferably a CDE or one who has special knowledge of and interest in diabetes).

Assessment

As part of the overall pre-education assessment, it is useful to obtain at least a general diet history and a report of the range of times of meals, medication, and exercise. Even if patients are to see a nutritionist at a future time, a diabetes educator can give patients some immediate feedback about their current dietary habits that may place them at risk for pronounced hyperglycemia or hypoglycemia. For example, frequent hyperglycemia may occur in patients who avoid sweets but who consume large quantities of juice or fruit or milk with the assumption that these healthy foods do not have a negative impact on blood glucose control. Conversely, patients may be in the habit of skipping certain meals or having a prolonged delay between medication and meals or exercising before (rather than after) a meal, and this practice may put them at risk for hypoglycemia.

When asking a patient about current eating habits, an accepting, nonjudgmental attitude promotes rapport and honesty. An educator can ask patients what they like to eat for breakfast, lunch, dinner, and snacks. If patients seem to be vague or seem to be describing a meal plan that may be what they think the educator wants to hear, it may be useful to obtain a 24-hour recall of food intake.

Reassurance by the educator is helpful—letting patients know that it is human nature to be imperfect and to go off the diet sometimes. This may be a good time to introduce the concept that the current approach to the diabetes diet is not to give patients a standard diet. Rather, the educator wants to help patients make a few adjustments in their current diet. Favorite foods need not be eliminated, but changes in portion size or food combinations or timing of certain food intake may be suggested. Reassure patients that dietary indiscretion that results in elevated blood glucose levels, although not advisable on a regular basis, does not cause immediate onset of long-term complications or hyperglycemic coma.

Basic Self-Management Education

For patients who are beginning oral agents or insulin and who seem overwhelmed with the diabetes treatment plan.

Provide a few general principles:

1. Limit concentrated sweets, juices, milk, and fruit.
2. Encourage patient to eat at least three meals a day, eating something, either a meal or snack, every 4 to 5 hours while awake. Explain that spacing food throughout the day is better to help maintain a healthy weight.
3. If a meal must be delayed, eat a small snack at the usual mealtime. If on a medication that increases insulin levels (some oral medications), do not.
4. Try to eat meals and snacks consisting of a mixture of different types of food (give patients examples):

a. Sandwich with fruit; low-fat cheese and crackers; cottage cheese with crackers or fruit; chicken or fish with rice.

b. Vegetables and starches; convenience foods—list specific meals readily available in your community

c. Limited amounts of sugar, honey, and candy are acceptable (as are products with sugar listed as an ingredient); the patient does not need to eliminate every source of sugar from the diet

5. For patients starting insulin or taking certain types of oral agents that increase insulin secretion (e.g. glyburide [Diabeta, Micronase], glipizide [Glucotrol], repaglinide [Prandin], nateglinide [Starlix], and so on), emphasize the importance of not skipping meals to prevent low blood sugar reactions.

6. Teach patients that it is better to eat a meal or snack that is less than ideal than to skip a meal altogether.

7. For all patients, unless contraindicated, encourage an increase in intake of water and vegetables.

8. For patients who need to lose weight, discuss decreasing portion sizes and overall fat intake. Reassure them that a moderate weight lost of 10 to 20 pounds irrespective of starting weight may have a beneficial effect on their blood glucose levels, blood pressure, and cholesterol levels.

Questions to Stimulate Discussion and Assess Patients' Comprehension

When reviewing the foregoing general guidelines with patients, test patients' comprehension by asking very practical questions. The following are examples:

Based on our discussion today, name three changes that you think you can make in your diet.

What would you like to eat for dinner tonight?

If you get hungry tomorrow between meals, what do you think would be a good snack?

When you go to the store, what types of fluids will you buy?

What do you think would happen if you ate a piece of cake?

Are you worried about the diet?

How do you feel about having to make some changes in the food you eat?

What is the food you fear you will miss the most? (Then try to help patients incorporate their favorite food back into their meal plan.)

Intermediate Self-Management Education

For patients who are able to absorb more than just the very basic information.

Explain to patients that the total amount of calories they need should be distributed between the carbohydrates, fats, and protein, and spread into meals and snacks. Introduce patients to the six different food groups—starch, fruit, milk and protein, vegetable, and fat (Table 12-3). One effective way to organize this information is to explain that the first three groups listed can be called sugar foods (i.e., contain the most carbohydrate) and the last three groups listed are nonsugar foods (i.e., contain less carbohydrate). At this point, the focus is on helping patients identify the groups to which their usual foods belong.

Explain to patients that even healthy foods such as fruit, bread, and nonfat milk cause the blood glucose levels to go up. This can be very confusing or surprising to many patients. Reassure them that they do not need to eliminate these foods, but they may need to eat starch, fruit, and milk in

TABLE 12-3 FOOD GROUPS	
Carbohydrate Food Groups (Will Affect Sugar)	**Non-Carbohydrate Food Groups (Minimum Effect on Sugar)**
Starch	Protein (meat)
Fruit	Vegetables
Milk	Fat
(Nutritive sweeteners, e.g., fructose, corn syrup, fruit juice)	(Nonnutritive sweeteners, e.g. aspartame, saccharin, acesulfame-K)

smaller portions at a time. Have patients identify the foods they ate in the preceding 24 hours that would be considered sugar foods.

If they are on oral agents that increase insulin secretion or fixed amount of insulin, emphasize the importance of concentrating or meal timing and keeping carbohydrates consistent. Explain that consistency will give them better and more stable blood glucose results and lead to better control. Help them problem solve how to be more consistent from meal to meal. If they are on flexible insulin dosage based on blood glucose and carbohydrate levels, explain that they can have more flexibility in the timing of their meals, and will learn how to vary the content of their meals and count carbohydrates. (Carbohydrate counting is discussing in Chapter 3. This is a very important tool for helping patients, especially those with type 1 diabetes, keep their blood glucose levels in the normal range.)

Encourage patients to eat plenty of vegetables and fruits as part of their carbohydrate allowance because they are rich in vitamins, minerals, and fiber. Advise them to eat less processed foods because they contain more fiber.

Introduce patients to the concept that the amount of starch, fruit, and milk that they will be able to consume depends on the degree of blood glucose rise after meals. An increase of up to 50 to 60 mg/dl 2 hours after a meal is considered acceptable. (The exact amount of increase considered acceptable may vary from setting to setting, but the general concept that food normally causes a rise in blood glucose can be universally taught.) Show patients sample blood glucose records with premeal and 2-hour postmeal pairs (Figure 12-4) and help them to identify the meals in which blood glucose increased more than 50 to 60 mg/dl. Have patients identify the foods in that meal responsible for the increase.

Teach patients that even though the nonsugar food such as proteins and fats have minimal impact on blood glucose levels, they need to be limited to avoid problems with cholesterol and heart disease. Explain that saturated fats increase blood cholesterol levels and cause damage to the blood vessels.

Because high blood pressure is more common in people with diabetes, advise patients to use salt in moderation. Suggest ways to cut down on salt such as avoiding foods that are canned, boxed, or frozen with extra salt, trying the "no salt added" varieties, and using herbs, spices, and salt-free seasoning instead of salt mixes for added flavor.

Reassure patients that experimenting with food is essential to help establish a sound meal plan. Patients are sometimes more willing to limit or eliminate certain foods once they have discovered on their own just how much their blood glucose increases after consuming these foods. Encourage them to bring labels from commonly used food and menus from frequently used restaurants to evaluate understanding and help problem-solve unusual situations.

For patients who choose to drink alcohol, advise them to do so in moderation (no

Date	Breakfast Before	Breakfast 2 Hours After	Lunch Before	Lunch 2 Hours After	Dinner Before	Dinner 2 Hours After	Comments
				Blood Glucose Tests			
Monday	135	182					
	2 eggs, 2 sausages, 1 biscuit, coffee						
Tuesday			166	244			
			2 bread, pork, corn, milk				
Wednesday					198	195	
					chicken, stuffing, vegetables		Exercised after dinner
Thursday	149	186					
	½ grapefruit, 1 toast, cheese, coffee						
Friday			139	192			
			tuna sandwich, salad, diet soda				
Saturday					146	271	
					salad, spaghetti, bread, apple		
Sunday	158	280					
	milk, cereal, banana 1 toast, OJ						

FIGURE 12-4. Sample blood glucose record.

more than one drink per day for women and two drinks for men). They should discuss with their physician how to safely include alcoholic beverages in their meal plan. Alcohol can dangerously lower blood glucose levels in patients who take insulin or certain oral diabetes medication and may be contraindicated in people taking certain diabetes oral agents such as metformin (Glucophage). Pregnant women should avoid alcoholic beverages.

Self-Management Education for Previously Diagnosed Patients with Diabetes

1. To establish knowledge level: After taking a 24-hour (or typical daily) food history, ask patients to identify the foods eaten that would cause a rise in the blood glucose levels (a 2-day food history can be very helpful in assessing meals consistency). Ask patients to identify the foods eaten that would increase the body weight or blood glucose and serum lipid levels. If patients are not able to answer these questions appropriately, instruct them as described earlier.

2. To identify behavioral issues: Ask patients to identify their trouble spots in terms of diet. Ask them which part of the diet is most challenging or where they think they have room for improvement. Find out if family, friends, or coworkers help or hinder them when it comes to diet. Negotiate a plan involving a few behaviors that

address patients' trouble spots. For example, if patients consume a high-fat and/or high-sugar snack daily, would they consider a lower-fat, sugar-free alternative and/or reducing the portion size of their usual snack and/or reducing the frequency of the snack to every other day. Working with patients to consider several options may promote behavior change more effectively than telling patients that they must completely eliminate the snack in question.

INCORPORATING PHYSICAL ACTIVITY INTO LIFESTYLE

Exercise is an integral part of diabetes management. In the preinsulin era, exercise was recommended along with carbohydrate restriction to control blood glucose levels. The general increase in the popularity of exercise and conditioning has created an awareness of the importance of exercise in the treatment of diabetes. Regular exercise is beneficial to almost everyone, although contrary to popular misconception, it does not by itself cause weight loss. To lose weight, patients must decrease their caloric intake relative to how many calories they burn each day. The benefits are primarily the same for patients with diabetes, with a few added benefits and some risks. The mechanisms by which exercise influences glucose levels are discussed in Chapter 9.

Benefits of Exercise

1. Results in increased efficiency of the heart and lungs.
2. Results in decreased "bad" cholesterol (low-density lipoprotein [LDL]) and triglyceride levels, which increase the risk for coronary artery disease, and increased "good" cholesterol (high-density lipoprotein [HDL]), which decreases the risk for coronary artery disease.
3. Causes changes in body composition that cause an increase in muscle mass and a decrease in body fat. Increased energy expenditure causes a decrease in weight if there is no compensatory increase in caloric intake.
4. Causes decreased blood glucose levels during and after exercise. (However, the effect on overall glucose control may be only slight if not combined with weight loss.)
5. Causes increased sensitivity of muscle and fat tissue to insulin.
6. Results in improved self-image and stress management.

General Guidelines

1. *Consult a physician* to determine whether a patient has any medical problems that are a contraindication to certain forms of exercise. These include heart disease, poor diabetic control, proliferative diabetic retinopathy, untreated hypertension, or hypoglycemia unawareness. A heart stress test (treadmill test) may be required for evaluating cardiac function.
2. *Select an appropriate exercise program.* An appropriate exercise program is one that patients will adhere to and that conforms to their life style. Some patients may be best suited to an individual exercise program; others may prefer group activities. For many, walking is the most convenient, safest, and most economic form of exercise. It is also a good starting point for the initiation of a more rigorous exercise program. If patients have no special exercise limitations, they should contact community facilities such as the YMCA/YWCA and senior citizen centers. Some hospitals offer low-impact aerobic classes, and some cardiac rehabilitation programs have excellent exercise facilities. Also, of course, private health clubs abound in most of the country and can be joined for a fee.
3. *Follow a specific exercise plan.* Regardless of the form of exercise, the exercise session should start with a warm-up period,

which is followed by the main intense (aerobic) exercise activity, and ends with a cool-down phase. A 5- to 10-minute warm-up is used to stretch the muscles that will be used in the exercise session (e.g., leg muscles for jogging or tennis; arm and shoulder muscles for swimming). This reduces the risk of tendon and muscle injury. The main activity should consist of 20 to 30 minutes of aerobic exercise. (Brisk walking, jogging, bicycling, and swimming all are forms of aerobic exercise.) This is defined as exercise that requires the use of extra oxygen to meet the energy demands of the muscles. Less intense exercise (such as golf, strolling) is called *anaerobic,* and the energy demands are met without the utilization of extra oxygen. Aerobic exercise is the form associated with cardiovascular fitness, increased sensitivity to insulin, and improved health. It is important to incorporate a cool-down period, which should begin 2 to 3 minutes after the exercise is completed and should last for approximately 5 minutes. It consists of gently stretching the muscle groups used during the aerobic activity.

4. *Encourage commitment to the exercise program.* To achieve health benefits, the aerobic activity must be performed a minimum of five times a week, for a continuous 20 to 30 minutes at each session.

SPECIAL CONSIDERATIONS AND RISK FACTORS FOR EXERCISE

FOOT PROBLEMS

Patients who have peripheral neuropathy may not be candidates for high-impact weight-bearing exercises such as jogging and high-impact aerobics. These may increase the risk of trauma to patients with insensitive feet. Swimming or cycling may be the best exercise.

PROLIFERATIVE RETINOPATHY

Patients with proliferative retinopathy should be evaluated on an individual basis. Some vigorous exercises can increase the blood pressure and put added stress on already weakened vessels in the retina, causing hemorrhage. In general, if recent photocoagulation procedures (laser) have been carried out, exercise may be contraindicated for several weeks. Exercise at any time that involves forceful holding of the breath (e.g., weightlifting) as well as jarring exercises (e.g., high-impact aerobics) may be contraindicated. Patients with proliferative retinopathy should check with their ophthalmologist for specific recommendations.

HYPERGLYCEMIA

Exercising when the blood glucose level is >250 to 300 mg/dl may lead to further increases in the blood glucose level. It may also lead to ketonuria in patients with type 1 diabetes (see the exercise section in Chapter 9).

HYPOGLYCEMIA

For insulin-treated patients, hypoglycemia is a potential problem and *specific measures* should be taken to prevent hypoglycemia. Hypoglycemia may occur when unusual exercise is performed without adjustment in food intake or insulin dosage. This occurs primarily because of increased absorption of the injected insulin. To help prevent the development of hypoglycemia, the following suggestions should be followed:

1. Exercise after meals (45 to 60 minutes after the meal), when the meal carbohydrate has been absorbed into the bloodstream and glucose levels are higher.
2. Carry concentrated glucose preparations during exercise (e.g.,

glucose tablets or gels) to consume if symptoms of hypoglycemia develop.

3. For prolonged and high-intensity exercise, a snack food (e.g., fruit, fruit juice, skim milk, bread products) should be consumed just before and/or at intervals during the exercise to help prevent hypoglycemia.

4. Wear identification (Medical Alert bracelet or necklace) and exercise with someone else when possible.

5. Perform blood glucose monitoring before and after exercise to evaluate the blood glucose response to exercise and to check for impending hypoglycemia.

6. Be aware of the phenomenon of postexercise late-onset hypoglycemia. This hypoglycemia occurs 6 to 15 hours after strenuous and prolonged activity and therefore may happen in the evening or overnight. If this proves to be a problem, a reduction in insulin doses that peak at these times may be required. Increased frequency of blood glucose monitoring and food intake after exercise may also be indicated.

7. Exercise should be avoided at the time of the peak action of insulin unless food is also eaten just before exercise (e.g., if regular insulin is given before breakfast, do not exercise just before lunch).

8. Insulin should not be injected into the primary exercising part of the body (e.g., if jogging, do not use the leg for injection, especially for regular insulin). Injections given in the abdomen may not be as affected by exercise as injections given in other sites.

9. Insulin doses should not be omitted, but the dose may need to be decreased or food intake increased (see Chapter 3).

MONITORING BLOOD GLUCOSE AND URINE KETONES

MEASUREMENTS OF GLYCEMIC CONTROL

Monitoring diabetes control means evaluating the therapeutic response to the treatment plan. In most illnesses, a physician monitors the results of the treatment and a patient is the passive consumer. In marked contrast, patients with diabetes must assume responsibility for management and control of their disease, and methods and tools such as self-monitoring of blood glucose (SMBG) or testing urine samples are required. Table 12-4 lists the ADA recommendations for treatment goals for patients with diabetes.

Two basic methods for assessing diabetic control exist, both short-term tests (including SMBG, urine glucose testing, and blood glucose measurement in the laboratory) and longer-term tests (such as A1C or fructosamine levels). The short-term tests, especially SMBG, are performed by patients in their own environment and can be used by patients (particularly patients taking insulin) to make immediate adjustments in insulin or diet. The longer-term tests are generally used by diabetes health care professionals (and the results shared with patients) to assess patients' progress and determine whether or not changes in the overall treatment plan need to be undertaken.

SELF-MONITORING OF BLOOD GLUCOSE

SMBG is one of the most significant developments in diabetes management since the discovery of insulin. It has allowed much greater interaction and teamwork between patients and health care providers in blood glucose management. For patients taking insulin, SMBG results are used to adjust

TABLE 12-4	BIOCHEMICAL INDICES OF GLYCEMIC CONTROL	
Biochemical Index	**Normal**	**Goal**
Fasting/preprandial glucose	<115 mg/dl (<6.4 mmole)	<120 mg/dl (<6.7 mmole)
Bedtime glucose	<120 mg/dl (<6.7 mmole)	100-140 mg/dl (<5.6-7.8 mmole)
AIC level*	<6%	<7%

*Referenced to a nondiabetic range of 4%-6% (mean 5%, standard deviation 0.5%).

American Diabetes Association: Management of Non-Insulin-Dependent (Type II) Diabetes, 3rd ed. American Diabetes Association, Alexandria, VA, 1994.

insulin doses, and for patients with a sophisticated understanding of diabetes control, SMBG can help patients maintain a more flexible life style and diet without severely compromising glucose control.

For all patients with diabetes (including those who do not use insulin), SMBG is a valuable tool in teaching the glycemic effects of various foods as well as increasing patients' involvement in overall evaluation of the diabetes treatment plan. In addition, SMBG has become a vital part of detecting and treating acute diabetic complications of hypoglycemia and hyperglycemia. This is especially important during times of diet or medication changes such as during illness, during the perioperative period, during fasting (e.g., for outpatient procedures), or after medication changes (e.g., changes in diabetic medication or drugs such as glucocorticoids that alter blood glucose levels).

Description

The two main categories of glucose-monitoring meters currently available are meters using reflectance technology, and those using sensor technology. In both meter types, patients must obtain a drop of blood and apply it to the reagent pad on a strip or on the sensor pad of a test strip. A result is obtained after the blood has remained on the strip for a certain time.

Reflectance Meters

With the reflectance meter, the strip is inserted over an electronic sensor area in the meter. After application of the blood sample, the glucose in the blood reacts with an enzyme on the test strip, causing a color change. The meter shines a light on the test strip through the sensor area to measure the color change and give a numeric readout based on the amount of light reflected back on the sensor (light reflectance). The darker the color change on the test strip, the less light reflected back, indicating a higher glucose level in the sample.

Meter with Sensor Technology

In a meter with sensor technology, the test strip usually has an electrode-type connector at the end that should be inserted, and most of the strip is outside the meter. The reaction between the glucose from the blood sample and on the enzyme in the test strip generate an electrical charge. That charge is measured by the meter and converted into a numeric readout of the blood glucose level. These types of meters usually require a smaller sample size, and give a faster reading than the reflectance meters.

Because patients and health care providers rely on the blood glucose monitoring values to make treatment decision, accuracy of the meters is critical for successful patient management. With appropriate education, regular evaluation of technique, and regular laboratory assessment (e.g., glucose concentration measured simultaneously with the SMBG test), most methods of SMBG can yield clinically useful results.

Choosing a Glucose-Monitoring Technique

Assisting patients in selecting a glucose-monitoring technique is a very important aspect of DSME. It is easiest for a diabetes educator to have a simple choice of only one or two systems from which patients may select. This may indeed be the situation if institutional or insurance controls are imposed on the equipment patients may receive. However, to promote long-term commitment to glucose monitoring, it is important for patients to have as much choice as possible so that their goals and characteristics can be matched with the various glucose-monitoring systems. Diabetes educators can be of most help when they have personal experience using various techniques and have evaluated the results by testing the meters in the laboratory or at least have collected data from other patients who have checked meters against laboratory values.

In terms of selecting a monitor, the following variables may be considered: accuracy, size, cost, memory, ease of use, coding, cleaning, computer compatibility, language capability, and company support. (For a detailed description of different monitoring systems, see the current year's ADA (e.g. "Resource Guide 2003." Diabetes Forecast (Suppl) 56: Jan 2003))

Accuracy

Most of the monitors have the capability of giving results that are within 15% of a matching laboratory test, provided the following guidelines are observed:

- The general technique for using the monitor is accurate.

- Strips are current and have been stored properly (inside the vial or foil wrapping) at appropriate temperatures.
- The meter is calibrated to the correct lot number of strips.
- The meter is clean (this mainly applies to reflectance-type meters).
- Sufficient blood was applied.
- The patient was fasting and the fingerstick blood glucose sample was taken minutes before or after the laboratory test.
- The finger was clean and dry before puncture.

Consideration must be made regarding plasma referenced meters versus whole blood reference meters. Meters who read whole blood may yield glucose values that are 11% to 15% lower than the laboratory value and the value of other meters that report plasma values. Educators may receive information from various companies claiming improved accuracy of one system over another. It is best if educators can formulate their own opinions through personal experience with different systems. Most importantly, explain to patients that all systems are capable of producing accurate results and all systems are capable of producing erroneous results. Explain to patients that it is important to check their monitor and technique on a regular basis and that the best system is the one that they are most willing to use most often based on other characteristics. Inform patients on the types of meter they have and the possible difference in results if they used two meters that report plasma or whole blood results. Because most meters are calibrated to report as plasma values, the ADA has revised the suggested blood glucose premeal target results from 80 to 120 mg/dl (4.4 to 6.7 mmol/L) to 90 to 130 mg/dl (5.0 to 7.2 mmol/L).

Advantages and Disadvantages

The main advantage of SMBG is that it gives immediate feedback. Patients who are educated can make a decision in terms of insulin, diet, and/or exercise that immediately affects the glucose results. This, in turn, may give patients more of a sense of control over their diabetes and may allow them to adapt the diabetes treatment plan to their life style rather than vice versa.

Providing regular results to a physician allows more frequent adjustments of the medication and can thus improve symptoms and diabetic control more effectively, especially in an outpatient setting.

For less sophisticated patients, SMBG may promote greater awareness and acceptance of the diagnosis of diabetes, recognition of the impact of certain behaviors (eating, drinking, skipping medication), and more of a sense of personal responsibility. Diabetes can become less a condition for the doctor to manage and more of an issue calling for self-ownership.

The main disadvantages of SMBG are cost, discomfort, and inconvenience (e.g., having to interrupt one's usual activities to do it). In addition, some patients experience a feeling of frustration at seeing high blood glucose results when they expected lower readings based on adherence to the diabetes treatment plan or based on a sense of physical well-being. As some patients state, "The good thing about blood testing is that I know what my sugar is, and the bad thing about glucose testing is that I know what my sugar is. It can ruin my mood if I think I have a 'good' sugar and then I discover that my reading is high."

Self-Management Education

Introducing Patients to Self-Monitoring of Blood Glucose

To help patients feel comfortable with their decision to learn SMBG, it is important to illustrate how the information will be used. Adults are more inclined to try it if they believe that the information is relevant to them on an immediate basis. Show patients sample blood glucose records that illustrate the effects of food, exercise, and/or med-

ication on blood glucose (see Figure 12-4). Introducing SMBG in conjunction with diet education is very useful. If patients want to find out how much of a certain food they can consume, show them records of pre-meal and 2-hour postmeal SMBG. Supply examples from other patients in whom variations in glucose results directly correlated with changes in carbohydrate consumption. For patients starting insulin treatment, show a sample record illustrating gradual dose changes based on SMBG results.

For most patients, teaching all aspects of SMBG in one session is not advisable. If at all possible, educators should plan to meet with patients more than once, focusing first on obtaining a large drop of blood and on basic meter use. Then follow up with instruction on meter maintenance, calibration, and alarms.

If it is not possible to meet with patients a second time, it is still advisable to limit the information presented at one time, placing emphasis on drop size and on the importance of periodic meter checks in the laboratory. Patients can become overwhelmed with information on control solution and meter cleaning at the first session and may be disinclined to use the meter, assuming it is too confusing. All meters have a toll-free information line that patients can use to review questions.

Instruction in Self-Monitoring of Blood Glucose

Many patients have minimal difficulty learning basic meter functioning, especially with the newer, nonwipe meters. Each meter comes with its own set of instructions, which may include written guidelines and (sometimes) videotape instructions. However, regardless of the simplicity of the basic technique, hands-on instruction on obtaining the drop of blood is important in promoting accurate blood testing. (This type of instruction is often not provided at local pharmacies where patients may purchase glucose meters.)

Tips for Obtaining a Large Drop of Blood. With the newer meters, a large drop of blood may not be needed. However, if a patient has trouble obtaining enough blood for a reading, the following may help:

1. Demonstrate how the drop typically clings to the finger and does not immediately fall so that they can continue to massage the finger as needed with the drop pointing toward the strip before applying it to the strip.
2. To promote greater blood flow, patients may be taught to wash and massage hands under warm water (finger must be dry for adequate drop size), shake the hand and hold it down at the side before performing the finger stick.
3. To increase drop size in patients who do not bleed easily, instruct patients to perform the finger stick and then immediately relax the arm and let the hand rest at the side for a few seconds without applying any pressure. Patients can wiggle their fingers while their hand hangs down to promote blood flow. After 5 to 10 seconds, teach patients to position the hand parallel to the table with the puncture site facing downward and begin to apply pressure at the base of the finger (near the knuckle). Hold the pressure firmly and steadily for about 5 seconds. Then reposition the hand so that pressure is now applied to the middle of the finger—again with steady pressure for about 5 seconds. Advise patients that there may appear to be no results at all from this technique. The blood is moving toward the tip, and when pressure is finally applied at the tip of the finger, a larger drop forms.
4. Encourage patients to try different surfaces of different fingers.
5. Encourage patients to try different finger-lancing devices and lancets.
6. Teach patients that most finger-stick devices come with different tips or gauges that allow for shallower or deeper puncture if needed.

Teaching Meter Maintenance and Calibration

Each monitoring system has a unique set of instructions for cleaning the meter, testing the meter with a check strip, and testing the strips and technique with glucose control (sugar-water) solutions. Some of the non-wipe meters require no special cleaning at all because the blood is applied on the end of a strip that has no direct contact with the meter. Other meters have a fairly simple cleaning routine that involves removing the part of the meter that holds the strip. Patients may mistakenly think that cleaning simply involves tidying up the outer surfaces of the meter and may be totally unaware that some meter parts are removable.

Many of the meters have an alarm indicating when the meter needs to be cleaned. In general, it is advisable to teach patients to clean the meter on a regular basis (according to the manufacturer's recommendations) rather than to wait for dust, lint, or blood to accumulate to such a degree that the alarm is triggered.

Most meters have a check strip or device that is included with the purchase of the meter. Patients need to use this regularly (e.g., once a week or as recommended by the manufacturer) to make sure that the meter gives an appropriate reading when the checking device is inserted. In addition, all meter purchases include glucose solutions, called *control solutions*, which can be used to check the accuracy of the strips, meter, and technique. Patients perform a test with the meter with the usual technique, substituting the glucose solution for blood. Provided on the container, strips, or control solution is a range of glucose values within which the control solution test results should fall. If results are out of range, the educator should check for meter cleanliness, appropriate technique, and expiration date of the strips and control solution. Manufacturers provide a toll-free number for assistance in case problems with the meter have no obvious explanation.

Although usually done less frequently than a test using control solution, the most important and reliable test for meter accuracy is a meter comparison of a blood test result from the meter with a laboratory result obtained at the same time.

The manuals that are supplied with each meter contain a list of possible alarms that should be reviewed (e.g., for very high or very low values), but it is also important to explain that poor technique can sometimes bypass the alarms and give inaccurate results. Again, periodic (every 6 to 12 months) comparisons of the meter with laboratory results are important.

Working with a Veteran User of SMBG/Evaluating Accuracy

The three main approaches to evaluating meter accuracy are (1) observation of patients' technique, (2) meter check (comparison with laboratory testing of glucose), and (3) A1C level.

Observation of Patients' Technique

1. Check the equipment for cleanliness—especially accumulation of dust, cotton, tissue fibers, or blood in the area where the strip is placed and read by the meter.
2. Ask patients when they last cleaned the meter and watch their meter-cleaning technique.
3. Check that the meter is programmed for the code number on the current batch of strips.
4. Check the low-battery alarm.
5. Check the expiration date of the strips and make sure the strips are securely stored in the vial or foil. Any exposure to

light or air renders most strips inaccurate (falsely low readings result).
6. Question patients about any extremes of temperature to which the strips or meter was exposed (e.g., leaving the equipment in a car on a hot day).
7. Check meter and strip accuracy with the check strip and control solutions. Expected ranges are provided with all meter equipment.
8. Observe the patients performing a test—pay close attention to drop size and placement (did the patient smear or mash the drop onto the strip?).

Meter Check. Have the patient bring the meter and strips to the laboratory to perform a finger stick (fasting blood glucose is recommended by most manufacturers) within a few minutes of a venipuncture for plasma glucose determination. Results should be within 15% of each other for whole-blood–referenced meters and closer for plasma-referenced meters. (Note: It is possible for the check strip and control solution to be within the manufacturer's recommended range while meter comparison with laboratory results is >15%.) The laboratory meter check is the single most reliable test of meter and technique accuracy and should be performed when problems are reported by patients or meter inaccuracy is suspected.

A1C Level: The A1C test is described in more detail later. It reflects overall blood glucose control during the prior 8 to 12 weeks. If this test result is not consistent with reported SMBG results, one possibility is that the patient has a problem with the SMBG technique. The guidelines described earlier help detect possible errors in SMBG results. Another possibility is that only preprandial blood glucose values are being tested, and postprandial blood glucose values are too high, contributing to poor overall glucose control. In some cases, patients write down fabricated blood glucose levels, making blood glucose levels appear falsely normal. If a patient's meter has a memory, real values can be downloaded and compared with those written in the patient's SMBG record book.

Computer Downloading

Using various software programs (including some that are supplied by the meter manufacturers), it is now possible to download many meters onto the internet or into a computer, which can then print out lists of results, including various graphic representations of the blood glucose values. This information can be helpful in analyzing trends of blood glucose values. Patients often rely on the meter to store all of their blood glucose values instead of writing them down. This can be a problem if patients do not store their insulin doses and note changes in diet and exercise patterns in either their meter memory (if possible) or their written record as well.

Patient Situations/Questions

Situation 1—Fabricated Results

If fabricated results are suspected on the basis of a disparity between the meter memory and the results recorded in a patient's monitoring book, these differences should be discussed in as direct and nonjudgmental a manner as possible. Calmly instruct patients on using the memory. Have the patient measure his or her blood glucose level and then immediately check the memory to provide reassurance that the memory is working properly. (Patients who have fabricated or deleted results typically feel guilty and uncomfortable when they realize that you are checking the memory. This makes a direct confrontation counterproductive.) A sensitive and understanding approach is best for most patients. Let them know that diabetes management is difficult and that

the health care providers would prefer no information or high glucose results to results that are not authentic.

In certain circumstances, such as pregnancy, repeated problems with fabricated results, or repeated episodes of DKA, a more direct, confrontational approach may be necessary. However, this may undermine the rapport that has been established between the diabetes educator and the patient, and it may be advisable to enlist the help of the patient's physician in this process.

Situation 2—Patients Who Experience Discomfort Performing SMBG

Some patients are able to perform multiple daily tests with minimal discomfort, but others experience extreme discomfort with each test. There is not always a logical explanation for the difference. To help reduce discomfort, try the following:

1. Use different finger-stick equipment.
2. Teach arm testing technique.
3. Try the techniques listed earlier for improving blood flow (especially allowing the hand to relax at the side for a few seconds after the puncture and before applying the pressure).
4. Encourage use of the sides of the fingers that are used infrequently for activities of daily living.
5. Try different rotation patterns; some patients prefer to use different surfaces of different fingers with each stick. Some prefer to use different surfaces of the same finger. Some prefer to use the same one or two fingers all the time.
6. Reduce the number of tests requested. This may promote more long-term commitment to at least a limited SMBG schedule.
7. Have open discussions with patients to help them come to terms with this uncomfortable but useful aspect of diabetes management (especially

patients taking multiple insulin injections). Reinforce the usefulness of the results and discuss with patients the potential consequences of performing no glucose monitoring at all or of using only urine testing results.

Situation 3—Timing of Tests

Patients frequently inquire about the best time to test. They have often been taught that they simply need to test first thing in the morning, and they assume that if these results are in an acceptable range that overall control is adequate. Morning tests alone, however, do not reflect problems of postprandial hyperglycemia or preprandial hypoglycemia, especially in the late afternoon.

For patients taking insulin injections, physicians typically request specific times for blood tests throughout the day to help with ongoing evaluation of doses. For sophisticated patients, frequent premeal testing is used to help adjust daily insulin doses.

Patients who are taking oral medication and who have a A1C level within the desired range may be instructed to alter the times of the tests—especially focusing on times at which hypoglycemia risk is the highest (before meals, after a long delay in meals, before and after exercise, before a long drive, or to assess postprandial blood glucose control). Simply checking at different times on 3 or 4 days a week may be sufficient for patients to make sure that control is maintained. Other patients may prefer to test more often because it provides pressure or external motivation to stay on the diet and exercise routine.

For patients who are on diet or oral agents and who have elevated A1C results, testing in premeal and postmeal pairs is useful for encouraging patients' awareness of the effect of various food combinations. Depending on the patient and the financial and insurance circumstances, testing around just three or four meals a week may

be enough to provide knowledge and motivation. Other patients may opt to increase testing at a certain meal for a specified time while they experiment with different menus.

CONTINUOUS BLOOD GLUCOSE MONITORING

Even with intensive testing of four times or more a day, traditional SMBG only allows the patient to see a few blood glucose points in time. Although this information is important in making gross adjustments in the patient's treatment plan, it does not provide a complete picture of the daily high and low blood glucose values during normal daily activities. The Food and Drug Administration (FDA) has approved two devices and many more are in various stages of clinical trials to help continuously measure the blood glucose level on a minute-to-minute basis to evaluate trends. One device, the Continuous Glucose Monitoring System is currently available to health care professionals. It is worn by the patient for 72 hours and continuously measures the glucose in the interstitial fluid. The information is then downloaded into a computer in the physician's office to provide useful information that can help in identifying problem areas and fine-tuning of the insulin dosing, meals composition, and exercise program. These devices can be useful to assess patients such as those with erratic blood glucose levels, recurrent or severe hypoglycemic events, and hypoglycemia unawareness. The analysis and utilization of the results can lead to improvements in overall blood glucose control and fewer hypoglycemic events.

Ketone Testing

Blood or urine testing should be performed by patients with type 1 diabetes to test for the presence of ketones under specific situations. All patients with type 1 diabetes should have nonexpired blood strips for measuring urine ketones at home and should be educated about their use. Blood ketones levels can be checked by using a specially designed meter for self-monitoring of both glucose and ketone levels. All patients should be advised to test their blood or urine ketones during illness or if on a restricted-calories diet for weight loss. Patients with type 1 diabetes should test for ketones when blood glucose level is over 240 mg/dl. Pregnant women with diabetes should be advised to test the ketones level in their first urine voiding to assess for adequacy of food intake and to avoid starvation ketosis

TESTS OF LONG-TERM DIABETES CONTROL

The A1C level test is a blood test that indicates the percentage of total hemoglobin to which glucose is attached. The higher the blood glucose level and the longer it has been elevated, the higher is the percentage of glucose that attaches to the hemoglobin. Hemoglobin is a substance (a protein) inside red blood cells that carries oxygen from the lungs to the body cells. On each hemoglobin molecule are several sites that attract sugar. An analogy is made with the product called Velcro. One side is smooth, and one is rough. The hemoglobin molecule could be compared with the rough side, the sugar with the smooth side. When the two attach to each other, they do not easily come apart. Therefore the A1C molecule has a memory that lasts for the life of the red blood cell. The memory remains until the red blood cells are replaced with new ones; this takes 2 to 3 months. Therefore this test reflects the average blood glucose level during the preceding 2 months. Consequently, it serves as a reliable assessment of the overall control during this period. For teaching purposes, patients should know the difference between SMBG and the A1C test. This has been described by Dr. Daniel L. Lorber, Professor of Clinical Medicine at the New York University School of Medicine in New York, as follows: "Imagine taking a train cross-country with all the curtains drawn except for one minute seven times a day, and trying to describe the countryside based on what you saw during those seven minutes. You can frequently come close, but not as close if you had had a panoramic view. The glycated hemoglobin is that panoramic view." Because laboratories use different assays, it is important to know which test your laboratory uses and what the normal range is. The best tests currently used include A1C levels and total glycated hemoglobin levels (measured by affinity chromatography). Patients should have the test every 2 to 3 months. Seeing the A1C level fall with treatment can be rewarding and motivating for patients (Figure 12-5).

Glucose also attaches to other proteins in the circulation. Tests for these measure glycated albumin, glycated serum proteins, and fructosamine. They furnish the same information as the A1C test, but show changes over a 3- to 4-week period. Again, the normal range of these test results from each laboratory differ, and the appropriate values must be used to compare with patients' results.

UTILIZING MEDICATIONS FOR THE TREATMENT OF DIABETES

Clinical experience has shown that in general, patients who take oral antidiabetic medications lack knowledge about diabetes and do not appreciate the importance of these medications in the control of blood glucose. Some of these patients may not even consider themselves as having diabetes. Rather, they may assume that only people who require insulin injections actually have diabetes. Table 12-5 lists the currently available oral medications for treating diabetes.

SULFONYLUREA AGENTS

Sulfonylurea agents are not insulin itself but act to stimulate the pancreas to secrete more

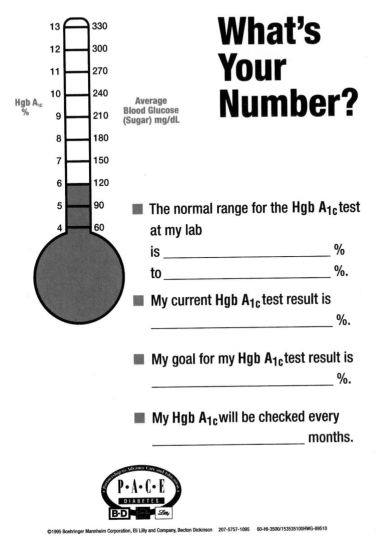

FIGURE 12-5. Patient teaching form for AIC levels.

insulin to lower blood glucose levels in patients with type 2 diabetes. By definition, they do not work in patients with type 1 diabetes, because these patients do not secrete any insulin. These drugs are often effective after diet therapy fails, although patients often gain some weight (4 to 6 pounds) when started on these agents. In addition, they sometimes cause the pancreas to secrete too much insulin, leading to hypoglycemia.

The sulfonylurea agents all have a similar mechanisms of action and therefore cannot be combined with each other. Chlor-propamide has a very long duration of action and can cause a low serum sodium level (especially in older adults) and therefore should not be used in patients older than 65 years of age. Chlorpropamide (Diabinese), glyburide (Micronase, DiaBeta, or Glynase), and glipizide (Glucotrol or Glucotrol XL), glimepiride (Amaryl) all are similarly effective. Choosing which agent to use depends largely on cost, a patient's age (no chlor-propamide if older than 65 years of age), and compliance (some patients are more compli-ant with once-a-day medications such as

TABLE 12-5 SELECTED CHARACTERISTICS OF ORAL ANTIDIABETIC MEDICATIONS

Generic Name	Trade Name	Tablet Size (mg)	Usual Daily Dose Range (mg)	Maximal Dose (mg)	Duration of Action (h)
Chlorpropamide	Diabinese*	100, 250	100–500 (single)	750	60
Glyburide	Micronase,[†] DiaBeta[††]	1.25, 2.5, 5.0	2.5–10 (single or divided)	20	12–24
	Glynase[†] (micronized glyburide	1.5, 3.0, 6.0	1.5–6.0 (single or divided)	12	12–24
Glipizide	Glucotrol[§]	5, 10	5–20 (single or divided)	40	10–24
	Glucotrol XL (long-acting glipizide)[§]	5, 10	5–10 (single)	20	24–48
Glimepiride	Amaryl[††]	1, 2, 4	1–4	8	~24
Metformin	Glucophage[‖]	500, 850	1000–2000 (divided)	2500	6–12
	Glucophage XR (long-acting metformin)[‖]	500	1000–2000	2550	~24
Acarbose	Precose[¶]	25, 50, 100	75–150 (divided)	300	Not absorbed
Miglitol	Glyset	25, 50, 100	75–150 (divided)	300	Not absorbed
Rosiglitazone	Avandia	4, 8	4–8 (single or divided)	8	6–24
Pioglitazone	Actos	15, 30, 45	30–45	45	24
Repaglinide	Prandin	0.5, 1, 2	1–2 mg AC meals TID	12	4–6
Nateglinide	Starlix	60, 120	120 mg AC meals TID	360	4
Combination Pills					
Glyburide/metformin)	Glucovance	1.25/250, 2.5/500	5/500	20/2000	
Rosiglitazone/metformin	Avandamet	2/500, 1/500, 2/500, 4/500, 2/1000, 4/1000	2/1000, 4/500	8/2000	
Glipizide/metformin	MetaGlip	2.5/250, 2.5/500	5/500	20/2000	

*Pfizer, Inc., New York, NY.

[†]Upjohn Co., Kalamazoo, MI.

[††]Hoechst-Roussel Pharmaceuticals, Somerville, NJ.

[§]Pratt Pharmaceuticals, New York, NY.

[‖]Bristol-Myers Squibb Company, Princeton, NJ.

[¶]Bayer Corp., Tarrytown, NY.

glimepiride [Amaryl] or glipizide [Glucotrol XL]).

Adverse Events

Side effects caused by sulfonylurea agents occur in less than 5% of patients. The first two in the following list are by far the most common.

1. Skin rashes
2. Gastrointestinal (GI) symptoms (loss of appetite, nausea with occasional vomiting, heartburn, feelings of abdominal fullness)
3. Flushed feeling after drinking alcohol (chlorpropamide only)
4. Mental status changes resulting from low sodium level (chlorpropamide only)
5. Dark urine, light-colored stools, yellowing of eyes or skin (drug-induced liver damage—very rare)

Hypoglycemia can be a serious adverse effect of sulfonylurea agents. It is more likely to develop when patients (often older adults) eat irregularly or consume less food than usual. It is also more likely to occur in patients with renal insufficiency. Patients taking glipizide (Glucotrol XL) and glimepiride (Amaryl) may have fewer episodes of hypoglycemia when compared with an agent such as glyburide. Because of the duration of effect of the oral agents, patients with severe hypoglycemia must be monitored carefully for a recurrence. Patients who are taking oral agents and who develop severe enough hypoglycemia to cause mentation changes should be hospitalized to receive continuous intravenous dextrose. Patients taking oral agents need to be educated about the signs, symptoms, and treatment of hypoglycemia.

BIGUANIDES

Biguanides (metformin [Glucophage]) lower glucose concentrations without stimulating the pancreas to secrete more insulin. Their mechanism of action is still controversial, but involves the liver (decreasing glucose output), muscle and fat (possibly increasing glucose utilization), and the GI tract (decreasing absorption of glucose into the bloodstream). Because its action in the body differs from that of the sulfonylurea agents, it can be used in combination with a sulfonylurea agent when a patient is failing to respond to maximal doses of one agent and needs insulin therapy. Its benefits are that it does not cause weight gain (which often occurs with sulfonylurea agents) or hypoglycemia and it improves the lipid profile. However, it must be taken two to three times per day, GI side effects are common, and lactic acidosis can occur in patients with contraindications to its use (discussed later). Therefore it must be used with careful consideration of its risks and benefits in each patient. An obese patient with diabetes is an appropriate candidate for metformin as a first-line drug, although others may benefit as well.

A longer-acting version of metformin, Glucophage XR, has been developed. It is taken only once a day and may cause fewer GI side effects when compared with shorter-acting Glucophage. A glyburide/metformin combination pill (Glucovance) exists, which combines a fast-acting form of glyburide along with metformin. This may be useful in patients who prefer to take fewer pills; however, some of the benefits of using metformin alone may be lost.

Adverse Events

Patients taking metformin commonly experience GI side effects such as cramping, diarrhea, nausea, vomiting, anorexia, metallic taste, and flatulence. These side effects usually are self-limited and improve after 1 to 2 weeks on the drug (or on the new dose). These side effects can be lessened by starting with small doses of the drug (500 or 850 mg per day), increasing the dose no more often than every other week, and giving the metformin with food. Lactic acidosis (a serious buildup of lactate levels in the blood) can occur in patients taking metformin, although only if the patient has a contraindication to its use. These contraindications include abnormal renal function (defined as a serum creatinine level above 1.5 mg/dl in males and 1.4 mg/dl in females), liver function abnormalities, excessive alcohol use, chronic or acute acidosis, and situations of possible hypoxia (e.g., congestive heart failure, pulmonary insufficiency). Any serious medical situation, especially one in which renal function might deteriorate, such as during an angiographic dye study or during a myocardial infarction, requires that metformin use be temporarily discontinued. Furthermore, serum vitamin B_{12} and folate levels can fall, and therefore patients must be monitored to ensure that anemia secondary to the medication does not occur (which is rare).

α-GLUCOSIDASE INHIBITORS

The α-glucosidase inhibitors work by a mechanism completely different from other oral medications for diabetes. These drugs inhibit the action of GI tract α-glucosidase and α-amylase enzymes that digest carbohydrates—that is, the breakdown of the carbohydrates in the meal to glucose is delayed. (Fortunately, the enzyme that digests the carbohydrate in milk is not affected much, which means that lactose intolerance is not a problem.) When the delay of carbohydrate digestion in the GI tract occurs, the rise of glucose in the circulation after the meal is blunted and less postprandial hyperglycemia is noted. Because of this mechanism of action, the α-glucosidase inhibitors, acarbose (Precose) and miglitol (Glyset), should be taken with the first bite of each meal. Some of the carbohydrate in the meal is not digested and reaches the large colon, where bacteria and other enzymes form gaseous products. Therefore a common side

effect of this drug is flatulence. However, if it is started in small doses and increased slowly, this side effect becomes less, although some patients choose not to take the drug because of it. The α-glucosidase inhibitors can be used as initial therapy in patients with type 2 diabetes or added to sulfonylurea agents or insulin. If patients are taking a combination of α-glucosidase inhibitors and a sulfonylurea agent or insulin, they must take a commercial preparation of glucose or milk to treat hypoglycemia. Because GI side effects are also common with metformin, experience with the combination of α-glucosidase inhibitors and metformin is scarce. Because they work by different mechanisms, however, an additive effect should occur when they are used together. Finally, α-glucosidase inhibitors can be added to insulin therapy in patients with type 1 diabetes. Patients should not be given this class of drug if they have a history of small bowel obstruction or inflammatory bowel disease. They are also contraindicated in patients with a serum creatinine level greater than 2.

THIAZOLIDINEDIONES

The thiazolidinediones (TZDs) are also called *insulin sensitizers* or *glitazones*. The medications in this class include pioglitazone HCl (Actos) and rosiglitazone (Avandia). Their main action is to decrease insulin resistance in the muscles and adipose tissue, and to a lesser extent to reduce glucose output in the liver. By reducing insulin resistance, they decrease the burden on the pancreas and lower blood glucose levels while lowering insulin levels. They do not cause hypoglycemia. In addition to their effects on glucose, they may have important effects on vascular factors. Both pioglitazone (Actos) and rosiglitazone (Avandia) raise HDL (good) cholesterol levels, which may lower the risk of heart disease. Pioglitazone also lowers triglyceride levels, although rosiglitazone does not.

The glitazones are used in the treatment of type 2 diabetes as monotherapy, or in combination with other oral agents such as sulfonylureas, meglitinides, and biguanides. The glitazones are very effective when used with insulin.

Adverse Events

Patients taking TZDs may experience weight gain, mild to moderate edema, and a slight decrease in hemoglobin levels as a result of plasma volume expansion. Because of the rare occurrence of idiosyncratic liver damage that occurred with troglitazone, a related compound, liver function tests should be normal at baseline and then tested every 2 months for the first year and periodically thereafter. The drug should be discontinued if the alanine aminotransferase level increases to greater than 2.5 times the upper limit of normal. Advise patients to notify their health care provider if they experience muscle aches, abdominal pain, jaundice, nausea, or vomiting. Because of the increase in plasma volume that can occur with these agents, they should be used with caution or not at all in patients with conditions such as class III or IV congestive heart failure. A glitazone may be used in renal insufficiency, as long as volume overload is not a problem.

MEGLITINIDES

Meglitinides are a new class of nonsulfonylurea oral hypoglycemic agents that are believed to bind to pancreatic β-cell receptor sites to produce a rapid and short release of insulin. The meglitinides, benzoic acid derivative (repaglinide/Prandin) and D-phenylalanine derivative (nataglinide/Starlix), are taken with meals to increase insulin levels for a short period. They are effective in helping to decrease postmeal blood glucose levels and should not be taken if meals are skipped. They can be used alone, or in combination with a metformin or a glitazone. Because they are taken with meals, patients have more flexibility in meal timing. However, the frequency of administration of the drugs, three times a day, may increase the risk for skipped dosages. Hypoglycemia is the most common adverse effect. The meglitinides are not indicated in patients who are susceptible to hypoglycemia such as older adult, debilitated, malnourished patients, or those with conditions such as adrenal, pituitary, or hepatic deficiency.

DRUG INTERACTIONS

Patients should be told that whenever they take more than one medication, one medication might interact with another one. Some medications, such as sulfa-based antibiotics, can directly potentiate (increase) the effects of the sulfonylurea agents and lower blood glucose levels further. Other drugs affect glucose levels by themselves (i.e., not by interacting with sulfonylurea agents). These include thiazide diuretics, glucocorticoids (e.g., prednisone), estrogen compounds, and phenytoin (Dilantin), which may *increase* blood glucose levels, and salicylates, propranolol, and pentamidine, which may *decrease* blood glucose levels. (Propranolol and other β blockers may also mask symptoms of hypoglycemia.)

Self-Management Education

Patients who start using oral antidiabetic medications need to be informed (1) about what type of diabetes they have (type 2), (2) about how to take the medications, (3) that they must be alert to any symptoms of hypoglycemia (if taking a sulfonylurea agent or meglitinide) and must report these episodes to their health care provider if they occur, (4) that these medications are not a substitute for a diabetic diet, (5) that they must be aware of the risks associated with the development of lactic acidosis (if on metformin—these include abnormalities of kidney or liver function, excessive use of alcohol, and any operation or medical test that requires that metformin use be discontinued temporarily), and (6) that they must be monitored closely for their diabetic control and for side effects of the drug. As with insulin, the goal of therapy is to keep blood glucose levels close to the normal range, which means at least a fasting glucose level <140 mg/dl and an A1C level of 7.0% or lower. SMBG may be helpful for detecting hypoglycemia and hyperglycemia (especially during illness).

Patients taking sulfonylurea agents should be advised to eat meals regularly to avoid hypoglycemia. The sulfonylurea agents can be taken just before, during, or after meals. Metformin, however, should always be taken with meals (after the patient has ingested some food) to decrease GI side effects. The glucosidase inhibitors should be taken with the first bite of the meal to maximize its effectiveness.

Patient Situations/Questions

If I am supposed to take my medication only once per day, does it matter when? (For sulfonylurea agents glitazones and glucophage XR, no; for metformin and α-glucosidase inhibitors, yes.)

If I have a low blood sugar reading on my meter, should I still take my medication? (Yes, but be sure to eat your meal. If on a meglitinide maybe not, depending on the setting)

If I have a treadmill test or GI study and am told not to eat in the morning or to delay eating, but am told to take all of my usual medications, should I take my diabetes pill? (Take it with the first meal that day.)

Is it all right to take a combination of pills or to combine insulin and pills? (Yes, if your physician has prescribed a combination you can always verify it with your pharmacist.)

INSULIN

Insulin is necessary to achieve blood glucose control in patients with type 1 diabetes and patients with type 2 diabetes who fail to respond satisfactorily to maximal doses of oral antidiabetic medications. The need to take insulin, especially daytime doses or mixed doses that affect meal timing, markedly increases the amount of information that a patient must master. In addition, the use of insulin in the diabetes treatment plan may be the focus of much fear and anxiety on the part of diabetes patients and their significant others.

Three main areas of instruction need to be addressed when patients start insulin treatment. These are practical issues (procedure for drawing up and injecting insulin), theoretic issues (how insulin works, timing of insulin, troubleshooting for missed or delayed doses), and emotional issues (dealing with the meaning of insulin treatment to the patient and significant others). In all three areas of discussion, it is important to assess and dispel any misconceptions about insulin treatment while respecting the unique set of experiences, expectations, and cultural beliefs that patients describe.

GENERAL ASSESSMENT

A helpful starting point when working with patients who need to learn about insulin is to allow patients to feel comfortable about expressing their fears: "Most people have fears or concerns about giving insulin shots. What concerns do you have about it?" Depending on the responses, an educator can begin instruction right away in the area of greatest concern to a patient. It is important for an educator to be flexible enough to allow discussion of information that may not necessarily follow a logical flow.

For example, if a patient's main concern surrounds the injection itself, the educator can start the lesson by having the patient self-inject saline first. If a patient's main concern is about accuracy of doses, start the lesson by having the patient locate different doses with an empty syringe. If a patient expresses concern about insulin storage and travel, address these issues at the beginning of the lesson. It is often helpful to ask patients how they feel about starting insulin so that their fears can be expressed openly. Also helpful is inquiring about the reaction of the patient's family and friends because these people can offer patients important support.

If a patient seems totally overwhelmed or consumed with anxiety, it may be best for the educator simply to start the hands-on lesson—kindly but firmly guiding the patient through a practice injection. Once this is completed, a more open, patient-guided discussion can take place. Table 12-6 lists some concerns or misconceptions that patients have when starting insulin.

MEDICAL ASSESSMENT

Determine the Type of Diabetes That the Patient Has

Patients with type 1 diabetes are at risk for DKA and may even have experienced it. Issues of concern to patients must be addressed, but educators may need to exert more influence over the flow of information to ensure that the first lesson covers the basics of giving insulin and avoiding hypoglycemia.

For patients with type 2 diabetes in poor control complicated by infection, corticosteroid treatment, anticipated surgery, or worrisome symptoms, the educator may need to use an approach similar to that for type 1 patients. There may be less opportunity to address all of patients' concerns at the initial teaching session. However, reassure patients that the insulin treatment may be temporary and that further teaching sessions will address other information, including reverting to oral antidiabetic medications.

For patients with type 2 diabetes without symptoms or coexisting illness, an educator has more latitude in negotiating the insulin treatment plan with a patient. Perhaps a patient could be given the option of starting with one injection instead of two or postponing the insulin treatment or asked to agree to a trial of 1 or 2 months on insulin with the chance to discontinue the insulin at the end of the trial. Educators need to be sure that patients understand the consequences of their decision.

Determine Adequacy of Visual/Hearing Skills

Patients with decreased visual acuity need to be taught methods for magnifying the marks on the syringes (discussed later) and strategies for insulin administration (such as use of insulin pens or having a family member assist). Patients with significant hearing deficits need to be taught in a quiet room, and much of the information provided may need to be written down.

SELF-MANAGEMENT EDUCATION

The following sections are divided into basic and comprehensive levels of information. A basic level of information is intended to provide patients with enough information to be safe users of insulin even if they never receive or are unable to comprehend more comprehensive insulin instruction. Focusing solely on the basic information is useful when working with patients who are very anxious, when time for the lesson is limited, and when patients have a limited capacity to comprehend complex information.

TABLE 12-6 MISCONCEPTIONS RELATED TO INSULIN

Misconception	Educator's Response
Once insulin injections are started (for treatment of type 2 diabetes), they can never be discontinued.	During periods of acute stress (such as illness, infection, or surgery) or when receiving certain medications that cause elevations in blood glucose, some patients with type 2 diabetes require insulin. If the diabetes had previously been well controlled with diet alone or diet with oral hypoglycemic agents, patients should be able to resume previous methods for control of diabetes when the stress is resolved. In addition, insulin is sometimes used to control blood glucose levels in obese type 2 diabetic patients who have been unsuccessful at weight loss. If patients are able to lose weight after insulin therapy is initiated, the insulin doses may be tapered and patients may be able to switch to diet and exercise alone or with oral hypoglycemic agents for control of blood glucose. (For patients with type 1 diabetes, insulin is needed on an ongoing basis. For thin patients with type 2 diabetes, once insulin has to be started, it is usually required permanently).
If increasing doses of insulin are needed to control the blood glucose, the diabetes must be getting "worse."	Explain to patients that unlike other medications that are given in standard doses, there is not a standard dose of insulin that is effective for all patients. Rather, the dose must be adjusted according to blood glucose test results. If the initial insulin dose prescribed for a patient does not adequately decrease the glucose level, the patient may assume that he or she has a "bad" case of diabetes or that the diabetes is getting worse. It is important to instruct patients that many different factors may affect the ability of insulin to lower the glucose, including obesity, puberty, pregnancy, illness, and certain medications. In addition, to avoid hypoglycemia, physicians frequently initiate insulin therapy with smaller doses than will eventually be needed. The doses are then increased in small increments until blood glucose levels are in the desired range.
Insulin causes blindness (or other diabetic complications).	When patients have a diabetic acquaintance in whom the initiation of insulin therapy happened to coincide with the onset of diabetic complications, the patient may view insulin as the cause of complications such as blindness or amputation. In these situations, the acquaintance probably had type 2 diabetes that was no longer controllable with diet and oral hypoglycemic agents. It must be explained to patients that factors such as elevated blood glucose and elevated blood pressure levels (and not insulin therapy) contribute to some of the diabetic complications. Furthermore, emphasize that insulin is a natural hormone present in every person's body, that it helps control blood glucose levels, and that it definitely does not cause long-term complications of diabetes.
Insulin must be injected directly into the vein.	When patients first learn that one area used for insulin injections is the arm, they may envision inserting the needle directly into a vein in the antecubital area as in

TABLE 12-6	MISCONCEPTIONS RELATED TO INSULIN—cont'd
Misconception	**Educator's Response**
	blood withdrawal. Patients must be reassured that insulin is injected into the fat tissue on the *back* of the arm (or on the abdomen, thigh, or hip) and that the needle is much shorter than that used for venipuncture.
There is extreme danger in injecting insulin if there are any air bubbles in the syringe.	Patients may have a fear of dying if air bubbles are injected with a syringe. (This may be related to the misconception that insulin is injected directly into the vein). Reassure patients that the main danger in having air bubbles in the insulin syringe is that the amount of insulin being injected is less than the required dose. It is often difficult to remove every small "champagne" bubble from the syringe. Thus patients should be reassured that injection of insulin when these bubbles are present does not cause any harm.
Insulin always causes people to have bad (hypoglycemic) reactions.	First, make sure that patients are aware that low blood sugar reactions are often related to an imbalance with the insulin, food, and activity and can often be avoided. Thus, before starting on insulin, patients should discuss their usual schedule of meals and activities as well as the content of meals with the health care team. Make sure that patients are aware that various different insulins and insulin schedules can be used to try to allow patients to maintain some of their usual life style habits. Reassure patients that avoiding hypoglycemic reactions is a high priority for the diabetes team. In addition, tell patients of the importance of reporting any hypoglycemic reactions to the health care team immediately so that early adjustments can be made in the insulin dosage. Focus early insulin education on treatment and prevention of hypoglycemia.
People who take insulin must travel only where there is a refrigerator to store the insulin.	Insulin bottles in use may be kept at room temperature. Therefore, for most business trips or vacations, keeping the insulin in a purse or brief case (or special diabetes supply case) is acceptable. If a prolonged trip is planned (more than 2 to 3 months), patients may want to consult the pharmacist or insulin manufacturer for suggestions. Most importantly, emphasize with patients that taking insulin should never deter them from pursuing activities they enjoy.

The educator can set up a follow-up appointment to review the basic information and to introduce the comprehensive information as appropriate. Some patients are able to receive comprehensive information from the beginning and wish to do so. The educator's assessment is helpful in determining the degree of difficulty of information to present.

BASIC INSULIN INSTRUCTION— PRACTICAL ISSUES

1. *Gather and identify supplies,* including alcohol, insulin, syringe, and cotton or tissue. Locate on the insulin label the *letter* or *number* indicating the type of insulin (e.g., NPH [N], regular [R], 70/30 mixture Humalog, Novolog, Lantus, etc). Note

the *color* of the insulin (white or clear). Identify the *size* of the syringe by looking at the highest number of units that the syringe can hold (e.g., 25, 30, 50, 100). Explain that one bottle holds enough insulin (1000 U) to last for 1 to 2 months.

At the basic level, it is not critical that a patient recite the full name for the insulin or identify the syringe by volume. Patients simply need to be able to correctly identify the insulin and syringes that they are supposed to be using.

2. *Open the supplies.* Flip off the cap on the insulin bottle. Carefully remove the needle cover and plunger cap (if present) from the syringe. At this point, patients can practice pulling and pushing the plunger of the syringe while locating different doses.

If patients are totally incapable of accurately positioning the plunger at this stage, the educator may need to make other arrangements for drawing up the insulin. For example, syringes can be prefilled by a member of the diabetes treatment team, a family member can be taught how to draw up the insulin, home health visits can be arranged, or the use of a prefilled insulin pen can be considered. Most patients can still be taught to give the injection, even if they are not able to draw up their own doses.

3. *Draw up the insulin* (Figure 12-6).
   • Wipe the bottle top with alcohol.

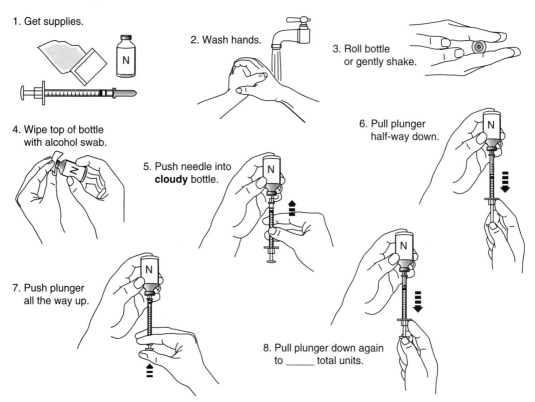

1. Get supplies.

2. Wash hands.

3. Roll bottle or gently shake.

4. Wipe top of bottle with alcohol swab.

5. Push needle into **cloudy** bottle.

6. Pull plunger half-way down.

7. Push plunger all the way up.

8. Pull plunger down again to _____ total units.

FIGURE 12-6. Technique for withdrawing insulin from a single bottle. (Injecting air into bottle not shown.) (See text for description.)

- Mix all cloudy insulin by gently shaking or rolling the bottle.
- Insert the needle through the rubber stopper.
- Position the bottle upside down, making sure the needle is completely covered with the insulin solution.
- Pull the plunger approximately half-way down the syringe and then push it all the way back up, squirting all the insulin back into the bottle.
- Pull the plunger down again and locate the prescribed number of units.
- Remove the syringe from the bottle; avoid touching the needle.
- Holding the upside-down bottle and syringe in one hand while manipulating the syringe plunger with the other hand can be very awkward for new patients. They can be shown various bottle-holding devices such as

the Becton Dickinson Magni-Guide or Diabetic Insulcap (see Appendix), or the educator can assist by holding the bottle for the patient at first. Another option is simply to tape the bottle to a vertical surface (e.g., a wall, refrigerator, or door) in an upside-down position.

4. *Give the injection* (Figure 12-7).
- Bunch up the skin of the abdomen (pinch up a fold about 1 inch thick).
- Insert the needle straight in with a dart action.
- Inject the insulin with slow, steady pressure on the plunger.
- Remove the needle, let go of the pinch (can be done in reverse order), and apply pressure to the site with dry cotton or tissue.
- Basic instruction need not cover elaborate injection site rotation

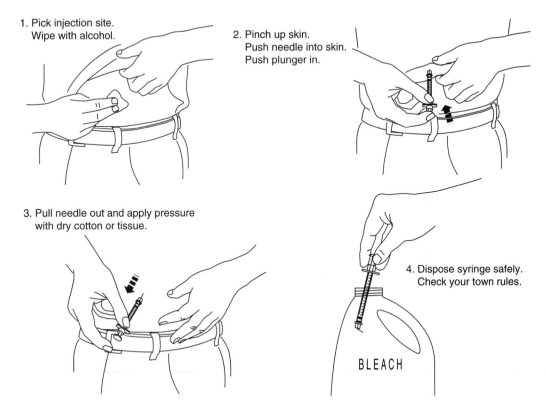

1. Pick injection site. Wipe with alcohol.

2. Pinch up skin. Push needle into skin. Push plunger in.

3. Pull needle out and apply pressure with dry cotton or tissue.

4. Dispose syringe safely. Check your town rules.

BLEACH

FIGURE 12-7. Technique for self-injection of insulin.

patterns. It is simplest to teach one area for injection—preferably the abdomen, because it offers the most consistent absorption, is easy to reach, and typically has the most subcutaneous tissue. In addition, patients who are taught to use only the arms or legs first are often quite fearful of trying the abdomen at a later date (whereas the reverse is not necessarily true).

- Advise patients to use a new site about 1 inch away from the previous site— moving sites down and across the entire abdomen, avoiding the area around the umbilicus.

5. *Discard the syringe.* ADA and Environmental Protection Agency recommendations include placing the entire uncapped syringe into a puncture-proof container such as an empty bleach or detergent bottle. It is helpful to have patients discard the syringe in such a bottle during the teaching session. Once full, the bottle may be discarded with the regular garbage— although the educator should check for any specific city or state regulations.

6. *Store the bottles of insulin.*
   - According to the insulin manufacturers, insulin bottles in use can be stored at room temperature for 1 month.
   - Insulin bottles should be kept out of direct sunlight.
   - Unopened bottles should be refrigerated and can be stored until they expire.
   - If bottles are refrigerated, they can be removed before the injection to allow them to return to room temperature. Be sure not to let the insulin freeze.

COMPREHENSIVE INSULIN INSTRUCTION—PRACTICAL ISSUES

1. *Gather and identify supplies.* Rather than simply identifying the insulin by reading the label, patients prepared for more advanced instruction can be introduced to four main differentiating characteristics of insulin: type, species/source, manufacturer, and concentration.

- *Type*—Bolus insulin is a kind of insulin that acts quickly to decrease the blood glucose level. It is usually taken before meals or to correct high blood glucose levels. Bolus insulins are divided into two types: rapid-acting insulins, lispro (Humalog) and insulin aspart (Novolog), and short-acting insulin, R. Basal or background insulin is slowly released in the blood stream throughout the day to help control the blood glucose. It is generally taken once or twice a day. They include intermediate-acting insulins (neutral protein hagedorn NPH [N] or lente [L]), and long-acting insulin ultralente (UL) and glargine (Lantus). It is helpful to have sample bottles of different types of insulin available to show patients. Patients can be introduced to the approximate time course of action (Table 12-7), although it is often best to introduce this information from a practical perspective rather than having patients memorize onset, peak, and duration. For example, rapid-acting insulin goes to work on the meal consumed right after the injection, whereas NPH insulin is time released and goes to work on a later meal or overnight (Figure 12-8). (For patients using premixed insulin, see the later discussion.)

- *Species* (or origin)—The currently available insulin source is mostly human (synthetic). A small supply of pork insulin is available upon request. Reassure patients that human insulin is produced in a laboratory to look just like human insulin and is not derived from humans, so there is no risk of being infected with hepatitis or acquired immune deficiency syndrome (AIDS).

TABLE 12-7	TIME COURSE OF ACTION OF INSULIN		
Insulin	**Onset of Action**	**Peak**	**Duration**
Rapid Acting (clear color)			
Lispro (Humalog)	5–15 min	30–75 min	2–4 hrs
Aspart (Novolog)	5–15 min	1–2 hrs	2–4 hrs
Short Acting (clear color)			
Regular insulin (R)	30–45 min	2–3 hrs	4–8 hrs
Intermediate Acting (cloudy)			
NPH	2–4 hrs	4–8 hrs	10–16 hrs
Lente	2–4 hrs	4–8 hrs	10–16 hrs
Long Acting			
Ultralente (cloudy)	3–5 hrs	8–12 hrs	18–20 hrs
Glargine (Lantus) (clear)	4–8 hrs	none	24 hrs
Insulin Mixtures (cloudy)			
70/30 (70% NPH, 30% R)	30–60 min	2–12 hrs	~18 hrs
50/50 (50% NPH, 50% R)	30–60 min	2–12 hrs	~18 hrs
75/25 (75% Humalog, 25% NPL—similar to NPH)	5–15 min	1–12 hrs	~18 hrs

- *Manufacturers*—Eli Lilly, Aventis, and Novo Nordisk are the three companies currently supplying insulin in the United States. Teaching patients about the company names is helpful in terms of learning to differentiate insulins. Patients often identify their insulin type simply with their brand names such as Humulin or Novolin. They need to understand that these are simply trade names for the whole series of human insulins and do not describe the type of insulin used. Patients should be taught, for example, that the name *Humulin N* indicates the Lilly brand of human NPH or that *Novolin R* is the Novo Nordisk brand of human regular insulin.
- *Concentration*—The usual concentration of insulin in the United States is U-100. Patients who travel, use insulin pumps, or are very inquisitive can be educated about different insulin concentrations such as U-40. Patients should be taught that this refers to the number of units of insulin per milliliter. Patients can be shown that the concentration noted on the bottle should match that noted on the syringe. Make patients aware that U-100 syringes are available in various sizes (e.g., 30 U, 50 U, 100 U) and that syringe size does not denote a different concentration. Also, needle sizes vary in gauge and length and patients should use the smallest needle size possible to reduce injection-related pain.

Show patients syringes of different sizes, pointing out that the main difference is that the 100-U (1-ml) syringes are typically marked in 2-U increments. Allow patients to practice drawing up insulin using different syringes so that they can appreciate the different sizes of syringes and are able to select the most appropriate size when new supplies are obtained.

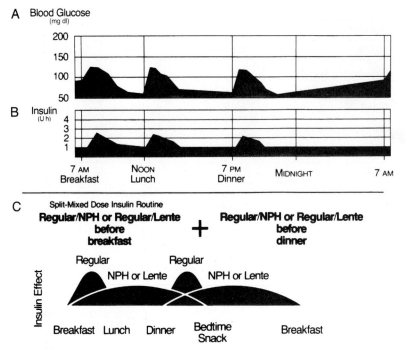

FIGURE 12-8. A: The normal rise in blood glucose level that occurs after meals. **B:** The normal increase in insulin release that occurs at mealtime. **C:** A twice-daily insulin injection regimen using two injections of neutral protein hagedorn (NPH) (or lente) mixed with regular "covers" breakfast; prebreakfast NPH covers lunch and afternoon snack; predinner regular covers dinner; predinner NPH covers bedtime snack and overnight.

2. *Equipment issues: flocculation, needle size and syringe reuse.* Patients prepared for more advanced information can be taught about insulin flocculation and syringe reuse.

   • *Flocculation:* White, cloudy insulins can develop a frosted appearance stuck to the inside of the insulin bottle, called *flocculation.* These white clumps may also appear in the insulin solution (Figure 12-9). This is more common if the insulin has been kept at room temperature for a prolonged time (>2 to 3 months). Frosted insulin is inactive and should be discarded. However, reassure patients that if they inadvertently use insulin that has gone bad, they will not harm themselves, but will have elevated blood glucose levels because their insulin is not working properly. (It is helpful for the educator

to have frosted bottles of insulin on display. The educator can keep one or two sample bottles of insulin at room temperature for a prolonged period to create the frosted appearance.)

   • *Needle size:* Most syringes and pen needles are now available in normal length of 12 mm or short length of 8 mm. The short needles can be used effectively for patients who are thin or of average weight, and those that are very muscular.

   • *Syringe reuse:* Studies that have been conducted have shown that reuse of insulin syringes is safe. The ADA Position Statement on Insulin Administration states, "For many patients, it appears both safe and practical for the syringe to be reused if the patient so desires. The syringe

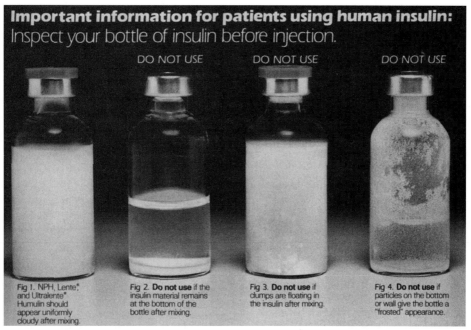

Important information for patients using human insulin:
Inspect your bottle of insulin before injection.

DO NOT USE   DO NOT USE   DO NOT USE

Fig 1. NPH, Lente,* and Ultralente* Humulin should appear uniformly cloudy after mixing.

Fig 2. **Do not use** if the insulin material remains at the bottom of the bottle after mixing.

Fig 3. **Do not use** if clumps are floating in the insulin after mixing.

Fig 4. **Do not use** if particles on the bottom or wall give the bottle a "frosted" appearance.

FIGURE 12-9. Important information for patients using human insulin: Inspect your bottle of insulin before injection. NPH, neutral protein hagedorn.

should be discarded when the needle becomes dull, has been bent, or has come into contact with any surface other than the skin; if reuse is planned, the needle must be recapped after each use." For patients using very fine needles, it may not be advisable to reuse their syringes because they may easily bend and break under the skin.

3. *Draw up the insulin.* In this stage of the insulin protocol, several variations in the technique are taught by diabetes educators and promoted by printed instructional material. The steps described previously in the basic section represent one approach to drawing up insulin. Beginning learners are best served by being taught a simple technique that achieves the basic objective of getting insulin from the bottle into the syringe with as few steps as possible. Unfortunately, many patients with diabetes harbor unwarranted anxiety about making any minor

changes in the protocol that they were initially taught. At the more advanced level of teaching, patients with diabetes can be exposed to several variations in the insulin protocol and allowed to select the steps that are most comfortable to them.

Injecting air into the vial—vacuum prevention: Injecting air into the vial of insulin is thought to eliminate the formation of a vacuum caused by repeated withdrawal of insulin from the closed vial. The most common technique is to inject air into the vial before each injection in a volume equivalent to the amount of insulin to be withdrawn. Variations are as follows:

- Inject an entire syringe full of air on a regular basis (e.g., every other day or once a week) rather than with each injection.
- Remove the plunger completely from a syringe and insert the empty syringe

barrel into the insulin bottle, allowing the pressure inside the bottle to equalize for a few seconds.

• The simplest technique is to completely eliminate all steps relative to injecting air.

Little if any scientific evidence shows that vacuum formation in insulin bottles is problematic. In fact, one study measured this phenomenon and found little support for the common and, for many patients, confusing steps of injecting exact quantities of air into bottles. Even if a vacuum does develop, it will not necessarily impair a patient's ability to draw up an appropriate dose. Patients capable of learning more comprehensive insulin information can be given a demonstration of all the different approaches to dealing with the vacuum and can be allowed to select the technique of their choice. For patients who are not capable of comprehending more than the basic insulin information, it may be safer to risk vacuum

formation than to risk confusion in preparing the dose.

4. *Give the injection.* Variations in injection technique can be introduced at the comprehensive level of education.

Injection Sites (Figure 12-10)

The first insulin instruction session can involve demonstration of just one injection area (preferably the abdomen). Follow-up comprehensive sessions can include information on the other possible sites, with discussion of site rotation and consequences of changing injection areas. *Abdominal* sites are located in a wide area from under the ribs, down to the hip line, and out to the side of the abdomen. *Arm* sites are located on the fleshy back surface of the upper arm, one hand's width down from the shoulder and one hand's width up from the elbow. A common error is for patients to use the deltoid area, just down from the shoulder, because the fleshy back surface is too hard to reach.

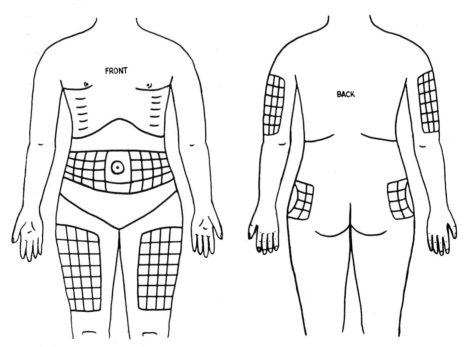

FIGURE 12-10. Injection sites for insulin.

This may cause inadvertent intramuscular injections, especially in a thin person. Intramuscular insulin injections may be more painful and can cause rapid absorption of the insulin. *Leg* sites are located one hand's width down from the groin and one hand's width up from the knee on the top surface of the thigh. *Hip* sites are located in the upper outer area of the buttocks. Research has shown that absorption is quickest from the abdomen and is progressively slower from the arm, leg, and hip sites.

Site Rotation

Insulin should not be repeatedly injected in exactly the same site. If the same injection point is used, the skin may develop *lipohypertrophy*, a fatty, spongy area of increased fat deposition, or *lipoatrophy*, a pitting or dimpling of the skin because subcutaneous fat is lost. Injections in these areas may lead to erratic absorption of the insulin. It is important to note that the absorption of the rapid-acting insulins is not affected by the injection site, thus they can be given at any site without causing erratic blood glucose levels, unless of course there is increased physical activity affecting the injection site.

Rotation of injection sites within one area is carried out by measuring one to two fingers' widths (½ to 1 inch) away from the most recent injection site. To avoid skin changes, patients should be advised to avoid injecting at the same site more than once in 2 to 3 weeks. If lipohypertrophy has occurred, it will resolve if no injections are given in the area until the skin resumes a normal contour.

Developing a systematic approach to site rotation, such as giving injections in a horizontal or vertical line pattern, helps to avoid repeated injections at the same site. Two different approaches that may be used for rotation of injection sites are as follows:

Use injection sites on the abdomen exclusively (most patients can rotate sites within the abdomen without using the same site in 2 to 3 weeks).

Use injection sites in one area at the same time of day (e.g., use the abdominal area every morning and the arm every evening). Patients who are having problems with early peaking of intermediate-acting insulins (NPH or lente) may benefit from using the leg or hip sites to prolong insulin action.

These approaches to rotation of injection areas provide the greatest consistency in absorption and effectiveness of insulin. They differ from previous methods of teaching rotation of injections, which included using a new area of the body for each injection. Patients who have been taking insulin for many years may need to be updated on this newer approach to injection rotation.

Stabilizing Skin

Patients may choose between *bunching* the skin or *spreading* it before inserting the needle. Bunching the skin helps to avoid injection into the muscle, which is especially important in thin patients. Spreading the skin is helpful if the skin tends to give during needle insertion and for inserting the Teflon catheters used with insulin pumps.

Angle of Insertion

A 90-degree angle is desirable in most patients to ensure delivery of insulin into the subcutaneous tissue instead of into the intradermal tissue. Also, injecting straight in promotes consistency from injection to injection. Very thin patients and children may prefer injecting at a 60- to 90-degree angle to avoid intramuscular injection. In general, patients can be reassured that if they can pinch an inch of fat between their fingers, they can inject straight in without a problem, because most needles are ½ inch or less in length.

Skin Problems

Bruises, leaking, and lumps are the skin problems most commonly described by insulin users. Less commonly, insulin users describe burning, itching, or redness at the site. Potential causes and preventive measures are described next.

Some patients may develop *bruises* when the needle has nicked a superficial blood vessel or if the angle of the needle has shifted during insertion or withdrawal of the needle. Reassure patients that although bruises pose a cosmetic problem, they are not hazardous from a health standpoint. To prevent bruises, encourage the use of a 90-degree angle with swift, darting action used for needle insertion and swift, straight pulling outward for needle withdrawal. In addition, pressure should be applied to the injection site using dry cotton or tissue. Advise patients to avoid rubbing the area with cotton or an alcohol swab because this may promote bleeding or bruising.

Patients may develop *leaking or skin lumps* from injections that are too rapid, too large (volume), or too shallow. Encourage the use of a 90-degree angle with slow injection of the insulin and release of the skin bunch as the injection is finishing. Patients using large doses of insulin may try dividing the injection and giving it in two different sites.

Patients may develop *burning, itching, and redness* from alcohol that is still wet at the time of needle insertion or from insulin that is too cold at the time of injection. Because of the increased acidity of the solution, glargine (Lantus) insulin may cause a mild burning sensation that should be quickly dissipated. Allowing the alcohol to dry on the skin before injection and using insulin at room temperature may resolve the problem. If not, patients may be having a reaction to the insulin preservative or to the needle. If the problem does not resolve with the use of different brands of insulin or syringes, patients may have an insulin allergy (see Chapter 5).

5. *Storing the bottles of insulin.* Patients who plan to carry insulin with them during the day or when traveling can consult the *ADA Yearly Buyer's Guide to Diabetes Supplies* and other diabetes publications or stores for various tote bags and insulin or syringe carrying cases. For patients who want to carry one or two prefilled syringes for a planned meal away from home, a simple solution is to use a toothbrush holder or a long, thin box such as a necklace or a watch box.

6. *Combining two types of insulin—basic technique.* Before starting the procedure for drawing up two insulins, have patients write down or verbalize the two dose markings that will be used—the dose of the first insulin to be drawn up and then the *total* dose of both insulins (add the two individual doses together). It is important to note that glargine (Lantus) insulin should never be mixed with any other insulin or be drawn in a syringe that was used to prepare another insulin. Doing so will cause the glargine (Lantus) insulin to precipitate and have unpredictable action. Mixing the insulins is carried out as follows (Figure 12-11):

- Wipe both bottle tops with alcohol.
- Insert the needle through the rubber stopper of the short- or rapid-acting insulin.
- Position the bottle upside down (and make sure the tip of the needle remains covered by solution).
- Pull the plunger approximately halfway down the syringe and then push it all the way back up, squirting all the insulin back into the bottle.
- Pull the plunger down again to the prescribed number of units of the regular or rapid-acting insulin.
- Remove the syringe from the bottle.
- Mix the cloudy insulin by gently shaking or rolling the bottle.
- Insert the needle through the rubber stopper of the longer-acting (cloudy, white, NPH, or Lente) insulin.
- Pull the plunger down to the total dose calculated by adding the two doses together.
- Remove the syringe from the bottle.

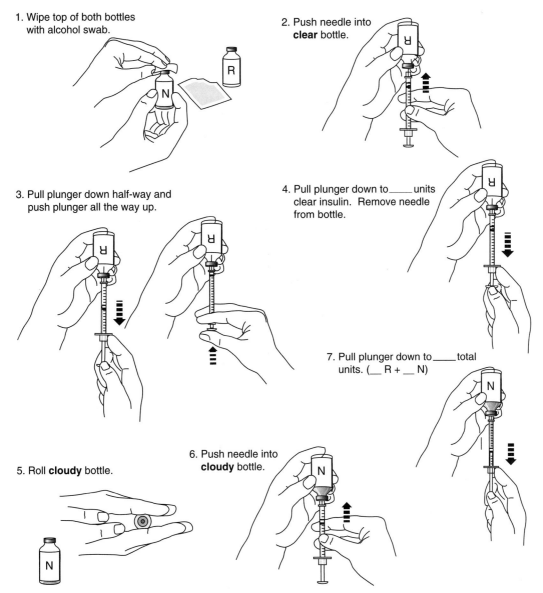

1. Wipe top of both bottles with alcohol swab.

2. Push needle into **clear** bottle.

3. Pull plunger down half-way and push plunger all the way up.

4. Pull plunger down to ____ units clear insulin. Remove needle from bottle.

5. Roll **cloudy** bottle.

6. Push needle into **cloudy** bottle.

7. Pull plunger down to ____ total units. (__ R + __ N)

FIGURE 12-11. Technique of withdrawing two different insulins from separate bottles into one syringe. (Injecting air into bottles not shown.) (See text for description.)

Variations in the Technique of Combining Insulins

Troubleshooting for Error in Technique

Demonstrate for patients an error in technique in which the amount of the second insulin accidentally exceeds the correct total dose. Explain that the only option at that point is to squirt out all the insulin, discard it, and start over. Simply squirting out the excess insulin into the air or back into the bottle is not appropriate because it would result in an incorrect ratio of the two insulins.

Altering the Order of Insulin Withdrawal

Generally, the short- or rapid-acting (clear) insulin is drawn up first because accidental injection of a cloudy, delayed-acting insulin into the bottle of short- or rapid-acting insulin may alter the time course of action of insulin remaining in the bottle. However, if patients have previously been taught to draw up the cloudy insulin first, they may continue to prepare the insulin this way provided the correct doses of both insulins are drawn up and the bottle of short- or rapid-acting insulin appears clear and uncontaminated by cloudy insulin.

Premixed Insulins. If a patient is unable to mix insulins, the physician may prescribe premixed insulins such as 70/30 or 50/50 with a set ratio of NPH and regular in the insulin bottle (provided the ratio of insulins appropriately matches the patient's insulin needs). Additionally, premixed insulins with rapid-acting insulin and NPH are available.

Prefilled Syringes. Another option for patients unable to draw up insulin properly is to have family members or neighbors prefill 1 to 2 weeks' worth of syringes. These syringes can be stored in the refrigerator. Patients should be made aware that the insulin in the syringe settles and that rolling the syringe in the hands before the injection remixes the insulins and warms the syringe.

Adding Regular or Rapid-Acting Insulin to the Lente Series. Regular or rapid-acting insulin added to NPH insulin has its usual time course of action. When regular insulin is added to Lente or Ultralente insulin, the time course of action is delayed. Patients having problems with blood glucose control because of delayed action of regular insulin mixed with a Lente insulin may need to take two separate injections rather than mix.

Glargine (Lantus) insulin should not be mixed with any other insulin.

BASIC INSULIN INSTRUCTION

THEORETICAL ISSUES

The theoretical information about insulin that patients need to learn includes understanding how insulin works, how insulin relates to other variables that affect blood glucose control, and troubleshooting when there are changes in routine. This information can be quite complex and difficult for some patients to understand. Much of the information revolves around prevention of problems (such as hypoglycemia) that patients may never have experienced. The less that patients seem able to comprehend theoretic information, the more practical and directed the information needs to be.

Start by asking questions such as, "What does insulin do?" If this is too broad, ask more specifically, "Does insulin make your blood sugar go up or down? Can you name one thing that could make your sugar go down?" (Answers are exercise, missed meal, delayed meal, or too much insulin.) "Can you name one thing that could make your sugar go up?" (Answers are too much food, illness, or too little insulin.) Alternatively, ask, "Does food make your sugar go up or down? Does exercise make your blood sugar go up or down?"

If patients are unable to answer the most basic questions, they need to be given very specific daily living and troubleshooting guidelines:

1. Take insulin at _____ (try to give a range of times).
2. Eat meals and snacks at _____ (again, give a range).
3. Don't skip meals—eat anything, even junk food, if you can't eat your normal meal on time.

4. If you miss your shot, just skip it. "When in doubt, leave it out."[*]

5. If you are supposed to skip a meal for medical reasons, call your doctor for advice. (If you can't reach your doctor, it is safer to miss one insulin shot.[*])

Keep in mind that these recommendations are intended for the initial basic or survival education. During follow-up visits or phone calls, many patients can be taught a more flexible problem-solving approach to managing variations in schedule.

COMPREHENSIVE INSULIN INSTRUCTION

THEORETICAL ISSUES

If patients seem comfortable describing the basic variables that cause an increase or decrease in blood glucose levels, they may then be ready to learn more sophisticated troubleshooting information.

Insulin Timing

A practical approach to teaching the time course of insulin action is to identify which periods during the day are covered by the different insulin doses (see Figure 12-8). For example, for regular and NPH injections taken before breakfast and supper, the morning regular covers the breakfast to lunch period, morning NPH the lunch to supper period, and evening regular the sup-

per to bedtime snack period. Evening NPH works overnight.

If patients take only one or two of the four components of the insulin regimen listed earlier, the same information can be taught, making them aware of the periods during the day that are not covered by the insulin taken.

To test patients' understanding of insulin timing and other variables, ask questions requiring application of knowledge, such as the following:

If you were going to exercise between breakfast and lunch, which insulin should be decreased? (Answer: morning regular)

If you got a low blood sugar reaction in the afternoon, which insulin would you blame? (Answer: morning NPH)
If you had to skip breakfast for a short morning dental appointment, which insulin could you skip? (Answer: morning regular)
To help reduce your high fasting blood sugars, which insulin dose should be increased? (Answer: evening NPH)

TIMING OF MEALS AND INJECTIONS

More sophisticated patients can be given a more flexible routine in terms of insulin and meal timing. Rather than giving specific times always to eat or take injections, teach relationships between insulin timing and meals. For example, regular insulin is generally given 20 to 30 minutes before a meal. Rapid acting insulin can be given immediately before or after a meal NPH insulin in the morning has a delayed and prolonged action that requires carbohydrate intake approximately every 4 to 5 hours during the day. NPH insulin in the evening helps control the body's own (liver) production of glucose during the night and is best taken

---

[*]These last recommendations may need to be altered for certain patients, especially those with type 1 diabetes. Usually, however, the acute complication of most concern with insulin-treated patients is hypoglycemia. Although hyperglycemia associated with missed doses is certainly a problem, one missed dose of insulin is less likely to cause DKA or hyperosmolar nonketotic syndrome (HNKS) than one poorly timed dose of insulin is to cause hypoglycemia.

approximately 8 to 10 hours before the anticipated time of arising in the morning. Thus if patients plan to sleep late, the insulin could be given at a later time the night before. If the blood glucose level is low at bedtime, a snack is usually required to prevent hypoglycemia in the middle of the night when the NPH starts to peak. Lantus insulin is a peakless basal insulin in many patients so adjustments for sleeping late or missing meals may not be needed.

If patients stay up late or start their day later on days off, guidelines can be given for simply taking insulin doses at a later time, provided that the general guidelines for meal timing are followed. Patients who are taught how to vary their schedule need to understand clearly that avoidance of hypoglycemia is the main priority on days that follow a highly unusual pattern for them.

DELAYED/MISSED INSULIN DOSES

Teach patients what to expect if insulin doses are delayed or missed and how to adjust the insulin dosing. Refer to the original teaching approach of associating each insulin dose with a different period of the day. It is important to avoid having two insulin doses that cover the glucose level or peak during the same period. For example, two NPH doses that are closer than 8 hours apart may overlap in terms of their hypoglycemic effect. Therefore, if a morning NPH injection is missed, it may be best to take regular insulin alone at lunchtime rather than give the forgotten NPH dose at lunchtime because this late NPH dose may peak at night when the evening NPH and short- or rapid-acting insulin doses are acting. A missed dose of short- or rapid-acting insulin in a patient on fixed dosage regimen should generally be skipped entirely, although rapid-acting insulin can be given after eating in certain circumstances. Patients on flexible regimen or insulin pump can be instructed on how to give

doses after meals, and on how to give a correction dosage for hyperglycemia.

INJECTING WHEN HYPERGLYCEMIC

To test patients' understanding, ask questions that require application of their knowledge. The following is an example:

> If your blood sugar is high at the time of the injection, what could you do to help lower your blood sugar level? (Answer[s]: Delay the meal for 1 hour after the injection, take extra short- or rapid-acting insulin according to your physician's guidelines, or reduce the intake of carbohydrate at the meal.)

If patients are not able to answer such a broad question, specific situations can be discussed. The following are examples:

> If your sugar is high, do you think it's best to eat sooner than usual or to delay the meal longer than usual? (Answer: Delay the meal.)

> If you cannot delay your meal more than usual, which of your usual breakfast foods might you eliminate from the meal? (Answer: Carbohydrate-containing foods, such as cereal or toast.)

Most importantly, explain to patients that all guidelines are personalized on the basis of frequent glucose monitoring, recording information, and reviewing information with their diabetes team.

INJECTING WHEN HYPOGLYCEMIC

Many patients assume that if their blood glucose level is low (<100 mg/dl) before a meal, they do not need to take any insulin. To assess this, ask patients what they would do if their blood glucose levels were low and it was time to take insulin. Explain that it is normal for blood glucose levels to increase after meals. If patients are taking only NPH insulin, the prolonged nature of the insulin action gives them plenty of time to eat an extra snack or consume extra carbohydrate at the meal to prevent a decline in blood glucose level when the NPH insulin starts to work in 3 to 4 hours. If patients are taking short- or rapid-acting insulin alone or combined with NPH insulin, they can either reduce their short- or rapid-action dose based on guidelines provided by their physician, or they can eat a snack before the dose.

To help patients think of a solution, the following line of questioning may help: "At what blood sugar level do you feel comfortable taking your shot?" If patients cannot answer, be more specific. "If you had a blood sugar level of 150 mg/dl in the morning, would you take your usual shot? 130 mg/dl? 100 mg/dl?" Help patients identify the lowest blood glucose level at which they would take their injection. Then ask, "If you woke up with a reading of 75 mg/dl and you prefer to be over 120 mg/dl before taking your shot, what could you do to increase your blood sugar to 120 mg/dl?" This type of interaction helps patients to come up with their own solution and helps with applying this line of reasoning to other unexpected situations.

INJECTING FOR EXTRA FOOD INTAKE

Patients should be encouraged to find out which foods cause their highest blood glucose levels. Ask questions to help them discover their options for avoiding food-related hyperglycemia. Also, review the advantages and disadvantages of each option. The following are examples:

Option 1

Increase premeal short- or rapid-acting insulin by learning to match insulin to carbohydrate intake (carbohydrate counting).

Advantages

Option 1 allows more variable food intake with less hyperglycemia and gives patients a feeling of more flexibility and control.

Disadvantages

Option 1 requires extra education, thinking, and awareness with each meal; it requires extra blood testing and documentation to test appropriateness of dose changes; it may lead to weight gain owing to more relaxed approach to food intake.

Option 2

Restrict or eliminate foods that cause excessive hyperglycemia.

Advantages

Option 2 requires less thought and separate planning for different meals.

Disadvantages

Option 2 may cause feelings of deprivation and less enjoyment of meals.

Option 3

Eat as desired; make no changes.

Advantages

Option 3 provides more flexibility, less preplanning, and fewer feelings of deprivation.

Disadvantages

Poor glucose control may lead to immediate symptoms such as fatigue or increased urination after the meal, and may increase the chances of long-term diabetic complications.

The role of the diabetes educator within the empowerment approach is to help patients discover options available and to make sure patients are aware of the potential consequences of each course of action.

SPECIAL OCCASIONS

Holidays and family celebrations are frequently times when larger amounts of food and special desserts are eaten. More sophisticated patients can be guided through a series of questions to help them discover the various options available and the associated advantages and disadvantages as described earlier.

Less sophisticated patients are typically aware that avoidance of sweets and excess portions of fatty foods is advisable. If possible, direct patients to sources that can provide options for holiday foods that contain less fat and less sugar. Otherwise, patients can be greatly relieved of their anxiety and guilt by letting them know that one day of poor eating usually does not lead to immediate diabetic complications. Patients can be advised to attempt to take a walk and to increase water intake (to compensate for possible polyuria) after excessive food consumption. The educator may be able to advise a one-time insulin increase according to a physician's recommendation. Patients can be taught to reduce consumption of other carbohydrates, including healthy foods such as fruit or bread or potatoes, when a dessert is planned.

Some educators are concerned that teaching patients about this type of behavior and allowing it on special occasions may encourage more frequent dietary indiscretions. However, many patients with diabetes choose to indulge whether or not they have discussed it with the diabetes team. An open discussion encourages better understanding of some immediate behaviors that help minimize the effect of dietary indiscretion and promotes more honesty and rapport in the relationship with patients and families.

INTENSIVE INSULIN THERAPY

For more sophisticated patients who wish to have greater flexibility in meal timing and content, along with improved glycemic control, a number of intensive insulin regimens are available. Generally, the more injections per day and the more doses of regular insulin that are used, the more flexible a patient's life style can be. Another intensive insulin regimen involves use of an insulin pump (discussed later). It is outside the scope of this chapter to expand on the different intensive insulin regimens. Educators interested in this topic should read Chapter 5 and information located in books and magazines listed in the Appendix.

ALTERNATIVE METHODS OF INSULIN DELIVERY

Several devices have been developed in an attempt to simplify the procedures involved in drawing up and injecting insulin. These devices may be especially useful for patients injecting insulin several times per day.

Injection Ports

These devices are similar in concept to intravenous ports used for intravenous piggyback medications in hospitalized patients. However, they are inserted by patients into the subcutaneous tissue and remain in place for 2 to 3 days. The Button Infuser has a 27-gauge needle attached to a resealable injection port. Another device called the Insulfon has a flexible Teflon catheter with an injection port attached. Inside the Teflon catheter, this device has an introducer needle that is removed once the catheter is in place. Patients then give their insulin injections through the resealable port rather than puncture their skin many times daily. One company, Disetronic, Inc., is working at developing a port for insulin pump delivery. The port is inserted surgically under the skin of the peritoneum. A catheter is positioned to float in the peritoneal cavity to deliver the insulin. The catheter of the external continuous infusion pump can be connected to the external port to deliver the insulin in a fashion mimicking an implantable insulin pump.

Insulin Pens

These devices use small (200-U) prefilled insulin cartridges that are housed in a pen-like holder. A disposable needle is attached to the device for injection of the insulin. Insulin is delivered by dialing in a dose and/or pushing a button for every 1- or 2-U increment given. The insulin pen eliminates the need to draw up insulin before each injection. These devices are most useful for patients who need to inject only one type of insulin each time (e.g., premeal rapid-acting insulin three times a day and bedtime NPH) or who use premixed insulin.

Jet Injectors

As an alternative to needle injections, jet injection devices deliver insulin through the skin under pressure in an extremely fine stream. These devices are more expensive than the other alternative devices mentioned earlier and require thorough training and supervision when first used. In addition, patients should be cautioned that absorption rates, peak insulin activity, and insulin levels may be different when switching to a jet injector. (Insulin given by jet injector usually works faster.)

Insulin Pumps

Small, externally worn pump devices attempt to mimic the functioning of the normal pancreas by supplying insulin in a similar manner. Insulin pumps contain a syringe attached to a long (42-inch), thin, spaghetti-like tube with a needle or Teflon catheter attached to the end. Patients insert the needle or catheter into the subcutaneous tissue (usually on the abdomen) and secure it with tape or a transparent dressing. The needle or catheter is changed at least every 2 to 3 days. The pump is then worn either on a belt or in a pocket. Some women keep the pump tucked into the front or side of their bra or wear it on a garter belt on the thigh.

The pump delivers only short- or rapid-acting insulin, which is delivered in two different ways. First, a continuous amount of insulin, the basal rate, is typically infused at a rate of 0.5 to 2.0 U/hr. Then, before each meal, patients activate the pump (through a series of button pushes) to deliver a bolus dose of insulin. Patients can decide on the amount of insulin bolus to give on the basis of blood glucose levels. For some patients,

anticipated food intake and activity level also influence that decision. Multiple companies currently manufacture insulin pumps in the United States, they include: Medtronic MiniMed, Disetronic, Animas and Deltec. The educator can play an active role in helping patients in the decision making process. Comparison of pump features can be found on the internet at sites such as www.Childrenwithdiabetes.com, or the yearly Buyers Guide published by the ADA.

Intensive training and follow-up are necessary for successful insulin pump therapy. Patients interested in this method of insulin administration should be referred to a diabetes program with a health care team experienced in the use of insulin pumps.

PREVENTING, DETECTING, AND TREATING ACUTE COMPLICATIONS

HYPOGLYCEMIA

Definition

Hypoglycemia is defined as a blood glucose level less than 50 to 60 mg/dl, often associated with symptoms (although some patients with diabetes lose their hypoglycemic warning signs, which is known as *hypoglycemia unawareness*). It can occur suddenly and is caused by an imbalance between the amount of insulin available (including increased insulin secretion caused by sulfonylurea agents or meglitinides), food eaten, and activity. Some patients, however, may experience signs and symptoms of hypoglycemia when the blood glucose level is much higher than 50 to 60 mg/dl. These patients have been in poor control previously and have accommodated to higher blood glucose levels. More normal glucose concentrations are perceived as too low. Patients may take several weeks to accommodate to these new, lower glucose levels. Other terms that patients may use to refer to hypoglycemia include *insulin shock* and *insulin reactions*. Insulin-treated patients who maintain near-normal blood glucose levels may experience two to three mild (easily recognized and treated) episodes of hypoglycemia per week.

Signs and Symptoms

The body has two main responses to hypoglycemia. First, several hormones (glucagon, epinephrine, growth hormone, and cortisol) are released into the bloodstream to help increase the amount of circulating glucose. The former two hormones act rapidly to bring blood glucose levels back up to normal. Epinephrine causes the autonomic (adrenergic) symptoms of hypoglycemia, which include weakness, sweating, nervousness, anxiety, tachycardia, shakiness, tingling of the mouth or fingers, and hunger.

The second type of response to hypoglycemia results from a decreased level of glucose in the brain. These symptoms are called *neuroglucopenic* and may include headache, visual disturbances, mental dullness, confusion, amnesia, seizures, or coma. Patients who have had type 1 diabetes for longer than 5 years have lost their ability to secrete glucagon in response to hypoglycemia, and some patients (after having diabetes for a longer duration) lose their ability to secrete epinephrine as well. Therefore those patients who have lost both hormonal responses have no immediate defense against hypoglycemia, do not experience the autonomic symptoms of hypoglycemia, and develop only the much more serious neuroglucopenic symptoms. Tight control of blood glucose levels can lower the threshold for sensing hypoglycemia. In addition, hypoglycemia on one day can cause a decrease in hypoglycemic symptoms on the next day.

Causes

The main causes of hypoglycemia in patients with diabetes include too much insulin (if taking insulin), sulfonylurea agents, too little food (carbohydrate), a delayed or missed meal, or excessive physical activity. Alcohol consumption may contribute to hypoglycemia if patients miss meals. In many cases, however, the exact reason why the hypoglycemia occurred is impossible to determine.

Inadequate Food Intake

When patients are initially started on insulin, the insulin doses are chosen to match their anticipated meal plan. Therefore, if patients' food intake decreases, that usual insulin dose may be excessive. This can occur when patients miss a meal, attempt to reduce their caloric intake, or choose to eat less for a given meal. Patients on intensive insulin regimens can reduce their premeal insulin dose, but those without this flexibility may develop hypoglycemia. If changes in the meal plan are persistent, the physician should alter the patient's insulin regimen (or sulfonylurea agent or meglitinide dose). If patients must delay a meal, they should be instructed to eat a small snack containing carbohydrate at the usual mealtime to prevent the occurrence of hypoglycemia (or delay taking their meglitinide until the actual mealtime).

Insulin

Accidental injection of too much insulin may lead to hypoglycemia. Patients need to be as precise as possible in drawing up insulin. If visual problems develop, the patient's diabetes health care team should be notified. Additionally, any planned changes in diet or physical activity should be discussed with the physician so that insulin dose changes can be made.

The area into which insulin is injected may occasionally contribute to hypoglycemia. For example, exercise increases the blood flow to the area of the body being used. If insulin is injected into the thigh and the patient then performs exercises using the thigh (e.g., running), the increased blood flow to this area may cause insulin to be absorbed into the bloodstream more rapidly. Similarly, insulin injected into muscle rather than fat tissue may be carried into the bloodstream more rapidly, causing hypoglycemia.

Exercise

During exercise, the muscles use up glucose, which can decrease the level of glucose in the bloodstream, especially if pre-exercise glucose levels are normal to low. If patients using insulin do not eat extra carbohydrate before strenuous exercise, they may develop hypoglycemia. It is important to realize that any physical activities (including those not typically viewed as exercise) may cause hypoglycemia. These include gardening, cleaning, shopping, vacuuming, and moving furniture. Increasing food intake before these activities (or planning physical activity immediately after scheduled meals or snacks, when the glucose level is the highest) is important. A more detailed discussion of how exercise causes hypoglycemia can be found in Chapter 9, and an approach to preventing exercise-induced hypoglycemia in Chapter 3.

Alcohol

Although a moderate amount of alcohol may be safely added to the diet if taken with meals, it can contribute to hypoglycemia if patients eat irregularly when drinking alcohol. Normally, when a person is not eating, the liver produces glucose to prevent hypoglycemia. Alcohol interferes with the ability of the liver to produce glucose (specifically, it inhibits gluconeogenesis). If a patient with diabetes is taking insulin or a sulfonylurea agent, has not eaten for a while, and then drinks alcohol, hypoglycemia may occur if the individual does not eat for several more hours.

Treatment (Patient Conscious)

The treatment of hypoglycemia is to eat some form of sugar. The amount of sugar recommended for treating hypoglycemia varies from 10 to 20 g of glucose. Patients may use commercial preparations of glucose, such as glucose that comes in 3- and 5-g tablets. These are chewable tablets that dissolve rapidly when eaten, and some

brands are available in various flavors. Also available are glucose gels. Other sources of concentrated sugar include juice, soda (nondiet), table sugar, honey, and LifeSavers (see Table 9-3). It is preferable to use commercial preparations of glucose because they provide a precise amount of glucose, are rapidly absorbed, and may offer less temptation to patients to overtreat hypoglycemia. *If patients are taking acarbose (Precose)or miglitol (Glyset), an oral antidiabetic medication, they must take a commercial preparation of glucose or milk to treat hypoglycemia.* These alpha-glucosidase inhibitors block the digestion of most carbohydrates such as table sugar, those in fruit and juice, and starches. Therefore eating these carbohydrates does not correct low blood glucose levels.

After taking approximately 10 to 15 g of glucose, patients should wait 10 to 15 minutes for the symptoms to resolve. If they have no improvement, they should take another 10 g of glucose. Once symptoms begin to resolve, a small snack should be eaten to prevent the recurrence of hypoglycemia. This snack should include a small amount of starch (one bread exchange) and 1 to 2 ounces of protein. Examples include cheese and crackers, milk and crackers, or half of a sandwich. If the next meal is to be eaten in 30 to 60 minutes, the snack is not necessary.

The use of dessert foods such as candy, cookies, and ice cream for treatment of hypoglycemia should be avoided. These foods are high in calories and may not work as rapidly to increase the blood glucose level because of the high fat content (which delays absorption of carbohydrate). In addition, it is difficult for many patients while experiencing hypoglycemic symptoms to limit the amount of sugar eaten in this form. From a psychologic perspective, dessert foods may be seen as a reward for experiencing hypoglycemia. This may limit patients' perception of the seriousness of this diabetic emergency and the importance of recognizing and treating hypoglycemia.

To avoid delays in treatment of hypoglycemia, patients should always carry some form of sugar and always wear and carry some form of identification (see Appendix). If patients taking insulin experience unusual symptoms at any time, it is always safer to treat the symptoms as if hypoglycemia has occurred rather than delay treatment because of uncertainty about the cause of symptoms. On the other hand, if they have the opportunity, patients may wish to measure the blood glucose level to document hypoglycemia. However, transient hyperglycemia does not create the same danger as worsening hypoglycemia.

Treatment (Patient Unconscious or Unwilling to Eat)

The commercial preparations and foods discussed earlier are effective only when swallowed. Therefore they cannot be used if patients are unconscious.

An injection of glucagon (1 mg) should be given to persons who lose consciousness because of a severe hypoglycemic reaction or who, after repeated attempts, absolutely refuse to take sugar by mouth (the irrational behavior is usually a result of the hypoglycemia). As discussed earlier, glucagon (a hormone that is made by the β cells in the islets of Langerhans in the pancreas) raises the blood glucose level by causing the liver to produce more glucose. It is sold as a prescription drug for emergencies and is a powder. A solution (diluent) to mix with the powder is provided in the package, either in a separate bottle or in a prefilled syringe. If in a bottle, draw up the liquid in the patient's (1 ml) insulin syringe. The liquid must be mixed with the powder until the resulting solution is clear (which occurs rapidly). All of the solution is then drawn up in the syringe provided or in the patient's (1 ml) insulin syringe and injected.

After the injection, turn the head of an unconscious patient to the side to avoid choking in case vomiting occurs when consciousness is regained. The glucagon may require 15 to 20 minutes to take effect. When patients regain consciousness, give them sugar and a snack for prevention of another hypoglycemic reaction. If no response occurs within 15 to 20 minutes, paramedics should be called.

The technique for drawing up and injecting glucagon should be taught to a family member, coworker, neighbor, or other person who spends time with the patient. It is sometimes helpful to encourage patients to allow this person to draw up and inject insulin on a periodic basis to maintain confidence in the skills required to use a syringe and give an injection under emergency conditions.

Hypoglycemia: Self-Management Education

Until patients actually experience hypoglycemic symptoms, it may be difficult for them to comprehend or memorize the symptoms and treatment for hypoglycemia. Simply giving patients a list or pamphlet describing the symptoms (especially if low and high blood glucose levels are addressed in the same pamphlet) does not usually ensure comprehension. Patients may be confused to find some similarities in the list of symptoms for low and high glucose levels (headache, fatigue, weakness, blurry vision). Patients may feel undue pressure to be able to differentiate hypoglycemia from hyperglycemia before treating themselves with carbohydrate consumption. Thus, for safety purposes, it is important for the educator of new patients with diabetes to emphasize the more serious nature of low sugar (as compared with high sugar) and to reassure patients that eating sugar when it was not really low does not have serious consequences for a hyperglycemic patient. Emphasize that problems resulting from low blood glucose levels can develop rapidly (minutes to 1 hour), whereas problems caused by high blood glucose levels take much longer to develop (days to weeks).

Basic Teaching Guidelines

Listed next are some basic facts to address with both newly diagnosed patients with diabetes and veteran patients with diabetes, especially if a sulfonylurea agent or insulin has been added to the regimen. In addition to reviewing the symptoms, emphasize the following:

- Low blood sugar is an emergency.
- If you feel any unusual symptoms, test your blood sugar immediately.
- To treat low blood sugar, or hypoglycemia, we want you to eat the type of foods that you usually are supposed to avoid.
- Carry some form of sugar (sugar packets, LifeSavers, raisins, dextrose tablets) at all times.
- Don't worry about making a mistake. If you are not sure that you are having a low sugar reaction, eat sugar anyway.
- Low blood sugar is more of an emergency than high blood sugar, except in rare cases.
- It's important to learn to avoid low blood sugar by eating snacks and extra food. Even though a low sugar reaction might not feel very serious, it can cause terrible problems if it happens in a dangerous place (like when you are driving).

Teaching Tips for All Patients

To reinforce the importance of carrying some form of sugar and identification, ask patients at each visit to show the nurse the sugar source being carried for treatment of hypoglycemia and identification tags or cards. If possible, keep a supply of sample glucose products available to give patients who are not carrying any sugar. Be sure to explain to patients that it is not safe to plan on purchasing soda or juice as needed whenever hypoglycemia occurs. Rather, encourage patients to carry the sugar constantly, especially when driving or participating in physical activity.

Prevention

Many patients may be tempted to increase their dose of oral agent or insulin on finding an elevated glucose result. They should not do this on the basis of one result only (unless given guidance on using extra amounts of short- or rapid-acting insulin to compensate). In addition, patients taking medication need to understand that it is not safe to assume that they will always feel a low blood sugar reaction in an appropriate location and time frame to prevent a serious problem. Thus, rather than waiting until the symptoms occur, prevention is crucial.

1. Consistent technique of insulin injection and rotation of sites are important (see the earlier section on insulin).
2. Insulin dosage should be adjusted only according to a physician's guidelines.
3. If meals are going to be more than 4 to 5 hours apart, a snack should be eaten, unless on a flexible insulin regimen with a basal insulin dose.
4. Monitor blood sugar before, during, and after exercise. Depending on the type and duration of exercise, additional carbohydrates may need to be ingested (or insulin dose decreased).
5. When patients are sick and normal intake of food is decreased (but the insulin dose remains the same), they should eat any form of carbohydrate (e.g., regular soda, Jell-O, ice cream) (see the later section on sick day rules).

HYPERGLYCEMIA

The syndromes of hyperglycemia (high blood glucose level) are (1) diabetes out of control, (2) DKA, and (3) hyperosmolar nonketotic syndrome (HNKS).

Diabetic control is a term used to describe a patient's usual blood glucose concentrations.

Poor control signifies marked hyperglycemia; strict or tight control implies glucose levels more near normal. Uncontrolled diabetes leads to the symptoms of polyuria, polydipsia, and nocturia. An explanation of both normal and abnormal glucose metabolism follows to provide a detailed understanding of the processes that lead to hyperglycemia.

Postprandial (After Eating)—Normal State

After GI absorption of the carbohydrate contained in a meal, plasma glucose levels rise. This stimulates insulin secretion from the pancreatic β cells located in the islets of Langerhans. After its release, insulin binds to specific receptors located on the cell surfaces of liver, muscles, and fat tissue, where it exerts an effect for several hours after its binding. This results in the storage of the carbohydrate from the meal largely as glycogen (the storage form of glucose). In persons without diabetes, glucose levels rise between 20 and 50 mg/dl 1 to 2 hours after a meal and return to baseline before the next meal.

Postabsorptive (Fasting)—Normal State

In the postabsorptive state (i.e., after all of the food from meals has been absorbed and stored in the tissue); glucose concentrations are regulated within a narrow range (70 to 100 mg/dl). This is accomplished by very precise mechanisms by which the liver releases almost the exact amount of glucose that the tissues require. The glucose is produced by the liver through two separate pathways, *glycogenolysis* (breakdown of glycogen) and *gluconeogenesis* (synthesis of new glucose from other molecules). The control of glucose production by the liver is regulated by the balance between insulin (which inhibits production of glucose) and glucagon (which stimulates production of glucose).

Postprandial Hyperglycemia

When carbohydrate metabolism begins to deteriorate, diabetes starts to develop. Postprandial blood glucose concentrations fail to return to normal before the next meal. Once glucose levels exceed the kidneys' ability for glucose reabsorption, glucose is lost in the urine and urine test results for glucose become positive (glucosuria). This usually occurs at glucose levels above 180 mg/dl. Patients often have minimal or no symptoms at this time, although they may complain of mild fatigue.

Fasting Hyperglycemia

The next stage of worsening carbohydrate metabolism is the loss of normal regulation of glucose production by the liver. This leads to fasting hyperglycemia, which leads to even higher preprandial and postprandial blood glucose levels. When blood glucose levels become higher, usually above 180 mg/dl (or higher in older patients), they exceed the renal threshold for glucose. This means that sugar is lost in the urine. When glucose is in the urine, water is drawn out with it; hence, patients start to urinate frequently (polyuria)—especially noticeable at night (nocturia)—and drink increasing amounts of fluids (polydipsia). As insulin becomes increasingly unavailable and/or ineffective, the body is unable to utilize sufficient calories. This leads to weight loss even though patients usually have increased hunger (polyphagia).

The phenomenon of diabetes out of control can usually be treated in the outpatient setting with close follow-up. Patients with type 2 diabetes may either be relatively asymptomatic and may have had a blood glucose level measured for other reasons or may have sought medical attention for symptoms of poorly controlled diabetes (polyuria, polydipsia, nocturia, and/or unintentional weight loss). For patients with type 2 diabetes, outpatient treatment may involve initiating diet measures and starting or increasing oral diabetes medication. It is imperative that patients be able to retain fluids. If patients are vomiting and/or unable to drink fluids, then hospitalization is often needed because they are at risk for developing severe dehydration or HNKS (described later).

Diabetes out of control in patients with type 1 diabetes may be a more serious situation because it can rapidly progress to DKA, which, if untreated, can render patients seriously ill. If patients are newly diagnosed with type 1 diabetes or are vomiting and unable to drink fluids, hospitalization is often needed.

Ketosis

In patients whose diabetes is out of control and in whom the amount of effective insulin becomes very low or absent (usually only in type 1 diabetes), an increase in ketone body formation, or ketosis, can occur. This occurs because without insulin, the body cannot utilize glucose effectively. Therefore fat breakdown occurs to provide extra energy. A byproduct of increased fat breakdown is ketone body formation (by the liver). If patients do not receive insulin (and the pancreas is not able to produce insulin, as in type 1 diabetes), ketone body production increases, causing an acid-base imbalance called DKA.

Diabetic Ketoacidosis

If a patient develops DKA and is not treated quickly and appropriately, coma and eventually death ensue. The biochemical hallmarks of DKA are electrolyte depletion, dehydration, and acidosis (see Chapter 6 for a detailed discussion of DKA).

Symptoms. The signs and symptoms of DKA result from the high levels of blood glucose and ketone bodies (Figure 12-12). In

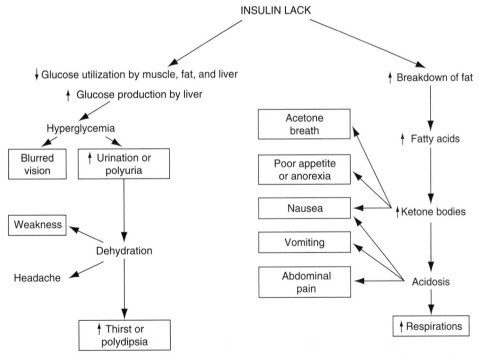

FIGURE 12-12. Abnormal metabolism that causes signs and symptoms of diabetic ketoacidosis. ↑, increased; ↓, decreased.

an attempt to rid the body of the excess glucose, the kidneys excrete extra glucose and water. Both urination and thirst increase. In addition, high blood glucose levels and dehydration can lead to headache, weakness, and fatigue.

The acidosis caused by the ketone bodies produces an additional set of symptoms. Most importantly, patients often have abdominal pain, nausea, and vomiting and are unable to ingest the fluids necessary to prevent worsening dehydration. Symptoms of acidosis often include difficulty in catching one's breath, rapid or deep breathing, headache, and a sweet or fruity smell on the breath.

Causes. A common cause of DKA is illness. During illness, insulin resistance tends to increase, with a subsequent increase in blood glucose levels. It is important that patients do not omit insulin injections when ill, even if regular meals are not being eaten. Patients also must receive prompt medical treatment for any infectious process that may develop to avoid triggering DKA. Stopping insulin injections or inappropriately decreasing the dose of insulin can cause DKA in patients with type 1 diabetes. All of the causes of DKA listed earlier can largely be prevented if patients are treated appropriately with adequate insulin therapy throughout periods of illness as well as health. However, some patients (often children) who do not know they have diabetes first come to the attention of their physicians with DKA as the initial manifestation of their disease.

Treatment. In the early stages of DKA, treatment includes adjustment or initiation (if DKA is the initial sign of diabetes) of insulin therapy and drinking large quantities of salt-containing fluids. For more advanced cases, especially if nausea and vomiting prevent oral intake of fluids, hospitalization is necessary to institute treatment. In the hospital, patients are given a large volume of intravenous fluids for the first several hours, along with potassium and other electrolytes. In addition, insulin is given in an intravenous solution. DKA is usually resolved within 24 hours, although treatment sometimes takes longer. It is important to treat the underlying cause of the DKA if one is present. Once patients have recovered from their DKA, subcutaneous insulin injections must be started when the intravenous insulin infusion is stopped. Otherwise, patients could become insulin deficient again and have a another episode of DKA.

Prevention and Education. The most important way for patients to prevent DKA is to take insulin every day and to call their medical care provider if they become ill with elevated blood glucose levels, particularly if they have nausea and vomiting. If a patient becomes ill, sick day rules (discussed later) should be followed to avert the development of DKA.

HYPEROSMOLAR NONKETOTIC SYNDROME

In patients with type 2 diabetes, some insulin is still being produced by the pancreas (even if patients have to take insulin to help control blood glucose levels) and prevents the development of ketoacidosis. However, symptomatic hyperglycemia can occur in patients with type 2 diabetes, especially during periods of illness or stress. In a few patients (often older adults), the polyuria and polydipsia are ignored, and symptomatic hyperglycemia is tolerated for many weeks. In this situation, hyperglycemia can become so profound and prolonged that patients can experience extreme dehydration with glucose levels exceeding 1000 mg/dl. This causes decreased mentation that can progress to coma. This is called *hyperosmolar nonketotic coma.*

Symptoms

The symptoms are similar to those of DKA, except that overbreathing and a fruity odor on the breath do not occur. The GI symptoms (nausea, vomiting, abdominal pain) usually are less severe or are absent. Increased urination and thirst are most prominent. Patients may have seizures or symptoms similar to having a stroke (e.g., slurred speech, weakness of an arm or leg).

Causes

HNKS is often associated with an illness or infection. It is important for patients with type 2 diabetes to realize that illness can cause increases in blood glucose levels and that communication with a physician during times of illness is important. The general sick day rules should be followed, as indicated. Patients with type 2 diabetes do not need to test their urine for ketones, but blood (or urine) glucose monitoring, eating and drinking properly, and notifying a physician of symptoms are important. Some patients with type 2 diabetes may temporarily require insulin during illness or other stressful situations, such as surgery, to avoid severe hyperglycemia or HNKS.

Treatment

The treatment of HNKS is similar to that of DKA, although the dehydration may be more severe and patients (who tend to be older adults) may tolerate vigorous fluid replacement poorly. Treatment of HNKS usually takes several days longer than treatment of DKA, because patients with HNKS tend to be sicker and to have more severe hyperglycemia. Unlike patients with DKA, however, patients with HNKS may not need insulin when they leave the hospital (i.e., they can be treated with diet alone or in combination with oral diabetes medications). It is very important to search for the cause of patients' HNKS because many have an underlying infection, myocardial infarction, or other illness that requires treatment in addition to the treatment of HNKS.

SICK DAY RULES

When teaching a patient about sick day rules, it is important to differentiate between patients with type 1 diabetes and type 2 diabetes (even though some may be treated with insulin). This was discussed earlier, but is particularly important in this section because patients with type 1 diabetes can develop DKA in the absence of adequate intake of carbohydrate and injection of insulin, whereas sick patients with type 2 diabetes with a decreased caloric intake may not require any insulin at all. In patients with type 1 diabetes, testing for urine ketones (Figure 12-13) is necessary during periods of illness because hyperglycemia with negative urine ketones is not as serious a condition as hyperglycemia in the presence of small to moderate urine ketones, which could portend the development of DKA.

SELF-MANAGEMENT EDUCATION: HYPERGLYCEMIA

Patients can become confused or forgetful if they are simply given a list of symptoms of hyperglycemia. They may notice that some of the symptoms are similar to those associated with hypoglycemia, such as fatigue, drowsiness, or blurred vision. To assist learning, the educator can provide an image or "anchor" with which patients can associate hyperglycemia. If patients have already had the experience of symptomatic hyperglycemia, ask them to describe the feelings in their own words. Make sure they are aware that these are the symptoms to associate with high blood glucose levels. For sophisticated patients, the educator could

How To Test

You can buy a ketone testing kit at your pharmacy. You don't need a prescription. Don't wait until you're sick to get one—keep one in your house and check the expiration date every six months.

Urine tests for ketones come in three forms: test strips, tapes, and tablets. To test:

1. Dip the strip or tape in your urine, or put drops of urine on a tablet.

2. Wait. The directions tell you how long—from 10 seconds to 2 minutes, depending on the brand you're using.

3. Match the color of the strip, tape, or tablet to the color chart on the package.

Results will be negative, trace, small, moderate, or large.

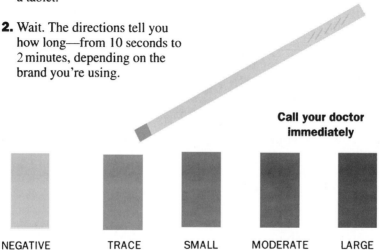

Call your doctor immediately

NEGATIVE   TRACE   SMALL   MODERATE   LARGE

FIGURE 12-13. Patient instructions for urine testing for ketones. *(From Lebovitz HE: Keeping clear of ketoacidosis. Diabetes Forecast 48:20, 1995.)*

describe the progression of hyperglycemia as presented earlier in this section.

If patients have not experienced symptomatic hyperglycemia and need a simplified explanation, the educator could use an image such as, "When your blood sugar is high, the blood is filled with sugar and is very sweet and sticky. This makes you move slowly (like honey) and feel tired. Your body wants to get rid of the sugar or clean it out, so it pushes the sugar out into your urine and this makes you urinate a lot. Your body also tries to get more water to water down all the extra sugar, so it takes water from your tongue and mouth (dry mouth, thirst), and

from your eyes (blurry vision)." Learning is most effective if the educator involves patients in the discussion by asking questions during the explanation (e.g., "When your body wants to get rid of the extra sugar, how can the sugar escape from your body? If your body takes a lot of water from your mouth and tongue, how does it make you feel?").

HYPERGLYCEMIA/SICK DAY RULES—TYPE 2 DIABETES

1. *Hyperglycemia may not always cause dramatic (noticeable) symptoms.* Therefore, after dia-

betes is diagnosed, it is important to have regular doctor appointments and blood tests even if you feel well.

2. *Symptom education/recognition.* Symptoms of hyperglycemia include fatigue, thirst, excess urination, blurry vision, vaginal infections, and sores that heal slowly over a period of a few days or weeks. (At this point, have a discussion with patients in which they describe past experiences of hyperglycemia, or give patients an anchor story as described earlier.)

3. *Causes of hyperglycemia.* Blood sugar levels may increase in certain situations, such as increased stress, illness, or surgery. Certain medications, such as asthma medicine or steroids, may cause very high blood sugar levels. Increases in blood sugar levels may also result from an inadequate dose of diabetes medication, especially when combined with problems with diet recommendations or a decrease in exercise.

4. *Treatment of hyperglycemia.* Drink fluids, test your blood sugar level (if you have the equipment), and stay in touch with your diabetes health care professional. To avoid dehydration, *drink extra fluids* (at least one glass every hour) even if you are not thirsty. Good choices include water, broth, decaffeinated tea, diet soda, diet iced tea, diet Kool-Aid, and sugar-free Popsicles. *Take all diabetic medications.* However, sometimes your diabetes health care provider may tell you to change the amount of medication. Also, the doctor may prescribe antibiotics if you have an infection—be sure to take all of the antibiotic pills, even if you are feeling better.

5. *Sick day rules: Appetite normal or slightly reduced.* If you are sick and your appetite is normal, be sure to take all of your diabetic medication and drink extra fluids. If you are sick and your appetite is less than normal, take all your diabetic medication and eat smaller meals every few hours, along with extra fluids. Avoid foods that are high in fat content and avoid dairy products if you have diarrhea.

6. *Sick day rules: Appetite poor or unable to eat solid foods.* In this situation, the ability to monitor blood sugar levels at home can be useful in making decisions about what to eat and what medication to take. It is important to continue drinking fluids and to communicate with your diabetes health care provider. If your blood sugar levels are high (>250 mg/dl), drink sugar-free fluids as listed earlier, and if they are low (<150 mg/dl), drink sugar-containing fluids. In some instances, it may be necessary to decrease your diabetes medication (especially if symptoms of low blood sugar levels develop). In other circumstances, no dose change should occur. Be sure to continue taking your diabetes medication as prescribed until you speak with your diabetes health care provider, who can give you advice and follow you through your illness. It is particularly important to do this if your blood sugar levels remain above 300 mg/dl or below 100 mg/dl.

7. *Signs of severe dehydration.* If you become sick and unable to eat or drink, you can become dehydrated. If this occurs, you or your family must call your doctor or you must be taken to the hospital, especially if you become confused or sleepy or cannot be awakened.

HYPERGLYCEMIA/SICK DAY RULES—TYPE I DIABETES

1. *Insulin: Never stop taking insulin.* Patients with type 1 diabetes should take their usual dose of insulin when they are ill (including short- or rapid-acting insulin), unless instructed by their physician to do otherwise. For patients with type 1 diabetes, insulin is needed even if food intake is decreased. Illness tends to raise blood sugar levels, and thus the same dose or even more insulin usually is safe. Patients with type 2 diabetes who require insulin may be able to lower the dose if food intake is markedly decreased. A physician's guidance is often needed (see

number 3, following, for guidelines for eating).

2. *Monitoring: Check the blood sugar* at least four times a day. In patients with type 1 diabetes, blood or *urine testing for ketones* should occur several times per day, especially when blood sugar levels are above 250 mg/dl in association with illness. *Notify your physician* if the urine ketones become more than trace positive and/or the blood glucose level is above 300 mg/dl (or urine sugar levels are 1% to 2%).

3. *Eating:* If the normal meal pattern cannot be followed, eat soft foods or drink liquids instead. It may by necessary to eat soft foods or drink liquids that contain sugar to avoid hypoglycemia. Having food and liquids with salt and minerals is also important. Table 12-8 contains a list of foods commonly used for carbohydrate replacement during an illness. Some examples of soft foods include ⅓ cup regular gelatin, 1 cup cream soup, ½ cup custard, and three squares of graham crackers. Eat these six to eight times per day until the regular diet is resumed. Examples of liquids include ½ cup regular cola, ½ cup orange juice, 1 cup Gatorade, and ½ cup broth. Drink these every hour if you have vomiting, diarrhea, or a fever. It is important to drink liquids whenever you have an illness. However, if soft foods or the normal foods can be eaten, limit liquids to broth, tea, water, and diet drinks (i.e., limit the source of carbohydrates to the more slowly absorbable foods rather than the more rapidly absorbed liquids).

4. *Reporting symptoms: Keep your physician informed!* It may be possible to prevent ketoacidosis and avoid hospitalization. Report nausea, vomiting, and diarrhea to your physician, especially if it has not been possible to retain fluids for 3 to 4 hours. Also report any symptoms of possible DKA, such as abdominal pain, fruity breath, or inability to catch your breath. It is usually necessary for persons who have type 1 diabetes and who are unable to retain fluids to be hospitalized to avoid severe dehydration and ketoacidosis.

PREVENTING (THROUGH *RISK REDUCTION* BEHAVIOR), DETECTING, AND TREATING CHRONIC COMPLICATIONS

The long-term complications of diabetes are considered part of the diabetes syndrome, and in many cases, preventing these complications is the primary goal of diabetes treatment. The classification of the complications is summarized in Table 12-9 (see Chapter 7 for a more detailed discussion).

QUESTIONS TO TEST KNOWLEDGE/STIMULATE THOUGHTS

When teaching patients about diabetic complications, it is helpful first to ask them if they are aware of any problems or complications that can happen to people who have diabetes. The diabetes educator should take some time to find out if patients have any particular fears or worries based on past experiences with relatives or acquaintances who suffered a diabetic complication. It is important to try to instill a sense of hope and optimism about the ability of the patient and the health care team working together to prevent diabetic complications. The educator needs to acknowledge that this is not easy to do and requires some work and commitment.

Some patients may be confused by the seemingly unrelated list of problems that can result from diabetes. A simplified introductory explanation may help. Patients can be taught that high blood glucose levels can damage very small blood vessels of the body (such as those found inside the eyes and kidneys) and the nerves (such as those found in the feet and legs). The problem is that the

TABLE 12-8 SICK DAY DIET

Stage	Symptoms	Foods	Frequency
1	Severe nausea, vomiting, severe diarrhea, fever	Orange juice, grapefruit juice, tomato juice, broth, strong tea, coffee, cola, soft drinks.	Sip a tablespoon of liquid every 10 to 15 minutes. Advance to stage 2 when the nausea and the diarrhea have stopped or almost stopped and you are no longer vomiting.
2	Little or no appetite, occasional diarrhea, fatigue, fever	Cream soup, mashed potatoes, cooked cereal, plain yogurt, banana, ice cream, fruit-flavored gelatins, juice, broth, regular soft drinks.	Take ½ cup to 1 cup of food or liquid every 1 to 2 hours. Advance to stage 3 when you have eaten this amount of food several times and your symptoms are improving.
3	Limited appetite but can tolerate small meals, sluggish, slight fever can be sitting up and walking	Food choices are selected using your diabetic meal plan (if you do not have one, talk to a dietitian or diet counselor). At this stage, you do not have to eat your protein and fat food choices. If you feel up to it, advance to stage 4.	Eat as many meals and snacks as planned in your meal plan. This usually means three meals plus an evening snack.
4	General sick feeling; heavy or spicy foods are upsetting	Use your food lists and follow your regular meal. Choose foods that do not give you problems (avoid spicy or high-fat foods). For protein choices, you might want to choose scrambled or soft boiled eggs, cottage cheese, broiled fish, or baked chicken. Eat fruit, vegetables, starch, and protein in moderate amounts according to your usual meal pattern.	Eat at regular meal and snack times. Advance to your regular diabetic meal plan if you have no problems with the easier-to-digest foods for a day. If at any stage your symptoms get worse and you cannot tolerate the described foods, drop back one stage until you feel better.

From Getting Started—Answers to Questions About Sick Days. Becton Dickinson Consumer Products, Becton Dickinson Company, Rochelle Park, NJ, 1995.

TABLE 12-9 LONG-TERM COMPLICATIONS OF DIABETES MELLITUS
Macrovascular (large vessel or atherosclerosis)
Coronary artery disease (angina, myocardial infarction)
Cerebrovascular disease (stroke)
Peripheral vascular disease
Microvascular (small vessel)
Retinopathy (eye)
Nephropathy (kidney)
Neuropathic
Peripheral neuropathy
Autonomic neuropathy

damage does not show up immediately, and when damage to the eyes, kidneys, and nerves does begin, patients may not even know it because often there are no symptoms. People with diabetes can also develop problems with the large blood vessels in the body. Depending on the location of the damage, different problems can occur, such as damage to blood vessels in the heart (heart attack), in the brain (stroke), and in the legs (sores and possibly gangrene).

To prevent the complications, there are things that patients need to do at home and there are things that the health care professionals must do in the office. For example, patients have the job of working on control of blood sugar, blood pressure, and cholesterol levels through diet, exercise, medication, and monitoring. The health care team has the job of looking for any problems with the eyes, kidneys, heart, and so forth by performing certain laboratory tests, physical examinations, and check-ups. It is important to emphasize to patients that even if they have been feeling well or if they have had no problems in carrying out self-care activities at home, they will still benefit greatly from keeping appointments at which the health care team can monitor diabetic complications.

MICROVASCULAR COMPLICATIONS

Diabetic Retinopathy

Diabetic eye disease, commonly called *diabetic retinopathy* (although other structures are sometimes involved), is a potentially very serious complication. Although only 1% to 2% of patients with diabetes become blind, diabetes is so common that it is the leading cause of blindness in persons between the ages of 20 and 74 years.

Background retinopathy, which is characterized by microaneurysms, hemorrhage, and exudates (see Chapter 7 for a description), usually takes approximately 10 years to occur after the onset of diabetes. As many as 80% of patients may eventually develop it. This form of retinopathy does not impair vision unless the area of the eye necessary for central vision (the macula) is involved, resulting in macular edema. Background retinopathy can progress to a more serious form, called *proliferative retinopathy*, in 5% to 10% of patients, most often the ones who maintain poor diabetic control. In this form of retinopathy, new vessels grow (proliferate) on the retina and extend toward the middle of the eye. If they break, the large amounts of blood released into the eye obscure vision, often resulting in permanent visual damage. Fortunately, laser treatment is helpful in forestalling visual loss in both macular edema and proliferative retinopathy. To be most effective, treatment must be given early to prevent damage. Therefore the ADA recommends that patients with type 1 diabetes be monitored yearly with a dilated funduscopic examination (usually performed by an ophthalmologist), beginning 5 years after the onset of diabetes. Patients with type 2 diabetes should be examined yearly from the time of diagnosis. As many as 25% of patients have some degree of retinopathy at the time of diagnosis owing to the hiatus of several years between the development of type 2 diabetes and its diagnosis.

The Lens

Visual impairment secondary to changes in the lens is also more common in patients with diabetes. The shape of the lens can be temporarily distorted owing to hyperglycemia, with resultant blurring of vision until blood glucose levels are normalized. The lens is also more prone to cataract formation in patients with diabetes. Although cataracts may not be more common in the diabetic population, they are approximately five times more likely to develop at a younger age than in the nondiabetic population. Diabetic control (as reflected in glucose levels) does not seem to have a role.

SELF-MANAGEMENT TRAINING

As part of teaching patients prevention of eye complications, the educator should encourage patients to keep a record of the dates of all eye examinations performed by the eye doctor. It should be emphasized that the eyes must be dilated and examined by a specialist. Clarify for patients that an optical examination for new prescription lenses or an examination by their regular physician (especially through undilated eyes) is not sufficient. Emphasize that permanent diabetic eye damage typically does not cause any symptoms in the early stages, when it could be treated. It is thus important to have yearly eye examinations even when vision is fine. It is possible, however, for very low or very high blood glucose levels to cause blurred vision temporarily, but this should resolve when levels become stable. Remind patients that to prevent eye damage, control of blood glucose levels and blood pressure are crucial.

DIABETIC NEPHROPATHY

Diabetic kidney disease (diabetic nephropathy) can be divided into five stages. *Stage I*

occurs at the onset of the disease and is characterized by an increase in kidney size and function. These changes usually return to normal within a few weeks to a few months with treatment that lowers glucose levels.

In *stage II*, kidney size and function are normal (regardless of the duration of diabetes). The kidneys normally excrete a very small amount of albumin (<30 mg/24 hr). Neither the usual laboratory dipstick test for protein nor the more recently developed very sensitive ones detect this amount. Therefore stage 2 is characterized by the urinary excretion of a tiny normal amount of albumin.

Stage III, or incipient diabetic nephropathy, is characterized by an amount of urinary albumin that is greater than normal but still less than the amount detected by the usual laboratory dipstick test for urinary protein. Patients who excrete this amount of albumin, between 30 and 300 mg/24 hr, are said to have *microalbuminuria*. Of these patients, 60% to 80% eventually progress to the next stage if they remain in poor control (e.g., A1C >8% to 9%), compared with only 5% of those without microalbuminuria. Controlling elevated blood pressure, returning glucose levels to near normal, using angiotensin-converting enzyme inhibitors (ACEIs), and/or ingesting a low-protein diet can decrease or possibly reverse microalbuminuria. Some evidence suggests that this may prevent progression of the kidney disease to the next stage.

Stage IV, or overt diabetic nephropathy, is characterized by clinical proteinuria (i.e., a level of urinary albumin [>300 mg albumin per 24 hours] that is detectable [dipstick positive] by tests routinely performed in clinical laboratories). Kidney function starts to decline during this stage, and hypertension is very common. Overt diabetic nephropathy is usually asymptomatic and can take years to progress to a point at which symptoms of renal insufficiency (fatigue, nausea, vomiting) start to occur. Although returning glucose concentrations to near normal does not affect the rate of decrease of kidney function, controlling hypertension, use of ACEIs, and possibly a low-protein diet help preserve kidney function during this stage.

Stage V, or end-stage renal disease, is similar to kidney failure resulting from any other cause. Treatment is usually by hemodialysis or peritoneal dialysis. At present, one third of all patients starting dialysis have kidney failure secondary to diabetic nephropathy. An alternative to dialysis is kidney transplantation if a suitable donor can be found. Because patients with diabetes generally fare worse on dialysis than do patients without diabetes, kidney transplantation is usually preferred, if possible.

Self-Management Education

As part of teaching patients how to prevent kidney damage, the educator should explain that it is important to accurately perform annual urine collection tests (either overnight or 24-hour) if ordered by the physician. If patients do not understand the directions or if they make a mistake and forget to save all the urine requested, encourage them to discuss the situation with the laboratory personnel or the doctor's office and to reperform the test if necessary. Remind patients that even though this type of urine collection is inconvenient, it is very important in detecting any signs of kidney damage before there are ever any symptoms of a problem. Emphasize that control of blood glucose levels and blood pressure are crucial for prevention of diabetic kidney damage.

NEUROPATHY

Diabetic neuropathy is a common long-term complication of diabetes and is the source of severe discomfort for many patients. The two types of neuropathy are peripheral and autonomic. Patients more commonly complain of symptoms associated with peripheral neuropathy than with autonomic neuropathy.

Peripheral Neuropathy

Symptoms of peripheral neuropathy consist of burning sensations, tingling, numbness, and pain in the lower extremities, especially starting in the feet. The pain can become very severe; it sometimes is relieved by walking and is often worse at night. Loss of feeling may occur eventually. This can be dangerous for patients because they cannot appreciate any external trauma to the feet, and they thus must take the appropriate measures either to prevent it from occurring or to treat the initial lesions. If skin breakdown should occur, infection is likely. If foot ulcers are not treated appropriately, amputation may be needed. The combination of a foot infection and impaired circulation resulting from peripheral vascular disease is extremely dangerous. Of all lower extremity amputations in this country, 50% to 75% are performed on patients with diabetes (who make up only 6% of the population). It is estimated that at least half of these amputations could have been avoided. Peripheral neuropathy can also involve the upper extremities. Patients may suffer burns, especially from cooking and smoking, because of the decreased sensation. Muscle atrophy (wasting), which also can occur in the feet, leads to weakness and impairs patients' ability to use their hands normally.

Self-Management Training

Working with patients suffering from the pain of peripheral neuropathy focuses mostly on pain relief measures. Patients first must understand that complete pain relief is often not possible, but measures can be taken to improve their ability to participate in normal activities. For some patients, the pain disappears spontaneously after 6 to 12 months. Persistent neuropathy pain may be treated with oral medications such as antidepressants or anticonvulsants. Another option is use of a topical cream derived from chili peppers (capsaicin). Some patients may benefit from a nondrug method of pain control using a transcutaneous electronic nerve stimulator (TENS) unit. TENS units work by stimulating pain-blocking nerves. In some patients, it may also be possible to improve the symptoms of peripheral neuropathy through improvement in blood glucose control.

Patients who have developed loss of sensation because of neuropathy must be instructed on safety measures for prevention of burns and injuries. Patients need to be made aware that normal daily activities such as driving, walking, and household chores all can be affected by decreased sensation of pressure and decreased ability to appreciate the location of limbs relative to other objects. A referral for occupational therapy is helpful for promoting independence and safety. (Specific education about avoidance of foot problems is discussed later.)

DIABETIC FOOT LESIONS

Foot lesions in patients with diabetes occur frequently, especially in patients with peripheral neuropathy. Most foot lesions can be prevented by educated patients, and if they occur, early treatment is often effective. If the lesions are allowed to progress before therapy is started, the prognosis is much worse. Patients with diabetes are more vulnerable to foot lesions because of three contributory factors:

1. *Neuropathy:* A foot lesion develops when an injury occurs, causing a break in the skin. The skin is the first line of defense against infection, and if its integrity is altered, bacteria may invade and the infectious process is initiated. Neuropathy is often the inciting factor for repeated trauma. This is because of patients' inability to perceive pain or pressure or to distinguish temperatures. Loss of sensation can lead to burns by hot water soaks or baths. The inability to feel pain or pressure can cause patients to be

unaware of such things as blisters caused by ill-fitting or new shoes or foreign objects in a shoe. Wounds can be caused by home surgery on corns, calluses, and toenails.
2. *Vascular disease:* Once an injury occurs, effective circulation is required for the delivery of nutrients and antibiotics. If patients have vascular disease, the healing process is compromised and the injury can worsen, progressing to ulceration, infection, or even gangrene.
3. *Hyperglycemia:* In addition to contributing to vascular problems, hyperglycemia itself can depress the body's defenses against invading bacteria, thus adding to the seriousness of the foot lesions.

Because of these three contributing factors, a minor injury can rapidly become a serious lesion, often eventually requiring some degree of amputation.

Foot Care

Inspection

The key to foot care is to look at the feet. Foot-care education can take place while performing a foot inspection. Shoes and stockings obviously must be removed. Some patients may need to use a mirror to see their feet completely. A foot inspection form (Figure 12-14) provides a record for further visits. The office inspection should serve as a demonstration of self-inspection. In addition, the health care professional should assess patients for protective sensation using a 10-g monofilament (Figure 12-15). If patients are unable to perform self-inspection (e.g., have visual impairment or are obese), it is advisable to involve a family member or other support person in foot-care education. The use of a home health service may be indicated. The following should be carried out during a daily foot inspection (by the health care professional

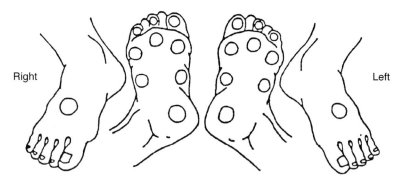

FIGURE 12-14. Foot assessment record.

or the patient). Foot care instructions for patients are summarized in Figure 12-16.

1. Inspect pressure points (Figure 12-17) for corns, calluses, blisters, or redness.
2. Inspect between toes for cracks, signs of fungus, blisters, or discoloration.
3. Inspect the skin for dryness, especially the heels.
4. If a clawfoot (Figure 12-18) or a hammertoe (Figure 12-19) is present, inspect for calluses or blisters on the prominent joints.
5. Call the patient's physician about any changes or signs of infection, such as tenderness, swelling, redness, or an injury that is not healing.

Hygiene

All patients must keep their feet clean and dry. The guidelines listed next should be followed.

1. Wash your feet with mild soap as part of a daily shower or tub bath.

2. Water temperature must not be too hot (test with elbow).
3. Patients who do not shower or bathe daily may clean their feet in a foot basin (if a basin is used, do not soak the feet for more than 10 minutes).
4. Dry carefully between the toes with a soft cloth.
5. Prevent dryness of the skin by applying a skin lubricant daily (e.g., Vaseline Intensive Care, Nivea, Alpha-Keri, Eucerin). Do not apply between the toes.
6. Prevent fungus by removing excess moisture. A small amount of talcum powder may be used between the toes. If a fungal infection develops, an appropriate medication to treat the fungus should be prescribed.

Prevention of Foot Injury

It is most important to emphasize these measures for patients with loss of protective sensation (i.e., cannot feel the 10-g monofilament). Prevent injury to the feet by being aware of

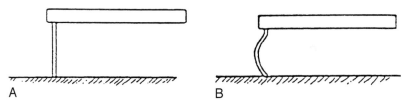

A   B

FIGURE 12-15. Technique of use of 10-g monofilament for foot assessment.

Foot Care for People with Diabetes

People with diabetes have to take special care of their feet.

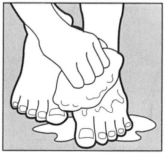
1 **Wash your feet daily** with lukewarm water and soap.

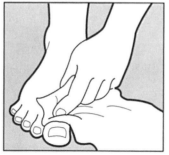
2 **Dry your feet well,** especially between the toes.

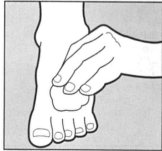
3 **Keep the skin supple** with a moisturizing lotion, but do not apply it between the toes.

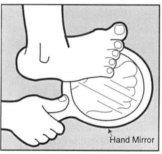
4 **Check your feet** for blisters, cuts or sores. Tell your doctor if you find something wrong.

Hand Mirror

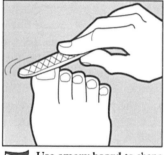
5 **Use emery board** to shape toenails even with ends of your toes.

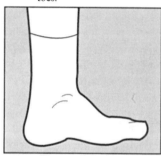
6 **Change daily** into clean, soft socks or stockings, not too big or too small.

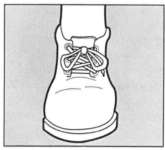
7 **Keep your feet warm and dry.** Preferably wear special padded socks and always wear shoes that fit well.

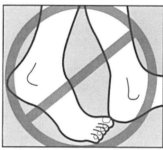
8 **Never walk barefoot** indoors or outdoors.

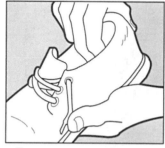
9 **Examine your shoes** every day for cracks, pebbles, nails or anything that could hurt your feet.

Take good care of your feet - and use them.
A brisk walk every day stimulates the circulation.

FIGURE 12-16. Foot-care instructions for patients. *(Courtesy of Nicole Hopkins.)*

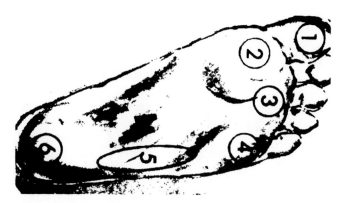

FIGURE 12-17. Pressure points on the bottom of the foot requiring daily inspection. *(From Reed JK: Footwear for the diabetic. In Levin M: The Diabetic Foot, 3rd ed. CV Mosby, St. Louis, 1983, p. 360.)*

potential injuries and practicing the following approaches in foot care:

1. Do not use hot water baths, heating pads, or other heating techniques to warm the feet.
2. Try to avoid placing the feet on or near heat registers, car heaters, or heat lamps.
3. Avoid sunburn.
4. Do not walk barefooted on hot sand or pavement (sandals or water shoes may be necessary).
5. In general, shoes should be worn at all times to protect the feet. Seek medical advice if special shoes or foot appliances are necessary (e.g., cocked-up toe problems). The toe box (toes area) of the shoe should allow for toe expansion. Break in new shoes gradually—initially wear them for only 2 hours at a time.
6. Remove the shoes and inspect the feet for areas of redness or irritation.
7. Use the hand to feel and inspect the inside of the shoes for rough areas, foreign objects, exposed nails, or other protruding surfaces.

Toenail Injuries

Toenail injuries are usually caused by incorrect cutting. The following guidelines should be followed to prevent difficulty:

1. If vision is impaired or if patients are obese and unable to reach their feet, have a podiatrist, physician, or other trained person cut the nails.

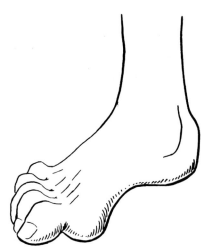

FIGURE 12-18. Clawfoot. *(From Larson CB, Gould M: Orthopedic Nursing, 9th ed. Mosby, St. Louis, 1978, p. 346.)*

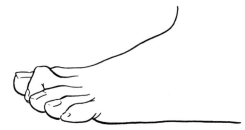

FIGURE 12-19. Hammertoe. *(From Larson CB, Gould M: Orthopedic Nursing, 9th ed. Mosby, St. Louis, 1978, p. 346.)*

2. Before cutting, soften the nails with soft brush, or cut after bathing.
3. Use a nail clipper to cut nails, not scissors, knives, or razor blades.
4. Cut nails straight across. Do not cut into the corners. File any sharp edges with an emery board.
5. Ingrown or thickened nails require special care and should not be self-treated.

Corns and Calluses

Corns and calluses indicate irritation and pressure on the skin and are potential areas for the development of an ulcer. Most ulcers start under a corn on the protruding part of a toe or under a callus on pressure areas of the foot. If the corn or callus is very prominent or if discoloration develops, seek medical advice. Otherwise, the following methods can be used to prevent buildup of a hard callus or cracking of the skin, which is a potential source of infection.

1. First, soften the corn or callus by soaking the feet in a foot basin filled with warm water (no longer than 10 minutes).
2. Rub the corn or callus gently with a soft brush, pumice, or cleansing sponge, and then apply lubricating material. Do not use any tools or commercial preparations for removing corns or calluses (e.g., preparations that contain iodine, bichloride of mercury, or phenol, or corn remedies, corn pads, or adhesives).
3. If corns are caused by overlapping of the toes, place a small amount of lamb's wool between them.
4. Moleskin may be used for protecting any protruding parts of the foot that are subject to irritations.

Circulation Problems

Improve circulation by walking or other physical activities that increase blood flow to the legs. Avoid behaviors or activities that decrease circulation, such as the following:

1. Smoking
2. Sitting with legs crossed at the knees
3. Exposure to extremes in temperature
4. Wearing "gathers" or knee-high stockings that have a narrow elastic top

AUTONOMIC NEUROPATHY

Autonomic neuropathy can involve the GI, genitourinary, and cardiovascular systems. In addition, it may cause hypoglycemia unawareness.

Gastrointestinal Tract

1. *Gastroparesis diabeticorum:* This form of autonomic neuropathy causes delay in the emptying of stomach (gastric) contents, which may lead to unpredictable absorption of food and thus may interfere with diabetic control. Symptoms include feeling full after eating only a small amount of food (early satiety), nausea, and vomiting. It is common for the vomitus to contain food eaten many hours before. Small frequent feedings are helpful, as are metoclopramide (Reglan) and erythromycin. Testing for gastric motility and bacterial overgrowth can be helpful in guiding therapy.
2. *Diabetic enteropathy:* Involvement of the nerves that control the intestinal function can cause either constipation or diarrhea. Constipation is more common. Some patients experience alternating constipation and diarrhea. The diarrhea may occur at night and may get better or worse for no apparent reason. Fecal incontinence occasionally occurs (especially at night) because the anal sphincter does not function normally. Treatment includes antibiotics and antidiarrheal drugs. Some patients with type 1 diabetes may also have celiac disease, and antibody

testing may be indicated in symptomatic patients

Self-Management Education— Gastroparesis

Education of patients with autonomic neuropathy affecting the GI tract focuses on symptom recognition and explanation of treatments as listed earlier. In addition, encouraging frequent glucose monitoring is important for avoidance of unexpected hypoglycemia when food absorption and times of peak insulin action do not match. Patients need to understand that previously taught insulin dose adjustments based on patterns of blood glucose results and/or dose adjustments in anticipation of diet changes may need to be altered in response to inconsistent food absorption. Sometimes postprandial insulin administration is useful. Goals of blood glucose need to be less strict, with emphasis on avoidance of hypoglycemia.

Genitourinary Tract

1. *Neurogenic bladder:* When the bladder expands, autonomic nerves located in the muscle wall give the signal for the bladder to contract, resulting in urination. If these nerves are affected by diabetic autonomic neuropathy, the urge to urinate is delayed until the bladder becomes very full. This process is slow and insidious, but patients may eventually notice infrequent urination. In addition, the strength of contraction is weakened, causing incomplete emptying of the bladder. The urine that remains is a potential source for bacterial growth. Therefore patients with neurogenic bladder often have urinary tract infections that start in the bladder but may ascend to the kidneys.

Treatment involves patient self-care strategies such as self-catheterization to help bladder emptying, drugs that promote bladder contraction, antibiotics, and, in advanced cases, surgery.

Self-Management Education— Neurogenic Bladder

Patients with neurogenic bladder should be instructed to do the following:

- Void frequently (every 2 to 4 hours) on a scheduled basis; this may necessitate use of a watch or clock with an alarm.
- Triple-void. This is a simple technique of voiding as much as possible, resting 1 minute and voiding again, and then repeating once again.
- Perform Crede's maneuver. Press the hands against the lower abdomen to increase the pressure and thereby empty the bladder.

Impotence

Impotence is the inability to complete the act of sexual intercourse successfully because of failure either to initiate or sustain an erection. An erection results from a reflex action that traps blood in the penile shaft. The reflex is transmitted through a group of autonomic nerves originating in the lower part of the pelvic area. As a result of autonomic neuropathy, these nerves are unable to respond to the appropriate stimuli, and an erection can either not take place or if initiated cannot be sustained. Impotence is estimated to be four or five times more common in male patients with diabetes older than 30 years than in nondiabetic individuals in the same age group. It may eventually affect as many as 50% of male patients with diabetes.

In some patients with diabetes, impotence may be due to macrovascular disease in the vessels supplying blood to the penis. Of course, nondiabetic causes of impotence (e.g., psychogenic causes, endocrine causes, drugs, alcohol) may also affect patients with diabetes and must be ruled out. Impotence resulting from diabetes can be treated with oral medications (usually a phophodieste-case-5 [PDE-5] inhibitor such as sildenafil, tadalafil, and vardenafil), vacuum tumescence devices, intrapenile injections, or penile implants.

Self-Management Education— Impotence

Discussion of sexual dysfunction is often a neglected area because both the patients and the health care providers may be embarrassed to address such issues. The educator must make a special effort to openly discuss this important matter with their male patients. It is important to make men with diabetes aware that controlling blood glucose levels and other risks factors such as blood pressure, cholesterol, excessive alcohol intake, and smoking cessation helps prevent impotence. In addition to discussing the various treatment options available, such as oral and injectable medications, devices to help achieve and maintain erection, and implants, the patient should be encouraged to consult a urologist to further discuss the various specific treatment options to help evaluate and resolve the problem.

CARDIOVASCULAR CONDITIONS

The autonomic nervous system is critically important for maintaining the blood pressure when one goes from lying down to standing up. A reduction in systolic blood pressure of 30 mm Hg 1 to 2 minutes after standing up defines orthostatic hypotension. Symptomatic orthostatic hypotension can be quite troublesome for patients with diabetes who have autonomic neuropathy. Treatment usually consists of administration of a salt-retaining hormone, but congestive heart failure is a possible side effect. In addition, patients with diabetes are more likely to have silent myocardial infarction (i.e., heart attacks without pain). This is because of autonomic neuropathy of the nerves innervating the heart so that the chest pain of the heart attack is not felt by patients.

Self-Management Education— Cardiac Autonomic Neuropathy

Patients need to be taught that nerve damage caused by cardiac autonomic neuropathy affects the ability of the heart and blood vessels to function normally. Patients with orthostatic hypotension should be taught to arise slowly from a standing or lying position (i.e., wait a minute or two at each position when moving from lying to sitting or from sitting to standing). Special elastic stockings that extend to the thigh or even waist may be used to help direct blood flow to the heart and brain and to prevent dizziness and falls. Some patients may need to use a wheelchair or walker to prevent falls. An evaluation of the home by an occupational therapist is important for promotion of safety and injury prevention.

Patients with cardiac autonomic neuropathy need to be taught to report any unusual symptoms such as shortness of breath, ankle swelling, or unusual fatigue. They may notice that they become short of breath during light physical activity. Explain to patients that these types of symptoms may be the only indication that they have had a heart attack. They need to understand the seriousness of the potential for a silent (painless) heart attack and the importance of immediately reporting these symptoms no matter how mild they may seem.

HYPOGLYCEMIA UNAWARENESS

One of the causes of hypoglycemia unawareness is autonomic neuropathy. In this situation, failure of the autonomic nervous system leads to impairment of the epinephrine and norepinephrine response to hypoglycemia. Therefore the autonomic symptoms of hypoglycemia are blunted or absent. Thus patients with autonomic neuropathy may be unaware of their low blood glucose level and fail to take appropriate steps to correct it. As the hypoglycemia continues to worsen, they suffer from the more severe signs and symptoms (e.g., visual changes, behavioral changes, confusion, lethargy, and possibly seizures and coma) of neuroglycopenia (see Chapter 6 for a more detailed discussion of this topic).

Self-Management Education

Patients who no longer feel the adrenergic symptoms of hypoglycemia need to understand the serious danger this can pose. Patients may mistakenly enjoy the fact that they can tolerate much lower glucose levels than they used to without the inconvenient symptoms of sweating, shakiness, nervousness, and so forth. Explain to patients that without these warning signs to alert the patient or family to get something to eat, the blood glucose level can drop so low that the brain no longer functions normally. Serious and possibly fatal damage can occur to patients or to people affected by patients if they are driving, operating machinery, walking alone, or supervising young children at the time of the low blood glucose level.

Prevention of low blood glucose levels is absolutely critical for these patients. Thus goals for blood glucose control should be set higher than usual. Extra blood glucose testing is necessary—especially before driving and other types of activities listed earlier. If patients are unable or unwilling to test their glucose levels more often, then more frequent eating of snacks and meals (not more

than about 3 hours between feedings) is required.

MACROVASCULAR COMPLICATIONS

Diseases of the large blood vessels are two (males) to four (females) times more common in patients with diabetes than in persons without diabetes. These conditions include coronary artery disease, peripheral vascular disease, and cerebrovascular disease. Diabetes is only one of the six independent risk factors for macrovascular disease in the general population (Table 12-10). The first four of these risk factors are reversible—that is, once they are eliminated, the risk disappears. As difficult as it may be, patients can quit smoking. Hypertension and hyperlipidemia can be successfully treated by diet and drugs. Although obesity itself is associated with three other risk factors (hypertension, elevated triglyceride levels, and diabetes), it has been identified as an independent risk over and beyond the ones with which it is associated. Like smoking, the treatment of obesity requires a life style change, which, although difficult, can be successfully accomplished.

Everyone inherits a certain likelihood of acquiring large vessel diseases independent of the other risk factors. The best evidence of this genetic tendency for an individual is a history of atherosclerosis in first-degree male relatives (e.g., father, uncles, brothers). If such a relative suffered an early coronary event, the genetic tendency for macrovascu-

TABLE 12-10 RISK FACTORS FOR MACROVASCULAR DISEASE	
Reversible	**Irreversible**
Smoking	Family history (genetic)
Hypertension	Diabetes mellitus
Hyperlipidemia*	
Obesity	

*Elevated cholesterol and/or triglyceride levels.

lar disease may be high. If these male relatives were free of coronary or other macrovascular disease until late in life, the inherited tendency is low. This risk factor is obviously an irreversible one.

Whatever the risk for macrovascular disease in an individual, the presence of diabetes approximately doubles it. Although blood sugar levels are only one part of the risk for macrovascular disease, increasing evidence suggests that strict diabetic control can help prevent or delay macrovascular disease. There may also be non–glucose-related components to diabetes that accelerate atherosclerosis.

Self-Management Education

It is beyond the scope of this chapter to provide in-depth information on cardiovascular risk factor modification. A few general pointers are provided here to help patients understand that effective diabetes management means more than just blood glucose level control.

Most DSME, especially for patients newly diagnosed with diabetes, focuses on blood glucose control. Improvements in blood glucose levels are relatively easy to achieve in a short time and can easily be appreciated by patients. Patients may either feel immediate improvement in symptoms (if they had been experiencing hyperglycemic symptoms), or they will detect improvement in blood glucose results obtained at home or at the medical office. Once improvement in blood glucose control is achieved, it is important to emphasize that the most common causes of death among people with diabetes are heart disease and stroke. These conditions require attention to matters other than blood glucose control—namely, blood pressure, cholesterol, and weight control.

To help patients deal with feeling overwhelmed by all the details of complications prevention, point out that the behaviors that improve blood glucose levels such as eating a healthy diet, maintaining a reasonable weight, and regular physical activity, usually also improve cardiovascular conditioning. Help patients identify whether they anticipate increased success with life style changes through small incremental changes or more drastic changes in health habits. Whatever approach patients choose, encourage them to celebrate successful behavior changes rather than to focus solely on end results.

To promote a sense of empowerment and optimism, help patients to consider that the diagnosis of diabetes is forcing them to pay much needed attention to their diet and health. Many people who do not have diabetes suffer from the same cardiovascular problems but do not make attempts to improve their health until after their first heart attack or surgery. Patients with diabetes are given special opportunities through education and increased medical follow-up to prevent cardiovascular problems before they occur. Patients should also expect that polypharmacy (5 to 9 drugs) is often required to treat the high glucose levels, abnormal lipids, and elevated blood pressure found in patients with diabetes. Although this may seem odious, it is also extremely fortunate that we can do so much to reduce the risk associated with diabetes.

PERSONAL HYGIENE

The hygiene needs of patients with diabetes do not differ from those of nondiabetic persons but must be attended to with more caution and diligence. Education should be directed toward preventive measures, especially during periods of high blood glucose levels, because this is the factor that interferes with the healing process. The three diseases discussed next require special care and are particular problems in patients with diabetes.

PERIODONTAL DISEASE

Diseases of the gums and surrounding tissues are estimated to occur three times more frequently in patients with diabetes who have elevated blood glucose levels than in patients without diabetes. Poor oral hygiene associated with hyperglycemia can cause gum (periodontal) infections. Teach patients to watch for the following symptoms:

1. Inflammation of gum tissue (red and swollen gums)
2. Easy bleeding of gums
3. Dental plaque and calculus accumulation
4. Increased spacing between teeth, receding gums, and loose teeth
5. Early loss of teeth resulting from primary gum disease

Teach Preventive Measures

Patients should be taught the following:

1. Maintain good control of blood sugar.
2. Clean the teeth at least twice a day with a soft toothbrush and toothpaste; frequently use dental floss.
3. Rinse mouth with water after using mouthwash.
4. Promptly see the dentist if experiencing bleeding gums, poorly fitting dentures, or sores in the mouth.
5. Examine the gums by pulling the lips apart and looking for inflamed tissue.

See a dentist on a routine basis at least every 6 months (excess dental plaque may need to be removed more frequently) and when abnormalities develop.

Goal Setting to Promote Health, and Problem Solving for Daily Living

To facilitate behavior change, in addition to helping patients set realistic goals, the educator must differentiate between short-term and long-term goals because short-term goals are steps toward achieving long-term goals. The educator can also help promote patients' self confidence by reinforcing their successful experience in self-management.

In addition, the patient should be given ample opportunity to discuss problem solving for practical situations and be encouraged to experiment and explore (e.g., by trying different foods, different medication schedules, different sleeping schedules, variable glucose-monitoring schedules), provided the behavior has no immediate detrimental consequences. This type of discovery learning is often the most powerful and motivating for patients. Even if a temporary worsening of blood glucose control results from experimentation, the benefits (i.e., lessons learned by the patient, feelings of more control, freedom to try new approaches, feelings of comfort with the diabetes team) usually outweigh the temporary risks.

Integrating Psychosocial Adjustment to Daily Life

Managing diabetes is demanding and unrelenting, and will undoubtedly affect the patient's quality of life. The educator must remember that for effective diabetes management, the patient must assume most of the self-management responsibility. Therefore one of the goals of self-management education is to help decrease the impact of diabetes on quality of life. Strategies such as helping patients to set realistic self-management goals and prioritize behavior change can help facilitate the integration of diabetes management into the patient's life.

In addition to the possible impact of negative coping mechanism such as denial on health outcome, in the last 2 decades growing attention has been given to the relationship between diabetes and psychosocial disorders such as depression and eating disorders. The educator must continuously evaluate adjustment by being alert to changes in self-management and by asking the patient to verbalize feelings about the different aspects of living with diabetes. Patients must periodically screen for possible psychosocial disorder. Preoccupation of a patient with type 1 diabetes with being thin could be a sign of eating disorder. Expression of decreased interest in usual activities, decreased ability to concentrate, depressed mood or feelings of worthlessness, sluggishness or unusual agitation, excessive sleep or lack of sleep, and statements such as "I might as well be dead" can be indicative of clinical depression and should be further evaluated. Referral should be made to mental health professional as appropriate.

SPECIAL SITUATIONS

Fasting

The most important thing to remember whenever fasting is necessary (e.g., for a blood test, dental appointment, outpatient surgical procedure, religious practices) is to speak to the diabetes health care professional who is assisting in the management of the diabetes. The main danger to be avoided is hypoglycemia, which may occur if the usual insulin or oral hypoglycemic medication is taken without eating. In general, having mild hyperglycemia for a few hours or for half a day is safer than risking hypoglycemia. More problem solving guidance will be needed for patients who are required to fast for more than a day.

In type 2 diabetes, the body is still able to produce some of its own insulin. As discussed earlier, this prevents the development of DKA. If patients must fast for only a few hours or half a day, the physician may have them omit or delay taking the oral hypoglycemic agent until they are eating again. For patients with type 2 diabetes taking insulin, the physician may have them decrease the dose or omit it entirely (and then resume insulin injections whenever the next dose is usually taken).

In type 1 diabetes, the body is not producing its own insulin, and omitting an insulin dose entirely may lead to DKA. Although delaying the dose for a few hours may be safe, the physician may also eliminate the short-acting (regular) insulin from the morning injection and have patients simply take a smaller dose of longer-acting (e.g., NPH or glargine) insulin alone. Patients on insulin pumps may be instructed to maintain or slightly reduce their basal rate, and take small correction boluses as needed. It is important to avoid injecting the usual morning dose of short- or rapid-acting insulin when patients have no plans to eat for several hours. In addition, if the morning injection was not taken at all, it may be unsafe to take the usual full morning dose at a later point in the day because it may peak at a time not covered by appropriate food intake.

Communication with the diabetes health care professional involved in management of the patient's diabetes is crucial.

Travel

To be a successful traveler, a patient with diabetes needs to be prepared and well supplied. Travel that involves changing time zones requires that insulin-requiring patients consult with their diabetes health care professional to formulate a plan for insulin dose adjustments. Many airlines do not serve meals or snacks during the flight. Patients should contact the airlines and find out if and how many in-flight meals and snacks will be served. If served, timing of meals is not always predictable. Patients are thus advised to be prepared with their own snacks or meals. For patients or a flexible intensive insulin regimen, the rapid-acting insulin doses are simply given before each meal and the basal insulin dose given on the new time zone schedule as soon as possible. For patients on a more fixed regimen, insulin should be given based on the original time zone and switched to the new time zone on the morning of the first day in the new location. What is most important is to avoid giving doses of intermediate or long-acting insulin too closely together, resulting in hypoglycemia. It is best to keep blood sugar levels slightly higher while traveling to avoid unexpected lows, which can occur because of increased exercise and/or decreased food intake. If needed, an extra injection of short- or rapid-acting insulin can be given to bridge the time until the dose of intermediate or long-acting insulin is given in the new time zone. Patients must also rely on SMBG to evaluate changes in their blood glucose levels and to assess the need for food or insulin dose adjustments. Using supplemental regular insulin during periods of high blood glucose levels as the adjustment to the new time zone occurs or during periods of illness can be useful.

Patients should carry all of the supplies they need to care for their diabetes during the duration of the trip. A good rule of thumb is to carry twice the number of supplies necessary for the length of the trip to avoid running out. Many items cannot be purchased abroad. In some foreign countries, U-100 insulin is not available. All of the diabetes-related supplies (and any other medications) should be packed in a carry-on bag, not put in luggage that is checked. It may be helpful to check with the ADA or Federal Aviation Administration (FAA) before going on a major trip, in case requirements for traveling with diabetic supplies have recently changed.

In the event that the insulin, syringes, or prescriptions are lost or stolen and U-100 insulin and syringes are not available, purchase U-40 or U-80 insulin with *syringes to match*. Give the *same number of units*. Do not try to compute insulin doses for a syringe that does not correspond (i.e., U-100 insulin in a U-40 syringe).

Patients taking oral diabetes medications must know the generic (chemical) name of the drug, because the brand name is different in foreign countries. This applies to all other medications as well. Medications should be transported in their original labeled bottles. As with insulin, take a liberal supply of all required oral medications.

In addition to a consultation with one's personal physician about diabetes management, other health care issues need to be addressed. If patients are going to a destination such as Africa or Asia, vaccinations must be updated (or given for the first time). Malaria prophylaxis may be required. For many destinations, it is useful to carry medication to treat nausea, vomiting, and diarrhea, should these symptoms develop. Sick day rules for food replacement in the event of GI upset should be reviewed.

As recommended in general, it is particularly important to wear clear Medical Alert tags identifying the diabetic condition. It is important to prevent development of hypoglycemia. Patients should carry a fast-acting glucose preparation and a long-acting carbohydrate at *all* times (even on the airplane), especially if they plan much walking. (For more information, refer to the section on prevention and treatment of hypoglycemia.)

Appropriate footwear should be worn. Constant walking may cause blisters and other foot problems. Bring moleskin to apply to areas of redness that develop as a result of pressure from shoes. Change shoes and socks or stockings frequently. If shoes are new, break them in before traveling. As always, do not wear new shoes more than 2 hours at a time.

Diabetes Packing Checklist
The following items must be kept in the carry-on luggage so that they are available at all times. Luggage that is checked may be delayed, lost, or even stolen.

Medications

Insulins or oral diabetes medications

Antinausea suppositories

Other prescription medications

Antibiotic ointment

Glucagon emergency kit (for patients taking insulin)

Supplies

Urine ketone test strips (for patients with type 1 diabetes)

Insulin syringes/pens/pen needles/pump supplies as indicated

Wallet medical identification card

Glucose meter with test strips

Lancets

Blood-sampling device and a spare (spring may break)

Alcohol wipes

Extra batteries (if patient uses a meter)

Cotton or facial tissues

Food

Quick-acting glucose preparation for reactions

Convenient snacks, such as cheese and cracker packets, granola bars, trail mix, or dried fruit to eat as a longer-acting carbohydrate

For long journeys, especially in developing countries, bring a spare meal to eat in case food is not readily available or safe to eat and carry bottled water

Airport Security

If traveling by plane, the FAA has implemented new security measures at the nation's airports, which may cause added inconvenience for individuals with diabetes who need to fly with their supplies and equipment within the United States.

1. Passengers may board with syringes or other insulin delivery systems only if they can produce a vial of insulin with in its original pharmaceutical pre-printed label that clearly identifies the medication. No exceptions will be made.
2. For passengers who do not require insulin, boarding with their lancets is acceptable as long as the lancets are

capped, and as long as the lancets are brought on with the glucose meter that has the manufacturer's name embossed on the meter (e.g., One Touch meters say "One Touch," Accucheck meters say "Accucheck").
3. Glucagon kit must be kept in its original preprinted pharmaceutically labeled plastic container or box.
4. Because of forgery concerns, prescriptions and letters of medical necessity will not be accepted as proof of diabetes.

The previous list of measures is a minimum requirement only, and air carriers may have other requirements that may affect a passenger's ability to board with diabetes equipment and supplies. Passengers should consult their individual air carrier at least 1 day in advance of his or her scheduled flight to confirm what that airline's policy is with regard to diabetes medication and supplies for most current domestic (US) and international travel regulations. Be advised that the FAA's policy and the policy of each airline are subject to change.

The ADA suggests that if a passenger is denied boarding a flight or is faced with any other unforeseen diabetes-related difficulty because of security measures, he or she should ask to speak to the security screener's supervisor or contact the FAA grounds security commissioner at the departing airport.

For more information contact the ADA at 703-549-1500 extension 2108 or the FAA at 1-866-289-9673.

Resources

In North America, contact the local ADA if problems occur.

In non–English-speaking countries, do the following:

1. Carry an index card with emergency phrases in the appropriate language. Essential phrases include "I have diabetes. Please call a doctor" and "I

have diabetes and I am having a low-sugar reaction. Please give me sugar."

2. If possible, have the name of English-speaking physicians in each city/country on the itinerary. A list of physicians may be available from the local American Embassy or Consulate, from foreign tourism offices in the United States, or from the International Association for Medical Assistance to Travelers, 417 Center Street, Lewiston, NY 14092.

3. Know where the Diabetes Association is located in each country. The International Diabetes Federation (IDF; 10 Queen Street, London W1M OBD, England) can supply names and addresses. The IDF also has information on diabetes medications and supplies. Other sources are (1) the IDF at the International Association Center (40 Washington Street, 1050 Brussels, Belgium) and (2) Intermedic (777 3rd Avenue, New York, NY, 10017, telephone 212-486-8976).

Useful Phrases in Foreign Languages

"I am diabetic."

French: "Je suis diabetique."

Spanish: "Yo soy diabetico."

German: "Ich bin zuckerkrank."

Italian: "Io sono diabetico."

"Please get me a doctor."

French: "Allez chercher un medecin, s'il vous plait."

Spanish: "Haga me el favor de llamar al medico."

German: "Rufen sie bitte einen Arzt."

Italian: "Per favore chiami un dottore."

"Sugar or orange juice, please."

French: "Sucre ou jus d'orange, s'il vous plait."

Spanish: "Azucar o un vaso de jugo de naranja, por favor."

German: "Zucker oder orangensaft, bitte."

Italian: "Zucchero or arancia succo, per favore."

SPECIAL POPULATIONS

VISUALLY IMPAIRED PATIENTS

Various degrees of visual impairment may affect patients with diabetes. Causes range from blurred vision resulting from hyperglycemia, especially in newly diagnosed patients, to cataracts and, more seriously, diabetic retinopathy. Retinopathy can lead to marked decreases in a patient's sight, from diminished vision to blindness.

The educator's role may vary from simple explanations, such as the cause of blurred vision, to demonstrations and discussions of ways and aids to facilitate independence in diabetes management. One of the most important roles may be to direct patients to resources for special assistance. Many communities have centers for educating and treating partially sighted and totally blind patients, and a referral to one of these institutions is often helpful because they have the resources to fully evaluate and treat patients with all degrees of visual impairments.

Assessment

1. Determine the degree of independence that patients want and the support system that is available to them. For example, if the support system performs blood glucose monitoring and prefills syringes, education should be directed toward members of the support system to ensure accuracy in the procedures involved.

2. Determine the patient's degree of visual impairment. Level 1: blurred vision and visual fluctuation, usually transient and

caused by fluctuations in blood glucose levels in patients with new-onset diabetes; level 2: usable vision, low vision, legally blind, or partially sighted; and level 3: functionally blind, totally blind. Classifying the patient's visual impairment is necessary so that the appropriate level of education can be provided (e.g., by a knowledgeable diabetes educator for levels 1 and 2 and by a center for the blind for level 3).

3. To assess the need for visual aids, check patients' vision in the following ways: Have patients use an insulin vial and insulin syringe. Can they read the labels on the insulin vial? Can they read the markings on the syringe? Can they insert the needle into the insulin vial without bending the needle? Can they read the blood glucose value seen on the meter?

Teaching Aids

Various aids can help patients with decreased vision. A discussion of these devices can be found in the current year issue of the *American Diabetes Association Buyer's Guide to Diabetes Supplies and Diabetes and Visual Impairment: An Educator's Resource Guide* (see Appendix).

To increase patients' function with diminished sight, the following may be helpful (see Appendix for more complete details):

Emphasize strong lighting for insulin injections and SMBG procedures.

Use the insulin syringe most closely suited for the insulin dose (e.g., for <30 U of insulin use a 30-U syringe).

Magnifying devices that slip over the syringe (such as the Becton Dickinson Magni-Guide) can double the size of the numbers; some patients may prefer to use a small pocket magnifier.

Use of prefilled syringes may be necessary.

Some patients benefit from use of insulin pens.

Blood glucose meters that have large displays or give audible instructions for the test procedure and that state the blood glucose result can be purchased.

Needle guides and vial stabilizers can be used to help guide the needle into the vial.

Devices are marketed for ensuring dose accuracy when a poorly sighted person is drawing up insulin into a syringe. It is helpful to mark the vials of insulin clearly if more than one type is used, with either a rubber band or a notch in the top.

PEDIATRIC PATIENTS

Educating children with diabetes and their families is a unique challenge. If at all possible, these families should be referred to a medical center, children's hospital, diabetes educator, and/or endocrinologist specializing in childhood and adolescent diabetes management. The specific information and diabetes treatment modalities are, for the most part, the same as those for adults with diabetes. However, a number of special issues must be considered in dealing with this population, such as dynamics of the relationship between parent-child, parent-parent, child-sibling, child-caretaker, child-school, and so on. When a child has recently been found to have diabetes, the parents may express a great deal of guilt, anger, or spousal blame in trying to understand "where the diabetes came from."

In the past, emphasis was placed on having the child or adolescent accomplish specific diabetes-related tasks by a certain chronologic age. Too much parental involvement was feared to foster lack of independence and poor control of diabetes. A child's inability to achieve certain tasks by a certain age could become a source of family conflict, cause parents to feel a sense of failure, and impede development of positive self-esteem in the child. Research now suggests promoting more of a parent-child team approach with flexible expectations. A child's ability to become more involved with diabetes management depends on cognitive and emotional maturity, external stressors (e.g., school, family, or social problems), and simple individual variations in growth and development. Table 12-11 provides a description of some general issues and tasks for parents and children with diabetes.

Special Considerations in Diabetes Treatment

Goals of Blood Glucose

The specific indices for control of blood glucose, lipids, and A1C are somewhat different for the pediatric population and the adult population. This is, in part, due to the difficulty associated with tight glucose control in developing children, as well as a lack of data on the outcomes of treatment of some of these metabolic abnormalities in children. An approach that is useful is to set blood glucose goals that are more flexible and that take into account other issues such as normally erratic eating habits, especially in very young children and adolescents. As with all patients with diabetes, striving for the best possible blood glucose control is of vital importance in preventing the long-term complications. If pursuit of unrealistic goals creates more parent-child tension and alienates the child or family from the diabetes team, however, the

TABLE 12-11	DEVELOPMENTAL ISSUES AND TASKS IN CHILDREN WITH TYPE I DIABETES
Infant (0–1 year)	Differentiate hypoglycemic reactions from "normal" distress. Parents may be overwhelmed by demands of diabetes. Identify and train trustworthy babysitters.
Toddler (1–3 years)	Differentiate misbehavior from hypoglycemia. Expect dietary inconsistency as child begins to feed self. Give child choices in food, injection, and finger-stick sites (avoid mealtime battles). Encourage child to report "funny" feelings (hypoglycemia). Let child begin to "help" with diabetes tasks.
Preschool (3–6 years)	Teach child to report hypoglycemia to adults in charge. Teach child what to eat when "low." Reassure child who may view finger sticks and injections as punishment and/or become overly fearful of procedures. Teach preschool teachers about diabetes. Encourage child to participate in simple diabetes tasks. Involve child in menu planning.
School age (6–12 years)	Teach all school personnel involved with child about diabetes. Manage diabetes to minimize school absences. Parents should foster age-appropriate independence. Parents and child should learn to adjust insulin and regimen to encourage participation in social and sports events. Encourage self-monitoring: recognize hypoglycemia, participate in meal planning, gradually learn to do own blood testing and injections—all activities to be supervised.

Adapted from Schreiner B, Pontious S: Diabetes mellitus and the preschool child. In Haire-Joshu D (ed): Management of Diabetes Mellitus: Perspectives of Care Across the Life Span. Mosby, St. Louis, 1992, pp. 362–398

ultimate outcome may be worse than accepting less than optimum diabetic control.

Hypoglycemia

Hypoglycemia is of special concern to parents of young children who are not yet able to clearly recognize and report the symptoms of hypoglycemia. Special education and attention should be given to conditions that may predispose children to hypoglycemia (e.g., unusual activity, missed snack, smaller than usual meal). Parents concerned about possible overnight hypoglycemia need to be alerted to watch the child for nightmares and sweating and to test the blood glucose level during the night. Parents and caretakers must be taught to use injectable glucagon (see previous section on hypoglycemia). For small children, half of the adult dose (0.5 mg) is usually sufficient.

Special attention to hypoglycemia is also important for adolescents learning to drive. Teaching adolescents to test their blood glucose level and to take a snack as needed every time they plan to drive promotes safe practices as adolescents become more independent.

Diet

The current approach to diabetes diet education and treatment promotes greater flexibility for all patients. This is especially helpful in reducing conflict in families of children and adolescents with diabetes. Substitution of sucrose-containing foods for other carbohydrates and education on age-appropriate foods and snacks (e.g., pizza and other fast foods) help the family and child with diabetes deal with the normal social aspects of growth and development.

Injection Sites

Pediatric (older than toddler) and adolescent patients are encouraged to use the same injection sites as recommended for adults. In infants and toddlers, the sciatic nerve is not well stabilized and injection in the buttocks is discouraged until children are walking. If possible, use of the abdomen is encouraged for older children and adolescents, especially to avoid resistance to using this area later in life. If arms and legs are used, a consistent rotation pattern (as described in the earlier insulin section) is especially important in this physically active group of patients. As with adults, avoid injecting into a limb that will be used during an activity.

Organizations/Support Groups/Camps

The ADA and Juvenile Diabetes Foundation are good sources of information for parents of children with diabetes. In addition, local hospitals or regional facilities specializing in the care of children with diabetes could provide information on local support groups, camps, and ongoing classes. Parents are encouraged to obtain written materials from diabetes organizations and diabetes lay magazines (see Appendix) to use in educating teachers and school staff on basic diabetes information—especially symptoms, treatment, and prevention of hypoglycemia. Encouraging contact between families with diabetic children and participation with diabetes camps can provide much needed support and guidance for families and can prevent feelings of isolation, especially in communities that do not offer formal pediatric diabetes services.

DEALING WITH DIABETES IN OLDER ADULTS

When dealing with older adult patients, assessment of patients' ability and willingness to learn diabetes self-management skills is important. With this group of patients, probably more than any other population, individualizing the treatment and teaching plans is essential for successful diabetes management and for assisting patients to maintain independence. Older adult patients represent a diverse population with self-care abilities that do not predictably correlate with a patient's age.

Factors that may impair older adult patients' ability to learn diabetes self-care skills include the following:

- Decreased vision and hearing
- Decreased fine motor coordination
- Tremulousness of hands
- Decreased range of motion (impaired ability to perform foot care)
- Impaired short-term memory

In addition, certain psychological issues such as loneliness, depression, and an unwillingness to change long-standing habits may negatively affect patients' desire to learn about diabetes. Other medical illnesses, financial limitations, and decreased ability to travel (to the clinic or office) may limit the amount of time and effort patients may put into diabetes management.

If patients are resistant to learning new information or have difficulty attending to details, the teaching sessions must be kept brief and limited in scope. If necessary, written teaching materials should be in large print with dark-colored lettering. A flexible approach to teaching is essential. A well-prepared and organized teaching plan may need to be changed several times during the teaching session to ensure that the basic information is understood by patients.

A sensitive but firm approach must be taken when asking patients who have managed their diabetes for many years to demonstrate skills of preparing and injecting insulin or measuring capillary blood glucose. A fear of loss of independence or of embarrassment may lead patients to feel insulted when asked to demonstrate skills learned many years earlier. It may be helpful for educators to explain to patients that they would like to show them new equipment or new techniques. Giving the appearance of an information-sharing session rather than a teaching or evaluation session may help patients feel less threatened. Using shortcuts such as eliminating the injection of air into insulin vials, using simpler blood glucose meters, or working with family members to prefill syringes is important in promoting continued independence in diabetes management.

Although the goal of diabetes control in older adults may be less strict than in younger patients, careful monitoring for diabetes complications must not be neglected. Hypoglycemia may be especially dangerous because of cerebral or coronary artery disease. Importantly, it may result in falls in older adults. Decreased appetite or irregular meals may increase the chances of hypoglycemia in this population. Dehydration is a concern in patients who have chronically elevated glucose levels because of the associated hyperglycemia-induced diuresis. Assessment for long-term complications such as eye and foot problems is important. Avoiding blindness and amputations through early detection and treatment of retinopathy and foot ulcers, respectively, may mean the difference between institutionalization and continued independent living for elderly patients with diabetes.

WOMEN'S ISSUES

Because of differences in anatomy, women with diabetes must cope with some special issues related to their sexual health. This section briefly addresses these special issues in the care of women with diabetes

Menstrual Cycle, Birth Control, and Safe Sex

Because estrogen and progesterone also affect blood glucose levels by blunting the effect of insulin and increasing hepatic glycogenesis, some patients experience an increase in their blood during ovulation when the levels of estrogen rise. It is important for the educator to discuss these changes with the patients, and help them make the appropriate changes in their blood glucose level monitoring frequency and medication if needed, to help them stay healthier during that period. Women who frequently monitor their blood glucose levels may notice trends of highs and lows during certain phases of their cycles and can be taught to adjust to compensate for them.

Birth control and safe sex are two important women's health issues to prevent unplanned pregnancy as well as sexually transmitted diseases. Although birth control choices are up to the patient and her partner, women with diabetes should be made aware that oral contraceptives may raise their blood glucose levels and blood pressure. Some gynecologists are under the impression that women with diabetes should not take oral contraceptives. This is not true—an individual evaluation should be made for each woman to assess risk and benefit. If blood glucose levels rise on one form of oral contraceptive, then another type can be tried.

Urinary Tract Infections

Because urinary tract infections are common in women with diabetes, the following special hygiene is indicated:

1. Clean the vagina and anus from front to back after urinating or defecating.
2. Urinate to empty the bladder after sexual intercourse.
3. If a patient has a neurogenic bladder, urinate on a schedule. It may be necessary to restrict fluids after midnight.
4. Report to the physician any symptoms of urgency, frequency, or painful urination.
5. Drink increased amounts of liquids and urinate every 3 to 4 hours during the day to help to irrigate the bladder and wash out bacteria.

Candida Skin Infections (Fungus Or Yeast Infection)

Fungal infections thrive in sweet, warm, moist areas, particularly in the vagina and genital region. They can also occur under the breasts and between other overlapping skin folds. Therefore this infection frequently affects overweight patients with blood glucose levels out of control. The risk increases after menopause, because of lack of estrogen to nourish and support the vaginal lining. Instruct patients to look for a white, cheesy vaginal discharge with a peculiar yeasty odor, vaginal itching, and redness and swelling of the upper thighs, beneath the breasts, or in the creases between the legs and abdomen (the intertriginous area). If patients find evidence for a *Candida* infection, they should seek medical care. Topical medications are effective, but blood glucose control is also extremely important.

Self-Management Education

Patients should be taught the following

- Keep diabetes in good blood glucose control.
- Bathe often to keep fecal bacteria from getting into the vagina.
- During periods of high blood glucose levels, cleanse the perineal and vaginal areas after urination to wash away any residual urine, which contributes to the *Candida* skin infection.
- Wear clean underclothes.
- Wear underclothing that does not promote or trap heat and moisture (e.g., wear cotton-crotch underwear, especially panty hose with a cotton crotch or cotton top).
- Eating a cup a day of low-fat yogurt that has "active cultures" may help battle yeast and prevent vaginitis.

Sexual Problems

Although both women with and women without diabetes have some sexual problems in common, we still do not know as much as we should about how diabetes affects women's sex lives. The possible manifestation of sexual problems in women include poor vaginal lubrication, a decrease in sexual desire, pain during sex, and trouble having an orgasm. Doctors are not sure how much diabetes affects women's sexual ability.

In addition to poor diabetes control and possible psychosocial problems such as poor communication or conflict with sexual partner, poor self-image, stress, depression, history of sexual abuse, several different physical factors may contribute to causing these sexual problems. These physical factors may include diabetes complications such as severe nerve damage causing loss of skin sensation around the genital area, and neurogenic bladder causing poor bladder control. In addition, low hormone levels exist in postmenopausal women, which can cause poor vaginal lubrication leading to vaginal irritation and pain during sex.

Difference seems to exist in the way women with type 1 and type 2 diabetes experience these problems. Women with type 2 diabetes seem to be more likely to have sexual problems than women of the same age without diabetes. Changes in blood vessels and nerve damage caused by diabetes may play a role in these problems. Although they may have some trouble with vaginal lubrication or suffer more frequent yeast infections if their diabetes is poorly controlled, women with type 1 diabetes who have not gone through menopause do not seem to have higher rates of sexual problems than other women.

As discussed previously, both patients and health care professionals are often uncomfortable addressing this important topic with patients. The educator needs to make a special effort to discuss the special concerns of women patients, including the possible psychosocial issues that are often associated with these problems for both men and women. Women should be made aware that factors such as poorly controlled diabetes, yeast infections, and urinary tract infections may increase the risk for sexual problems. If necessary, referrals can be made to the appropriate health care provider such as mental health professional, sex or marital therapist, or gynecologist.

Self-Management Education

Postmenopausal women should be encouraged to discuss hormone replacement with their gynecologist or internist. In addition, these simple strategies may be helpful in alleviating some of the problems:

- Use of a water-soluble vaginal lubricant.
- Learning to relax the muscles that surround the vagina (Kegel exercises: advise patient to practice by stopping the flow of urine while urinating, then let the muscles relax and feel the contrast)
- Try different positions such as sitting or kneeling over your partner or lying on your side and facing your partner
- Gentle touch or a hand-held vibrator on or around the clitoris can help a woman with decreased vaginal sensation reach orgasm more easily
- Emptying the bladder before and after sex
- Encouraging patients with decreased physical mobility to talk to a physical therapist about ways to be comfortable during sex

Promoting Preconception Care, Management During Pregnancy, and Gestational Diabetes Management

For a complete discussion of diabetes in pregnancy, see Chapter 11.

Diabetes Before Pregnancy

Strict control of blood glucose levels is essential for diabetic women at the time of conception and throughout the entire pregnancy. Fetal problems that have been associated with hyperglycemia include increased body fat (babies weighing >9 pounds at birth), often complicating vaginal delivery. After birth, these babies are at increased risk for neonatal hypoglycemia, hyperbilirubinemia, and hypocalcemia. In addition, hyperglycemia is thought to contribute to the increased rate of congenital malformations (noted in women with poor diabetic control during the first 2 months of pregnancy).

Women with diabetes should discuss plans to become pregnant with the physician helping to manage their diabetes (as well as with their obstetrician). Normalizing blood glucose levels before conception is important and may require several months of intensive monitoring, education, and diet counseling with follow-up. Women should also be counseled on the possible effects of pregnancy on maternal health. Women with advanced kidney and eye disease may experience worsening of these conditions during pregnancy and need to discuss these risks fully before becoming pregnant.

The goals of diabetic management during pregnancy are to maintain fasting blood glucose levels in the range of 60 to 90 mg/dl and 1-hour postmeal blood glucose values less than 140 mg/dl. Blood glucose levels must be monitored daily, usually at least four times per day. Insulin injections are taken a minimum of two and often three to four times per day. Because of the anti-insulin effects of the hormones of pregnancy, the insulin dose requirements may increase two- to threefold during the course of pregnancy. Women who have type 2 diabetes and who are taking oral antidiabetic agents before pregnancy must stop taking the oral agents (some evidence in animals suggests that they can be harmful for a fetus) and use insulin during the pregnancy for control of blood glucose levels. Monitoring for urine ketones during pregnancy should be performed every morning as well as during any sudden elevation of blood glucose value or during minor illness. An elevation in ketones levels must be reported immediately, because ketosis poses a danger to the fetus.

Gestational Diabetes

Of all (nondiabetic) women who become pregnant, 2% to 5% develop a temporary form of diabetes called *gestational diabetes.* During pregnancy, the amount of insulin produced by the pancreas of a pregnant woman normally increases. This occurs because the hormones that are produced by the placenta during pregnancy make it more difficult for the normal insulin in the body to control blood glucose levels. Therefore more insulin needs to be produced to counteract the effect of these hormones. If a woman's body is not able to produce enough extra insulin, the blood glucose values become elevated. This occurs mostly during the latter part of pregnancy, when placental hormone levels increase. Most pregnant women should be screened for gestational diabetes (with a 1-hour, 50-g glucose challenge test) at 24 to 28 weeks of pregnancy or even earlier if they are at high risk.

Women most at risk for gestational diabetes are obese, are older than 30 years, have a family history of diabetes, and/or have previously given birth to a baby weighing more than 9 pounds. Treatment includes diet, monitoring blood glucose levels and urine ketones, and, for some women, insulin injections. Because gestational diabetes is not usually a problem until later in pregnancy, congenital malformations are not usually associated with gestational diabetes. However, the other problems related to hyperglycemia that were mentioned previously do occur more frequently if gestational diabetes is not well controlled.

The diabetes usually resolves after delivery, although approximately 50% of women who have gestational diabetes develop overt type 2 diabetes within 5 to 15 years (especially if they are overweight).

The most important information to give to women dealing with pregnancy and diabetes is that (except for a slightly higher risk for congenital malformations) with optimal diabetes control, close monitoring, and teamwork on the part of these women and their health care providers, the chances of delivering a healthy baby are similar to those of any pregnant woman.

Menopause

Menopause may cause many physical changes in women. These changes include weight gain, skin wrinkling, breast tissue sagging, and for some, a decrease in sexual desire. For women with diabetes, it is important to know that menopause may also affect blood glucose levels. Because estrogen and progesterone also affect blood glucose levels by blunting the effect of insulin and increasing hepatic glycogenesis, when the level of these hormones drop with menopause, the action of insulin may go up, causing the blood glucose levels to be lower. Consequently, patients with type 2 diabetes on oral agents may need lower doses of medication, and patients on insulin may need a decrease their insulin dosage by up to 20%. However, weight gain and lack of exercise raise insulin needs and may often balance the dropping hormone levels. Therefore follow-up and treatment must be individualized.

Self-Management Education

Keep blood sugar in good control, and test regularly to monitor changes in blood sugar level.

Eat less and stay active to prevent excessive weight gain.

Eat soy and calcium-rich food.

Discuss hormone replacement therapy with your physician.

CONCLUSION

Working in the field of DSME can be a very challenging and rewarding experience. The most effective diabetes educators are those who keep abreast of new treatments and equipment available for diabetes care. In addition, successful DSME requires willingness to reevaluate teaching techniques and teaching tools continually to maximize patients' understanding and ability to apply concepts to daily living situations.

Helping patients and their families cope with the unrelenting and demanding routines and stresses of diabetes management is an important role of the diabetes educator. Diabetes educators are encouraged to read the literature available on motivation, coping, chronic illness, and relapse prevention.

Creative problem solving is very useful in motivating patients who have strayed from the diabetes program. One helpful technique for prevention of burnout among patients with diabetes is to suggest a monthly or biweekly diabetes vacation day—during which patients need not record blood glucose levels and can be more free with the diet (while maintaining basic safety precautions). Another suggestion is periodically to conduct a patient visit or at least a portion of the visit without looking at the blood glucose records or laboratory results. Simply allow patients to talk freely about how diabetes is affecting their life or about any other aspects of life. Spending some amount of time simply talking to patients helps them to appreciate that their personality and identity are not defined by the level of diabetes control and to learn to enjoy life no matter what their level of success with the diabetes program.

REFERENCES

1. Mensing C, Boucher J, Cypress M et al: National standards for diabetes self-management education programs. Diabetes Care 26(suppl 1): S149–156, 2003.
2. Ruggiero L: Helping people with diabetes change behavior: From theory to practice. Diabetes Spectrum 13:125, 2000.
3. Diabetes Control and Complications Trial Research Group: The effect of intensive treatment of diabetes on the long-term development and progression of long-term complications in insulin-dependent diabetes mellitus. N Engl J Med 329:977, 1993.
4. United Kingdom Prospective Diabetes Study Group: Intensive blood glucose control with sulphonylureas or insulin compared with conventional treatment and risk of complications in patients with type 2 diabetes. Lancet 352:837, 1998.

Appendix

PROFESSIONAL EDUCATION RESOURCES

American Association of Diabetes
Educators
100 West Monroe Street, Suite 400
Chicago, IL 60603
Phone: (800) 338-3633
www.aadenet.org

American Diabetes Association
National Call Center
1701 North Beauregard Street
Alexandria, VA 22311
Phone: (703) 549-1500 or (800) 342-2383
www.diabetes.org

American Dietetic Association
216 West Jackson Boulevard, Suite 800
Chicago, IL 60606-6995
Phone: (800) 877-1600
www.eatright.org

Centers for Disease Control and
Prevention
National Center for Chronic Disease
Prevention and Health Promotion
Mail Stop K-10, 4770 Buford Highway NE
Atlanta, GA 30341-3717
Phone: (770) 488-5000, (800) 311-3435,
or (877) 232-3422
www.cdc.gov/health/diabetes.htm

Children with Diabetes
5689 Chancery Place
Hamilton, OH 45011
Fax: (513) 755-6797
www.childrenwithdiabetes.org

Diabetes Exercise and Sports Association
(DESA)
P.O. Box 1935
Litchfield Park, AZ 85340
Phone: (623) 535-4593 or (800) 898-4322
Fax: (623) 535-4741
www.diabetes-exercise.org

International Diabetes Center (books
and other information on diabetes)
3800 Park Nicollet Boulevard
Minneapolis, MN 55416-2699
Phone: (952) 993-3393 or (888) 637-2675
Fax: (952) 993-1302
E-mail: idcpub@parknicollet.com
www.idcdiabetes.org

International Diabetes Federation
Avenue Emile De Mot 19, B-100
Brussels, Belgium
Phone: 32 2 538 5511
Fax: 32 2 538 5114
E-mail: idf@idf.org
www.idf.org

Juvenile Diabetes Foundation
120 Wall Street
New York, NY 10005-4001
Phone: (800) 533-2873
Fax: (212) 785-9595
www.jdf.org

Milner-Fenwick, Inc. (diabetes
educational videos)
2125 Greenspring Drive
Timonium, MD 21093-3113
www.milner-fenwick.com

National Diabetes Education Program
1 Information Way
Bethesda, MD 20892-3560
ndep.nih.gov

National Diabetes Information
Clearinghouse (NDIC)
1 Information Way
Bethesda, MD 20892-3560
Phone: (800) 860-8747
Fax: (301) 907-8906
E-mail: nidic@info.niddk.nih.gov
diabetes.niddk.nih.gov/about/index.htm

National Institute of Diabetes and
Digestive and Kidney Disease (NIDDK)
diabetes.niddk.nig.gov

National Certification Board for Diabetes
Educators (NCBDE) (CDE exam)
330 East Algonquin Road, Suite 4
Arlington Heights, IL 60005
Phone: (847) 228-9795
Fax: (847) 228-8469
E-mail: info@ncbde.org
www.ncbde.org

▼
MANUFACTURERS OF DIABETES MEDICATIONS AND SUPPLIES—PARTIAL LIST

Abbott Laboratories (MediSense
Products)
4A Crosby Drive
Bedford, MA 01730
Phone: (781) 276-6000 or (800) 527-3339
www.MediSense.com

Activa Brand Products, Inc.
(Jet Injectors)
36 Fourth Street
Charlottetown, PEI
Canada, C1E 2B3
(902) 566-3229 or (800) 991-4464
activa@ISN.net
www.advantajet.com

American Medical Identifications
4001 North Shepherd, Suite 100
Houston, TX 77018
www.americanmedical-id.com

Amylin Pharmaceuticals (pramlintide)
9360 Towne Centre Drive, Suite 110
San Diego, CA 92121
Phone: (858) 552-2200
Fax: (858) 552-2212
www.amylin.com

Animas Corporation (Animas Pump)
590 Lancaster Avenue
Frazer, PA 19355
Phone: (610) 644-8990 or (877)
YES-PUMP (937-7867)
Fax: (610) 644-8717
www.animascorp.com

Astra Zenica (Crestor)
Phone: (800) 236-9933
www.astrazeneca-us.com

Aventis Pharmaceuticals (Lantus insulin)
300 Somerset Corporate Boulevard
P.O. Box 6977 (required)
Bridgewater, NJ 08807-0977
Phone: (908) 243-6000 or (800) 981-2491
www.aventis.com

Bayer Corporation (Precose, Meters,
Levitra)
Diagnostics Division
511 Benedict Avenue
Tarrytown, NY 10591
Phone: (800) 348-8100
www.bayercarediabetes.com

BD (insulin syringes)
One Becton Drive
Franklin Lakes, NJ 07417-1883
Phone: (888) BD-CARES (232-1737)
www.bddiabetes.com

Bioject, Inc.
7620 Southwest Bridgeport Road
Portland, OR 97224
Phone: (503) 639-7221 or (800) 848-2538
www.bioject.com

Bristol-Myers Squibb (Pravachol/
metformin)
1350 Liberty Avenue
Hillside, NJ 07207
Phone: (800) 468-7746
www.bms.com

Cygnus, Inc. (Glucowatch)
400 Penobscot Drive
Redwood City, CA 94063-4300
Phone: (866)549-2842
Fax: (650) 599-2503
www.glucowatch.com

Deltec, Inc. (Deltec pumps)
1265 Grey Fox Road
St. Paul, MN 55112
Phone: (800) 426-2448
Fax: (651) 628-7485
www.delteccozmo.com

Disetronic Medical Systems, Inc.
(Disetronic Pumps)
5151 Program Avenue
St. Paul, MN 55112
Phone: (763) 795-5200 or (800) 280-7801
www.disetronic-usa.com

Eli Lilly and Company (Lilly insulins and
pens/Cialis)
Lilly Corporate Center
Indianapolis, IN 46285
Phone: (800) 545-5979
www.lillydiabetes.com

GlaxoSmithKline Pharmaceuticals
(Avandia, Levitra)
One Franklin Plaza
P.O. Box 7929
Philadelphia, PA 19101
Phone: (888) 825-5249
www.gsk.com

Goldware Medical ID Jewelry
P.O. Box 22335
San Diego, CA 92192
Phone: (858) 453-4005 or (800) 669-7311
www.goldware-id.com

Home Diagnostics, Inc.
2400 Northwest 55th Court
Fort Lauderdale, FL 33309
Phone: (954) 677-9201 or (800) 342-7226
www.prestigesmartsystem.com

ICN Pharmaceuticals, Inc.
3300 Hyland Avenue
Costa Mesa, CA 92626
Phone: (714) 545-0100 or (800) 556-1937
www.instaglucose.com
www.nitebite.com

Identi-Find Iron-On Labels
P.O. Box 567
Canton, NC 28716
Phone: (828) 648-6768
labels@identifind.com
www.identifind.com

LifeScan, Inc. (Lifescan meters)
1000 Gibraltar Drive
Milpitas, CA 95035-6312
Phone: (408) 263-9789 or (800) 227-8862
Fax: (408) 946-6070
lifescan@lfsus.jnj.com
www.lifescan.com

The Lighthouse Catalog (supplies for
individuals with decreased vision)
111 East 59th Street
New York, NY 10022
Phone: (800) 829-0500
www.lighthouse.org

Mead Johnson, Inc.
2400 West Lloyd Expressway
Evansville, IN 47721
Phone: (812) 429-5000
Fax: (812) 429-8994
www.choicedm.com
www.meadjohnson.com

Medical Alert Watch
P.O. Box 995
London, KY 40743-0995
Phone: (800) 722-6955
Fax: (606) 878-1567
www.medicalalertwatch.com

MedicAlert Foundation
2323 Colorado Avenue
Turlock, CA 95382
Phone: (209) 668-3333 or (800) 432-5378
customer_service@medicalert.org
www.medicalert.org

Medicool, Inc (sells a variety of diabetes supplies)
23520 Telo Avenue, Suite 6
Torrance, CA 90505
Phone: (310) 784-1200 or (800) 433-2469
medicool@medicool.com
www.medicool.com

Medtronic MiniMed (Minimed pumps and sensors)
18000 Devonshire St.
Northridge, CA 91325
Phone: (800) 646-4633
www.minimed.com

Merck Pharmaceuticals (Zocor)
One Merck Drive
P.O. Box 100
Whitehouse Station, NJ 08889-0100 USA
Phone: (908) 423-1000
www.merck.com

NeedleAid, Ltd.
21 Saratoga Drive
Dartmouth, NS
Canada, B2X 3P3
Phone: (902) 452-6085
Fax: (902) 434-2869
info@needleaid.com
www.needleaid.com

Novartis Pharmaceutical Corporation (Starlix)
1 Health Plaza
East Hanover, NJ 07936
Phone: (888) 669-6682
www.novartis.com

Novo Nordisk Pharmaceuticals, Inc.
(Novo insulins and pens/repaglinide)
100 College Road West
Princeton, NJ 08540
Phone: (609) 987-5800 or (800) 727-6500
www.novonordisk-us.com

Ortho-McNeil Phamaceutical, Inc.
1000 Route 202
P.O. Box 300
Raritan, NJ 08869-0802
Phone: (888) REGRANEX (734-7263)

Owen Mumford, Inc.(insulin pens)
1755-A West Oak Commons Court
Marietta, GA 30062
Phone: (770) 977-2226 or (800) 421-6936
E-mail: info@owenmumford.com
www.owenmumford.com

Pfizer Pharmaceuticals (Lipitor, Viagra)
www.pfizer.com/main.html

Pfizer Prescription Medicine
Phone: (800) TRY-FIRST (879-3477)

Pharmacia + Upjohn Company (Glyset)
100 Route 206 North
Peapack, NJ 07977
Phone: (908) 901-8000 or (888) 768-5501
www.pnu.com

Roche Diagnostics (Accuchek Meters)
9115 Hague Road
P.O. Box 50457
Indianapolis, IN 46250-0457
Phone: (800) 858-8072
www.roche.com
www.accu-chek.com

Roche Pharmaceuticals
340 Kingsland Street
Nutley, NJ 07110
Phone: (973) 235-5000 or (800) 526-6367
www.rocheusa.com

Takeda Pharmaceuticals
America, Inc.(Actos)
Millbrook Business Center
475 Half Day Road, Suite 500
Lincolnshire, IL 60069
Phone: (877) 825-3327
www.takedapharm.com

TheraSense, Inc.(Freestyle
Meters/Tracker Sensor)
1360 South Loop Road
Alameda, CA 94502
Phone: (888) 522-5226
www.TheraSense.com

UltiGuard
Insulin Syringe Dispenser and Disposal
Container
Phone: (877) ULTIMED (858-4633)
www.ulti-care.com

INDEX

Note: Page numbers in *italics* refer to illustrations; page numbers followed by t refer to tables.